The Shoulder

Jenny T. Bencardino
Editor

The Shoulder

Imaging Diagnosis with Clinical Implications

Springer

Editor
Jenny T. Bencardino
Penn Medicine Department of Radiology
Perelman School of Medicine at the
University of Pennsylvania
Philadelphia, PA
USA

ISBN 978-3-030-06239-2 ISBN 978-3-030-06240-8 (eBook)
https://doi.org/10.1007/978-3-030-06240-8

This Springer imprint is published by the registered company Springer Nature Switzerland AG
The registered company address is: Gewerbestrasse 11, 6330 Cham, Switzerland

Acknowledgements

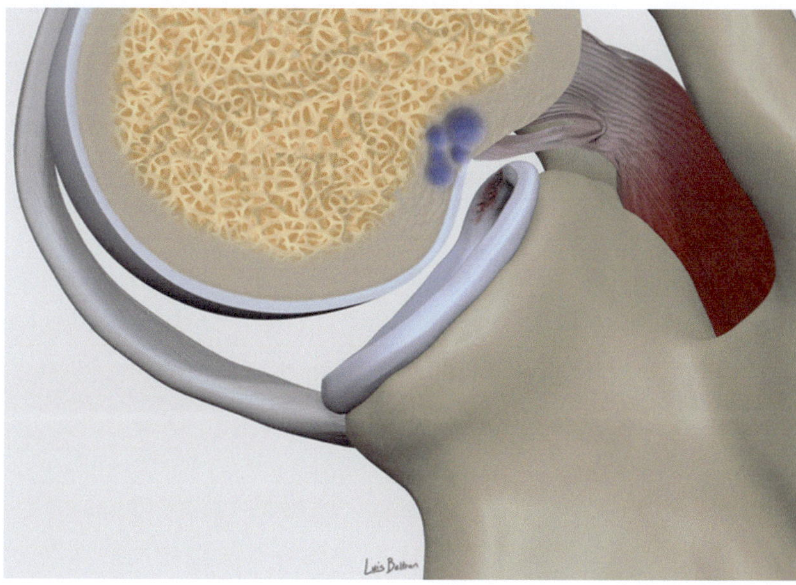

The art of publishing involves the orchestrated work of many individuals. The journey as the editor of *The Shoulder: Imaging Diagnosis with Clinical Implications* has been both inspiring and rewarding thanks to the outstanding contributions found in this book by so many renowned experts in the field of musculoskeletal imaging.

I am very grateful to Dr. Monica Tafur for her invaluable assistance in the preparation of this manuscript.

Dr. Luis S. Beltran is the mastermind behind the high-quality original illustrations found in this page and in the chapters devoted to the biceps tendon, rotator interval and glenohumeral instability.

I am also very thankful to Springer, in particular to Reshmi Rema, for seeing our project through to completion.

My utmost gratitude goes to my dearest husband Alvand and my sons Dario and Avan for their patience and unwavering support through the years that took to bring this book to fruition.

Contents

Contributors

Ronald S. Adler Department of Radiology, New York University Langone Health, New York, NY, USA

Sana Ali Department of Radiology, Maimonides Medical Center, Brooklyn, NY, USA

Javier Beltran Department of Radiology, Maimonides Medical Center, Brooklyn, NY, USA

Luis S. Beltran Department of Radiology, Brigham and Women's Hospital, Harvard Medical School, Boston, MA, USA

Jenny T. Bencardino Department of Radiology, New York University Langone Health, New York, NY, USA

Penn Medicine, Department of Radiology, Perelman School of Medicine at the University of Pennsylvania, Philadelphia, PA, USA

Miriam A. Bredella Division of Musculoskeletal Imaging and Intervention, Department of Radiology, Massachusetts General Hospital, Harvard Medical School, Boston, MA, USA

Eric Y. Chang Department of Radiology, VA San Diego Healthcare System, San Diego, CA, USA

Department of Radiology, University of California, San Diego Medical Center, San Diego, CA, USA

Christine B. Chung Department of Radiology, VA San Diego Healthcare System, San Diego, CA, USA

Department of Radiology, University of California, San Diego Medical Center, San Diego, CA, USA

Jorge Delgado Department of Radiology, Massachusetts General Hospital, Harvard Medical School, Boston, MA, USA

Alireza Eajazi Division of Musculoskeletal Imaging and Intervention, Department of Radiology, Massachusetts General Hospital, Harvard Medical School, Boston, MA, USA

James F. Griffith Department of Imaging and Interventional Radiology, Prince of Wales Hospital, The Chinese University of Hong Kong, Shatin, NT, Hong Kong

Mingqian Huang Department of Radiology, Stony Brook University Hospital, Stony Brook School of Medicine, Stony Brook, NY, USA

Diego Jaramillo Department of Radiology, Columbia University Medical Center, New York, NY, USA

Shefali Kothary Division of Ultrasound, Department of Radiology and Imaging, Hospital for Special Surgery, Weill Medical College of Cornell University, New York, NY, USA

Konstantin Krepkin Department of Radiology, New York University Langone Health, New York, NY, USA

Eric Ledermann Department of Radiology, Maimonides Medical Center, Brooklyn, NY, USA

Joyce H.Y. Leung Department of Imaging and Interventional Radiology, The Chinese University of Hong Kong, Shatin, NT, Hong Kong

Seema Meraj Zwanger-Pesiri Radiology, Lindenhurst, NY, USA

Theodore T. Miller Division of Ultrasound, Department of Radiology and Imaging, Hospital for Special Surgery, Weill Medical College of Cornell University, New York, NY, USA

Matthew J. Minn American Institute for Radiologic Pathology, Silver Spring, MD, USA

Mark D. Murphey American Institute for Radiologic Pathology, Silver Spring, MD, USA

Departments of Radiology and Nuclear Medicine, Uniformed Services University of the Health Sciences, Bethesda, MD, USA

Walter Reed Army Medical Center, Washington, DC, USA

Ogonna Kenechi Nwawka Division of Ultrasound, Department of Radiology and Imaging, Hospital for Special Surgery, Weill Medical College of Cornell University, New York, NY, USA

Jonelle Petscavage-Thomas Department of Radiology, Penn State Milton S. Hershey Medical Center, Hershey, PA, USA

Mark Schweitzer Department of Radiology, Stony Brook University Hospital, Stony Brook School of Medicine, Stony Brook, NY, USA

Monica Tafur Department of Radiology, Michael's Hospital, University of Toronto, Toronto, ON, Canada

Martin Torriani Division of Musculoskeletal Imaging and Intervention, Department of Radiology, Massachusetts General Hospital, Harvard Medical School, Boston, MA, USA

Michael J. Tuite Department of Radiology, University of Wisconsin School of Medicine and Public Health, Madison, WI, USA

Eric A. Walker Department of Radiology, Milton S. Hershey Medical Center, Hershey, PA, USA

Departments of Radiology and Nuclear Medicine, Uniformed Services University of the Health Sciences, Bethesda, MD, USA

Avner Yemin Envision Physician Services—Radiology Associates of Hollywood, Memorial Healthcare System, Hollywood, FL, USA

Joseph S. Yu Department of Radiology, The Ohio State University Wexner Medical Center, Columbus, OH, USA

Part I

Imaging Techniques

Current Protocols for Radiographic and CT Evaluation of the Shoulder

1

Joyce H.Y. Leung and James F. Griffith

1.1 Shoulder Pain

Shoulder pain is one of the most common musculoskeletal symptoms and a frequent indication for musculoskeletal imaging. Shoulder pain, compared to pain in smaller joints such as the elbow, wrist, or ankle, is usually not well localized and even when it is well localized may not necessarily correlate closely with the site of the pathology. There is considerable overlap in the clinical presentation of common shoulder conditions such as rotator cuff tendon tear, subacromial-subdeltoid bursitis, calcific tendinitis, superior labral tears, and adhesive capsulitis. The most likely reason for poor localization of shoulder pain is the expansive nature of the two main pain generators in the shoulder, namely the subacromial-subdeltoid bursa and the shoulder joint synovium/capsule.

This poor localization of shoulder pain clearly has implications for shoulder imaging since one has to consider a range of potential etiologies in most patients referred for imaging with shoulder pain. The most common causes of shoulder pain in clinical practice are rotator cuff tendinosis and subacromial-subdeltoid bursitis, rotator cuff tears, biceps tendinosis and tears, calcific tendinitis, superior labral tears, adhesive capsulitis, and acromioclavicular joint arthritis. These entities account for over 95% of patients with shoulder pain. Radiographs and computed tomography (CT) are not the primary imaging modalities used to evaluate these specific pathologies, which are best visualized by ultrasound and magnetic resonance imaging (MRI). Nevertheless, radiographs are still the primary imaging modality used to investigate a patient with shoulder problems. This is testament to the ease of availability of radiographs and their ability to provide a good overview of shoulder anatomy and pathology as well as helping to quickly exclude several serious shoulder pathologies such as tumor, dislocation, or fracture.

1.2 Radiography

Standard radiographic views of the shoulder are still very widely obtained. However, since the 1990s, with the emergence of supplementary imaging investigations (ultrasound, CT, MRI), specialized radiographic views of the shoulder are less frequently obtained. Increasingly, the tendency is to obtain an alternative investigation to show and grade features previously investigated by radiography such as Hill-Sachs deformity, or glenoid bone loss. This trend is

J. H.Y. Leung
Department of Imaging and Interventional Radiology, The Chinese University of Hong Kong, Shatin, NT, Hong Kong

J. F. Griffith (✉)
Department of Imaging and Interventional Radiology, Prince of Wales Hospital, The Chinese University of Hong Kong, Shatin, NT, Hong Kong
e-mail: griffith@cuhk.edu.hk

J. T. Bencardino (ed.), *The Shoulder*, https://doi.org/10.1007/978-3-030-06240-8_1

understandable and likely to continue, since in most instances these alternative investigations (US, CT, MRI) show the abnormality more reliably and to better effect than radiographs and also provide clinically relevant information on adjacent soft-tissue structures. Specialized radiographic views are technically more difficult to obtain especially in the acute trauma setting though also in the more chronic setting if there is limitation of shoulder movement. The net effect is that one encounters specialized views of the shoulder much less frequently than previously. As a consequence, when specialized views are requested, the technological nuance to achieve a high-quality specialized view is not always readily available.

1.2.1 Common Radiographic Views of the Shoulder

1.2.1.1 Anteroposterior (AP) View

This is the most common, and often the only, view obtained when screening for shoulder pathology. It is the easiest to perform, even in the setting of severe trauma.

Technique (Fig. 1.1a–c)

Patient Position:

- Standing or supine.
- Coronal plane of body parallel to cassette/image detector.
- Usually performed with the arm in a neutral position. The same view with the arm in internal rotation is used to reveal a Hill-Sachs deformity while in external rotation it can show the greater tubercle in profile.

Radiographic Beam:

- Directed in a true anteroposterior plane relative to the body. The scapula is in a coronal oblique plane (tilted about 40° anteriorly). The beam is centered medial to the glenohumeral joint.

Image Analysis and Clinical Benefit

On this image, one can see the glenohumeral joint, acromioclavicular joint, lateral clavicle, and scapula (Fig. 1.1d–f). The lateral border of the scapula and medial cortex of the proximal humerus forms a smooth arch known as scapulohumeral arch or Moloney's line. This is analogous to Shenton's line of the hip. The acromiohumeral interval can also be seen. This should normally be >7 mm. Superior migration of the humeral head which is a feature of severe rotator cuff tears, particularly of the supraspinatus tendon, leads to disruption of the scapulohumeral arch and narrowing of the acromiohumeral interval.

One can also appreciate that there is normally a slight overlap between the glenoid rim and the humeral head as the glenohumeral joint is normally tilted anteriorly by about 40°. As the projection is not tangential to the glenohumeral joint space, this joint space is not seen in profile. The anteroposterior view is particularly good for showing fractures of the proximal humerus, scapula, or clavicle (Fig. 1.1g–i), for showing dislocation of either the glenohumeral (Fig. 1.1j, k) or the acromioclavicular joints. It is also helpful for showing rotator cuff calcific tendinitis (Fig. 1.1k) or acromioclavicular joint arthritis. The AP view in internal rotation can show up to 92% of Hill-Sachs deformities [1], though not in the same detail as axillary or Stryker notch views.

1.2.1.2 Scapular Y-View

This view is used to show the relationship of the humeral head to the glenoid and also show the subacromial space.

Technique (Fig. 1.2a)

Patient Position:

- Standing or lying prone.
- Body is positioned in an approximate 45–60° anterior oblique position with the shoulder to be examined in contact with cassette/image detector.
- Arm in neutral rotation.

Radiographic Beam:

- Directed along the plane of the scapula (true lateral of scapula).

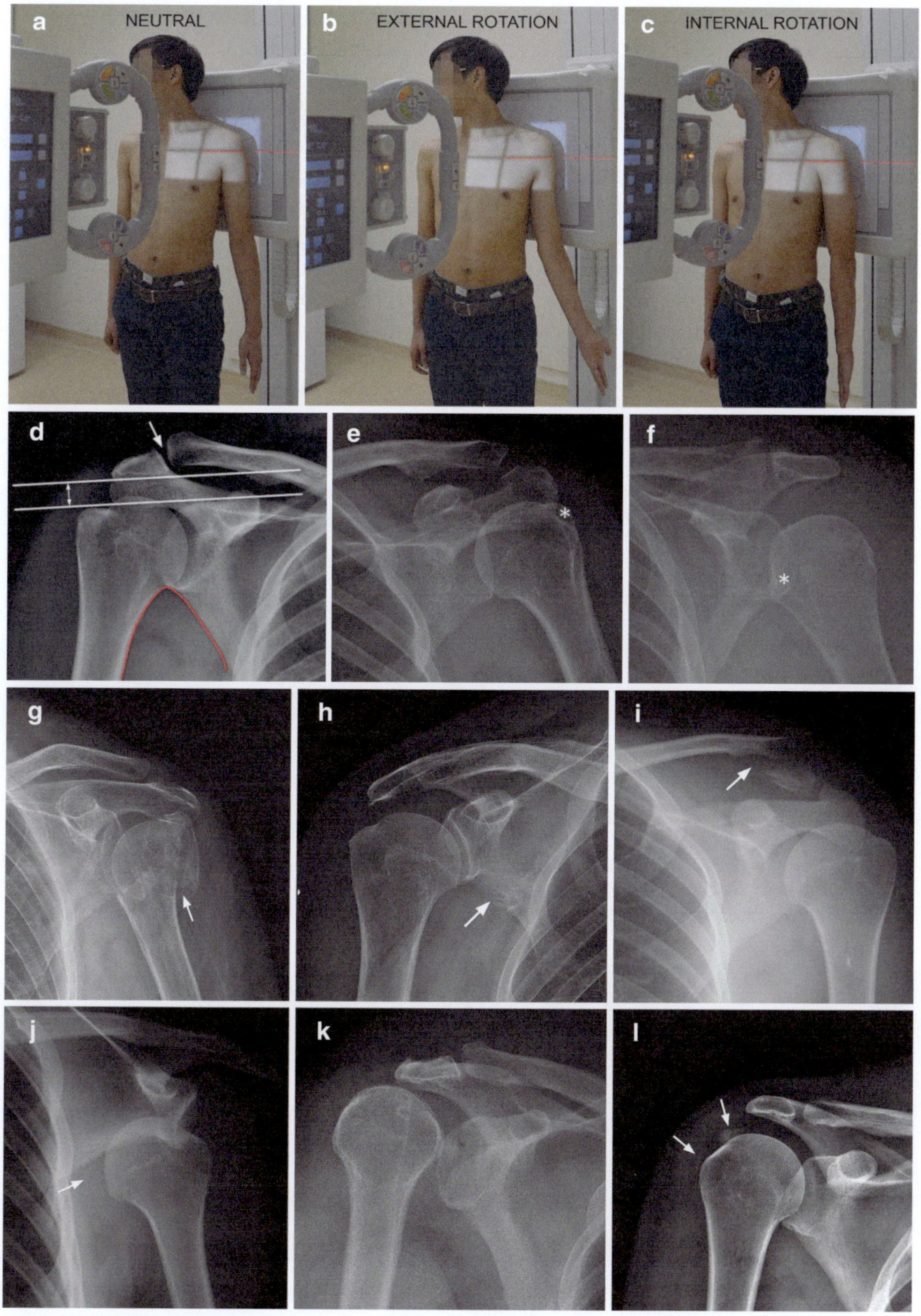

Fig. 1.1 Radiographic positioning for anteroposterior (AP) shoulder radiograph in (**a**) neutral, (**b**) external rotation, and (**c**) internal rotation positions. (**d–f**) Anteroposterior radiographs of the shoulder taken in the (**a**) neutral position showing the glenohumeral joint with overlap between the humeral head and the glenoid rim, a smooth scapulohumeral arch (red curve), and the acromioclavicular joint (arrow). The normal acromiohumeral internal (>7 mm) is also shown; (**b**) external rotation position showing the greater tuberosity (*) and (**f**) internal rotation position showing the lesser tuberosity (*). Anteroposterior radiographs of the shoulder showing a (**g**) proximal humeral fracture (arrow), (**h**) scapular blade fracture (arrow), (**i**) distal clavicular fracture (arrow), (**j**) anterior shoulder dislocation (arrow), (**k**) a posterior shoulder dislocation, and (**l**) supraspinatus tendon calcification (arrows)

Image Analysis and Clinical Benefit

On this image, you can appreciate that the scapular body is seen in tangent with the glenoid fossa seen en face as a Y-shaped intersection of the scapular body, acromion process, and coracoid process (Fig. 1.2b). The humeral head is centered over the glenoid fossa. The scapular Y-view is good for determining whether a shoulder dislocation is anteriorly or posteriorly located as well as revealing fractures of the coracoid process, scapula, acromion process, and proximal humeral shaft (Fig. 1.2b, d). This view is preferable to the axillary view when the patient has limited shoulder abduction [2].

1.2.1.3 Axillary View

This view provides a "top-down" view of the shoulder joint. It is a very useful view though it may be difficult to obtain in patients with severe shoulder pain following trauma, in children, or in uncooperative patients.

Technique (Fig. 1.3a, b)

Many variations of the axillary view exist. The most commonly used in the outpatient setting is as follows:

Patient Position:

– Erect.

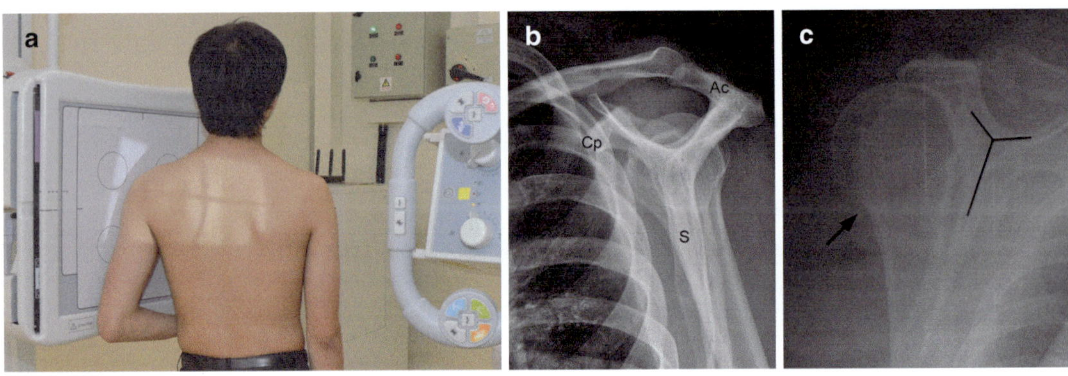

Fig. 1.2 (**a**) Radiographic positioning for scapular Y-view. (**b**) Normal scapular Y-view showing coracoid process (Cp), acromial process (Ac), and blade of scapula (S). (**b**). Note how the humeral head is centrically located over the glenoid. (**c**) Scapular Y-view showing anterior dislocation of humeral head

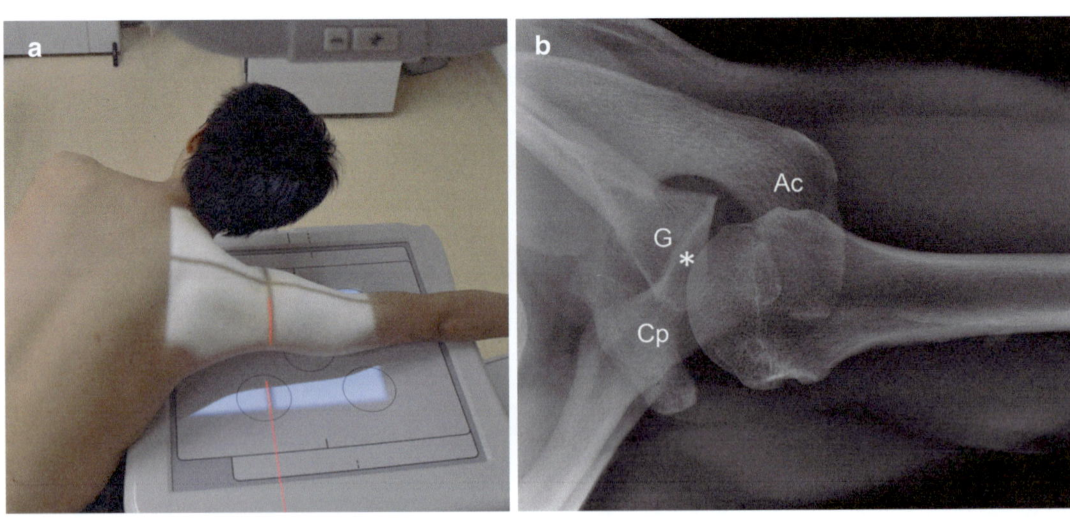

Fig. 1.3 (**a**) Radiographic positioning for axillary view. (**b**) Normal axillary view showing coracoid process (Cp), acromion (Ac), glenoid (G), and glenohumeral joint (*) which is almost but not quite in profile

Radiographic Beam:

- Patient leans laterally with arm abducted over the cassette/image detector which is centered under axilla. Beam is angled 5–15° (towards the elbow) centered at the shoulder joint.

Image Analysis and Clinical Benefit

This image provides a superior-inferior tangential view of glenohumeral joint. The humeral head to glenoid relationship can easily be ascertained. This view can also assess fractures of the anterior glenoid rim and Hill-Sachs deformities as well as fractures of the coracoid process and subscapularis calcific tendinitis. Glenoid version is not accurately assessed on axillary views when compared to CT [3].

In the acute trauma setting, one of the three modified axillary views can be used if the patient is unable to abduct the shoulder. All of these views can all be taken with the patient's arm in a sling, i.e., there is no need to abduct the arm, and are very useful at evaluating glenohumeral alignment.

1. Velpeau view [4]:
   (a) Patient leans 30° backwards (either sitting or standing) over horizontally placed cassette/image detector.
   (b) Radiographic beam angled vertically downwards through shoulder joint from above.
2. Wallace view [5]:
   (a) Upright sitting position.
   (b) Cassette/image detector placed horizontally on table behind humerus in contact with arm.
   (c) Patient rotated 30° so that scapula is parallel to the edge of image detector.
   (d) Radiographic beam angled downwards and posteriorly 30° from vertical, centered at glenohumeral joint.
3. Takahashi view [6]:
   (a) Upright sitting position.
   (b) Cassette/image detector placed on superoanterior aspect of shoulder, angled 25° anteroinferiorly.
   (c) Radiographic beam angled 25° upwards and anteriorly centered at glenohumeral joint.

1.2.1.4 Acromioclavicular (AC) Joint View

The oblique orientation of the acromioclavicular joints is such that either each joint can be radiographed in isolation or both joints can be radiographed in unison allowing ready side-to-side comparison. A weight-bearing (stress) view is sometimes performed to accentuate AC joint capsular laxity or mild subluxation, and to differentiate Rockwood classification of type II and III injuries.

Technique (Fig. 1.4a, b)

Patient Position and Beam:

- Single side: AP view with beam directed at the coracoid process.
- Both AC joints: AP view with beam directed at the sternal notch and coned to pass through both acromioclavicular joints (Fig. 1.4a).
- Weight-bearing AP view (Fig. 1.4b): As per AP view of both AC joints except that the patient holds a 5 kg weight in both hands.

Image Analysis and Clinical Benefit

This view is primarily used to evaluate AC joint subluxation (Fig. 1.4d, e). One can see both AC joints in profile. The normal width of the AC joint varies widely and can be up to 7 mm in normal subjects [7] with a normal coracoclavicular (CC) distance of 11–13 mm [8]. AC joint dislocation is suspected when radiographic measurements of the AC joint is >7 mm or coracoclavicular distance is >13 mm [9, 10]. In addition, to the width of the AC joint, one must also ensure that the inferior cortices of the clavicle and the acromion are aligned with each other. AC joint injuries are commonly radiographically graded using the Rockwood classification (Table 1.1).

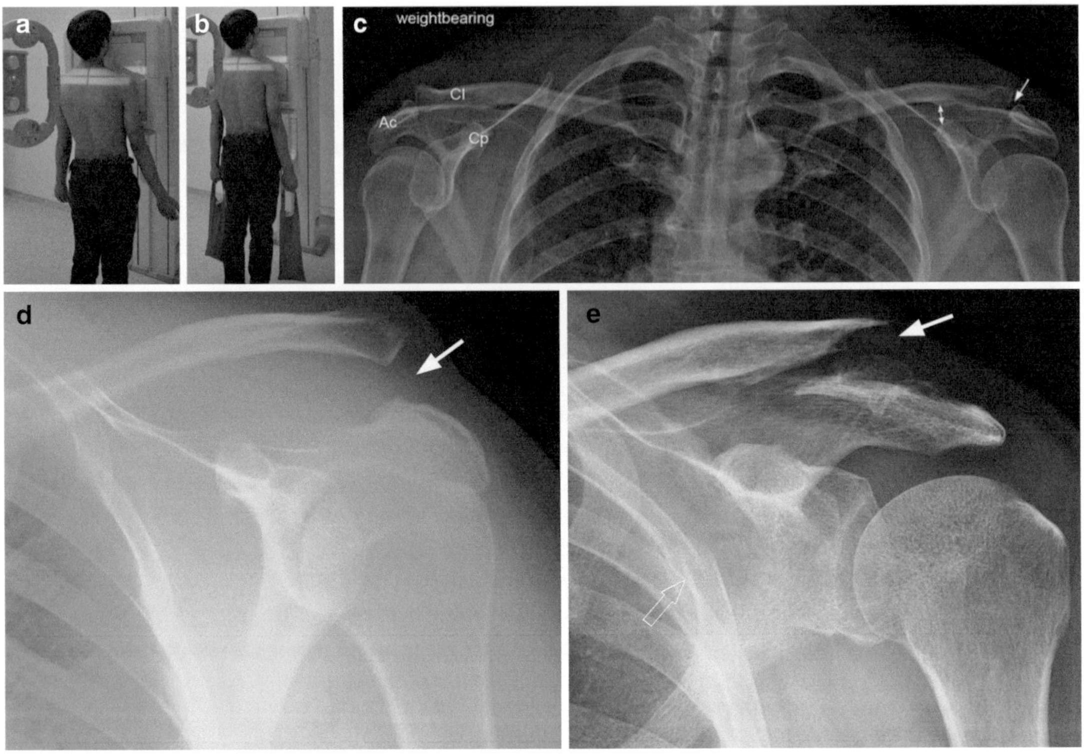

Fig. 1.4 (**a**) Radiographic positioning for acromioclavicular joint radiography: (**a**) non-weight bearing and (**b**) weight bearing. (**c**) Normal large-field-of-view image of both acromioclavicular joints with weight bearing showing coracoid process (Cp), acromion (Ac), and clavicle (Cl) on the right side. On the left side, the normal acromioclavicular joint space (→, up to 7 mm) and normal coracoclavicular distance (↔, 11-13 mm) are shown. (d,e). (**d**) Frontal AC view showing Rockwood grade III ACJ injury (arrow). (**e**) Frontal AC view showing distal clavicular fracture (arrow) with no acromioclavicular joint disruption

Table 1.1 Rockwood classification of ACJ injuries [11]

Type	Pathology	Radiographic findings
I	AC ligament partial tear and CC ligament intact	Normal
II	Complete tear AC ligament with partial tear CC ligament	<25% Superior elevation of distal clavicle
III	Complete tear of both AC and CC ligaments	25–100% Elevation of distal clavicle
IV	Type III + posterior displacement of clavicle (through trapezius muscle) Anterior dislocation of sternoclavicular joint can also occur	Posterior dislocation of clavicle behind acromion (best seen on axillary view)
V	Type III injury + disruption of deltoid and lateral trapezius muscle insertion as well as deltotrapezial fascia	>100% Elevation of distal clavicle. CC distance increased by 100–300%
VI	Distal clavicle is displaced inferior to the acromion or coracoid process	Distal end of clavicle located inferior to acromion or coracoid

AC Acromioclavicular, *CC* coracoclavicular

1.2.2 Specialized Radiographic Views of the Shoulder

1.2.2.1 Bernageau View

Technique (Fig. 1.5a)
Patient Position:

- Standing upright.
- Anterior oblique position with arm abducted at 135° so that the elbow is above the head.

Radiographic Beam:

- Directed to the posterior aspect of the shoulder.
- 30 degrees caudal tilt of radiographic beam
- Optimal angulation of the beam and rotation of the patient can be obtained under fluoroscopic guide.

Image Analysis and Clinical Benefit
The Bernageau view provides a true tangential view of the anterior rim of the glenoid (Fig. 1.5b). It is useful for assessing glenoid bone loss or fractures of the anterior rim of the glenoid in patients with anterior dislocation. The Bernageau profile view is a valid and reliable method for quantifying glenoid bone loss revealing glenoid bone loss with a sensitivity and specificity of >90% [12]. It can be used as an alternative to MR or CT assessment [13]. Bilateral examination for side-to-side comparison may help in assessing subtle change [12].

1.2.2.2 Stryker Notch View

Technique (Fig. 1.6a)
Patient Position:

- Supine or standing position.
- Arm extended overhead, elbow flexed, and palm placed on the back of head.

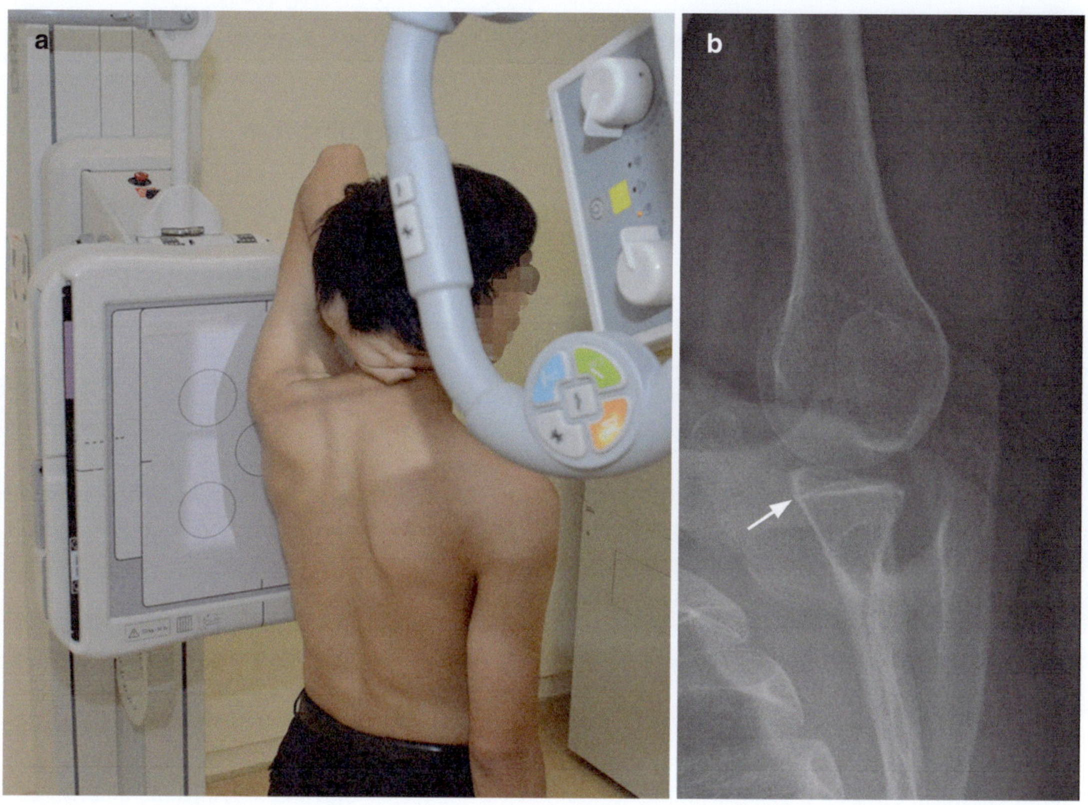

Fig. 1.5 (**a**) Radiographic positioning for Bernageau view. (**b**) Bernageau view showing normal anterior glenoid rim (arrow)

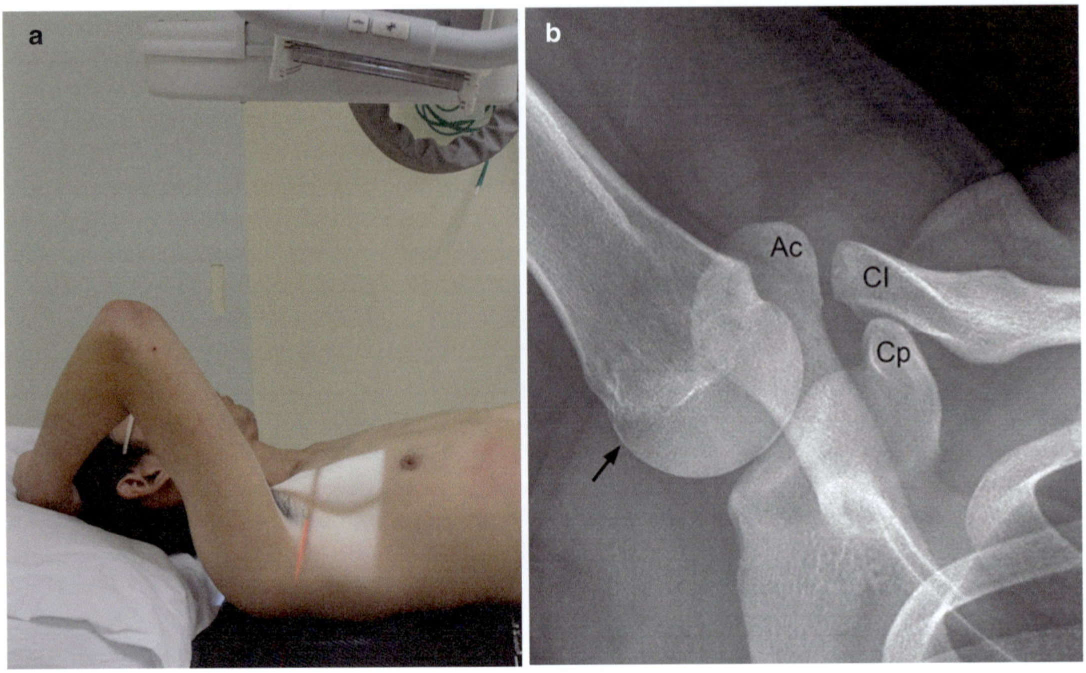

Fig. 1.6 (**a**) Radiographic positioning for Stryker notch view. (**b**) Stryker notch view showing how the posterolateral aspect (arrow) of the humeral head is well demonstrated. Ac: Acromion; Cl: clavicle; Cp: coracoid (*radiograph courtesy of Dr. Bill Morrison*)

Radiographic Beam:

- Directed to the coracoid process, 10° cephalad.

Image Analysis and Clinical Benefit

One can appreciate how well the Stryker notch view demonstrates the posterolateral aspect of the proximal aspect of the humeral head (Fig. 1.6b). As such, this view is mainly used to reveal Hill-Sachs deformity which it can detect with a sensitivity of >90% [1]. A Hill-Sachs deformity is a compression fracture of the humeral head caused by impaction of the humeral head against the anterior or anteroinferior aspect of the glenoid after anterior dislocation. Hill-Sachs deformity is seen as a diffuse flattening or a more angulated depression at the posterolateral aspect of the humeral head. Large or angulated Hill-Sachs deformities can engage with the glenoid rim during external rotation precipitating anterior dislocation. Comparison with the normal opposite side can be helpful in qualifying the size of defect present.

1.2.2.3 West Point view

Technique (Fig. 1.7a)

Patient Position:

- Prone.
- Arm abducted to 90° with forearm hanging over the edge of the examination table.

Radiographic Beam:

- Cassette/image detector placed against the top of shoulder, perpendicular to the table.
- Beam centered at axilla, with 25° downward angulation from horizontal and 25° medial angulation.

Image Analysis and Clinical Benefit

The West Point view is a modified axillary projection that similar to the Bernageau view demonstrates fractures or bone loss of the anterior glenoid rim (Fig. 1.7b) [14]. While on an axillary view the lateral clavicle overlaps the anterior rim of the glenoid, this is not a feature of the West Point view. The West Point view can identify

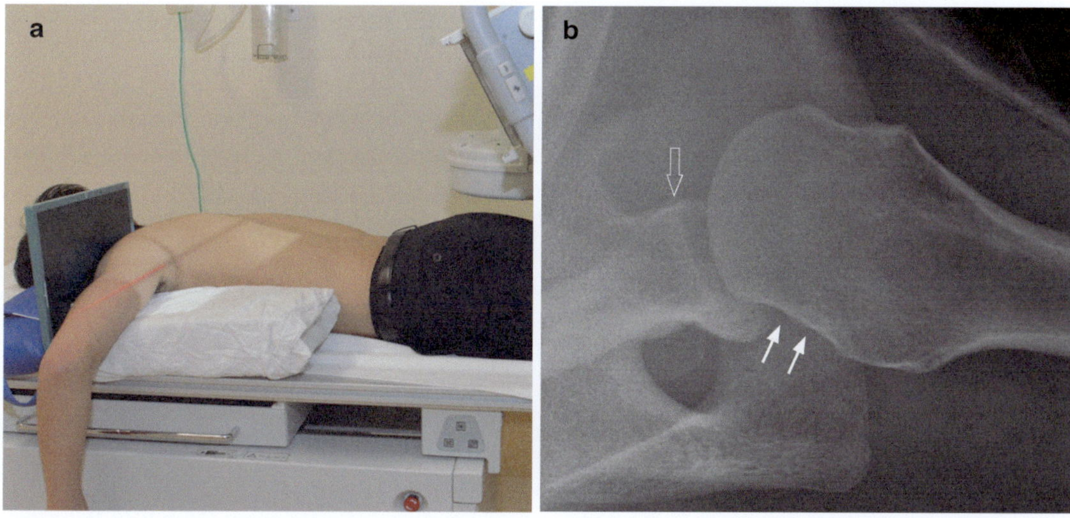

Fig. 1.7 (**a**) Radiographic positioning for West Point view. (**b**) West Point view is used to evaluate the anterior glenoid rim for fracture and anterior glenoid bone loss (open arrow). A medium-sized Hill-Sachs deformity is also shown (arrow) (*radiograph courtesy of Dr. Bill Morrison*)

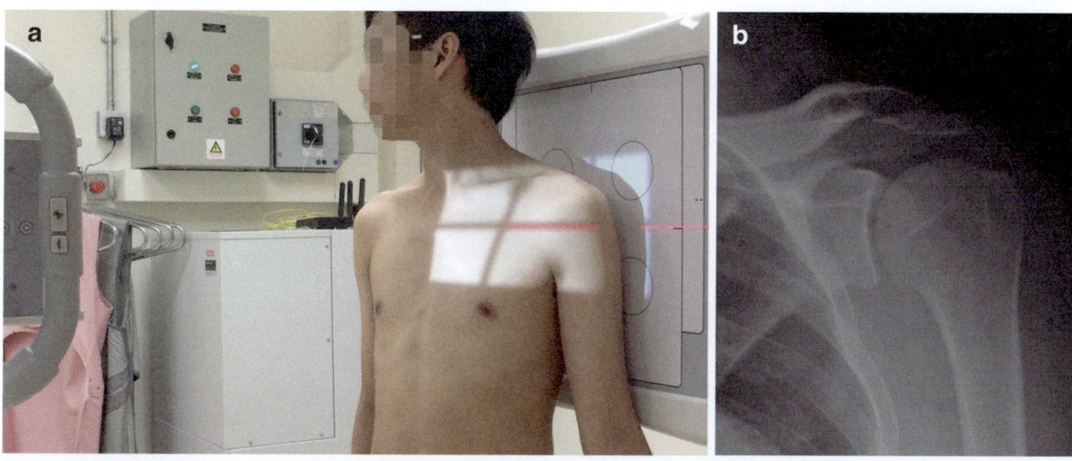

Fig. 1.8 (**a**) Radiographic positioning for Grashey view (**b**) The Grashey view provides a tangential view of the glenohumeral joint (*radiograph courtesy of Dr. Bill Morrison*)

anterior glenoid rim fractures with 70% sensitivity [14, 15].

1.2.2.4 Grashey View

Technique (Fig. 1.8a)
Patient Position:

- Patient's body angled 35°–45° with the scapula against and parallel to the cassette/image detector.

Radiographic Beam:

- Directed perpendicular to cassette/image detector and provide tangential view of glenohumeral joint.

Image Interpretation and Clinical Benefit
The Grashey view is a posterior oblique view with the glenoid articular surface in profile, i.e., it is a true AP view of the glenohumeral joint space and is used to evaluate widening or narrowing of this joint.

Other specialized view:

- **Garth view**: Radiographic beam is angled caudally 45° from that used to obtain the standard anteroposterior view of the shoulder joint. The beam is then tangential to the anteroinferior glenoid rim. The Garth view is used to detect Bankart fractures and Hill-Sachs deformity [16].

1.3 Computed Tomography of the Shoulder

CT of the shoulder is mainly used to:

(a) Diagnose and classify acute fracture (Fig. 1.9a, b).
(b) Quantify glenoid bone loss (Fig. 1.10a–d).
(c) Assess severe glenohumeral arthritis preoperatively (Fig. 1.11a, b).
(d) Assess fracture healing.
(e) Assess shoulder prostheses and internal fixation (Fig. 1.12).

1.3.1 CT Technique (64-Slice Multidetector CT)

Irrespective of the clinical indication for shoulder CT, the scanning protocol used is identical for all patients.

- Supine position.
- Shoulder close to gantry center.
- Upper arm close to body.

Parameters:

- Kv120kV.
- Effective mA: 300–400 mA.
- Detector collimation: 64 × 0.625 mm.
- Scan plane extends from the top of the acromion to below the glenoid.

1.3.2 Specific Clinical Indications for Shoulder CT

CT improves classification of proximal humeral [17] and glenoid/scapular neck [18, 19] fractures

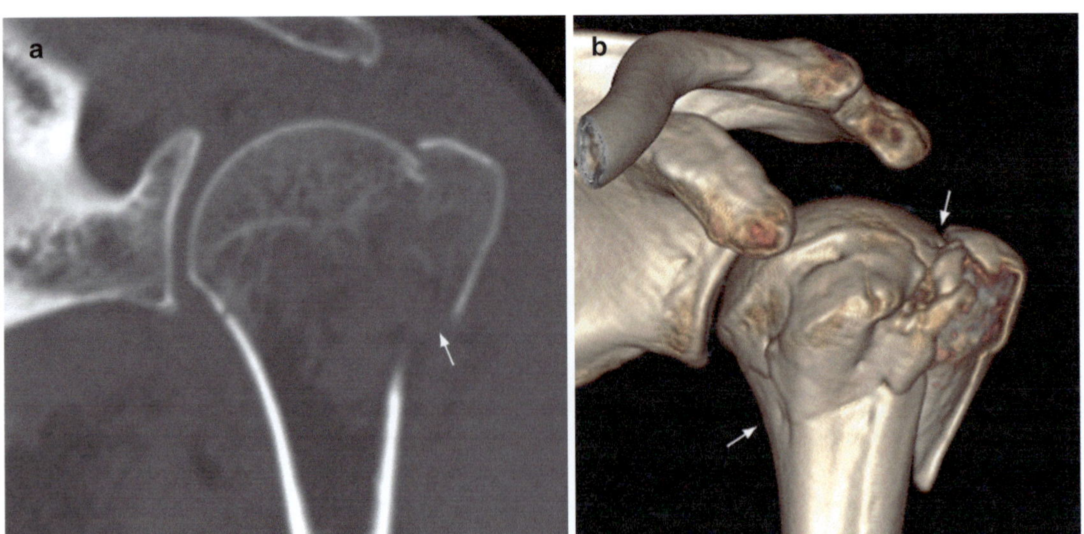

Fig. 1.9 Comminuted fracture of proximal humerus (arrows) shown on coronal (**a**) and three-dimensional (**b**) reconstruction

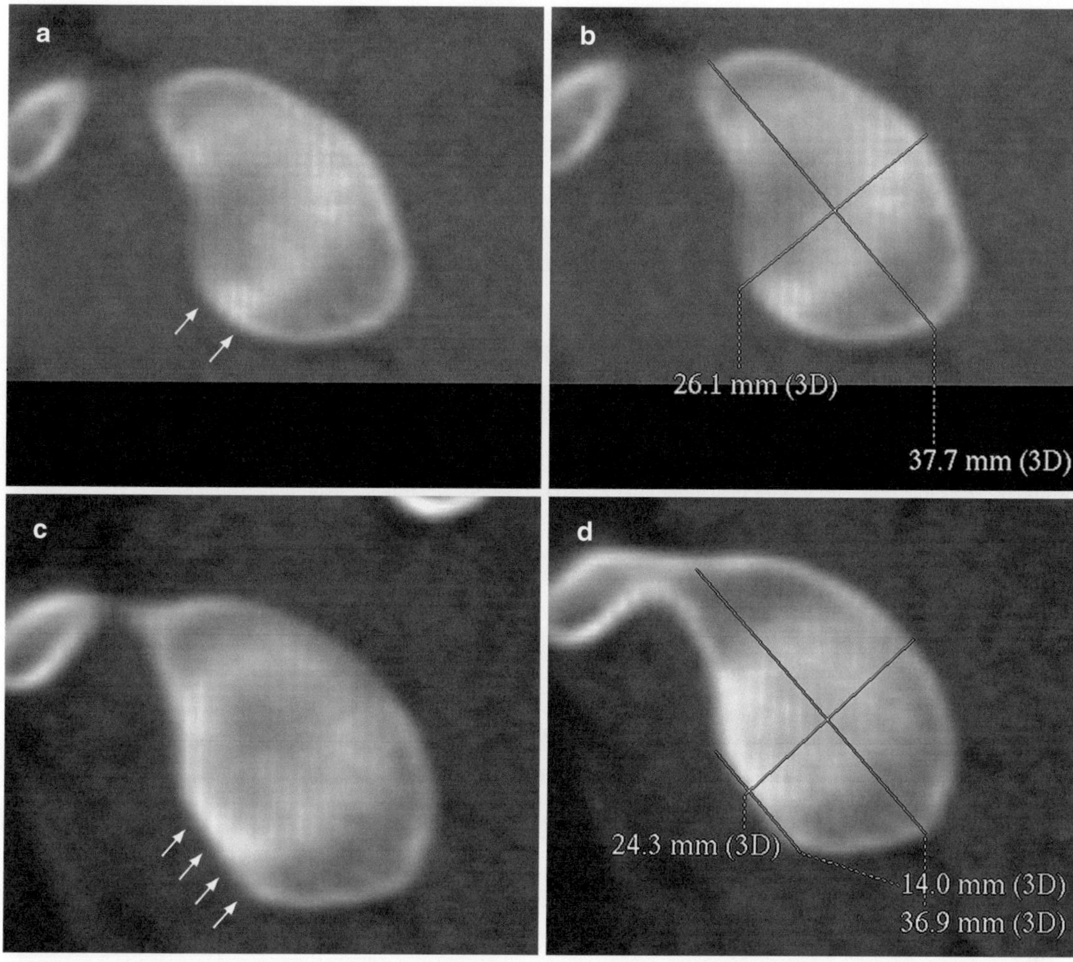

Fig. 1.10 CT of the normal (**a**, **b**) shoulder showing a normal curved anterior glenoid rim (arrows) with a glenoid width of 26.1 mm. On the contralateral shoulder (**c**, **d**) with recurrent dislocation, there is loss of the normal curvature with an anterior straight line (14 mm long) to the glenoid. The glenoid width is reduced to 24.3 mm. The glenoid bone loss is therefore 26.1–24.3 mm = 1.8 mm or alternatively 1.8/26.1 x 100 = 6.9%. This is considered to be mild glenoid bone loss

compared to radiographs allowing more accurate decisions to be made regarding the need for and form of operative treatment and fixation [20]. 3D CT reconstruction improves proximal humeral fracture classification (Neer or ATAO classification) compared to 2D reconstructions [17, 21].

CT examination is now almost a routine preoperative investigation for patients with severe glenohumeral osteoarthritis being considered for total shoulder arthroplasty (TSA) [22]. CT enables preoperative determination of glenoid retroversion, which is a common feature of the osteoarthritic shoulder, as well as estimation of premorbid glenoid bone stock and humeral head size (Youdarian AR 2013). Not recognizing glenoid retroversion can lead to a retroverted prosthesis and an increased risk of posterior instability. Prior to CT, glenoid version was measured on axillary view radiographs. Glenoid version is the angle between (a) a line drawn from the medial border of the scapula to the center of the glenoid and (b) a line perpendicular to the face of the glenoid on an axial CT image at or just below the tip of the coracoid process (Fig. 1.12b). The normal

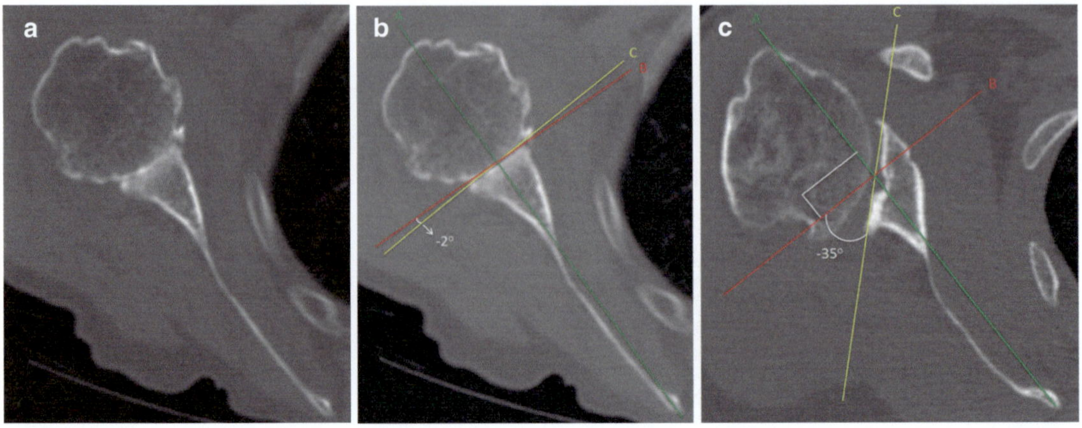

Fig. 1.11 (**a**) Axial CT of severe glenohumeral osteoarthritis. (**b**) The same image as A with measurement of glenoid version. To measure glenoid version draw a line from the medial border of the scapula to the center of the glenoid (line A). Draw a line perpendicular to this line (line B). Draw a line along the face of the glenoid (line C). Glenoid version is the angle between lines B and C. In this case, glenoid retroversion is −2° which is normal. (**c**) In this other case, glenoid version is −35° which is abnormal. Normal glenoid version is from +5° to −15°

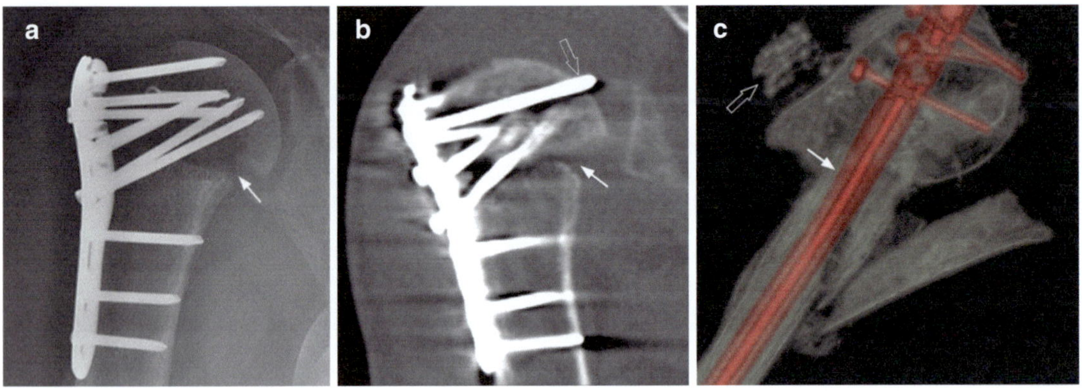

Fig. 1.12 (**a**) Radiograph of shoulder showing fracture proximal humerus postfixation. (**b**) 2D coronal reconstruction of same patient as previous image showing incomplete fracture healing with screw tip protruding across the articular surface. (**c**) 3D CT reconstruction of comminuted proximal humeral fracture in another patient with volume rendering and windowing designed to increase bone transparency allowing clearer view of metallic fixation devices (arrow). There are also some antibiotic beads in situ (open arrow)

glenoid version is from 5° anteversion to 15° retroversion.

Restoration of glenoid version to neutral is one's aim of TSA while premorbid head size estimation allows selection of the appropriate anatomically sized prosthetic head [23]. CT is also helpful in evaluating bone morphology, posterior or superior humeral head subluxation, subchondral bony resorption, and bone density—all of which help guide prosthesis shape selection and positioning as well as operative technique [24, 25].

Glenoid component failure is the most common complication of total shoulder arthroplasty. CT is more sensitive than radiography at revealing periprosthetic lucency, which is the cardinal sign of prosthetic loosening [26]. CT scanning in the lateral decubitus position with maximum forward flexion aligns the glenoid with the CT scan plane and thus helps to minimize metallic artifact around the glenoid prosthesis [26].

Assessment of glenoid bone loss (GBL) is a common indication for CT examination though this is likely to be increasingly undertaken solely

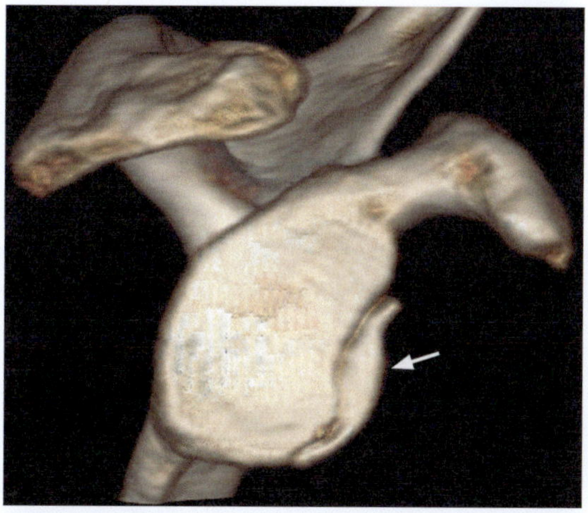

Fig. 1.13 3D CT reconstruction of shoulder in patient with anterior dislocation showing large fracture (arrow) of anterior glenoid rim. 3D allows very good perception of fracture fragments. The humeral head has been electronically disarticulated to allow an unobstructed clear en face view of the glenoid

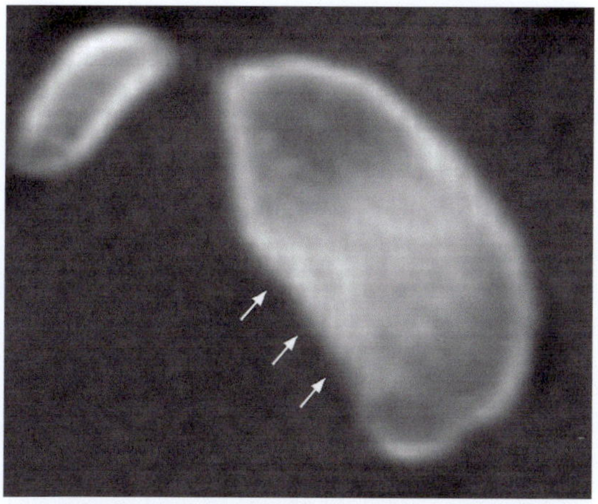

Fig. 1.14 2D double-oblique reconstruction en face to the glenoid. This shows severe glenoid bone loss with a concave rather than convex anterior curvature to the glenoid (arrows). An anterior concavity is normally associated with severe (>20%) anterior glenoid bone loss

by MR examination [27]. The following are 12 basic concepts regarding CT assessment of GBL [28–30]:

1. GBL after shoulder dislocation is very common (>80%).
2. Most (>90%) GBL is not associated with a glenoid rim fracture (Fig. 1.13).
3. GBL first affects the anterior rather than the anteroinferior aspect of the glenoid.
4. The earliest sign of GBL is an anterior straight line to the anterior glenoid rim. If an anterior straight line is not present, i.e., if the anterior glenoid rim is curved, then there is no GBL present.
5. Excellent side-to-side symmetry in glenoid shape and size exists such that the contralateral shoulder can be used as a template for initial glenoid size.
6. Mild GBL is <10% bone loss, moderate 10–20%, and severe >20% bone loss.
7. The most severe GBL is 33%.
8. With severe GBL, the anterior glenoid rim becomes concave (Fig. 1.14), rather than straight as seen in mild-to-moderate degrees of GBL.
9. Critical GBL is >15%. At this level, the frequency of anterior dislocations seems to increase.
10. A Hill-Sachs deformity ± some degree of GBL seems to be present in all patients with documented anterior shoulder dislocation.
11. CT has good agreement (r = 0.79) with shoulder arthroscopy regarding the severity of glenoid bone loss. That said, arthroscopy is not the perfect gold standard.
12. GBL can be assessed by radiography, MR, or CT. Of these approaches, CT with comparison of the opposite side seems to be the most accurate while MR seems to be the most practical.

1.3.3 How to Quantify GBL Using CT (Fig. 1.10a–d)

The best CT method is to compare both shoulders, i.e., the dislocating side with the non-dislocating side. For CT of a single shoulder, the contralateral shoulder will necessarily be included in the scan plane (i.e., irradiated) so it is best to employ a large field of view and use the information from the contralateral normal shoulder to your advantage. A double-oblique reconstruction technique is used to obtain an en face view of each glenoid articular surface. On this en face view, first note whether there is an anterior straight line present. If there is no anterior straight line, then there is no glenoid bone loss and it can be reported as such without any need to do additional measurements. If there is an anterior straight line present, the amount of glenoid bone loss should be quantified. This is done by first drawing a line along the long axis of the glenoid (Saller line). Glenoid width is then measured at right angles to the long axis of the glenoid at the midportion of the rounded inferior two-thirds of the glenoid. Absolute (in mm) and percentage (%) glenoid bone loss is then calculated as the difference between the width of the glenoid on the dislocating side compared to that of the contralateral normal glenoid. This method is applicable in all cases except when there is bilateral dislocation with bilateral GBL.

If there has been bilateral dislocation with bilateral GBL or if only a single shoulder has undergone CT examination, an alternative method is to use the best-fit circle method. This involves applying the smallest possible best-fit circle to the rounded inferior two-thirds of the glenoid. The margins of the circle should just contact the cortex of the glenoid except for along the anterior glenoid rim. The limitation of this technique is that the inferior two-thirds of the glenoid does not always have a completely circular shape. A noncircular configuration to the glenoid before bone loss will not be captured with the best-fit circle technique.

Hill-Sachs lesions are seen on CT in over 80% of patients with anterior dislocation [30] being, as expected, more frequent and larger in recurrent dislocation. Large or angulated Hill-Sachs deformities (known as "engaging" Hill-Sachs deformities) are a risk factor for recurrent dislocation (Fig. 1.15). CT will not demonstrate purely cartilaginous Hill-Sachs lesions though these are much less common and of little clinical significance [31].

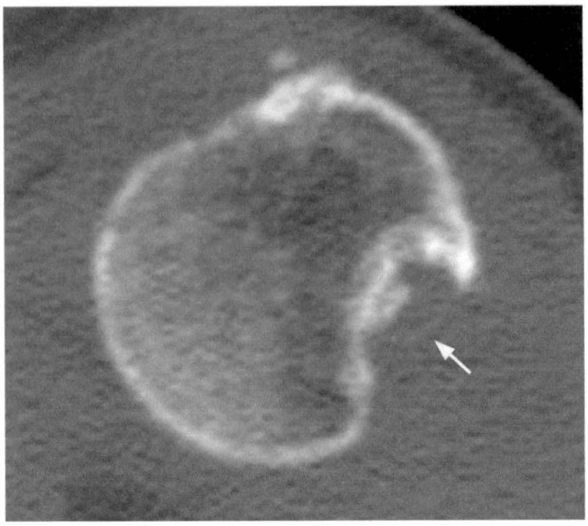

Fig. 1.15 Axial CT of the shoulder through the proximal aspect of the humeral head. There is a large angulated Hill-Sachs deformity (arrow) at the posterosuperior aspect of the humeral head. Such large, angulated deformities may "engage" with the glenoid rim during external rotation precipitating anterior dislocation

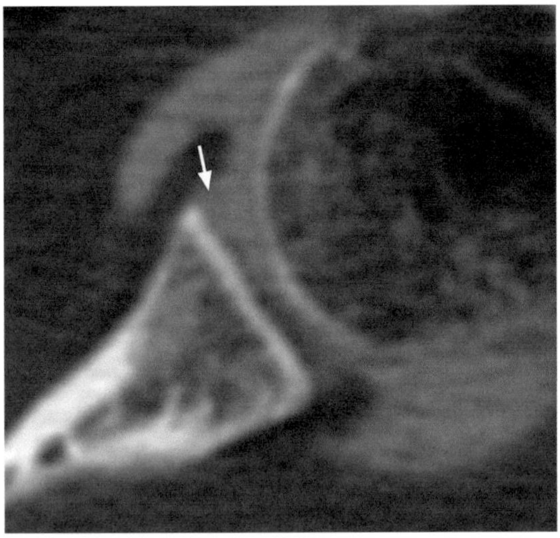

Fig. 1.16 Axial CT arthrogram in patient following anterior dislocation showing absence of the anterior labrum (arrow) which had retracted inferiorly

1.3.4 CT Arthrography

CT arthrography is not as commonly performed nowadays with the more widespread availability of MRI. CT arthrography is however a valid alternative for shoulder imaging of patients with contraindications to MRI or after failed MRI [32] (Fig. 1.16). CT arthrography is accurate for assessment of most intra-articular shoulder abnormalities and may become the imaging test of choice for evaluation of the postoperative shoulder [32].

1.3.4.1 Technique

For CT arthrography, intra-articular contrast injection is performed under either ultrasound or fluoroscopic guidance, most commonly using the anterior approach aiming at the rotator cuff interval. The patient is positioned supine with the hand fully supinated to achieve external rotation of the humeral head. A standard spinal needle (20–22 gauge) containing 12 ml of a solution of 5 ml normal saline, 10 ml Omnipaque 300, and 5 ml 1% lidocaine is used. The needle tip is advanced to the upper third of medial articular surface of humeral head prior to injection of this contrast medium solution into the glenohumeral joint. Local anesthetic (2% mepivacaine) does not seem to reduce post-arthrography pain [33]. Lowering tube voltage from 140 kVp to 120 kVp reduces the radiation dose by as much as 33% without significant loss of image quality [34].

One can also consider using a posterior approach to guide intra-articular injection as this seems to be easier with less risk of extravasation than the rotator cuff interval approach [35]. Also, abduction and external rotation (ABER) positioning before CT seems to improve dispersion of intra-articular contrast medium and increase the sensitivity to detection of rotator cuff tears [36] while external rotation and active supination performed during CT arthrography seems to improve detection of SLAP tears [37].

1.3.5 Clinical Uses of CT Arthrography

MDCT arthrography is a valid alternative for shoulder imaging of patients in whom MRI is contraindicated or after failed MRI. MDCT arthrography has comparable accuracy to MRI for identifying chondral, fibrocartilaginous, and rotator cuff tears [32, 38, 39] and may even be the imaging test of choice for evaluating the postoperative shoulder [32].

For glenohumeral cartilage defects, CTA has moderate diagnostic performance though it is more accurate than MR arthrography in this respect with improved inter-observer agreement ($\kappa = 0.63$) compared to MRA ($\kappa = 0.54$) for detection of modified Outerbridge grade ≥2 and grade 4 chondral defects [40]. Multidetector CT arthrography also shows high accuracy and good inter-observer reliability for diagnosis of superior labral anterior to posterior (SLAP) tears [41]. External rotation and active supination during CT arthrography seem to improve the SLAP tear detection compared with neutral-position CT arthrography [37]. The mean gap width of a SLAP tear was greater during CT arthrography with external rotation and active supination (ERAS) (3.98 mm ± 2.48 sd) compared to neutral CT arthrography (1.61 mm ± 1.11), while the mean gap depth did not alter significantly [37].

Multidetector CT arthrography also shows high accuracy for detection of rotator cuff tendon tears. Abduction and external rotation (ABER) positioning before CT seems to improve the delineation of partial rotator cuff tendon tears allowing demonstration of a higher number of tendon tears than CT in which no ABER positioning was performed beforehand [36]. Compared to arthroscopy, both CT arthrography and MR arthrography perform poorly in the detection of biceps tendon pathology (tendinosis, tendon subluxation, partial and complete tendon tears) [42]. CT arthrography was found to be more sensitive and specific than MRI in identifying biceps tendinosis [43]. Compared to arthroscopy however, both tests were not perfect. CT arthrography had a sensitivity of 71%, a specificity of 100%, positive predictive value of 100%, and negative predictive value of 68% for revealing biceps tendinosis [43].

Following total shoulder arthroplasty, CT arthrography has been used to assess prosthetic loosening with the cardinal sign being intra-articular contrast medium leaking deep to the polyethylene component. CT arthrography is, however, only moderately accurate at determining glenoid component loosening with a sensitivity of 70%, a specificity of 75%, a positive predictive of 87.5%, and a negative predictive value of 50.0% [44]. More studies and improved techniques to increase CT accuracy in this respect are required.

Following arthroscopic superior labrum anterior to posterior (SLAP) repair, superior labral clefts, defined by leakage of contrast medium between the superior labrum and the anchor site, are seen in almost 50% of patients on CT arthrography and do not seem to correlate with clinical outcome [45].

1.3.6 Dual-Energy CT (DECT)

DECT simultaneously irradiates the area under investigation with two X-ray beams of different KVp—typically 80 KVp and 120 KVp. This enables it to provide added information on the chemical composition of the tissues under interrogation, based on the differential X-ray attenuation. It can be used to assess bone marrow edema, bone mineral density, tendons, and ligaments and crystal deposition [46]. Many of these applications are currently being researched. Using virtual non-calcium images, generated by dual-energy subtraction of calcium, good interrater reliability ($k = 0.85$) in the detection of traumatic bone marrow edema in both other than those at the shoulder by dual-energy CT has been shown [47]. The CT value of traumatized proximal tibial bone marrow was -51.3 ± 30.2 HU while that of normal bone marrow was -104.7 ± 17.5 HU ($p < 0.0001$) [47]. DECT can use monoenergetic techniques to significantly reduce metallic beam hardening artifact [48]. This is clearly beneficial to the assessment of the shoulder following treatment with internal fixation or a prosthesis.

Phantomless DECT has the potential to provide a more accurate estimation of bone mineral density (BMD) than DXA or multidetector CT (MDCT) and has the added potential of providing a measure of marrow constituents as well as being able to provide marrow-free quantification of trabecular BMD. A deformable template mesh has been used to define trabecular bone on DECT [49]. Such information on bone quality is likely to become an increasingly utilized aspect of CT examinations providing added relevant information when CT is used to examine complex fractures around the shoulder. Early studies show poor correlation between DXA and DECT BMD measurements of the lumbar spine which is not surprising since the former is measuring integral BMD and the latter trabecular BMD [50]. DECT seems to provide a better estimation of bone strength correlating better the pullout strength used to extract pedicular screws than DXA. The most widely used application of DECT to date is its noninvasive and highly specific ability for confirming the presence of and quantifying the amount of monosodium urate deposits in patients with gout [46]. In a study of six cadaveric internally fixed humeri, both mono-energetic DECT and single-energy CT using an iterative-frequency split-normalized metal artifact reduction algorithm yielded improved image quality and a reduction of metal artifact when compared to filtered back projection on singe-energy CT [51]. Screw-tip position could be most confidently assessed using DECT [50].

1.3.7 Iterative CT

One of the latest developments in CT technology is "ultralow-dose CT" (256 ICT Brilliance) which employs a combination of vacuum slipring technology and an iterative model reconstruction (IMR). This helps to reduce noise (which will improve image quality), reduce radiation dose to only about 1/6 standard CT dose, and reduce metallic artifact. These advantages have been shown in the abdomen, coronary arteries, and thorax [52–54] though the shoulder region has not been specifically evaluated. Clearly it would be beneficial to shoulder imaging to reduce dose to the breast area and improve image resolution following internal fixation [52–54]. To reduce metallic artifact with iterative CT, imaging with a slightly higher KVp (140KVP) than usual (120KVp) is recommended. The acquired data is then subjected to an automatic post-processing algorithm which can yield significant improvement in image quality

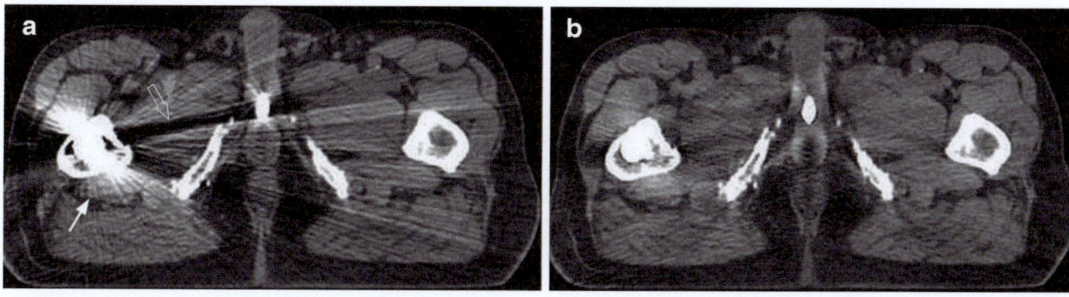

Fig. 1.17 (**a**) Original image showing streak (arrow) and darkening (open arrow) artifacts from hip prosthesis. (**b**) Corrected image following metallic artifact reduction shows significant improvement in diagnostic quality (image courtesy of Philips Health Systems)

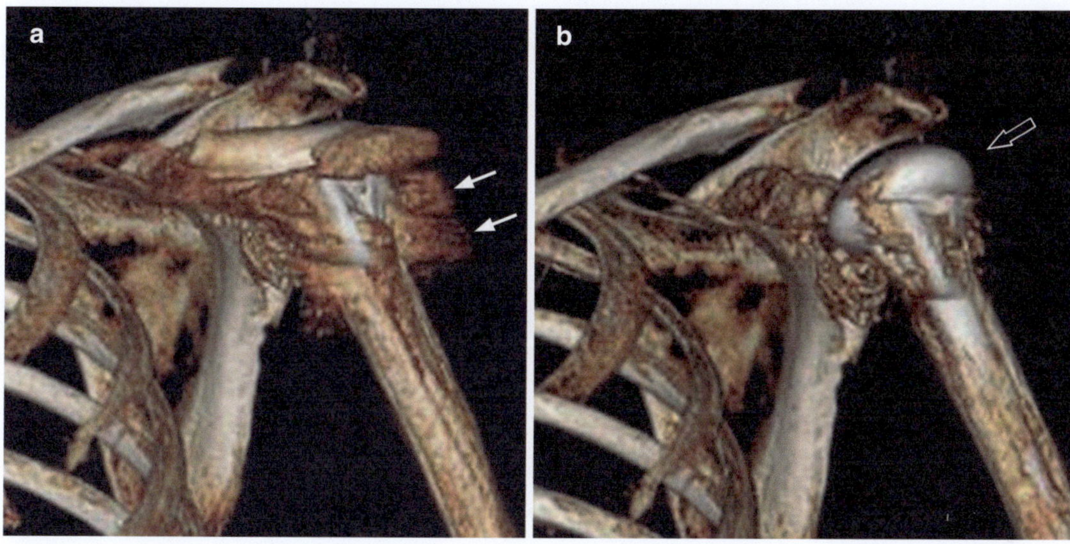

Fig. 1.18 (**a**) Original image showing noise (arrows) due to metal artifact from humeral head prosthesis. (**b**) Corrected image showing significantly reduced noise following application of metallic artifact reduction software allowing improved visibility of the humeral head prosthesis (open arrow) (image courtesy of Philips Health Systems)

particularly with large metallic implants such as hip or shoulder prostheses (Figs. 1.17 and 1.18).

Acknowledgement We wish to thank Ms. Judy Wong Yee Ha, radiographer, for her help and advice with selecting radiographs for this chapter.

References

1. Pavlov H, Warren RF, Weiss CB, et al. The roentgenographic evaluation of anterior shoulder instability. Clin Orthop Relat Res. 1985;194:153–8.
2. Rubin SA, Gray RL, Green WR. The scapular Y: a diagnostic aid in shoulder trauma [technical note]. Radiology. 1974;110:725–6.
3. Nyffeler RW, Jost B, Pfirrmann CW, et al. Measurement of glenoid version: conventional radiographs versus computed tomography scans. J Shoulder Elbow Surg. 2003;12(5):493–6.
4. Bloom MH, Obata WG. 1967 Diagnosis of posterior dislocation of the shoulder with use of Velpeau axillary and angle-up roentgenographic views. J Bone Joint Surg Am. 1967;49(5):943–9.
5. Wallace WA, Hellier M. Improving radiographs of the injured shoulder. Radiography. 1983;49:229–33.
6. Takahashi K, Kato K, Ishida H, Sai S, Nakazawa Y. Study of a new axial projection of shoulder

joint without abduction of upper extremity. Nihon Hoshasen Gijutsu Gakkai Zasshi. 2011;67(2):137–44. Japanese
7. Petersson CJ, Redlund-Johnell I. Radiographic joint space in normal acromioclavicular joints. Acta Orthop Scand. 1983;54(3):431–3.
8. Bearden J, Hughston J, Whatley G. Acromioclavicular dislocation: method of treatment. Am J Sports Med. 1973;1:5–17.
9. Mazzocca AD, Arciero RA, Bicos J. Evaluation and treatment of acromioclavicular joint injuries. Am J Sports Med. 2007;35(2):316–29.
10. Melenevsky Y, Yablon CM, Ramappa A. Clavicle and acromioclavicular joint injuries: a review of imaging, treatment, and complications. Skelet Radiol. 2011;40(7):831–42.
11. Rockwood CA Jr, Williams GR, Young CD. Injuries to the acromioclavicular joint. In: Rockwood Jr CA, et al., editors. Fractures in adults. Philadelphia: Lippincott; 1996. p. 1341–431.
12. Edwards TB, Boulahia A, Walch G. Radiographic analysis of bone defects in chronic anterior shoulder instability. Arthroscopy. 2003;19:732–9.
13. Pansard E, Klouche S, Billot N, et al. Reliability and validity assessment of a glenoid bone loss measurement using the Bernageau profile view in chronic anterior shoulder instability. J Shoulder Elbow Surg. 2013;22(9):1193–8.
14. Rokous JR, Feagin JA, Abbott HG. Modified axillary roentgenogram, a useful adjunct in the diagnosis of recurrent instability of the shoulder. Clin Orthop. 1972;82:84.
15. Itoi E, Lee SB, Amrami KK, et al. Quantitative assessment of classic anteroinferior bony Bankart lesions by radiography and computed tomography. Am J Sports Med. 2003;31(1):112–8.
16. Garth WP Jr, Slappey CE, Ochs CW. Roentgenographic demonstration of instability of the shoulder: the apical oblique projection. A technical note. J Bone Joint Surg. 1984;66A:1450–3.
17. Berkes MB, Dines JS, Little MT, Garner MR, Shifflett GD, Lazaro LE, Wellman DS, Dines DM, Lorich DG. The impact of three-dimensional CT imaging on intraobserver and interobserver reliability of proximal humeral fracture classifications and treatment recommendations. J Bone Joint Surg Am. 2014;96(15):1281–6.
18. Van Oostveen DP, Temmerman OP, Burger BJ, van Noort A, Robinson M. Glenoid fractures: a review of pathology, classification, treatment and results. Acta Orthop Belg. 2014;80(1):88–98.
19. Bartoníček J, Tuček M, Frič V, Obruba P. Fractures of the scapular neck: diagnosis, classifications and treatment. Int Orthop. 2014 Oct;38(10):2163–73.
20. Brorson S. Fractures of the proximal humerus. Acta Orthop Suppl. 2013;84(351):1–32.
21. Bruinsma WE, Guitton TG, Warner JJ, Ring D, Science of Variation Group. Interobserver reliability of classification and characterization of proximal humeral fractures: a comparison of two and three-dimensional CT. J Bone Joint Surg Am. 2013;95(17):1600–4.
22. Walch G, Mesiha M, Boileau P, Edwards TB, Lévigne C, Moineau G, Young A. Three-dimensional assessment of the dimensions of the osteoarthritic glenoid. Bone Joint J. 2013;95-B(10):1377–82.
23. Youderian AR, Ricchetti ET, Drews M, Iannotti JP. Determination of humeral head size in anatomic shoulder replacement for glenohumeral osteoarthritis. J Shoulder Elb Surg. 2014;23(7):955–63.
24. Terrier A, Ston J, Farron A. Importance of a three-dimensional measure of humeral head subluxation in osteoarthritic shoulders. J Shoulder Elb Surg. 2015;24(2):295–301.
25. Sharma GB, McMahon PJ, Robertson DD. Structure modeling of the glenoid: Relevance to shoulder arthroplasty. J Orthop Res. 2014;32(11):1471–8.
26. Gregory T, Hansen U, Khanna M, Mutchler C, Urien S, Amis AA, Augereau B, Emery R. A CT scan protocol for the detection of radiographic loosening of the glenoid component after total shoulder arthroplasty. Acta Orthop. 2014;85(1):91–6.
27. Lee RK, Griffith JF, Tong MM, et al. Glenoid bone loss: assessment with MR imaging. Radiology. 2013;267(2):496–502.
28. Griffith JF, Antonio GE, Tong CW, et al. Anterior shoulder dislocation: quantification of glenoid bone loss with CT. Am J Roentgenol. 2003;180(5):1423–30.
29. Griffith JF, Yung PS, Antonio GE, et al. CT compared with arthroscopy in quantifying glenoid bone loss. AJR Am J Roentgenol. 2007;189(6):1490–3.
30. Griffith JF, Antonio GE, Yung PS, et al. Prevalence, pattern, and spectrum of glenoid bone loss in anterior shoulder dislocation: CT analysis of 218 patients. Am J Roentgenol. 2008;190(5):1247–54.
31. Ozaki R, Nakagawa S, Mizuno N, Mae T, Yoneda M. Hill-Sachs lesions in shoulders with traumatic anterior instability: evaluation using computed tomography with 3-dimensional reconstruction. Am J Sports Med. 2014;42(11):2597–605.
32. Fritz J, Fishman EK, Small KM, Winalski CS, Horger MS, Corl F, McFarland E, Carrino JA, Fayad LM. MDCT arthrography of the shoulder with datasets of isotropic resolution: indications, technique, and applications. AJR Am J Roentgenol. 2012;198(3):635–46.
33. Choo HJ, Lee SJ, Kim DW, Choi SJ, Lee IS. Intra-articular local anesthesia: can it reduce pain related to MR or CT arthrography of the shoulder? AJR Am J Roentgenol. 2013;200(4):860–7.
34. Ahn SJ, Hong SH, Chai JW, Choi JY, Yoo HJ, Kim SH, Kang HS. Comparison of image quality of shoulder CT arthrography conducted using 120 kVp and 140 kVp protocols. Korean J Radiol. 2014;15(6):739–45.
35. Ogul H, Bayraktutan U, Ozgokce M, et al. Ultrasound-guided shoulder MR arthrography: comparison of rotator interval and posterior approach. Clin Imaging. 2014;38(1):11–7.
36. Cochet H, Couderc S, Pelé E, et al. Rotator cuff tears: should abduction and external rotation

(ABER) positioning be performed before image acquisition? A CT arthrography study. Eur Radiol. 2010;20(5):1234–41.
37. Choi JY, Kim SH, Yoo HJ, Shin SH, Oh JH, Baek GH, Hong SH. Superior labral anterior-to-posterior lesions: comparison of external rotation and active supination CT arthrography with neutral CT arthrography. Radiology. 2012;263(1):199–205.
38. De Filippo M, Bertellini A, Sverzellati N, Pogliacomi F, Costantino C, Vitale M, Zappia M, Corradi D, Garlaschi G, Zompatori M. Multidetector computed tomography arthrography of the shoulder: diagnostic accuracy and indications. Acta Radiol. 2008;49(5):540–9.
39. Lecouvet FE, Simoni P, Koutaïssoff S, Vande Berg BC, Malghem J, Dubuc JE. Multidetector spiral CT arthrography of the shoulder. Clinical applications and limits, with MR arthrography and arthroscopic correlations. Eur J Radiol. 2008;68(1):120–36.
40. Omoumi P, Rubini A, Dubuc JE, Vande Berg BC, Lecouvet FE. Diagnostic performance of CT-arthrography and 1.5T MR-arthrography for the assessment of glenohumeral joint cartilage: a comparative study with arthroscopic correlation. Eur Radiol. 2015;25(4):961–9.
41. Kim YJ, Choi JA, Oh JH, Hwang SI, Hong SH, Kang HS. Superior labral anteroposterior tears: accuracy and interobserver reliability of multidetector CT arthrography for diagnosis. Radiology. 2011;260(1):207–15.
42. De Maeseneer M, Boulet C, Pouliart N, et al. Assessment of the long head of the biceps tendon of the shoulder with 3T magnetic resonance arthrography and CT arthrography. Eur J Radiol. 2012;81(5):934–9.
43. Nourissat G, Tribot-Laspiere Q, Aim F, et al. Contribution of MRI and CT arthrography to the diagnosis of intra-articular tendinopathy of the long head of the biceps. Orthop Traumatol Surg Res. 2014;100(8 Suppl):S391–4.
44. Mallo GC, Burton L, Coats-Thomas M, Daniels SD, Sinz NJ, Warner JJ. Assessment of painful total shoulder arthroplasty using computed tomography arthrography. J Shoulder Elb Surg. 2015;31:S1058–2746.
45. Choi BH, Kim NR, Moon SG, Park JY, Choi JW. Superior labral cleft after superior labral anterior-to-posterior tear repair: CT arthrographic features and correlation with clinical outcome. Radiology. 2015;1:142431.
46. Nicolaou S, Liang T, Murphy DT, et al. Dual-energy CT: a promising new technique for assessment of the musculoskeletal system. Am J Roentgenol. 2012;199(5 Suppl):S78–86.
47. Cao JX, Wang YM, Kong XQ, et al. Good interrater reliability of a new grading system in detecting traumatic bone marrow lesions in the knee by dual energy CT virtual non-calcium images. Eur J Radiol. 2015;84:1109.
48. Coupal TM, Mallinson PI, McLaughlin P, et al. Peering through the glare: using dual-energy CT to overcome the problem of metal artefacts in bone radiology. Skelet Radiol. 2014;43(5):567–75.
49. Wichmann JL, Booz C, Wesarg S, et al. Quantitative dual-energy CT for phantomless evaluation of cancellous bone mineral density of the vertebral pedicle: correlation with pedicle screw pull-out strength. Eur Radiol. 2015;25(6):1714–20.
50. Wichmann JL, Booz C, Wesarg S, Kafchitsas K, Bauer RW, Kerl JM, Lehnert T, Vogl TJ, Khan MF. Dual-energy CT-based phantomless in vivo three-dimensional bone mineral density assessment of the lumbar spine. Radiology. 2014;271(3):778–84.
51. Winklhofer S, Benninger E, Spross C, Morsbach F, Rahm S, Ross S, Jost B, Thali MJ, Stolzmann P, Alkadhi H, Guggenberger R. CT metal artefact reduction for internal fixation of the proximal humerus: value of mono-energetic extrapolation from dual-energy and iterative reconstructions. Clin Radiol. 2014;69(5):e199–206.
52. Khawaja RD, Singh S, Blake M, et al. Ultra-low dose abdominal MDCT: using a knowledge-based Iterative Model Reconstruction technique for substantial dose reduction in a prospective clinical study. Eur J Radiol. 2015;84(1):2–10.
53. Matsuura N, Urashima M, Fukumoto W, et al. Radiation dose reduction at coronary artery calcium scoring by using a low tube current technique and hybrid iterative reconstruction. J Comput Assist Tomogr. 2015;39(1):119–24.
54. Khawaja RD, Singh S, Madan R, et al. Ultra low-dose chest CT using filtered back projection: comparison of 80-, 100- and 120 kVp protocols in a prospective randomized study. Eur J Radiol. 2014;83(10):1934–44.

2 Technical Update in Conventional and Arthrographic MRI of the Shoulder

Seema Meraj and Jenny T. Bencardino

Magnetic resonance (MR) is the imaging modality of choice for the evaluation of the shoulder, offering superior soft-tissue contrast while acquiring images in multiple planes. Various factors affect shoulder MR acquisition including the strength of the magnetic field, position of the patient, selection of imaging planes, and use of contrast.

2.1 Conventional MR Protocol

MR imaging of the shoulder is performed with the patient supine and the arm parallel to the long axis of the body, with the thumb facing up (Fig. 2.1). The upper extremity is held as close as possible to the body so that it is nearest to the center of the magnet, with the shoulder held in partial external rotation and placed in a dedicated shoulder coil. To ensure parallel positioning relative to the body, the patient's arm can be supported by weights and/or sandbags placed under the elbow. The shoulder is not held in internal rotation to avoid anterior capsular redundancy and to enable the discrete evaluation of the supraspinatus and infraspinatus tendons, which tend to overlap in this position [1]. Conversely, exaggerated external rotation can result in false-positive tendon tears because potential fluid signal within the biceps tendon sheath may blend with the anterior lateral supraspinatus tendon, mimicking tear [1]. A wide strap is then wrapped around the patient's shoulder and secured to the table to limit respiratory motion-related artifact.

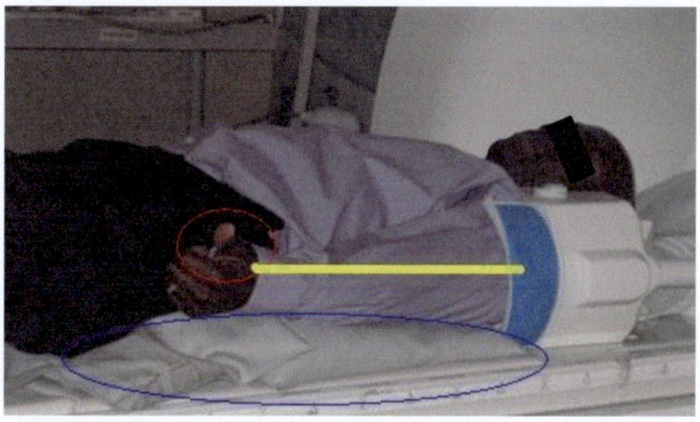

Fig. 2.1 *Patient positioning for conventional shoulder MR.* The patient is supine on the MRI table with the affected arm close to and parallel to the body (yellow line) and the thumb pointed up (red circle) so that the shoulder is held in slight external rotation within the shoulder coil. Note that the arm is propped with sandbags (blue circle) to ensure parallel positioning

2.1.1 Technique and Protocol

3.0T MR imaging is preferred in the evaluation of the shoulder because of the greater signal-to-

S. Meraj (✉)
Zwanger-Pesiri Radiology, Lindenhurst, NY, USA
e-mail: smeraj@zprad.com

J. T. Bencardino
Department of Radiology, New York University Langone Health, New York, NY, USA

Penn Medicine, Department of Radiology, Perelman School of Medicine at the University of Pennsylvania, Philadelphia, PA, USA
e-mail: jenny.bencardino@nyumc.org

J. T. Bencardino (ed.), *The Shoulder*, https://doi.org/10.1007/978-3-030-06240-8_2

noise ratio (SNR) and contrast-to-noise ratio (CNR) offered by higher field strengths due to faster acquisition time and thinner slice selection. Studies have shown that imaging the shoulder at higher field strengths allows for more accurate interpretation and can also affect management [2].

Once the localizer images are obtained, standard conventional MR imaging of the shoulder is acquired in three orthogonal planes: axial, coronal-oblique, and sagittal-oblique (Fig. 2.2). Axial sequences are imaged from the superior margin of the acromion through the inferior aspect of the glenoid. The coronal-oblique images are obtained from the infraspinatus to the subscapularis muscles, parallel to the course of the supraspinatus tendon on the axial images, such that the muscles of the rotator cuff can be seen in continuity. Finally, the sagittal-oblique images are obtained parallel to the glenoid surface, perpendicular to the coronal-oblique images from the level of the scapular neck to the greater tuberosity.

At our institution, five sequences are typically obtained: an axial proton density fat suppressed, coronal oblique proton density and T2-fat suppressed, and sagittal oblique T1 and T2 fat suppressed (Table 2.1). It is important for the sagittal-oblique images to be obtained in T1 or proton density/T2 with and without fat suppression in order to properly assess the osseous structures as well as fat, particularly when assessing for muscle atrophy in the setting of chronic rotator cuff tear or denervation-related muscle injury (Fig. 2.3).

2.1.2 Accuracy

Shellock and colleagues found that noncontrast MRI has a sensitivity of 89% and a specificity of 100% in the detection of rotator cuff tears, missing only partial tears, on a 0.2T extremity MRI system [3]. Noncontrast MRI is also accurate in the evaluation of cartilage lesions with a sensitivity and specificity of up to 53% and 93% for glenoid lesions, and 32% and 80% for humeral lesions, respectively, on 1.5T and 3T MRI scanners [4, 5].

Conventional noncontrast MR examinations of the shoulder are sensitive and accurate in the assessment of anterior labrum tears and less sensitive for superior labral tears [6, 7]. At 3.0T, Magee and Williams found a sensitivity and

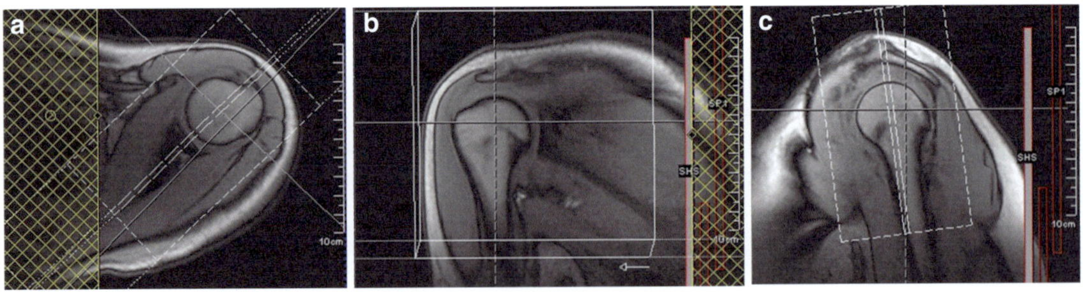

Fig. 2.2 *Imaging planes.* The imaging planes for conventional noncontrast imaging in the (**a**) axial, (**b**) coronal-oblique, and (**c**) sagittal-oblique planes

Table 2.1 Protocol for conventional noncontrast 3.0T MRI of the shoulder

Sequence	TR (ms)	TE (ms)	Slice thickness (mm)	FOV (mm)	Matrix (%)
Coronal PD	4500	32	2.0	140 × 140	320 × 75
Coronal T2 FS	3500	72	3.0	140 × 140	256 × 151
Sagittal T1	600	11	2.5	140 × 140	320 × 90
Sagittal T2 FS	5000	62	2.5	140 × 140	320 × 75
Axial PD	3030	33	2.0	140 × 140	256 × 100

PD proton density, *FS* fat suppressed

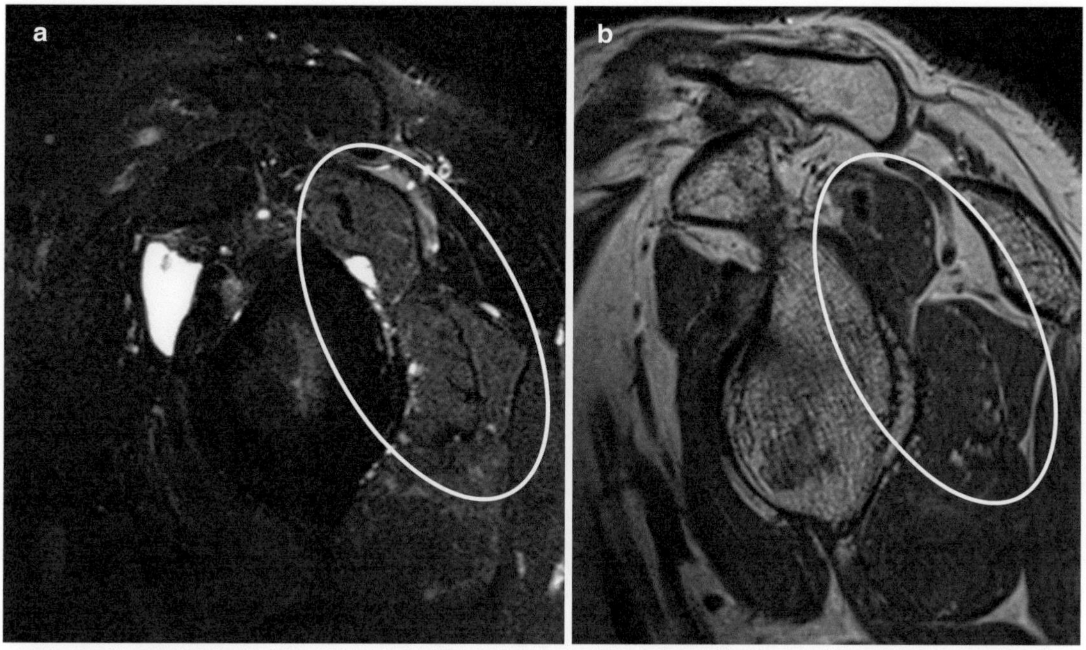

Fig. 2.3 *Rotator cuff denervation.* Sagittal oblique (**a**) T2-weighted fat-suppressed and (**b**) T1-weighted images of the shoulder demonstrating faint denervation edema -like changes and mild fatty infiltration of the supraspinatus and infraspinatus muscles (circled) as a result of suprascapular nerve impingement by a paralabral cyst in the suprascapular notch (not visualized)

specificity of 90% and 100%, respectively, in the detection of SLAP tears on conventional MRI, 89% and 100%, respectively, in the detection of anterior labral tears, and 86% and 100%, respectively, in the detection of posterior labral tears [8].

2.1.3 Provocative Positioning

Provocative positioning such as abduction external rotation (ABER), flexion-adduction internal rotation (FADIR), and adduction internal rotation (ADIR) have been shown to be helpful in the evaluation of the labroligamentous complex and in the detection of subtle labroligamentous injuries, particularly when using MR arthrography [9, 10] (refer to the "Arthrography" section of this chapter).

For the ABER view, the affected shoulder is abducted and externally rotated, with the forearm tucked behind the patient's head while lying supine (Fig. 2.4). The shoulder coil is placed anteriorly over the shoulder and scout images are obtained in a plane parallel to the long axis of the humerus, perpendicular to the glenohumeral articular surface. The images obtained are therefore axial to the scapula, but coronal to the humerus. ABER imaging aids in the assessment of the anteroinferior and posterosuperior labrum.

For imaging in the ADIR position, the arm is placed behind the patient's back with the patient in the supine position and the shoulder coil placed anterior to the shoulder. Although fewer studies have evaluated the efficacy of this position, it has been shown to aid in the diagnosis of anterior labroligamentous periosteal sleeve avulsion lesions (ALPSA) of the anteroinferior labrum and Bankart subtypes [11].

The arm is placed across the chest on top of the contralateral shoulder with the palm facing outward for the FADIR position. Imaging in the FADIR position has been shown to increase

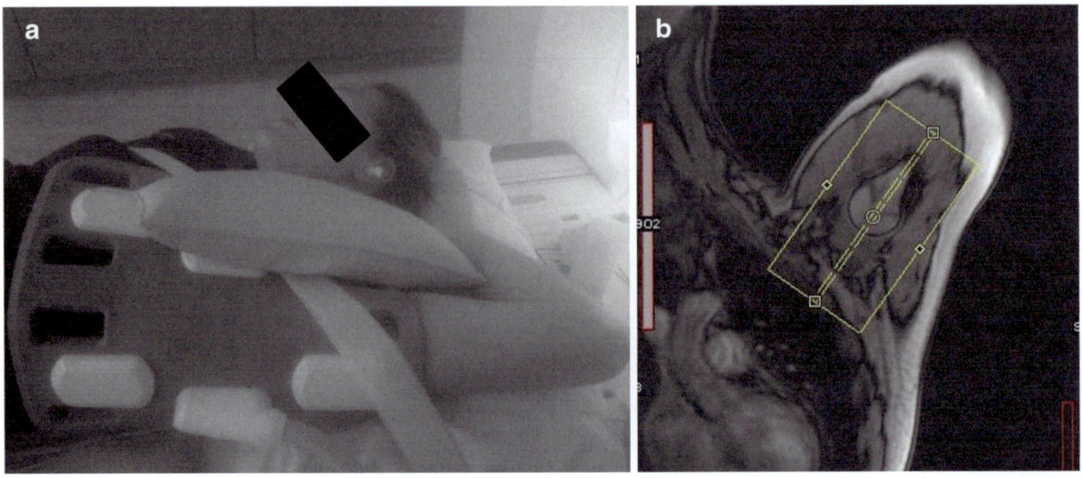

Fig. 2.4 *ABER position.* (**a**) The patient is supine with the elbow flexed and their hand behind the head. The coil is placed overlying the axillary region with a sandbag/weight to maintain position during the scan. (**b**) ABER MR images are prescribed from the coronal localizer along the long axis of the humerus to produce axial oblique images

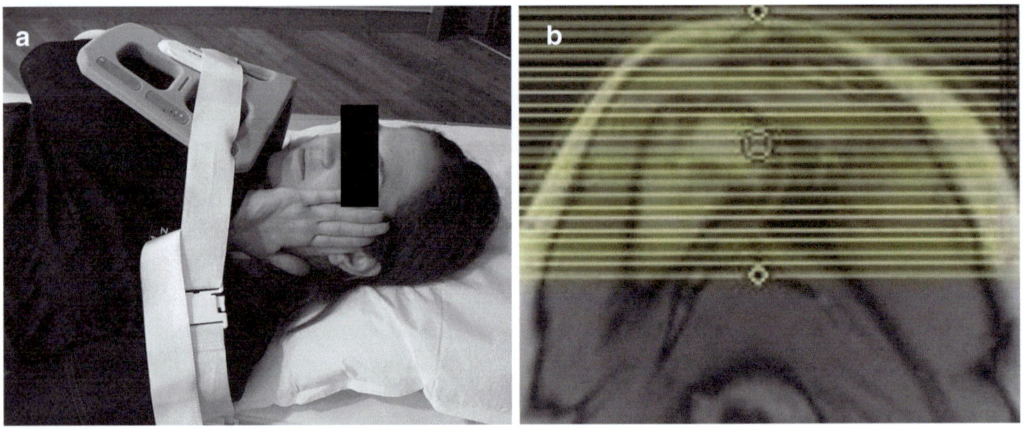

Fig. 2.5 *FADIR position.* FADIR MR images are prescribed from the coronal localizer to produce axial images

diagnostic confidence in the evaluation of the posteroinferior labrum (Fig. 2.5) [12].

In 1999, Wintzell and colleagues found that when the arm is abducted at 90° and maximally extended, capsulolabral lesions were better evaluated compared to ABER positioning [13]. SLAP lesions have been found to be better assessed when the arm is held in external rotation with traction using 3 kg weights [14]. Internal and external rotation has also shown to be helpful in the evaluation of subcoracoid impingement [15].

2.2 Normal MR Appearance of the Shoulder

2.2.1 Bones

The osseous structures imaged on a conventional shoulder MR examination are the clavicle, scapula, and humerus. Because of fat within marrow, the medullary cavity normally demonstrates hyperintense signal on T1-weighted images. After birth, hematopoietic red marrow converts into yellow fatty marrow, beginning in the

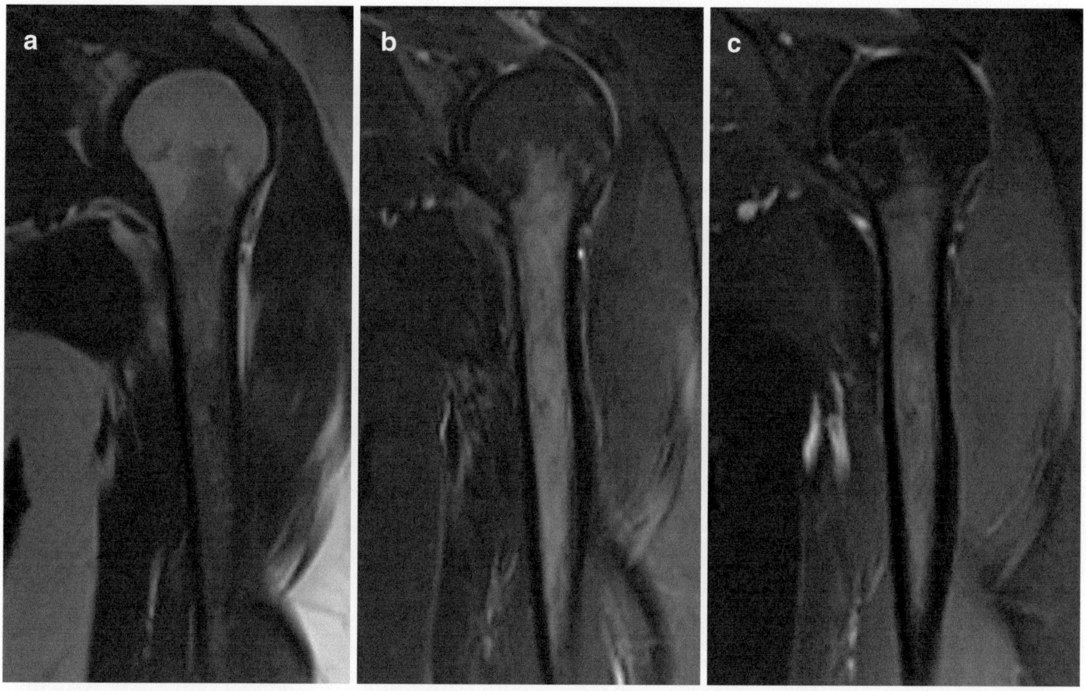

Fig. 2.6 *Normal marrow signal intensity.* (**a**) Coronal T1-weighted, (**b**) T2-weighted fat-suppressed, and (**c**) T1-weighted fat-suppressed post-contrast images of the proximal left humerus demonstrating diffusely T1 hypointense, T2 hyperintense signal within the proximal humeral metaphysis and extending into the imaged diaphysis with corresponding subtle enhancement, in keeping with red marrow reconversion

diaphysis of long bones including the humerus, followed by the distal metaphysis, and finally the proximal metaphysis [16]. Hematopoietic (red) marrow can be seen within the proximal humeral metaphysis to the epiphysis, with a curvilinear zone of transition between red and yellow marrow (Fig. 2.6). In one study, residual hematopoietic marrow was found in 99% of humeral metaphyses and extended to the epiphysis in 62% [17]. This pattern of marrow distribution is reached by the third decade, after which reconversion occurs, whereby red marrow is replaced by yellow marrow.

2.2.2 Tendons

Tendons, which attach muscle to bone, have high collagen content (mostly type I). Five confluent histologic layers have been described within the supraspinatus and infraspinatus tendons [18]. The most superficial layer, layer I, measures about 1 mm and is comprised of the coracohumeral ligament in addition to large arterioles. Layer II is the thickest layer, measuring 3–5 mm, and contains densely packed tendon fibers, which directly insert onto the greater tuberosity. Fibers from this layer also contribute to the roof of the biceps sheath. Layer III contains smaller bundles of collagen fibers oriented at a 45-degree angle to one another cross-linking measuring approximately 3 mm in thickness. Layer IV is a thin layer comprised of loose connective tissue and thick collagen fibers as well as the coracohumeral ligament. The deepest layer, layer V, is about 2 mm thick and is comprised of the joint capsule.

Collagen within a tendon is dense, restricting the Brownian motion of water molecules [19]. These collagen fibers are aligned with water molecules, causing dipole interactions and thus a shortened T2 of 1–2 ms. [20, 21] At 3.0T, T1 relaxation time is relatively short at 600 ms. [22] Normal tendons consequently demonstrate hypointense signal on all sequences (Fig. 2.7a). As the angle between the collagen fibers within a tendon and the static magnetic field (B_0) increases, the effects of dipole interactions are minimized and T2 increases, resulting in spurious signal alteration [23]. When the angle reaches 55°, T2 relaxation time is maximized and a normal tendon can demonstrate increased signal intensity known as the "magic angle" artifact (Fig. 2.7b) [24, 25]. T2-weighted images have been shown to be more dependent on fiber orientation than T1 [26]. Common sites of magic angle phenomenon in the shoulder include the critical zone of the supraspinatus, posterosuperior and anteroinferior labrum, and intra-articular long head of the biceps tendon proximal to the intertubercular groove [27]. Imaging with a longer echo time (TE greater than 37 ms) minimizes magic angle artifact; therefore this effect is not appreciated on T2-weighted and STIR sequences [28].

The primary shoulder tendons include the rotator cuff, comprised of the supraspinatus, infraspinatus, teres minor, and subscapularis tendons, as well as the long-head biceps tendon. When a tendon demonstrates increased signal intensity and magic angle artifact has been excluded as the cause, this can be indicative of tendinosis, particularly when the finding is associated with thickening (Fig. 2.8) [26]. The sensitivity of MRI in the detection of tendinosis has been shown to be up to 55%, with a specificity of up to 92.7% [29]. Pseudogap can be seen at the insertion of the supraspinatus tendon near the greater tuberosity, lateral to the myotendinous junction as a result of differing fiber orientation of the anterior and posterior bundles and their intrinsic tissue relaxation times (Fig. 2.9) [30]. Unlike magic angle artifact, pseudogap is present on all pulse sequences obtained in the coronal oblique plane.

Occasionally, tendinosis can be difficult to differentiate from partial-thickness tears [26]. Focal areas of fluid signal intensity along the articular or bursal surfaces or within the tendon substance on fat-suppressed T2 or STIR images are seen with partial-thickness tears (Fig. 2.10). Articular surface tears are the most common type of partial-thickness rotator cuff tears [31]. When a tendon is completely torn, the torn tendon fibers may be retracted. In chronic tears, scar tissue may

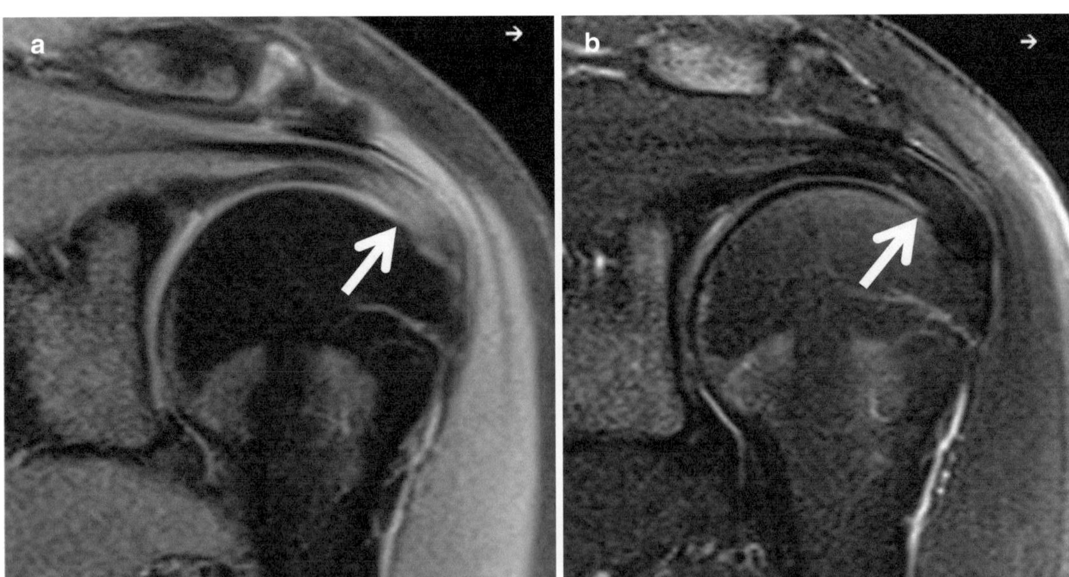

Fig. 2.7 *Magic angle artifact.* Coronal oblique MR images from the same patient demonstrate (**a**) increased signal intensity within the supraspinatus tendon (arrows) at a TE of 19 ms, (**b**) which resolves at a TE of 77 ms. The finding in (**a**) is a result of magic angle artifact given the short TE

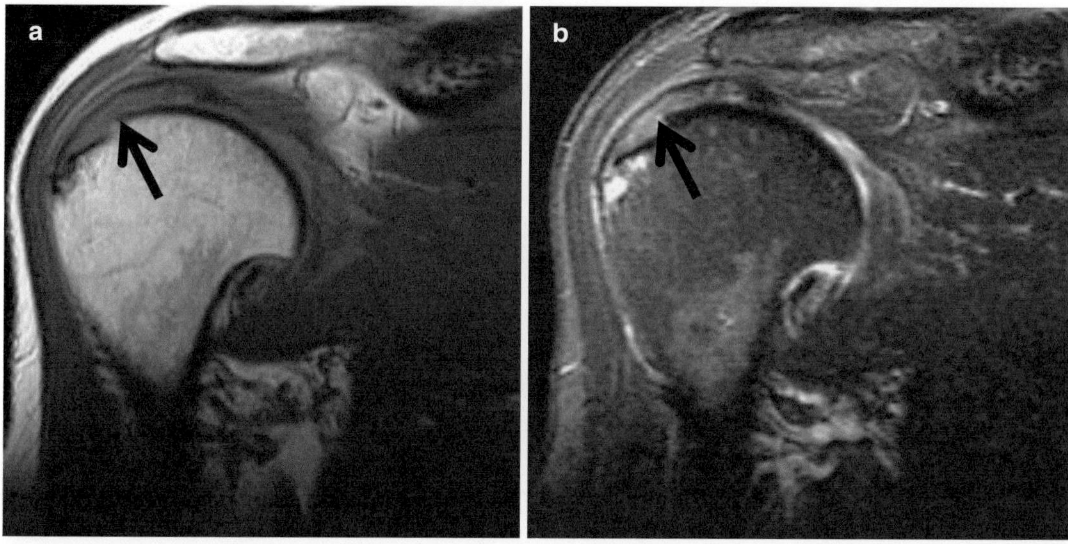

Fig. 2.8 *Tendinosis*. Coronal oblique proton density MR images (**a**) without and (**b**) with fat suppression demonstrate thickening and intermediate signal intensity of the insertional supraspinatus tendon fibers (arrows). No discontinuous fibers are seen. The findings are compatible with moderate-severe tendinosis

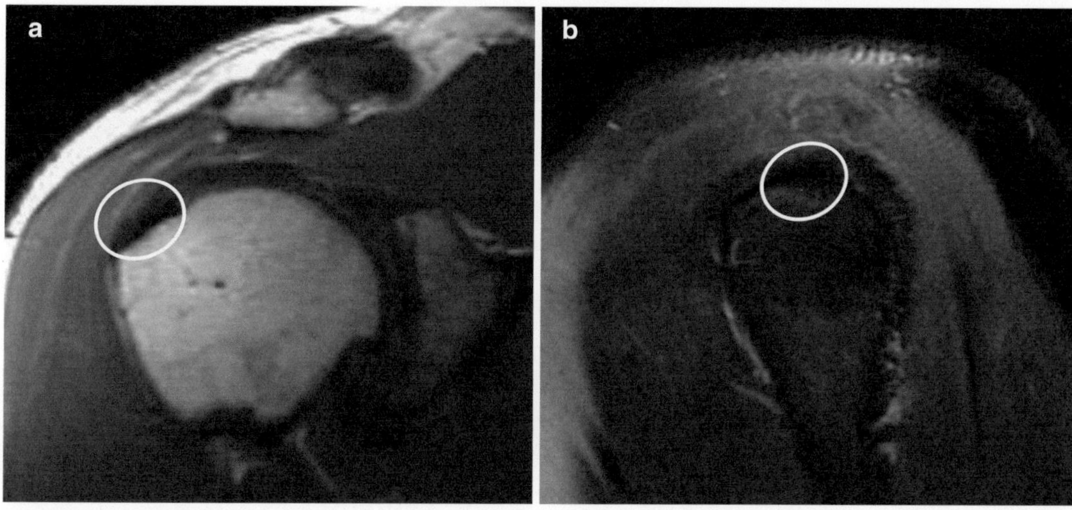

Fig. 2.9 *Pseudogap*. Coronal oblique proton density image on an asymptomatic patient demonstrating increased signal intensity of the supraspinatus tendon as it inserts onto the greater tuberosity (circled), (**b**) which resolves on the sagittal oblique T2-weighted fat-suppressed image. The findings in (**a**) correspond to pseudogap

develop at the site of the tear, resulting in low-to-intermediate signal intensity interposed between the torn tendon fibers on all pulse sequences (Fig. 2.11) [26]. The sensitivity of MRI in the detection of rotator cuff tears has been shown to be up to 92.1% and specificity up to 92.9% [29].

Traumatic tears commonly involve the supraspinatus tendon or rotator interval, whereas degenerative changes tend to occur at the junction of the supraspinatus and infraspinatus tendons [32, 33]. Studies have also reported that degenerative tears primarily involve the articular surface and the "critical zone," the area of vascular anastomosis just proximal to the rotator cuff insertion [34]. Both cadaveric and clinical studies found that decreased cellularity, fascicular thin-

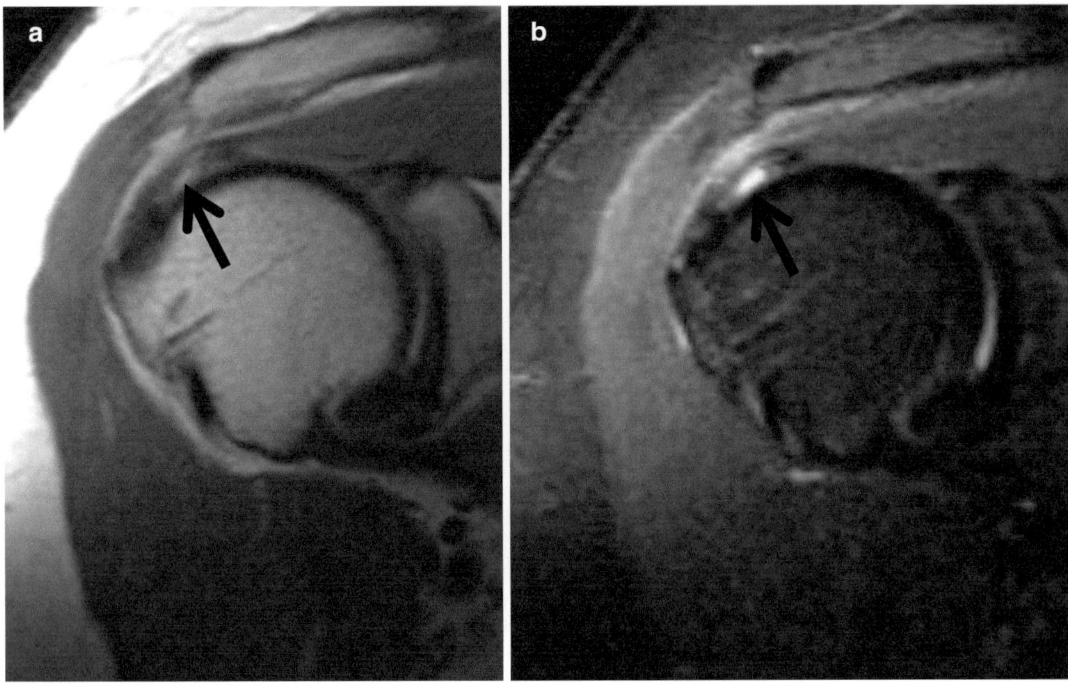

Fig. 2.10 *Partial-thickness tendon tear.* Coronal oblique (**a**) without and (**b**) with fat suppression demonstrates fluid-bright signal at the articular surface of the supraspinatus insertion (arrows) compatible with a partial-thickness tear

ning, disorganization of collagen fibers in layer III, and decreased vascularity in patients older than 40 years are all factors that predispose tendons to partial-thickness, articular-surface tears [35]. Intratendinous strain has additionally been described as an important factor in the development of partial-thickness tears, with secondary propagation of tears from the articular to bursal surface [36–39]. Extrinsic mechanisms of rotator cuff tearing include subacromial, coracoacromial, and internal impingement [40, 41].

2.2.3 Ligaments

Ligaments connect bone to bone and have high proteoglycan and water content and low collagen content [22]. Accordingly, ligaments are hypointense in signal on all pulse sequences. In the shoulder, the superior, middle, and inferior glenohumeral ligaments form the primary ligaments at the anterior aspect of the glenohumeral joint. The coracoacromial and coracoclavicular ligaments also have an important functional and anatomic significance, supporting the glenohumeral ligament superiorly. An additional accessory ligament known as the spiral ligament, ligamentum glenohumerale, or spirale fasciculus obliquus runs more obliquely along the anterior margin of the capsule from the lesser tuberosity and infraglenoid tubercle to the subscapularis tendon [42].

2.2.4 Labrum

The glenoid labrum rims the glenoid fossa and is predominantly comprised of fibrous connective tissue. At the junction of the labrum and hyaline cartilage is dense fibrocartilage tissue. As a result of the lack of mobile protons in such dense tissue, the normal glenoid labrum is hypointense on all pulse sequences (Fig. 2.12). Labral tears are classified by morphology, presence or absence of displacement, and location. When the labrum demonstrates surface irregularity, it may be frayed or torn. On MRI, fluid signal intensity

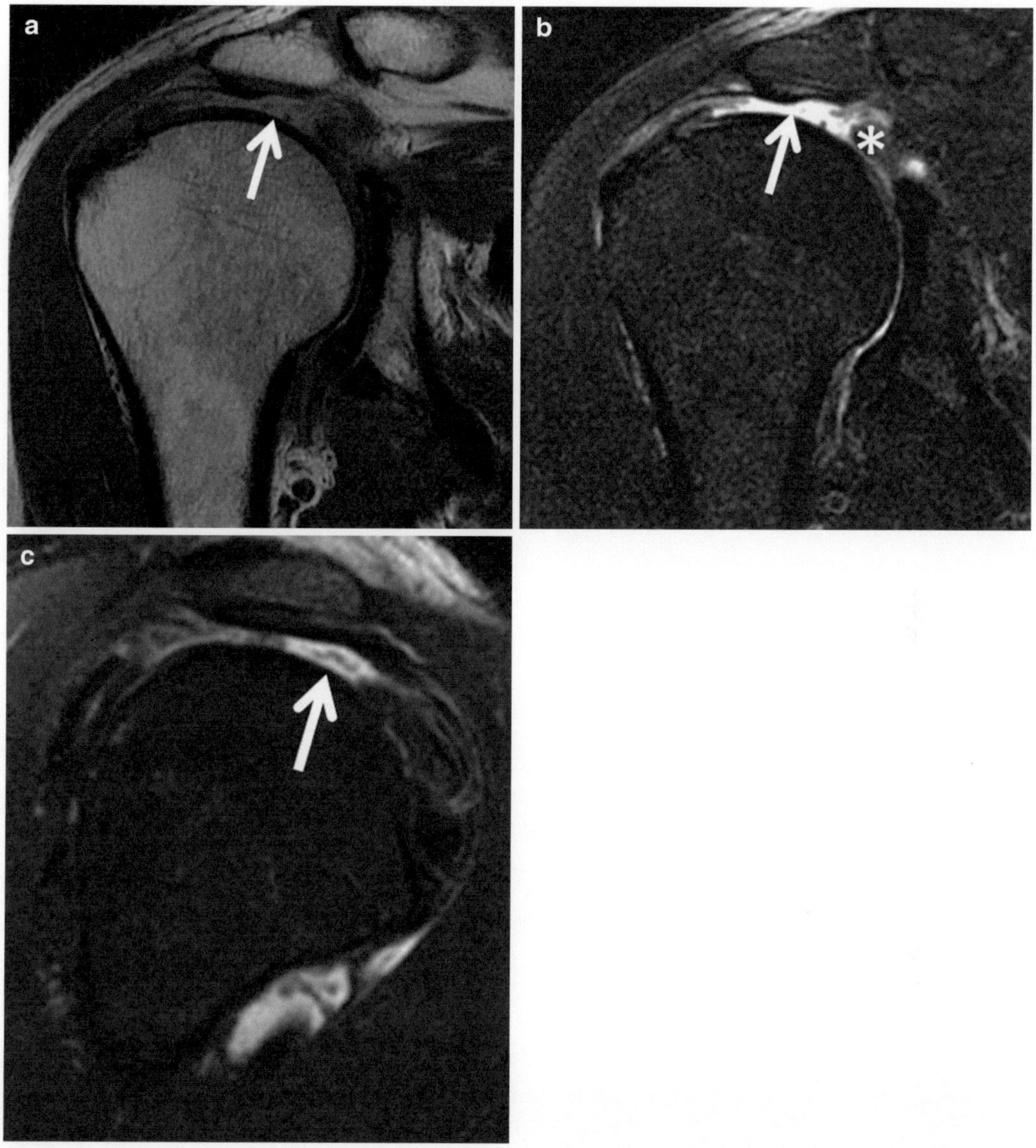

Fig. 2.11 *Full-thickness, full-width tendon tear.* Coronal oblique proton density (**a**) without and (**b**) with fat suppression, and (**c**) sagittal oblique T2-weighted fat-suppressed images on a patient with a complete tear of the supraspinatus tendon (arrows) evidenced by a full-thickness, full-width fluid-filled defect and discontinuity of the tendon. The torn tendon fibers are retracted to the level of the glenohumeral joint (asterisk)

within the labral substance extending to the surface or fluid signal/contrast imbibition within the labrum is diagnostic of tear (Fig. 2.13) [43, 44]. The labrum can also be avulsed. The findings may be seen in association with paralabral cyst formation, periosteal stripping or tearing, cartilage defects, and associated bone defects as in the setting of osseous Bankart lesions [45].

2.3 Artifacts/Pitfalls

The shoulder is best imaged in slight external rotation. However, both exaggerated external rotation and internal rotation are undesirable as the tendons shift in position with respect to the standard imaging planes. The tendons also overlap, resulting in false-positive tendon tears,

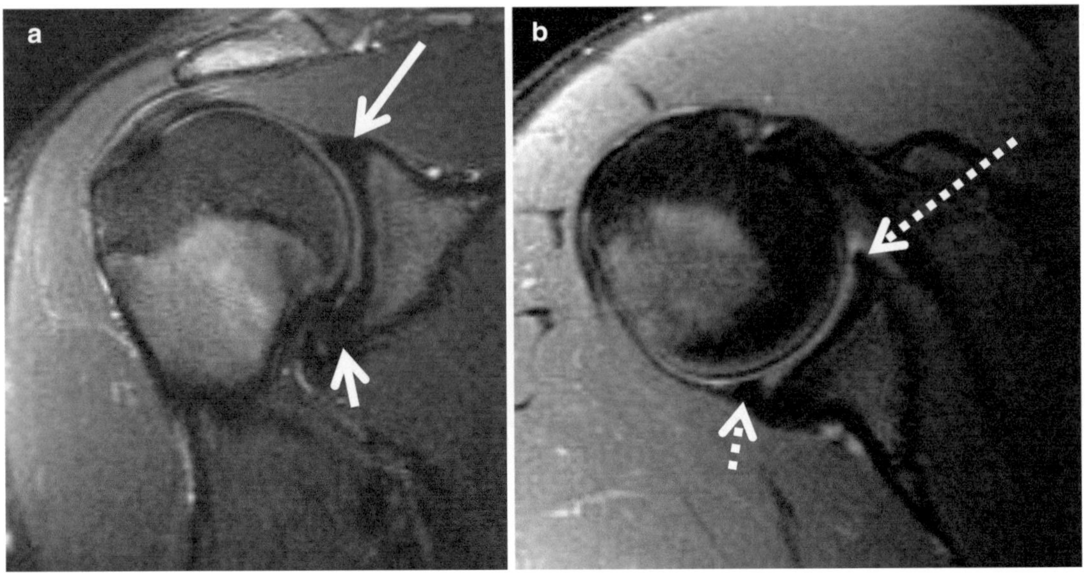

Fig. 2.12 *Normal glenoid labrum.* (**a**) Coronal oblique proton density fat-suppressed and (**b**) axial T2-weighted fat-suppressed (**b**) images demonstrating a normal hypointense triangular contour to the superior (long solid arrow), inferior (short solid arrow), and posterior (short dashed arrow) labrum. Note the somewhat more rounded configuration of the anterior labrum (long dashed arrow)

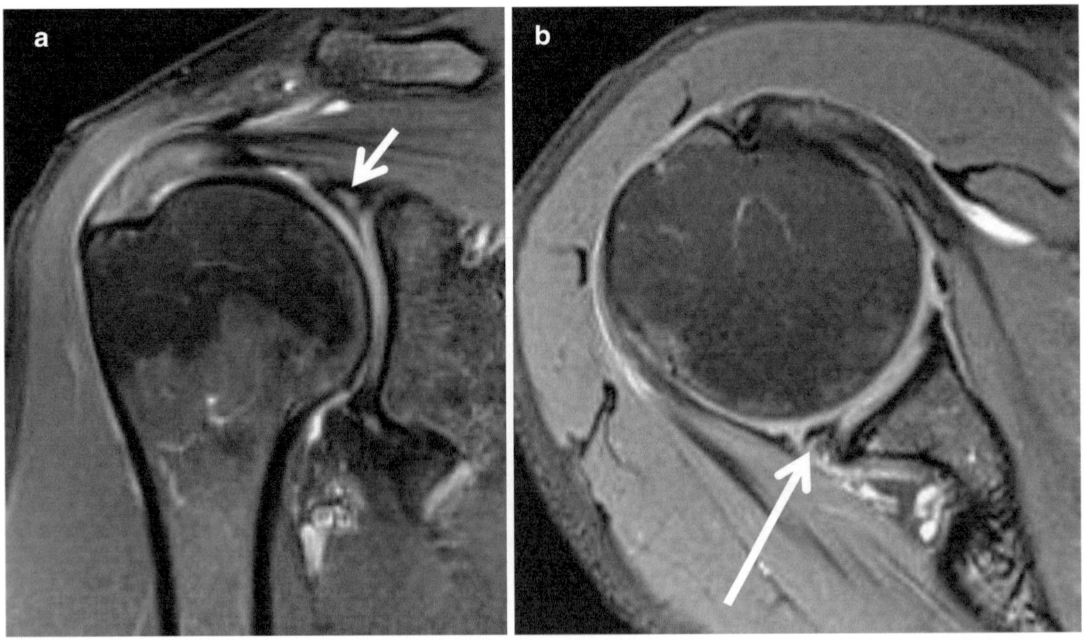

Fig. 2.13 *Labral tear.* (**a**) Coronal oblique proton density fat-suppressed and (**b**) axial T2-weighted fat-suppressed images from the same patient demonstrating linear fluid signal intensity within the substance of the superior (short white arrow) and posterior (long white arrow) labrum

particularly of the supraspinatus on the coronal images, where it can appear discontinuous and the capsule redundant (Fig. 2.14). The anterior structures may also overlap, resulting in abnormal signal intensity within the subscapularis, middle glenohumeral ligament, and capsular structures.

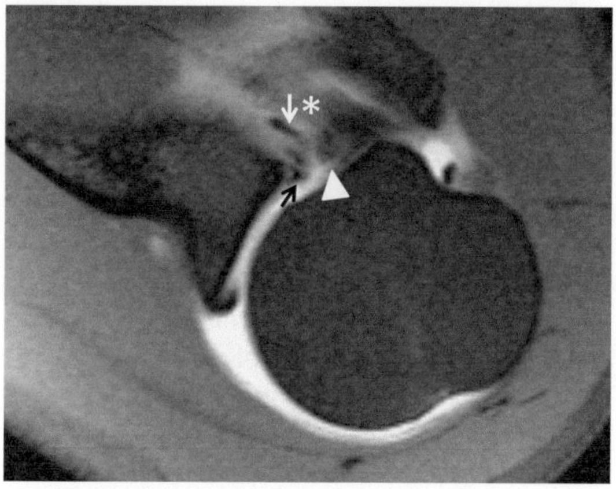

Fig. 2.14 *Internal shoulder rotation.* Axial T1-weighted fat-suppressed image of the shoulder in internal rotation following the intra-articular administration of contrast demonstrates medial migration of the middle glenohumeral ligament (white arrow), obscuration of the anterior labrum (black arrow), apparent thickening and redundancy of the anterior capsule (arrowhead), and increased signal intensity and thickening of the subscapularis tendon falsely suggesting tendinosis (asterisk)

2.3.1 Vacuum Phenomenon

When the shoulder is held in traction/extreme external rotation, gas has been shown to accumulate within the joint and referred to as vacuum phenomenon (Fig. 2.15) [46]. This finding may be related to the intra-articular accumulation of nitrogen in the setting of decreasing intra-articular pressure from traction separating the apposing articular surfaces [47]. Classically, curvilinear hypointense signal is seen superiorly in the absence of effusion or abnormal findings that could suggest septic arthritis. Differentiation of intra-articular gas from loose bodies, displaced labral/cartilage fragments, synovial tissue, metal, and chondrocalcinosis is of key importance.

2.3.2 Chemical Shift Artifact

In addition to the previously described magic angle phenomenon, another artifact commonly encountered on MR imaging of the shoulder is chemical shift artifact. This artifact occurs at the boundary between tissues containing high concentrations of fat and those containing high concentrations of water, such as within fluid-filled cysts and fat-containing lesions, and at the interface of

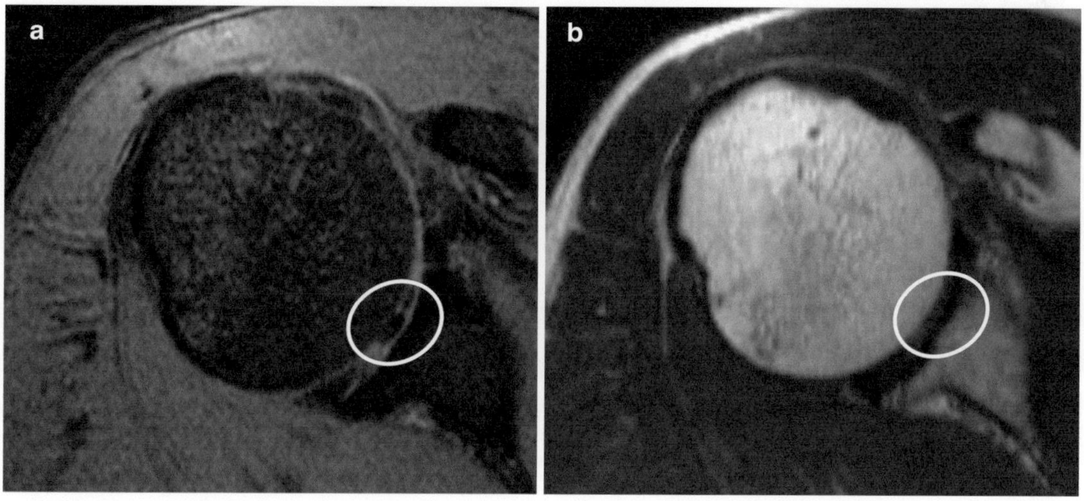

Fig. 2.15 *Vacuum phenomenon artifact.* (**a**) Axial gradient echo image demonstrates a hypointense focus within the glenohumeral joint (circled). (**b**) On the axial proton density sequence subsequently obtained, no corresponding hypointense focus is seen, in keeping with air in the setting of vacuum artifact and not intra-articular calcification

cartilage and bone marrow [48, 49]. It occurs because of the different resonance precession frequencies of fat and water, respectively, in the frequency-encoding direction, caused by inhomogeneity within the main magnetic field. This effect is exacerbated with increasing field strengths. In the shoulder, signal abnormality at the bone-cartilage interface of the glenohumeral joint can simulate full-thickness cartilage loss [50]. Knowledge of chemical shift artifact is thus essential in precluding misdiagnosis of glenohumeral cartilage wear. Chemical shift artifact may be reduced by suppressing fat or switching phase and frequency-encoding directions [51, 52]. Increasing bandwidth and utilizing lower field magnets are other alternatives.

2.4 Arthrography

MR arthrography (MRA) can be performed following the direct injection of dilute gadolinium or saline into the glenohumeral joint, or indirectly via intravenous injection of gadolinium. Structures that otherwise lie in close apposition separate due to distention of the capsule, allowing for better assessment.

2.4.1 Direct MR Arthrography

Over the past two decades, direct MR arthrography has been performed with increasing frequency [53, 54]. Direct arthrography outlines the fine intra-articular structures including the labrum, undersurface of the rotator cuff, and capsule by distending the joint [54–58]. It is most commonly performed on patients younger than 35 years or in the setting of prior surgery, shoulder instability, labral tear (particularly SLAP lesions), and to determine whether there is a partial- versus full-thickness rotator cuff tear when noncontrast MRI is inconclusive.

2.4.1.1 Gadolinium Dilution

Dilute contrast can be injected into the glenohumeral joint via a blind approach with palpation of anatomical landmarks, but variable rates of extra-articular injection ranging from 1% to 73% have been reported [59–61]. Ultrasound, CT, and fluoroscopy are effective modalities for image-guided techniques for direct MR arthrography [62, 63]. There are four primary image-guided techniques for direct MRA: (1) rotator interval approach under fluoroscopic guidance, (2) anterior approach under fluoroscopic guidance, (3) posterior approach under fluoroscopic guidance, and (4) posterior approach under ultrasound guidance (refer to Chap. 6—Image-Guided Procedures in the Shoulder).

Although intra-articular injection of gadolinium is not approved by the US Food and Drug Administration (FDA), direct arthrography is performed as an off-label technique. Gadolinium is diluted to a concentration of 1–2 mmol/L typically with saline to a volume of approximately 12 mL, although iodinated contrast can be added to confirm appropriate needle position when performing the study with fluoroscopic guidance [64–66]. While some studies found that the addition of iodinated contrast can compromise the signal intensity of gadolinium, others have shown that a 1:1 mixture of saline with iodinated contrast (for example 10 mL each) and 0.1 mL gadolinium does not result in significant dissociation of the gadolinium ion [10, 67–71]. The advantage of premixing the dilute gadolinium with iodinated contrast is that the chance of introducing bubbles of air when exchanging syringes is nonexistent. However, the addition of iodinated contrast further dilutes the gadolinium concentration, resulting in a lower signal intensity of the contrast [72]. This effect is exaggerated at 3.0T because the signal-to-noise ratio peak levels for iodinated contrast dilutions are relatively lower than at 1.5T. Although complications of direct MR arthrography are rare, infection, bleeding, allergic reaction, synovitis, and pain have been described.

2.4.1.2 Imaging Technique

Imaging can be performed up to approximately one hour following the shoulder injection. With dilute gadolinium, T1-weighted fat-suppressed images are commonly obtained, whereas intermediate and T2-weighted spin-

Table 2.2 Protocol for direct MR arthrography of the shoulder

Sequence	TR (ms)	TE (ms)	Slice thickness (mm)	FOV (mm)	Matrix (%)
Coronal T1 FS	400–800	Min	3.0–4.0	140 × 140	500 × 700
Coronal T2 FS	3500–5000	40–80	3.0–4.0	140 × 140	500 × 500
Sagittal T1	400–800	Min	3.0	140 × 140	500 × 500
Axial T1 FS	400–800	Min	3.0–4.0	140 × 140	500 × 700
ABER/ADIR	450–700	Min	4.0	140 × 140	500 × 700

FS fat suppression, *ABER* abduction external rotation, *ADIR* adduction internal rotation

echo sequences are performed following normal saline injection. At our institution, five sequences are typically obtained following intra-articular dilute gadolinium injection: axial and coronal oblique T1-weighted fat-suppressed, coronal oblique T2-weighted fat-suppressed, sagittal T1-weighted, and an axial T1-weighted fat-suppressed sequence in the abducted/externally rotated position (ABER view; Table 2.2).

Lee and colleagues advocate an additional gradient echo sequence in order to improve sensitivity for anterior and posterior labral tears relative to T1-weighted images alone, with sensitivities of 78% and 75% for the gradient echo sequences relative to 25% and 56% for T1-weighted images, respectively [73]. No significant difference was seen between the two sequences for superior labral tears in that study.

Direct gadolinium MR arthrography is preferred to direct saline injection because of significant improvement in image quality and signal-to-noise ratio of the T1 images obtained, compared to the T2-weighted images obtained in the saline injection studies. In addition, it is impossible to distinguish between injected saline and bursal fluid; as such, no diagnostic criterion exists to differentiate between partial- and full-thickness tears. Fat-suppressed images are preferred in direct gadolinium MR arthrography in order to distinguish fat within the subacromial-subdeltoid bursa and the intra-articular contrast, which would indicate a full-thickness rotator cuff tear (Fig. 2.16).

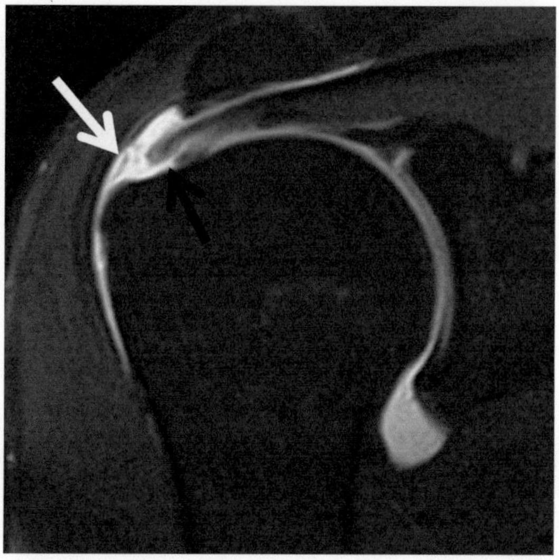

Fig. 2.16 *Full-thickness tendon tear on MR arthrography.* Coronal oblique T1-weighted fat-suppressed image following intra-articular administration of dilute gadolinium shows extravasation of contrast into the subacromial-subdeltoid bursa via a full-thickness tear at the insertion of the supraspinatus tendon (white arrow) with discontinuity and medial retraction of the torn tendon fibers (black arrow)

2.4.1.3 Provocative Imaging

Anteroinferior labral tears are more conspicuous on ABER views, particularly after the intra-articular administration of gadolinium because the anterior band of the inferior glenohumeral ligament is placed under tension (Fig. 2.17). ABER views also aid in the evaluation of superior and posterosuperior labral tears, partial-thickness articular surface tears of the insertional supraspinatus and infraspinatus tendons, suspected posterosuperior impingement, and subtle glenohumeral joint subluxations (Figs. 2.18 and 2.19). When used in conjunction with the standard direct MR arthrography protocol, the ABER view has been shown to increase sensitivity and specificity for anterior labral tear detection from 48% and 91% to 96% and 97%, respectively [10]. Studies have also shown that in patients who cannot tolerate long MR scans, the ABER view in a direct MR

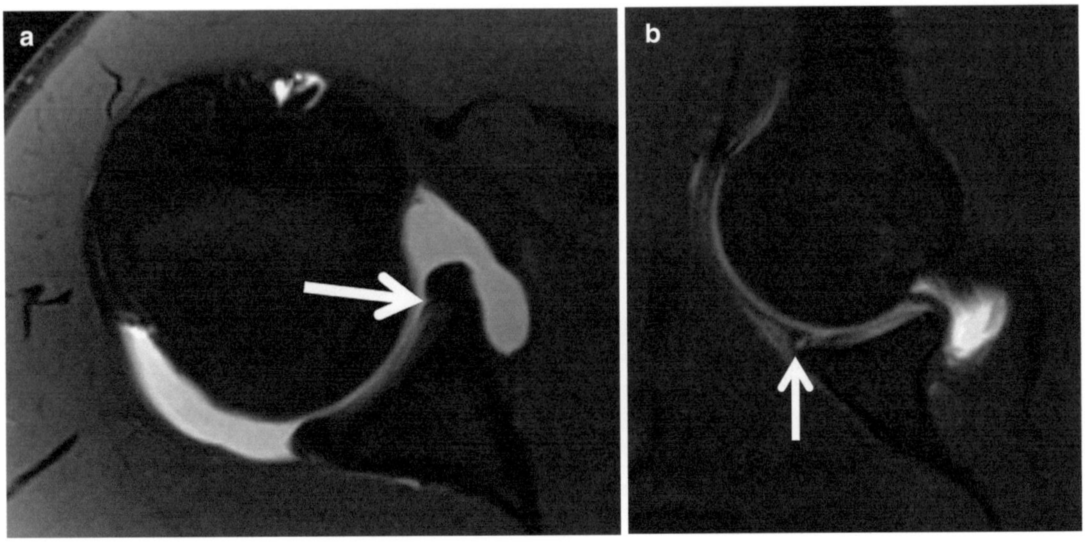

Fig. 2.17 *Anteroinferior labral tear on direct MR arthrography.* (**a**) Axial T1-weighted fat-suppressed image from a direct MR arthrogram demonstrates a normal-appearing labrum without contrast imbibition (arrow). (**b**) ABER image subsequently obtained on the same patient reveals a contrast-filled cleft at the chondrolabral junction of the anteroinferior labrum (arrow), reflecting tear

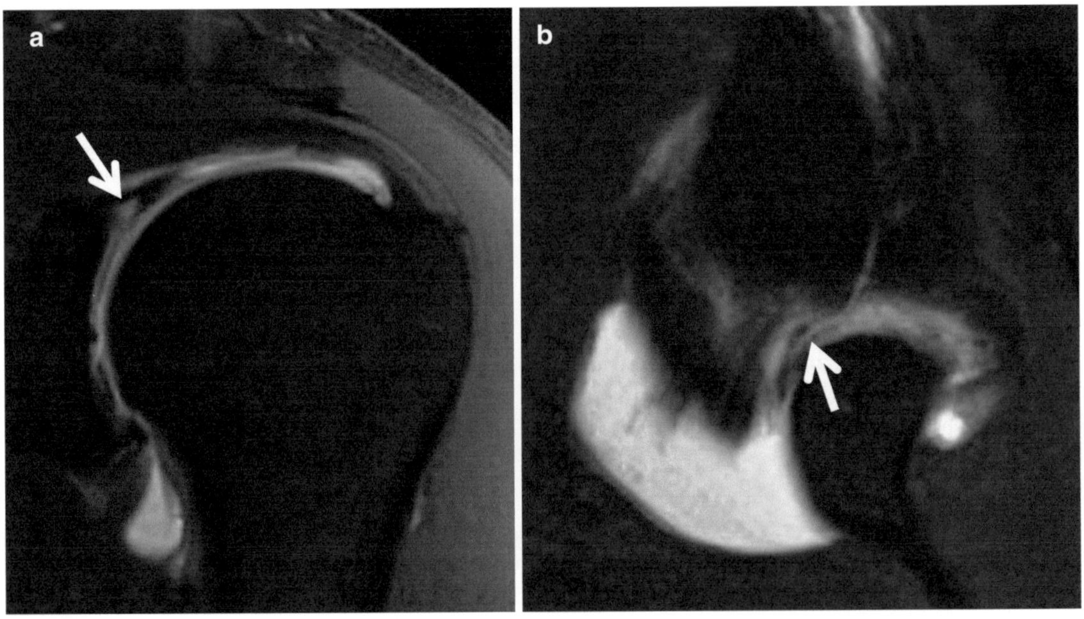

Fig. 2.18 *Superior labral tear on direct MR arthrography.* (**a**) Coronal oblique and (**b**) ABER T1-weighted fat-suppressed images following intra-articular administration of dilute gadolinium with contrast extension into the substance of the superior labrum (arrows), reflecting a nondisplaced labral tear

arthrogram alone is as accurate as an entire conventional MR arthrogram examination in the diagnosis of rotator cuff tear [74]. Additional FADIR MR imaging can increase conspicuity of posterior labral tears and improve assessment of the posterior joint capsule with intra-articular contrast distension (Fig. 2.20).

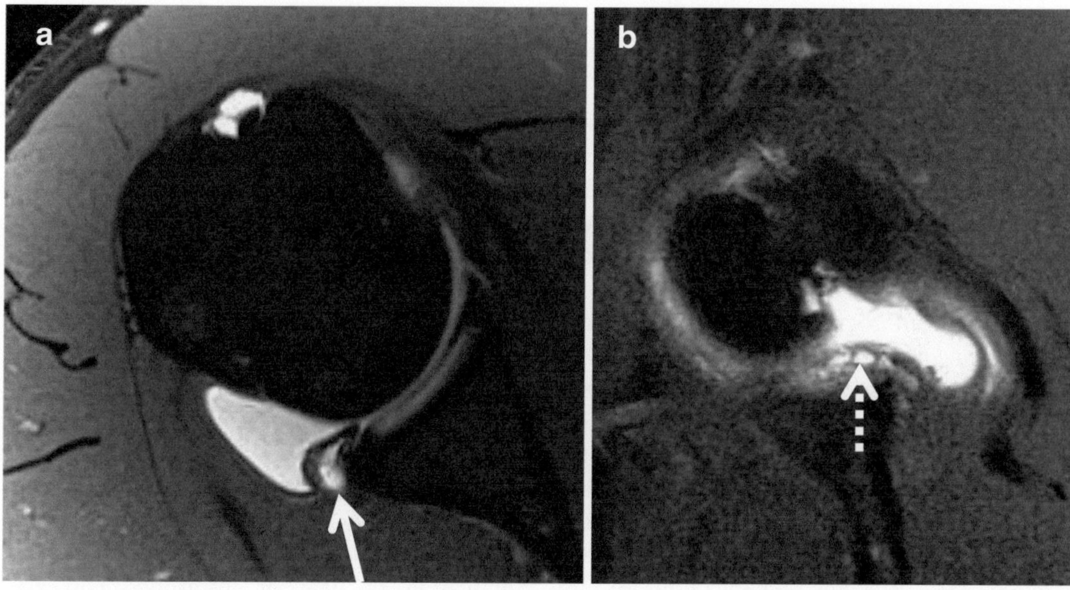

Fig. 2.19 *Posteroinferior labral tear on direct MR arthrography.* (**a**) Axial and (**b**) ABER T1-weighted fat-suppressed images following intra-articular administration of dilute gadolinium show extension of contrast at the posteroinferior chondrolabral junction in association with stripping of the periosteum from the posterior glenoid, which remains attached to the displaced labral tissue (solid arrow), in keeping with posterior labrum periosteal sleeve avulsion (POLPSA). Note that there is also a thin chain of paralabral cysts (dashed arrow)

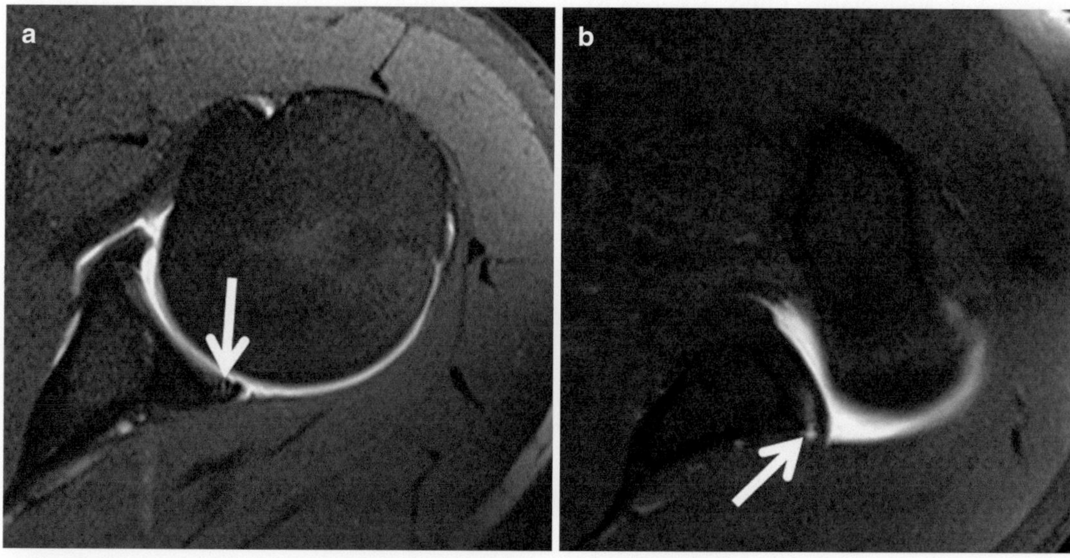

Fig. 2.20 *Posterior labral tear on FADIR direct MR arthrography.* (**a**) Axial T1-weighted fat-suppressed image following intra-articular contrast administration demonstrates subtle contrast imbibition within the posterior labrum (arrow) dissecting to the capsulolabral junction. (**b**) This finding is slightly more conspicuous on the FADIR image (arrow)

2.4.1.4 Advantages and Disadvantages

Compared to conventional noncontrast MR imaging of the shoulder, subtle tears within the rotator cuff are more conspicuous with direct MR arthrography [75]. MR arthrography has been shown to improve the accuracy of detection of supraspinatus and subscapularis abnormalities when compared with standard MR imaging [75, 76].

Waldt and colleagues demonstrated a sensitivity of 88%, specificity of 91%, accuracy of 89%, and negative and positive predictive values of 88 and 91%, respectively, with regard to direct MR angiography and detection of anteroinferior labral tears [77]. Using arthroscopy as the reference standard, direct MR arthrography showed a sensitivity of 82% and specificity of 98% in the identification of SLAP tears [78].

Direct MR arthrography has some disadvantages. Gianconi and colleagues studied 135 patients who underwent direct MR arthrography and found that 66% experienced transient but significant delayed-onset pain in the joint [79]. Nonspecific side effects such as allergic reaction to gadolinium or local anesthetic as well as vasovagal reactions and nausea have also been described [80]. Bleeding and infection are rare complications [80, 81].

2.4.2 Indirect MRA

Indirect MR arthrography offers a noninvasive alternative to direct MR angiography. It is based upon the concept that vessels and the intra-articular space enhance and demonstrate comparable signal intensity following the administration of intravenous contrast [82]. Because of the principles of bulk flow and diffusion, and lack of a basal membrane in the synovial lining, intravenous administration of gadolinium at a concentration of 0.1 mmol/kg eventually enters the joint space producing an arthrographic effect [83–86]. Since intravenous gadolinium diffuses from the capillary bed into the synovium and then enters the joint space over time, MR images are typically obtained after a delay of approximately 15 minutes.

The rate at which contrast leaks into the joint is dependent upon vascularity, synovial membrane permeability, and presence/absence of a joint effusion. In the setting of trauma, rheumatoid arthritis, or infection for example, the permeability of the synovial membrane is increased, resulting in halved transit time of contrast into the joint [82]. Conversely, synovial fibrosis would increase the time for contrast to enter the joint space. When a joint effusion is present, because of pressure differences, the rate at which contrast enters the joint space is decreased and imaging delay times may be increased by 50% when a hemorrhagic or septic effusion is present [54]. Some authors advocate exercise of approximately 10 minutes following the intravenous injection of contrast prior to imaging in order to promote blood flow to the joint [84, 87, 88]. Other studies have shown that application of heat or ultrasound can also increase the concentration of gadolinium within joints [89, 90].

2.4.2.1 Imaging Technique

At our institution, five sequences are typically obtained following a 10–15-minute period of exercise involving repetitive shoulder rotation, abduction, and adduction: axial and coronal oblique T1-weighted fat-suppressed, sagittal oblique T1-weighted, coronal oblique T2-weighted fat-suppressed, and an axial T1-weighted fat-suppressed sequence in the abducted/externally rotated position (ABER view, Table 2.3). As with direct MR arthrography, provocative imaging can be performed to increase diagnostic accuracy.

Imaging 15 minutes following intravenous injection of contrast material improves the sensitivity and detection of shoulder pathology [82, 84]. Studies have reported sensitivities and specificities ranging from 67% to 100% and 75% to 100%, respectively, in the assessment of supraspinatus and infraspinatus tears, with higher val-

Table 2.3 Protocol for indirect MR arthrography of the shoulder

Sequence	TR (ms)	TE (ms)	Slice thickness (mm)	FOV (mm)	Matrix (%)
Coronal T1 FS	400–800	8.6	4.0	140 × 140	500 × 500
Coronal T2 FS	3500–5000	55–80	4.0	140 × 140	500 × 500
Sagittal T1	400–800	9.4	4.0	140 × 140	500 × 500
Axial T1 FS	400–800	Min	4.0	140 × 140	500 × 500
ABER/ADIR	450–600	Min	3.0–4.0	140 × 140	500 × 700

ues seen for full-thickness supraspinatus tears and greater variation for partial-thickness tears [91–95]. High sensitivity and specificity have been reported for the evaluation of delaminating supraspinatus and infraspinatus tendon tears [96]. 64–67% sensitivity and 75–88% specificity have been reported for assessment of subscapularis tendon tears [94, 95]. As with direct MR arthrography, because of tension on the labrum with stretching of the inferior glenohumeral ligament in the ABER position, anteroinferior labral tears become more conspicuous as compared with neutral imaging. Herold and colleagues found that ABER views improved sensitivity and diagnostic confidence in the detection of partial-thickness supraspinatus tendon tears [92].

When compared to conventional noncontrast MRI, anterior labral tears can be more easily detected, although, studies have reported lower sensitivity and specificity in the detection of superior labral tears on indirect MR arthrography (Figs. 2.21 and 2.22) [95]. The diagnosis of labral tears on indirect MR arthrography can, however, be challenging due to the lack of capsular distension and is consequently highly dependent on the amount of native fluid within the joint for arthrographic effect. Fallahi and colleagues demonstrated 95–97% sensitivity for labral tear with indirect MRI versus 79–83% for conventional MRI. Diagnostic accuracy also increased from 84–86% to 93–95% from conventional to indirect MRI [97]. In one study, indirect MR arthrography had sensitivities and specificities comparable to those of direct MR arthrography in the assessment of labral tears [94].

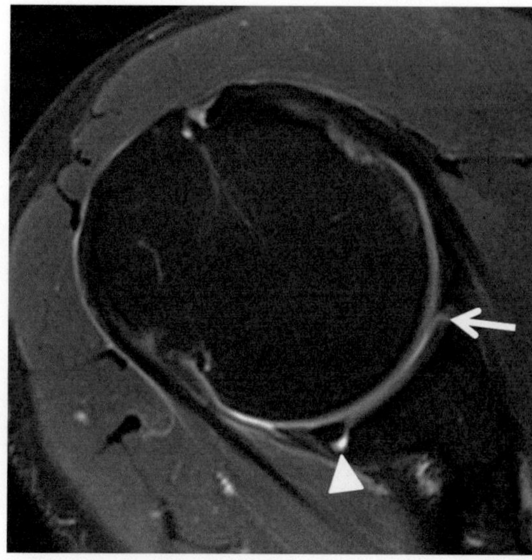

Fig. 2.21 *Labral tear on indirect MR arthrography.* Axial T1-weighted fat-suppressed image from an indirect MR arthrogram demonstrates slightly increased signal at the base of the anterior labrum, suggestive of tear (arrow). Without distension of the joint, it is unclear if this is indicative of a stable, healing tear with enhancing granulation tissue within the cleft versus an unstable lesion. Note that there is also linear enhancement at the base of the posterior labrum reflecting tear in this patient (arrowhead)

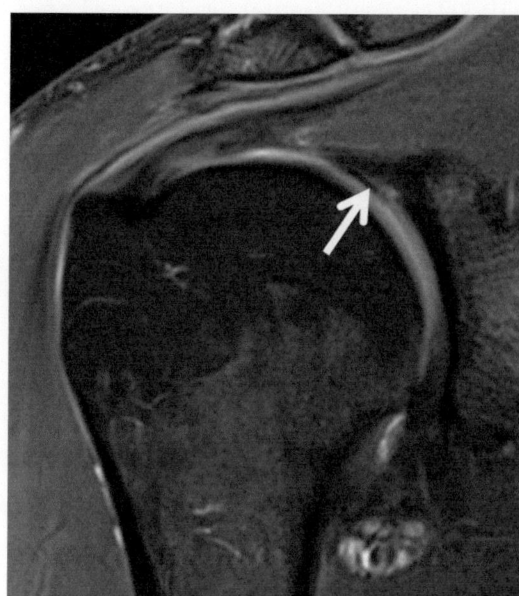

Fig. 2.22 *Superior labral tear on indirect MR arthrography.* Coronal oblique T1-weighted fat-suppressed image from an indirect MR arthrogram with linear enhancement within the substance of the superior labrum (arrow) reflecting a nondisplaced tear

2.4.2.2 Advantages and Disadvantages

There are several advantages to indirect MR arthrography. In comparison to direct MR angiography, it is less invasive and less time consuming, not requiring image guidance or iodinated contrast material.

Vessels, postoperative granulation tissue, tendon sheaths, and other synovial-lined structures including the shoulder bursae are some of the normally enhancing structures. Since the joint compartments also enhance, it is difficult to identify abnormal communication between them

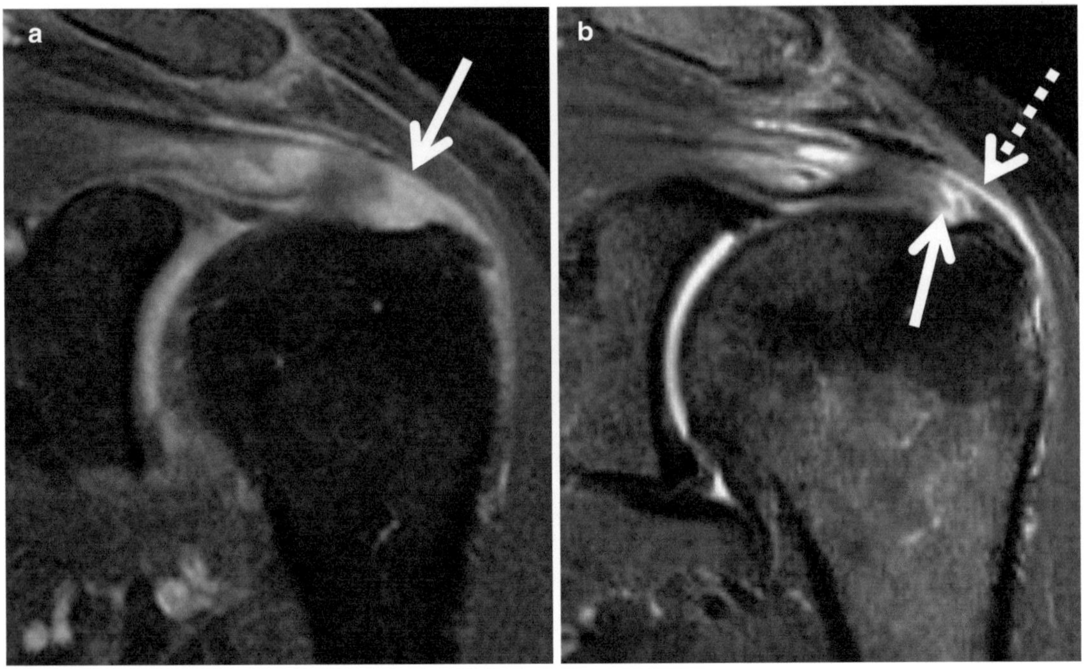

Fig. 2.23 *False-negative full-thickness supraspinatus tendon tear on indirect MR arthrography.* (**a**) Coronal oblique T1-weighted fat-suppressed image from an indirect MR arthrogram demonstrates enhancement without discrete continuous insertional supraspinatus tendon fibers and lack of the normal linear dark signal at the tendon margin, indicating a full-thickness tear (arrow). However, the corresponding (**b**) coronal oblique T2-weighted fat-suppressed image shows that the bursal surface fibers are actually intact and enables differentiation between the subacromial-subdeltoid bursa and torn tendon (arrow) by the intervening intact bursal surface fibers (dashed arrow)

resulting in the potential for misinterpretation [82]. As a result, unlike in direct MR arthrography, enhancement of the subacromial-subdeltoid bursa cannot be considered an indirect sign of full-thickness rotator cuff tear (Fig. 2.23) [54]. This fact makes identifying bursal sided partial tears easier [84, 92].

Because infection, inflammation, and tears all enhance, it is important to be able to distinguish between these three conditions. Song and colleagues found that the axillary joint capsule is increasingly thickened and demonstrates greater enhancement in the setting of adhesive capsulitis due to inflammation with resultant hyperemia and fibrosis [98]. Increased enhancement within the rotator interval has also been described (Fig. 2.24).

This method does not distend the joint capsule so indirect MR arthrography may suffer when there is scant native joint fluid. Furthermore, when compared with direct MR arthrography, the intra-articular fluid does not demonstrate as high of a signal intensity.

Side effects from intravenous gadolinium contrast are rare and the more common of these include nausea, vomiting, allergy, and hypersensitivity reactions [99]. This study is contraindicated in patients with poor renal function due to the risk of nephrogenic systemic fibrosis.

2.5 Three-Dimensional Imaging

With respect to the shoulder, 3D MR sequences have been utilized in the assessment of the articular cartilage typically using fast imaging with steady-state precession (FISP), double-echo steady-state (DESS), spoiled gradient recalled echo, and gradient echo sequences. 3D fast gradient echo isotropic images offer shorter scan times and have been shown to provide the same clinical information as conventional imaging [100].

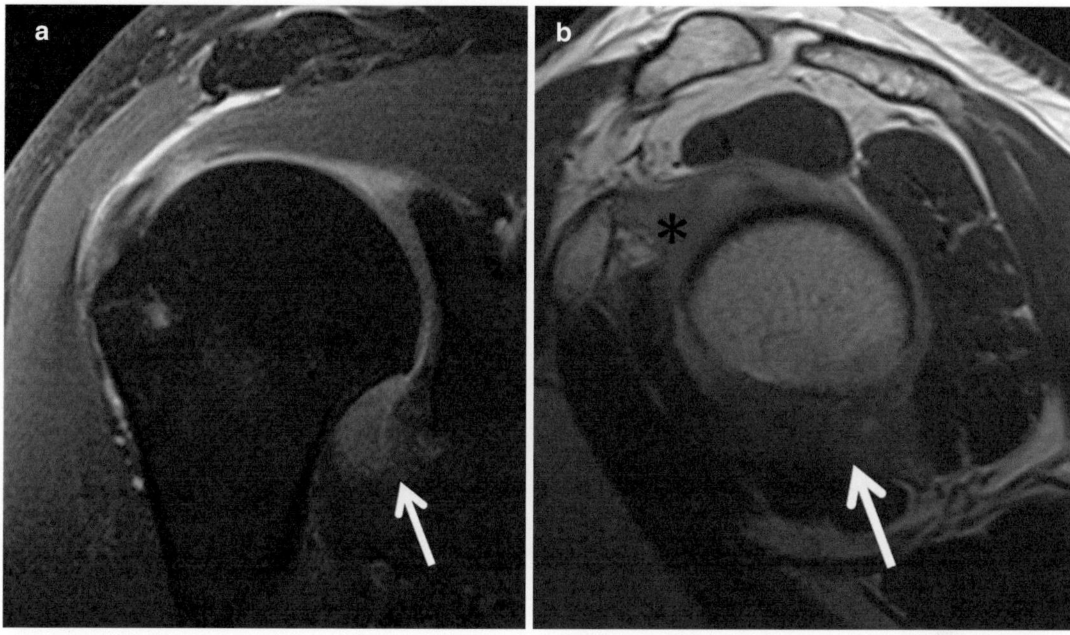

Fig. 2.24 *Adhesive capsulitis.* (**a**) Coronal oblique T1-weighted fat-suppressed and (**b**) sagittal oblique T1-weighted images from an indirect MR arthrogram demonstrate thickening and enhancement of the axillary pouch (arrows) with infiltration of the fat within the rotator interval (asterisk), which can be seen in the setting of adhesive capsulitis

Three-dimensional imaging has also been shown to be useful with MR arthrography. With direct MR arthrography, fat-suppressed gradient echo images have been found to be more sensitive than conventional spin-echo T1-weighted images in the detection of glenoid labral tears, particularly posterior labral tears [101]. Lee and colleagues found no statistical difference in the detection of superior labral tears. Jung and colleagues found no significant difference in diagnostic accuracy, sensitivity, or specificity of labral tear detection between 3D fat-suppressed fast GRE using an isotropic voxel size of 0.6 mm with an imaging time of 5 minutes 30 seconds and conventional fast spin-echo (FSE) sequences [102]. Magee showed that in addition to offering decreased scan times less than 3 minutes, 3D fast-spoiled gradient echo fat-suppressed isotropic (voxel size of 0.4 mm) imaging provided the same clinical information as conventional T1-weighted MR imaging at 3.0T [100]. In 3.0T indirect MR arthrography, Oh and colleagues found no statistically significant difference in sensitivity or specificity in the diagnosis of rotator cuff or labral tear when comparing 3D gradient echo isotropic and conventional FSE sequences.

Additionally, 3D MRI has been shown to be effective in the measurement of glenoid bone loss in the setting of anterior shoulder instability/dislocation (Fig. 2.25). Utilizing the best-fit circle method, Gyftopoulos and colleagues found no statistically significant difference between interpretation of axial 3D echo time T1-weighted FLASH sequences with Dixon-based water-fat separation for glenoid defect measurements relative to intraoperative findings [103]. In addition, no statistically significant difference was found between these 3D MR reconstructions and 3D CT reconstructions with respect to glenoid and humeral head bone loss [104].

2.5.1 The Postoperative Shoulder

Twenty five percent of patients who have undergone surgery to repair rotator cuff defects complain of persistent symptoms with a 20–47% prevalence of recurrent or persistent tearing

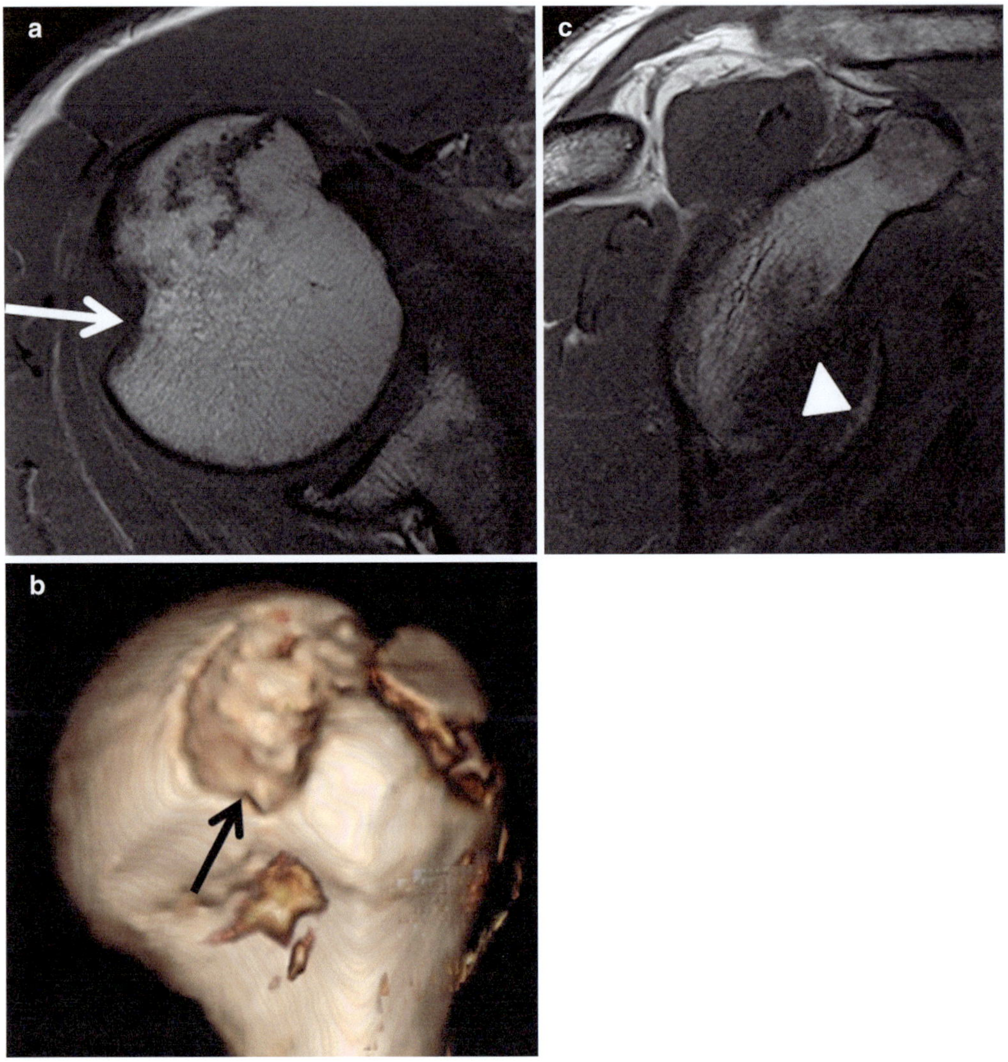

Fig. 2.25 *3D imaging.* (**a**) Axial T1-weighted and (**b**) 3D images demonstrating a large Hill-Sachs deformity (arrows) in this patient with recurrent anterior shoulder dislocations. Sagittal oblique T1-weighted sequence shows a corresponding osseous Bankart injury (arrowhead)

[105–109]. As one would expect, the larger the tear, the greater the symptoms [108–110]. These symptomatic patients tend to have a shorter interval between their initial presentation and surgical repair [111]. Zanetti and colleagues found that although 47% of symptomatic patients have postoperative rotator cuff tears, 21% of asymptomatic patients do, as well [105].

Radiographs and CT are the preferred initial imaging modalities for patients who have undergone surgery to identify the source of pain. Some postoperative complications include breakdown of repair, periprosthetic loosening and fracture, dislocation and instability, and scapular notching (in the setting of reverse total shoulder arthroplasty) [112–114]. Ultrasound can be used in isolation or as an adjunct to evaluate the adjacent soft tissues and evaluate for rotator cuff tear or nerve injury [115–117]. Nuclear medicine studies may also be performed in the setting of infection, although aspiration is recommended early in the diagnostic algorithm. Despite the fact that MR imaging offers superior contrast and spatial resolution, because of artifact related to the metallic hardware and residual metal shavings from the surgical instruments and postoperative anatomic distortion, it has not traditionally been used in post-arthroplasty patients.

2.5.1.1 Metal Reduction Protocols

One of the primary technical considerations when imaging postoperative patients is the presence or absence of hardware as well as its composition, as the degree of susceptibility artifact is dependent upon ferromagnetism. Because bioabsorbable suture anchors are nonmetallic, there is no associated susceptibility artifact. Some of the complications of these sutures include loosening/detachment, osteolysis, cyst formation, adjacent inflammation, and infection (Fig. 2.26) [118–120].

Most hardware currently used in arthroscopic shoulder surgeries is made of titanium. Metallic susceptibility artifact is most pronounced with ferromagnetic metals like cobalt-chrome and stainless steel, which were more commonly used in the past. These change the phase and frequency of local spins, causing a loss in signal and distortion along the frequency-encoding axis (Fig. 2.27a) [121]. Titanium and zirconium are paramagnetic metal alloys that are MR compatible, resulting in less metal-related artifact. With the advent of metal reduction protocols, MR imaging is an additional helpful imaging test, offering evaluation not only for capsular or nerve injury and tears of the rotator cuff, but also for hardware-related complications including osteolysis, fracture, and loosening [122, 123].

Metal reduction protocols minimize artifact by decreasing slice thickness and time to echo (TE), and increasing the matrix size and bandwidth [120]. Decreasing the TE offers less time for the protons to dephase, thereby preventing misregistration-related artifact [124]. Increasing the matrix size decreases the size of the pixels, which decreases the conspicuity of signal-related artifact. Swapping the phase and frequency-encoding gradients and aligning the frequency-encoding gradient along the longitudinal axis of the prosthesis are among some of the technical strategies utilized in MR imaging of hardware [125, 126]. While increasing the bandwidth decreases the interecho spacing, echo time and thus scan time, blurring, and chemical shift, it comes at a cost of compromising image quality by way of decreasing

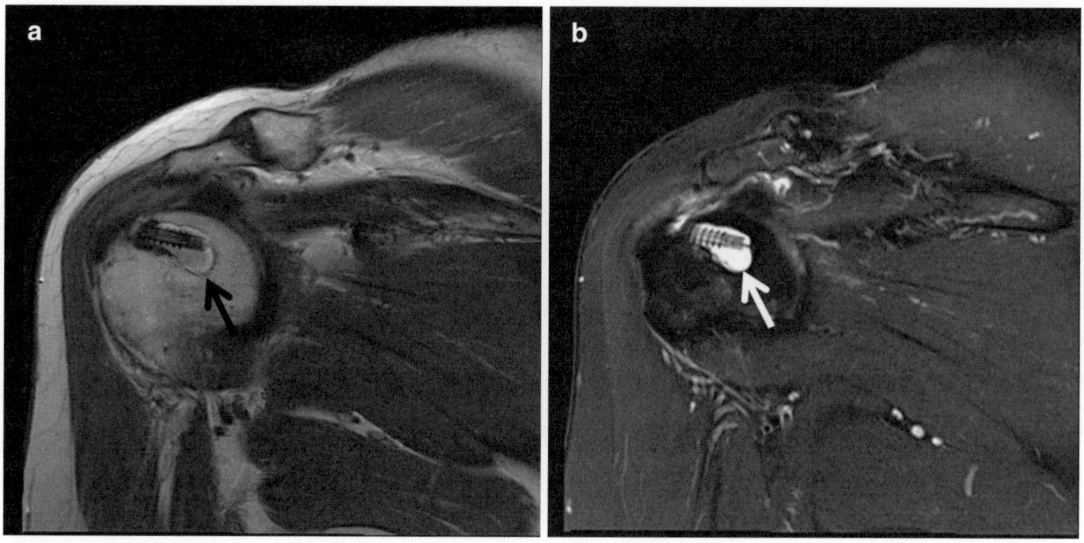

Fig. 2.26 *Bioabsorbable suture anchor.* (**a**) Coronal oblique proton density and (**b**) STIR MR images demonstrate lobulated signal hyperintensity (arrows) surrounding a bioabsorbable suture anchor within the humeral head that may be related to screw osteolysis versus granulation tissue, commonly seen following bioabsorbable suture anchor repair. Note that bioabsorbable suture anchors do not result in artifact severe enough to preclude appropriate diagnostic evaluation versus metallic suture anchors

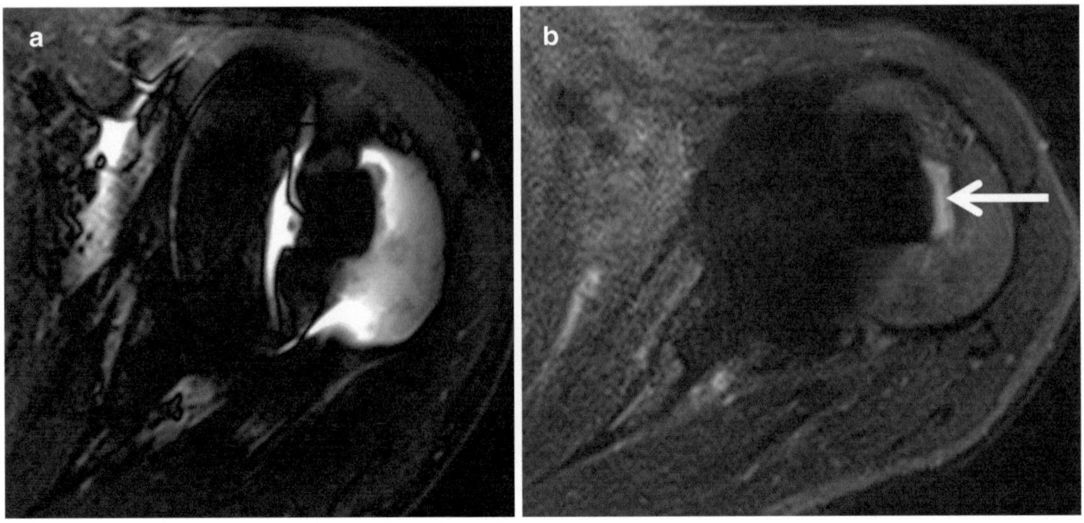

Fig. 2.27 *Loosening.* (**a**) Conventional axial STIR image in a patient status post-left total shoulder arthroplasty with shoulder pain and limited range of motion. Image interpretation is markedly limited due to susceptibility artifact from the metal hardware. (**b**) An axial STIR SEMAC image of the same patient has much less associated artifact and as a result a small amount of fluid signal intensity is more conspicuous along the lateral bone prosthesis interface (arrow), concerning for early loosening

the signal-to-noise ratio [125]. To compensate for this, the number of excitations (NEX) is concurrently increased. Because susceptibility artifact increases with increasing magnetic field strength, patients should not be imaged on 3.0T scanners. Susceptibility artifact is also exaggerated when the shoulder is eccentric to the isocenter of the bore of the magnet [122].

Gradient echo, chemical fat-suppressed, and spin-echo sequences should be avoided as these amplify susceptibility artifact. These sequences lack the 180-degree refocusing pulse, causing field inhomogeneity and distortion, and are prone to loss of signal intensity [127–130]. Fast spin-echo sequences may be used instead of standard spin-echo sequences. Short tau inversion recovery (STIR) sequences offer more homogeneous suppression of the fat adjacent to the metallic hardware and are the preferred fat-suppressed sequence in the postoperative patient [131].

Advanced MRI techniques for artifact reduction in high magnetic fields such as SEMAC (slice encoding for metal artifact correction), VAT (view angle tilting), and MAVRIC (multiacquisition variable-resonance image combination) enable useful imaging around implants (Fig. 2.27b) [128, 132–136]. SEMAC is a modified spin-echo sequence that extends VAT and slice-direction phase (z-phase) encoding to correct artifacts [128]. MAVRIC is a modified fast spin-echo sequence that acquires multiple image datasets at different frequency bands, offset from the dominant proton frequency. Both SEMAC and MAVRIC have shown to effectively reduce metal-related artifact when compared with fat spin-echo imaging [133]. The MAVRIC protocol has demonstrated improved imaging of the implant-bone and -soft tissue interfaces, enabling the diagnosis of synovitis, rotator cuff tears, and periprosthetic bone-related complications [122, 132]. Hybrid MAVRIC-SEMAC protocols have also been described [137].

2.5.1.2 Direct MR Arthrography

MR arthrography in the postoperative shoulder is useful for delineation of the labroligamentous structures, rotator cuff, and tendons [124]. Although conventional noncontrast MRI has an accuracy of 83–90% in the detection of full-thickness rotator cuff tears after repair, direct MR arthrography has been shown to improve diagnostic accuracy when compared with noncontrast MRI in the postoperative patient [138, 139].

Partial- and full-thickness rotator cuff tears are both reliably diagnosed in the postoperative shoulder after intra-articular distension of the joint, with contrast filling the partial-thickness defect or coursing through the full-thickness defect into the subacromial-subdeltoid bursa (Figs. 2.28 and 2.29) [140–142]. However, this is not always a reliable finding as sometimes postoperative scarring can prevent leakage of contrast into the bursa with full-thickness tears [143–145]. In the setting of full-thickness tears, MR arthrography more reliably identifies medial retraction of the torn tendon fibers [124].

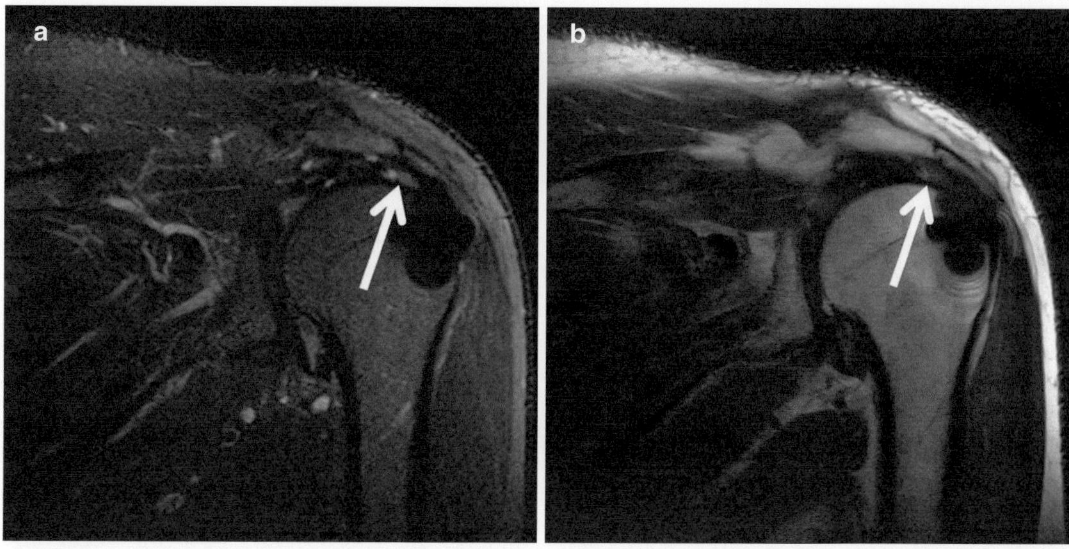

Fig. 2.28 *Postoperative partial-thickness rotator cuff tear.* (**a**) Coronal oblique STIR and (**b**) proton density MR images demonstrate fluid signal intensity and discontinuity of the articular sided insertional fibers extending to the intrasubstance fibers of the supraspinatus tendon (arrows) compatible with partial-thickness tear

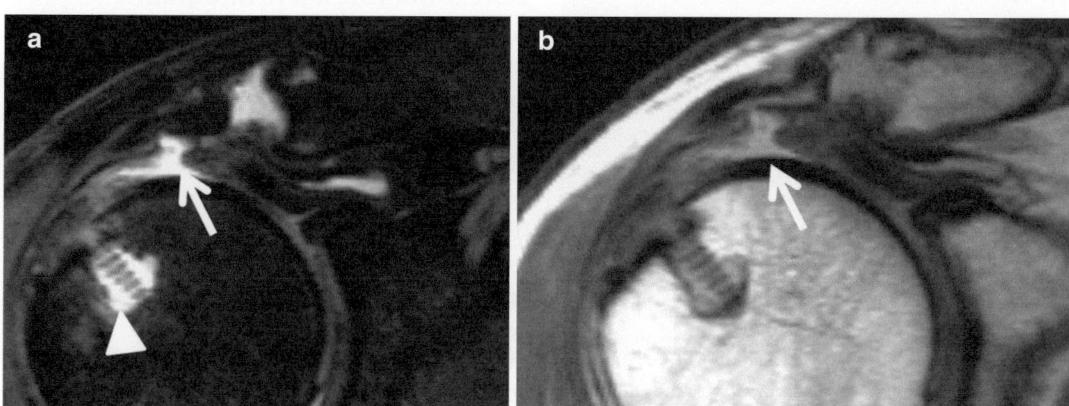

Fig. 2.29 *Postoperative full-thickness rotator cuff tear.* (**a**) Coronal oblique T2-weighted fat-suppressed and (**b**) T1-weighted images from a direct MR arthrogram in a patient status post-rotator cuff repair with recurrent shoulder pain and limited range of motion demonstrate a full-thickness tear of the supraspinatus tendon with discontinuous fibers and contrast extravasation via the defect into the subacromial-subdeltoid bursa (arrows). Note that there is increased signal surrounding the bioabsorbable suture anchor, which may reflect granulation tissue and/or osteolysis (arrowhead)

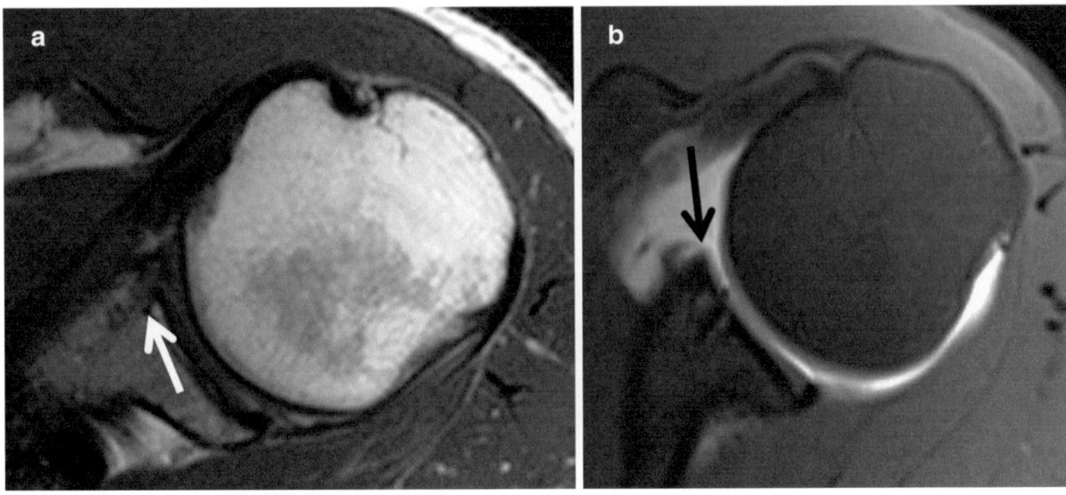

Fig. 2.30 *Postoperative anterior labral tear, noncontrast vs. direct MR arthrography.* (**a**) Axial proton density image from a noncontrast MRI in a patient status post-anterior labral debridement shows abnormal signal intensity of the subchondral bone (arrow) related to postsurgical changes from the suture anchor; however, lack of joint distension precludes assessment for retear/stability. (**b**) An axial T1-weighted fat-suppressed image from direct MR arthrogram on the same patient reveals absence of the anterior labrum due to tear with stripping of the anterior glenoid periosteum (arrow)

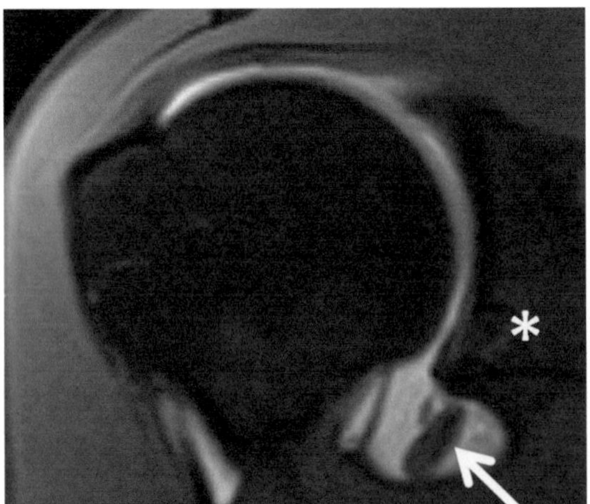

Fig. 2.31 *Displaced labral tear on direct MR arthrography.* Coronal oblique T1-weighted fat-suppressed image from a direct MR arthrogram in a patient status post anteroinferior labral repair (asterisk identifies the suture anchor) demonstrates a hypertrophied torn labral fragment (arrow) displaced into the inferior aspect of the joint, made conspicuous by the intra-articular contrast

Direct MR arthrography has shown 100% sensitivity in recurrent labral tear detection, compared to 71% in noncontrast MR, although the findings are less specific- 60% for direct MR arthrography and 80% for noncontrast MR (Figs. 2.30 and 2.31) [146].

2.5.1.3 Indirect MR Arthrography

Gadolinium is administered intravenously at a concentration of 0.1 mmol/kg and MR is performed following a delay of 30 minutes. Because postoperative granulation tissue enhances and the signal-to-noise ratio is lower with indirect MR arthrography, evaluation of the surgical bed can be challenging (Figs. 2.32 and 2.33). Wagner and colleagues studied 24 patients status post surgery for shoulder instability with symptoms of recurrent instability, and performed conventional noncontrast MR, direct MR arthrography, or indirect MR arthrography [146]. In this study, indirect MR arthrography was 100% accurate in identifying labral tears, greater than that for the other two imaging tests.

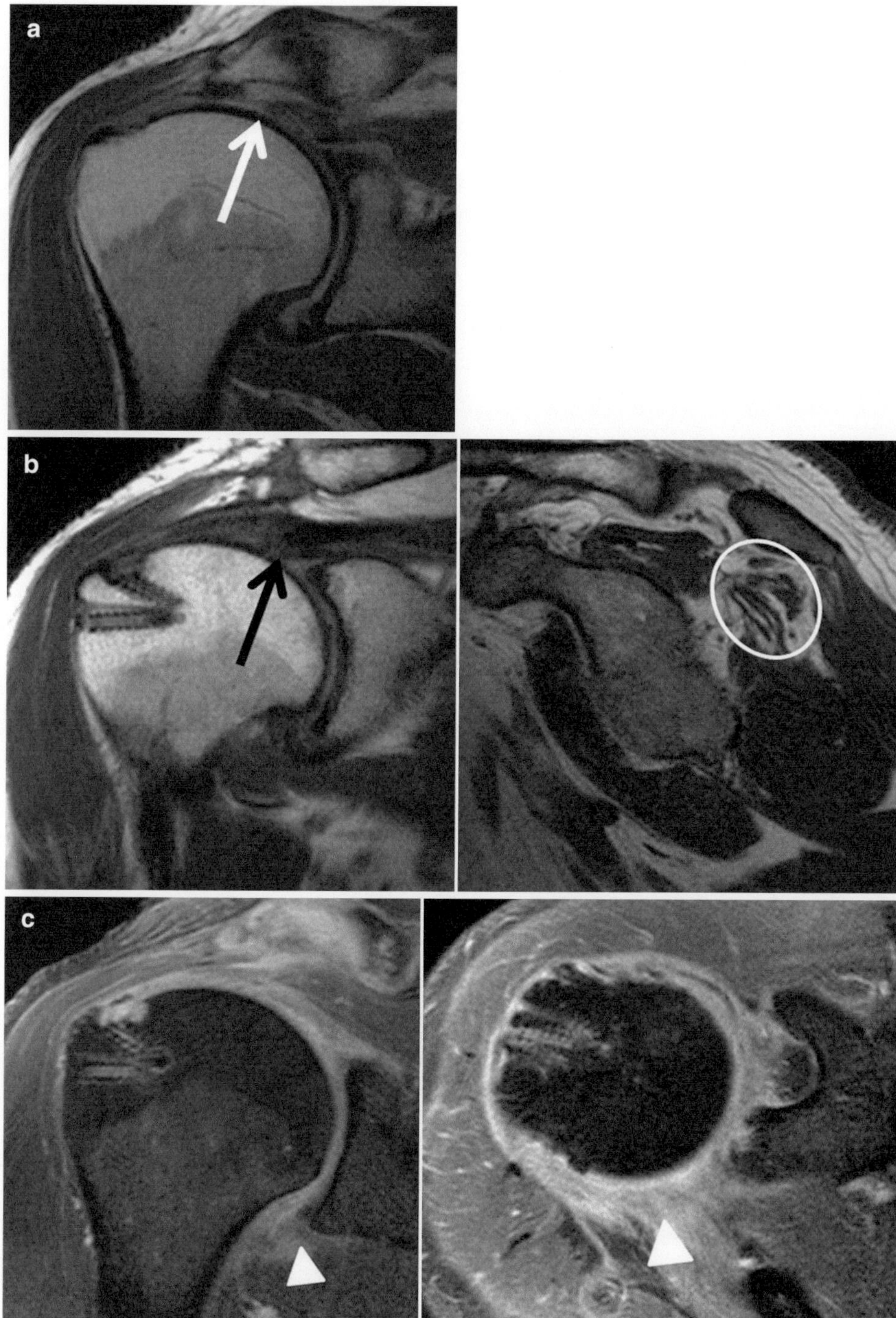

Fig. 2.32 *Postoperative indirect MR arthrography.* (**a**) Coronal oblique proton density image demonstrating a full-thickness tear of the supraspinatus tendon with retraction to the level of the glenohumeral joint (white arrow). A complete infraspinatus tendon tear was also present (not visualized). Five months following rotator cuff repair, the patient returned with complaints of shoulder pain and (**b**) coronal proton density (left) and sagittal T1-weighted (right) images obtained at this time redemonstrate full-thickness supraspinatus (black arrow) and infraspinatus tears (not shown) with high-grade fatty infiltration of the infraspinatus muscle (circled). (**c**) Subsequent coronal (left) and axial (right) T1-weighted fat-suppressed images from indirect MR arthrography show diffuse enhancement of the glenohumeral joint (arrowheads). Because both infection and inflammation enhance, it is difficult to distinguish between chronic synovitis and infection on indirect MR arthrography

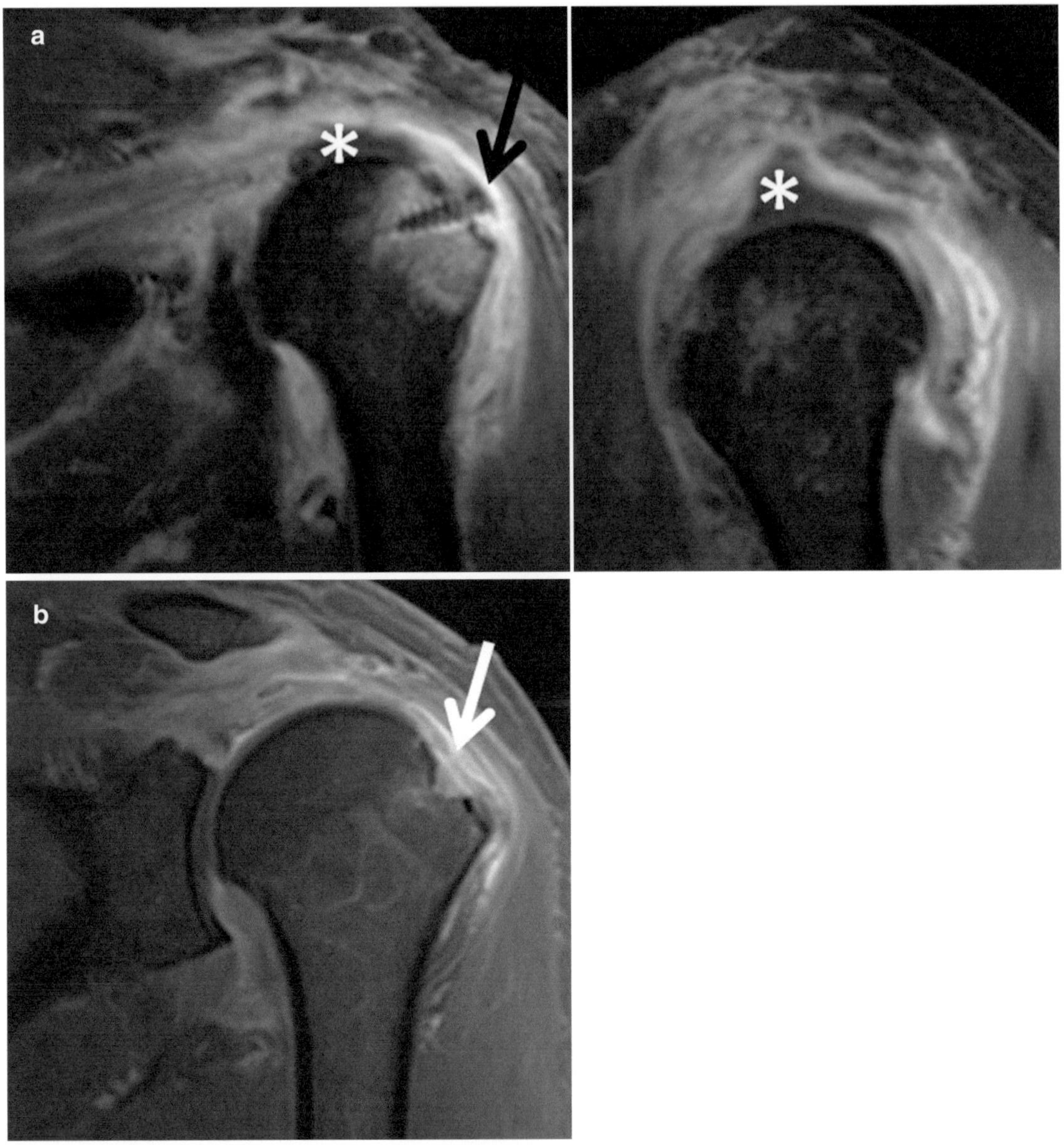

Fig. 2.33 *Postoperative infection.* (**a**) Coronal oblique (left) and sagittal oblique (right) T1-weighted fat-suppressed images from an indirect MR arthrogram in a patient status post-rotator cuff repair with pain and fever. The suture anchor (black arrow) protrudes beyond the cortex of the humeral head as a result of loosening in the setting of infection, with reactive marrow edema and pockets of peripherally enhancing fluid (asterisk) reflecting abscess formation and marked enhancement of the synovium. (**b**) Coronal oblique T1-weighted fat-suppressed image from an indirect MR arthrogram on the same patient two months following treatment demonstrates interval removal of the suture anchor (white arrow) with very little residual edema and enhancement at the suture track. The abscesses have also resolved

2.6 Biochemical Imaging

With recent advances in field strength and coil design, researchers are focused on using biochemical-based MRI to identify sensitive methods for detecting early changes in articular cartilage and fibrocartilage [66, 147]. Although much of the research has been focused on the knee given the presence of thick, flat cartilage and prevalence of knee osteoarthritis in the general population, there have been studies investigating the applicability of biochemical imaging to the glenohumeral cartilage and glenoid labrum [148–152]. In the clinical setting, these techniques may enable early diagnosis and management of osteoarthritis by targeting proteoglycan content as well as collagen orientation and concentration. Research has already demonstrated successful in vivo monitoring of collagen and proteoglycan content in patients who have undergone articular cartilage repair in the knee [153].

T1 rho, T2* mapping, sodium MRI, and delayed gadolinium-enhanced MRI of cartilage (dGEMRIC) are some of the techniques used to assess the ultrastructure of cartilage, detecting changes before gross morphological changes can be appreciated on conventional MRI. Both T1 rho and dGEMRIC evaluate the glycosaminoglycan content of articular cartilage.

For dGEMRIC studies, FSE IR T1-weighted MR imaging is performed on a 1.5T scanner 30 and 90 minutes following a double-dose intravenous injection of gadolinium at a dose of 0.2 mmol/kg and a brief period of exercise (approximately 10 minutes). The principle behind dGEMRIC studies is that negatively charged gadolinium replaces the extra-cellular negatively charged glycosaminoglycan molecules, which are depleted in early degeneration of cartilage. Thus, measuring T1 relaxation times following the intravenous administration of gadolinium creates a map of glycosaminoglycan depletion, with the concentration of gadolinium per voxel (T1gd or dGEMRIC index) being low in areas of low glycosaminoglycan content and vice versa. Wiener and colleagues found a decrease in T1gd 15 minutes after intra-articular injection of gadolinium, with increased uptake in hyaline versus labral cartilage [148].

T1 rho studies have demonstrated an inversely proportional relationship between T1 relaxation time in the rotating frame and glycosaminoglycan content [154]. T2* mapping takes advantage of the zonal structure of collagen to map out T2 values in articular cartilage. For example, collagen in the intermediate zone is organized in a random fashion, resulting in longer T2 values compared to the more organized collagen in the superficial and radial zones where T2 values are shorter. Studies have shown the feasibility of T2* mapping of cartilage in the glenohumeral joint [149]. Lee and colleagues demonstrated differences in T2 values not only between subjects with and without osteoarthritis, but also between primary and secondary osteoarthritis [155].

References

1. Davis SJ, Teresi LM, Bradley WG, et al. Effect of arm rotation on MR imaging of the rotator cuff. Radiology. 1991;181:265–8.
2. Magee T, Shapiro M, Williams D. Comparison of high-field-strength versus low-field-strength MRI of the shoulder. AJR Am J Roentgenol. 2003;181:1211–5.
3. Shellock FG, Bert JM, Fritts HM, Gundry CR, et al. Evaluation of the rotator cuff and glenoid labrum using a 0.2-Tesla extremity magnetic resonance (MR) system: MR results compared to surgical findings. J Magn Reson Imaging. 2001;14:763–70.
4. Spencer BA, Dolinskas CA, Seymour PA, Thomas SJ, Abboud JA. Glenohumeral articular cartilage lesions: prospective comparison of non-contrast magnetic resonance imaging and findings at arthroscopy. Arthroscopy. 2013;29:1466–70.
5. VanBeek C, Loeffler BJ, Narzikul A, et al. Diagnostic accuracy of noncontrast MRI for detection of glenohumeral cartilage lesions: a prospective comparison to arthroscopy. J Shoulder Elb Surg. 2014;23(7):1010–6.
6. Legan JM, Burkhard TK, Goff WB II, et al. Tears of the glenoid labrum: MR imaging of 88 arthroscopically confirmed cases. Radiology. 1991;179:241–6.
7. Phillips JC, Cook C, Beaty S, et al. Validity of non-contrast magnetic resonance imaging in diagnosing superior labrum anterior-posterior tears. J Shoulder Elb Surg. 2013;22(1):3–8.
8. Magee TH, Williams D. Sensitivity and specificity in detection of labral tears with 3.0-T MRI of the shoulder. AJR. 2006;187:1448–52.
9. Kwak SM, Brown RR, Resnick D, et al. Anatomy, anatomic variations, and pathology of 11- to 3-o'clock position of the glenoid labrum: findings on MR arthrography and anatomic sections. AJR. 1998;171:235–8.
10. Cvitanic O, Tirman P, Feller J, et al. Using abduction and external rotation of the shoulder to increase the sensitivity of MR arthrography in revealing tears of the anterior glenoid labrum. AJR. 1997;169:837–44.
11. Song JC, Lazarus ML, Song AP. MRI findings in Little Leaguer's shoulder. Skelet Radiol. 2006;35(2):107–9.
12. MM C, Harish S, Burr J. MR arthrographic assessment of suspected posteroinferior labral lesions using flexion, adduction, and internal rotation positioning of the arm: preliminary experience. Skelet Radiol. 2010;39(5):481–8.

13. G W, Haglund-Akerlind Y, Larsson H. Open MR imaging of the unstable shoulder in the apprehension test position: description and evaluation of an alternative MR examination position. Eur Radiol. 1999;9(9):1789–95.
14. Chan KK, Muldoon KA, Yeh L, et al. Superior labral anteroposterior lesions: MR arthrography with arm traction. AJR. 1999;173(4):111–1122.
15. Friedman RJ, Bonutti PM, Genez B. Cine magnetic resonance imaging of the subcoracoid region. Orthopedics. 1998;21:545–8.
16. Siegel MJ. MRI of bone marrow [PDF download]. American Roentgen Ray Society; 2005. http://www.arrs.org/shopARRS/products/pdf.cfm?theFile=s06p_sample.pdf.
17. Mirowitz SA. Hematopoietic bone marrow within the proximal humeral epiphysis in normal adults: investigation with MR imaging. Radiology. 1993;188:689–93.
18. Clark JM, Harryman DT. II: Tendons, ligaments, and capsule of the rotator cuff. Gross and microscopic anatomy. J Bone Joint Surg. 1992;74-A:713–25.
19. Erickson SJ, Cox IH, Hyde JS. Effect of tendon orientation on MR imaging signal intensity: a manifestation of the "magic angle" phenomenon. Radiology. 1991;181(2):389–92.
20. GuinelFilho H, Du J, Pak BC, et al. Quantitative characterization of the Achilles tendon in cadaveric specimens: T1 and T2* measurements using ultrashort-TE MRI at 3 T. Am J Roentgenol. 2009;192(3):W117–24.
21. Du J, Chiang AJ, Chung CB, Statum S, Znamirowski R, Takahashi A, et al. Orientational analysis of the Achilles tendon and enthesis using an ultrashort echo time spectroscopic imaging sequence. Magn Reson Imaging. 2010;28:178–84.
22. Hodgson RJ, O'Connor PJ, Grainger AJ. Tendon and ligament imaging. Br J Radiol. 2012;85(1016):1157–72.
23. Buck F, Grehn H. Degeneration of the long biceps tendon: comparison of MRI with gross anatomy and histology. Am J Roentgenol. 2009;193(5):1367–75.
24. Fullerton GD, Rahal A. Collagen structure: the molecular source of the tendon magic angle effect. J Magn Reson Imaging. 2007;25:345–61.
25. Hayes CW, Parellada JA. The magic angle effect in musculoskeletal MR imaging. Top Magn Reson Imaging. 1996;8:51–6.
26. Peto S, Gillis P, Henri VP. Structure and dynamics of water in tendon from NMR relaxation measurements. Biophys J. 1990;57(1):71–84.
27. Al-Riyami AM, Lim BK, Peh WC. Variants and pitfalls in MR imaging of shoulder injuries. Semin Musculoskelet Radiol. 2014;18:36–44.
28. Peh WCG, Chan JHM. The magic angle phenomenon in tendons: effect of varying the MR echo time. Br J Radiol. 1998;71:31–6.
29. Weinreb JH, Sheth C, Aposolakos J, et al. Tendon structure, disease, and imaging. Muscles Ligaments Tendons J. 2014;4(1):66–73.
30. Vahlensieck M, Pollack M, Lang P, et al. Two segments of the supraspinous muscle: cause of high signal intensity at MR imaging? Radiology. 1993;186(2):449–54.
31. Resnick D, Kang HS, Pretterklieber ML. Shoulder. In: Resnick D, Kang HS, Pretterklieber ML, editors. Internal derangements of joints. 2nd ed. Philadelphia, Pennsylvania: Elsevier; 2007. p. 713–1122.
32. Guckel C, Nidecker A. Diagnosis of tears in rotator-cuff injuries. Eur J Radiol. 1997;25(3):168–76.
33. Kim HM, Dahiya N, Teefey SA, et al. Location and initiation of degenerative rotator cuff tears: an analysis of three hundred and sixty shoulders. J Bone Joint Surg Am. 2010;92(5):1088–96.
34. Chansky HA, Iannotti JP. The vascularity of the rotator cuff. Clin Sports Med. 1991;10(4):807–22.
35. Matava MJ, Purcell DB, Rudzki JR. Partial-thickness rotator cuff tears. Am J Sports Med. 2005;33(9):1405–17.
36. Fukuda H, Hamada K, Nakajima T, Yamada N, Tomonaga A, Goto M. Partial-thickness tears of the rotator cuff: a clinicopathological review based on 66 surgically verified cases. Int Orthop. 1996;20:257–265.30.
37. Fukuda H, Hamada K, Yamanaka K. Pathology and pathogenesis of bursal-side rotator cuff tears viewed from en bloc histologic sections. Clin Orthop Relat Res. 1990;254:75–80.31.
38. Fukuda H, Mikasa M, Ogawa K, et al. The partial thickness tear of the rotator cuff. Orthop Trans. 1983;173:70–7.
39. Reilly P, Amis AA, Wallace AL, Emery RJ. Supraspinatus tears: propagation and strain alteration. J Shoulder Elb Surg. 2003;12:134–8.
40. Neer CS II. Anterior acromioplasty for the chronic impingement syndrome in the shoulder: a preliminary report. J Bone Joint Surg Am. 1972;67:41–50.
41. Ozaki J, Fujimoto S, Nakagawa Y, Masuhara K, Tamai S. Tears of the rotator cuff of the shoulder associated with pathological changes in the acromion: a study in cadavers. J Bone Joint Surg Am. 1988;70:1224–30.
42. Kolts I, Busch LC, Tomusk H, et al. Anatomical composition of the anterior shoulder joint capsule. A cadaver study on 12 glenohumeral joints. Ann Anat. 2001;183(1):53–9.
43. Park YH, Lee JY, Moon SH, Mo JH, Yang BK, Hahn SH, Resnick D. MR arthrography of the labral capsular ligamentous complex in the shoulder: imaging variations and pitfalls. AJR. 2000;175:667–72.
44. Snyder SJ, Karzel RP, Del Pizzo W, et al. SLAP lesions of the shoulder. Arthroscopy. 1990;6:274–9.
45. Maffet MW, Gartsman GM, Moseley B. Superior labrum-biceps tendon complex lesions of the shoulder. Am J Sports Med. 1995;23:93–8.
46. Patten RM. Vacuum phenomenon: a potential pitfall in the interpretation of gradient-recalled-echo MR images of the shoulder. AJR. 1994;162(6):1383–6.

47. Stallenberg B, Madani A, Burny F, et al. The vacuum phenomenon: a CT sign of nonunited fracture. AJR. 2001;176(5):1161–4.
48. Dwyer AJ, Knop RH, Hoult DI. Frequency shift artifacts in MR imaging. J Comput Assist Tomogr. 1985;9:16–8.
49. Rosen BR, Wedeen VJ, Brady TJ. Selective saturation NMR imaging. J Comput Assist Tomogr. 1984;8:813–8.
50. Guntern DV, Pfirmann CWA, Schmid MR, et al. Articular cartilage lesions of the glenohumeral joint: diagnostic effectiveness of MR arthrography and prevalence in patients with subacromial impingement syndrome. Radiology. 2003;226:165–70.
51. Frahm J, Haase A, Hanicke W, et al. Chemical shift selective MR imaging using whole body magnet. Radiology. 1985;156:441–4.
52. Haase A, frahm J, Hanicke W, et al. 1H NMR chemical shift selective (CHESS) imaging. Phys Med Biol. 1985;30:341–4.
53. Osinski, et al. Magnetic resonance arthrography. Orthop Clin N Am. 2006;37:299–319.
54. Steinbach LS, Palmer WE, Schweitzer ME. Special focus session: MR arthrography. Radiographics. 2002;22:1223–46.
55. Chandnani VP, Yeager TD, DeBerardino T, Christensen K, Gagliardi JA, et al. Glenoid labral tears: prospective evaluation with MR imaging, MR arthrography, and CT arthrography. AJR. 1993;161:1229–35.
56. Beltran J, Bencardino J, Mellado J, Rosenberg ZS, Irish RD. MR arthrography of the shoulder: variants and pitfalls. Radiographics. 1997;17(6): 1403–12.
57. Shankman S, Bencardino J, Beltran J. Glenohumeral instability: evaluation using MR arthrography of the shoulder. Skelet Radiol. 1999;28:365–82.
58. Palmer WE, Brown JH, Rosenthal DJ. Labral ligamentous complex of the shoulder: evaluation with MR arthrography. Radiology. 1994;190:645–51.
59. Sethi PM, Kingston S, El Attrache N. Accuracy of anterior intra-articular injection of the glenohumeral joint. Arthroscopy. 2005;21:77–80.
60. Catalano OA, Manfredi R, Vanzulli A, et al. MR arthrography of the glenohumeral joint: modified posterior approach without imaging guidance. Radiology. 2007 Feb;242(2):550–4.
61. Porat S, Leupold JA, Burnett KR, Nottage WM. Reliability of non-imaging-guided glenohumeral joint injection through rotator interval approach in patients undergoing diagnostic MR arthrography. AJR. 2008;191(3):W96–9.
62. Zwar RB, Read JW, Noakes JB. Sonographically guided glenohumeral joint injection. AJR. 2004;183:48–50.
63. Mulligan ME. CT-guided shoulder arthrography at the rotator cuff interval. AJR. 2008;191:58–61.
64. Kopka L, Funke M, Fischer U, et al. MR arthrography of the shoulder with gadopentetate dimeglumine: influence of concentration, iodinated contrast material, and time on signal intensity. AJR. 1994;163(3):621–3.
65. Engel A. Magnetic resonance knee arthrography. Enhanced contrast by gadolinium complex in the rabbit and in humans. Acta Orthop Scand Suppl. 1990;240:1–57.
66. La Rocca Vieira R, Rybak LD, Recht M. Technical update on magnetic resonance imaging of the shoulder. Magn Reson Imaging Clin N Am. 2012;20:149–61.
67. Masi JN, Newitt D, Sell CA, Daldrup-Link H, Steinbach L, Majumdar S, et al. Optimization of gadodiamide concentration for MR arthrography at 3 T. AJR. 2005;184:1754–61.
68. Montgomery DD, Morrison WB, Schweitzer ME, Weishaupt D, Dougherty L. Effects of iodinated contrast and field strength on gadolinium enhancement: implications for direct MR arthrography. J Magn Reson Imaging. 2002;15:334–43.
69. Jacobson JA, Lin J, Jamadar DA, Hayes CW. Aids to successful shoulder arthrography performed with a fluoroscopically guided anterior approach. Radiographics. 2003;23:373–8.
70. Brown RR, Clarke DW, Daffner RH. Is a mixture of gadolinium and iodinated contrast material safe during MR arthrography? AJR. 2000;175:1087–90.
71. Sanders TG, Tirman PF, Linares R, Feller JF, Richardson R. The glenolabral articular disruption lesion: MR arthrography with arthroscopic correlation. AJR. 1999;172:171–5.
72. Masi JN, Newitt D, Sell CA, et al. Optimization of gadodiamide concentration for MR arthrography at 3 T. AJR. 2005;184:1754–61.
73. Lee MJ, Motamedi K, Chow K, et al. Gradient-recalled echo sequences in direct shoulder MR arthrography for evaluating the labrum. Skelet Radiol. 2008;37(1):19–2.
74. Schreinemachers SA, van der Hulst VP, Willems WJ, Bipat S, van der Woude HJ. Detection of partial-thickness supraspinatus tendon tears: is a single direct MR arthrography series in ABER position as accurate as conventional MR arthrography? Skelet Radiol. 2009;38:967–75.
75. Hodler J, Loredo RA, Longo C, Trudell D, Yu JS, Resnick D. Assessment of articular cartilage thickness of the humeral head: MR–anatomic correlation in cadavers. AJR. 1995;165:615–20.
76. Pfirrmann CW, Zanetti M, Weishaupt D, Gerber C, Hodler J. Subscapularis tendon tears: detection and grading at MR arthrography. Radiology. 1999;213:709–14.
77. Waldt S, Burkart A, Imhoff AB, et al. Anterior shoulder instability: accuracy of MR arthrography in the classification of anteroinferior labroligamentous injuries. Radiology. 2005;237:578–83.
78. Waldt S, Burkart A, Lange P, Imhoff P, Rummeny EJ, Woertler K. Diagnostic performance of MR arthrography in the assessment of superior labral anteroposterior lesions of the shoulder. AJR. 2004;182:1271–8.

79. Giaconi JC, Link TM, Vail TP, et al. Morbidity of direct MR arthrography. AJR. 2011;196:868–74.
80. Newberg AH, Munn CS, Robbins AH. Complications of arthrography. Radiology. 1985;155:605–6.
81. Hugo PC 3rd, Newberg AH, Newman JS, Wetzner SM. Complications of arthrography. Semin Musculoskelet Radiol. 1998;2:345–8.
82. Vahlensieck M, Sommer T, Textor J, et al. Indirect MR arthrography: technique and applications. Eur Radiol. 1998;8:232–5.
83. Vahlensieck M, Lang P, Sommer T, Genant HK, Schild HH. Indirect MR arthrography: techniques and applications. Semin Ultrasound CT MR. 1997;18:302–6.
84. Vahlensieck M, Peterfy CG, Wischer T, et al. Indirect MR arthrography: optimization and clinical applications. Radiology. 1996;200(1):249–54.
85. Drape JL, Thelen P, Gay-Depassier P, Silbermann O, Benacerraf R. Intra-articular diffusion of Gd-DOTA after intravenous injection in the knee: MR imaging evaluation. Radiology. 1993;188:227–34.
86. Winalski CS, Aliabadi P, Wright RJ, Shortkroff S, Sledge CB, Weissman BN. Enhancement of joint fluid with intravenously administered gadopentetate dimeglumine: technique, rationale, and implications. Radiology. 1993;187:179–85.
87. Allmann KH, Schaefer O, Hauer M, et al. Indirect MR arthrography of the unexercised glenohumeral joint in patients with rotator cuff tears. Investig Radiol. 1999;34(6):435–40.
88. Zoga AC, Schweitzer ME. Indirect magnetic resonance arthrography: applications in sports imaging. Top Magn Reson Imaging. 2003;14:25–33.
89. Kaura DR, Sceweitzer ME, Weishaupt D, et al. Optimization of indirect arthrography of the knee by application of external heat: initial experience. J Magn Reson Imaging. 2005;22(6):810–2.
90. Weishaupt D, Schweitzer ME, Rawool NM, et al. Indirect MR arthrography of the knee: effects of low-intensity ultrasound on the diffusion rate of intravenously administered Gd-DTPA in healthy volunteers. Investig Radiol. 2001;36(8):493–9.
91. Yagci B, Manisali M, Yilmaz E, et al. Indirect MR arthrography of the shoulder in detection of rotator cuff ruptures. Eur Radiol. 2001;11:258–62.
92. Herold T, Bachthaler M, Hamer OW, Hente R, Feuerbach S, Fellner C, et al. Indirect MR arthrography of the shoulder: use of abduction and external rotation to detect full- and partial-thickness tears of the supraspinatus tendon. Radiology. 2006;240:152–60.
93. Van Dyck P, Gielen JL, Veryser J, et al. Tears of the supraspinatus tendon: assessment with indirect magnetic resonance arthrography in 67 patients with arthroscopic correlation. Acta Radiol. 2009;50(9):1057–63.
94. Jung JY, Yoon YC, Yi SK, Yoo J, Choe BK. Comparison study of indirect MR arthrography and direct MR arthrography of the shoulder. Skelet Radiol. 2009;38:659–67.
95. Oh DK, Yoon YC, Kwon JW, Choi S-H, Jung JY, Bae S, et al. Comparison of indirect isotropic MR arthrography and conventional MR arthrography of labral lesions and rotator cuff tears: a prospective study. AJR. 2009;192:473–9.
96. Choo HJ, Lee SJ, Kim JH, et al. Delaminated tears of the rotator cuff: prevalence, characteristics, and diagnostic accuracy using indirect MR arthrography. AJR. 2015;204:360–6.
97. Fallahi F, Green N, Gadde S, et al. Indirect magnetic resonance arthrography of the shoulder; a reliable diagnostic tool for investigation of suspected labral pathology. Skelet Radiol. 2013;42(9):1225–33.
98. Song KD, Kwon JW, Yoon YC, et al. Indirect MR arthrographic findings of adhesive capsulitis. AJR. 2011;197(6):W1105–9.
99. Murphy KP, Szopinski KT, Cohan RH, Mermillod B, Ellis JH. Occurrence of adverse reactions to gadolinium-based contrast material and management of patients at increased risk: a survey of the American Society of Neuroradiology Fellowship Directors. Acad Radiol. 1999;6:656–64.
100. Magee T. Can isotropic fast gradient echo imaging be substituted for conventional T1 weighted sequences in shoulder MR arthrography at 3 Tesla? J Magn Reson Imaging. 2007;26:118–22.
101. Lee MJ, Motamedi K, Chow K, Seeger LL. Gradient-recalled echo sequences in direct shoulder MR arthrography for evaluating the labrum. Skelet Radiol. 2008;37:19–25.
102. Jung JY, Yoon YC, Choi SH. Three-dimensional isotropic shoulder MR arthrography: comparison with two-dimensional MR arthrography for the diagnosis of labral lesions at 3.0 T. Radiology. 2009;250(2):498–50.
103. Gyftopoulos S, Yemin A, Mulholland T, et al. 3D MR osseous reconstructions of the shoulder using a gradient-echo based two-point Dixon reconstruction: a feasibility study. Skelet Radiol. 2013;42:347–52.
104. Gyftopoulos S, Beltran LS, Yemin A, et al. Use of 3D MR reconstructions in the evaluation of glenoid bone loss: a clinical study. Skelet Radiol. 2014;43:213–8.
105. Zanetti M, Jost B, Hodler J, Gerber C. MR imaging after rotator cuff repair: full-thickness defects and bursitis-like subacromial abnormalities in asymptomatic subjects. Skelet Radiol. 2000;29(6):314–9.
106. Wolfgang GL. Surgical repair of tears of the rotator cuff of the shoulder. Factors influencing the result. J Bone Joint Surg Am. 1974;56(1):14–26.
107. Knudsen HB, Gelineck J, Sojbjerg JO, Olsen BS, Johannsen HV, Sneppen O. Functional and magnetic resonance imaging evaluation after single-tendon rotator cuff reconstruction. J Shoulder Elb Surg. 1999;8:242–6.
108. Harryman DT, Mack LA, Wang KY, Jackins SE, Richardson ML, Matsen FA III. Repairs of the rotator cuff. Correlation of functional results with integrity of the cuff. J Bone Joint Surg Am. 1991;73:982–9.

109. Gazielly DF, Gleyze P, Montagnon C. Functional and anatomical results after rotator cuff repair. Clin Orthop Relat Res. 1994;304:43–53.
110. Galatz LM, Ball CM, Teefey SA, Middleton WD, Yamaguchi K. The outcome and repair integrity of completely arthroscopically repaired large and massive rotator cuff tears. J Bone Joint Surg Am. 2004;86-A:219–24.
111. Gerber C, Fuchs B, Hodler J. The results of repair of massive tears of the rotator cuff. J Bone Joint Surg Am. 2000;82:505–15.
112. Bohsali KI, Wirth MA, Rockwood CA Jr. Complications of total shoulder arthroplasty. J Bone Joint Surg Am. 2006;88:2279–92.
113. Merolla G, Di Pietto F, Romano S, et al. Radiographic analysis of shoulder anatomical arthroplasty. Eur J Radiol. 2008;68:159–69.
114. Ha AS, Petscavage JM, Chew FS. Current concepts of shoulder arthroplasty for radiologists: part 2—anatomic and reverse total shoulder replacement and nonprosthetic resurfacing. AJR. 2012;199:768–76.
115. Ives EP, Nazarian LN, Parker L, et al. Subscapularis tendon tears: a common sonographic finding in symptomatic postarthroplasty shoulders. J Clin Ultrasound. 2013;41(3):129–33.
116. Hennigan SP, Iannotti JP. Instability after prosthetic arthroplasty of the shoulder. Orthop Clin North Am. 2001;52:649–59.
117. Neer CS 2nd, Watson KC, Stanton FJ. Recent experience in total shoulder replacement. J Bone Joint Surg. 1982;64(3):319–37.
118. Magee T, Shapiro M, Hewell G, et al. Complications of rotator cuff surgery in which bioabsorbable anchors are used. AJR. 2003;181:1227–31.
119. Nusselt T, Freche S, Klinger HM, et al. Intraosseous foreign body granuloma in rotator cuff repair with bioabsorbable suture anchor. Arch OrthopTrauma Surg. 2010;130(8):1037–40.
120. Beltran LS, Bencardino JT, Steinbach LS. Postoperative MRI of the shoulder. J Magn Reson Imaging. 2014;40:1280–97.
121. Lee M, Kim S, Lee S, et al. Overcoming artifacts from metallic orthopedic implants at high field-strength MR imaging and multidetector CT. Radiographics. 2007;27:791–803.
122. Sperling JW, Potter HG, Craig EV, Flatow E, Warren RF. Magnetic resonance imaging of painful shoulder arthroplasty. J Shoulder Elb Surg. 2002;11: 315–21.
123. Eustace S, Goldberg R, Williamson D, et al. MR imaging of soft tissues adjacent to orthopaedic hardware: techniques to minimize susceptibility artifact. Clin Radiol. 1997;52:589–94.
124. Mohana-Borges AVR, Chung CB, Resnick D. MR imaging and MR arthrography of the postoperative shoulder. Radiographics. 2004;24:69–85.
125. Suh JS, Jeong EK, Shin KH, et al. Minimizing artifacts caused by metallic implants at MR imaging: experimental and clinical studies. AJR. 1998;171:1207–13.
126. Frazzini VI, Kagetsu NJ, Johnson CE, Destian S. Internally stabilized spine: optimal choice of frequency-encoding gradient direction during MR imaging minimizes susceptibility artifact from titanium vertebral body screws. Radiology. 1997;204:268–72.
127. Naraghi AM, White LM. Magnetic resonance imaging of joint replacements. Semin Musculoskelet Radiol. 2006;10(1):98–106.
128. Lu W, Pauly KB, Gold GE, et al. SEMAC: slice encoding for metal artifact correction in MRI. Magn Reson Med. 2009;62:66–76.
129. Guermazi A, Miaux Y, Zaim S, Peterfy CG, White D, Genant HK. Metallic artefacts in MR imaging: effects of main field orientation and strength. Clin Radiol. 2003;58:322–8.
130. Peh WC, Chan JH. Artifacts in musculoskeletal magnetic resonance imaging: identification and correction. Skelet Radiol. 2001;30(4):179–91.
131. F DG, Santini F, Herzka DA, et al. Fat-suppression techniques for 3-T MR imaging of the musculoskeletal system. Radiographics. 2014;34(1):217–33.
132. Hayter CL, Koff MF, Shah P, et al. MRI after arthroplasty: comparison of MAVRIC and conventional fast spin-echo techniques. AJR. 2011;197(3): W405–1.
133. Chen CA, Chen W, Goodman SB, et al. New MR imaging methods for metallic implants in the knee: artifact correction and clinical impact. J Magn Reson Imaging. 2011;33:1121–7.
134. Toms AP, Smith-Bateman C, Malcolm PN, et al. Optimization of metal artefact reduction (MAR) sequences for MRI of total hip prostheses. Clin Radiol. 2010;65:447–52.
135. Kolind SH, MacKay AL, Munk PL, et al. Quantitative evaluation of metal artifact reduction techniques. J Magn Reson Imaging. 2004;20:487–95.
136. Nwawka OK, Konin GP, Sneag DB, et al. Magnetic resonance imaging of shoulder arthroplasty: review article. HSS J. 2014 Oct;10(3):213–24.
137. Koch KM, Brau AC, Chen W, et al. Imaging near metal with a MAVRIC-SEMAC hybrid. Magn Reson Med. 2011;65:71–82.
138. Owen RS, Iannotti JP, Kneeland JB, Dalinka MK, Deren JA, Oleaga L. Shoulder after surgery: MR imaging with surgical validation. Radiology. 1993;186:443–7.
139. Magee TH, Gaenslen ES, Seitz R, Hinson GA, Wetzel LH. MR imaging of the shoulder after surgery. AJR. 1997;168:925–8.
140. Stoller DW, Wolf EM. The shoulder. In: Stoller DW, editor. Magnetic resonance imaging in orthopaedics and sports medicine. 2nd ed. Philadelphia, PA: Lippincott-Raven; 1997. p. 597–742.
141. Zlatkin MB. MRI of the postoperative shoulder. Skelet Radiol. 2002;31:63–80.
142. Resnick D. Shoulder. In: Resnick D, Kang HS, editors. Internal derangements of joints: emphasis on MR imaging. Philadelphia, PA: Saunders; 1997. p. 163–333.

143. Calvert PT, Packer NP, Stoker DJ, Bayley JI, Kessel L. Arthrography of the shoulder after operative repair of the torn rotator cuff. J Bone Joint Surg Br. 1986;68:147–15.
144. DeOrio JK, Cofield RH. Results of a second attempt at surgical repair of a failed initial rotator-cuff repair. J Bone Joint Surg Am. 1984;66:563–56.
145. Duc SR, Mengiardi B, Pfirmann CW, et al. Diagnostic performance of MR arthrography after rotator cuff repair. AJR. 2006;186:237–41.
146. Wagner SC, Schweitzer ME, Morrison WB, Fenlin JM, Bartolozzi AR. Shoulder instability: accuracy of MR imaging performed after surgery in depicting recurrent injury—initial findings. Radiology. 2002;222:196–203.
147. Jazrawi LM, Alaia MJ, Chang G, et al. Advances in magnetic resonance imaging of articular cartilage. J Am Acad Orthop Surg. 2011;19(7):420–9.
148. Wiener E, Hodler J, Pfirrmann CW. Delayed gadolinium-enhanced MRI of cartilage (dGEMRIC) of cadaveric shoulders: comparison of contrast dynamics in hyaline and fibrous cartilage after intra-articular gadolinium injection. Acta Radiol. 2009;50(1):86–92.
149. Maizlin ZV, Clement JJ, Patola WB, et al. T2 mapping of articular cartilage of glenohumeral joint with routine MRI correlation–initial experience. HSS J. 2009;5(1):61–6.
150. La Rocca Vieira R, Pakin SK, de Albuquerque Cavalcanti CF, et al. Three-dimensional spin-lock magnetic resonance imaging of the shoulder joint at 3 T: initial experience. Skelet Radiol. 2007;36(12):1171–5.
151. Bittersohl B, Miese FR, Dekkers C, et al. T2* mapping and delayed gadolinium-enhanced magnetic resonance imaging in cartilage (dGEMRIC) of glenohumeral cartilage in asymptomatic volunteers at 3 T. Eur Radiol. 2013;23(5):1367–74.
152. Iwasaki K, Tafur M, Chang EY, Statum S, Biswas R, Tran B, Bae WC, Du J, Bydder GM, Chung CB. High-resolution qualitative and quantitative magnetic resonance evaluation of the glenoid labrum. J Comput Assist Tomogr. 2015;39(6):936–44.
153. Chang G, Sherman O, Madelin G, et al. MR imaging assessment of articular cartilage repair procedures. Magn Reson Imaging Clin N Am. 2011;19(2):323–37.
154. Keenan KE, Besier TF, Pauly JM, et al. Prediction of glycosaminoglycan content in human cartilage by age, T1ρ and T2 MRI. Osteoarthr Cartil. 2011;19(2):171–9.
155. Lee SY, Park HJ, Kwon HJ, et al. T2 relaxation times of the glenohumeral joint at 3.0 T MRI in patients with and without primary and secondary osteoarthritis. Acta Radiol. 2015;56(11):1388–95.

Sonographic Evaluation of the Shoulder

3

Avner Yemin and Ronald S. Adler

3.1 Introduction

Diagnostic shoulder sonography has been well documented and established as an accurate tool for evaluation of shoulder pathology. In fact a meta-analysis study has shown the sensitivity and specificity of diagnostic ultrasound to be comparable to those of conventional MRI [1]. However, the diagnostic accuracy of shoulder sonography has been shown to depend on the experience and skill of the sonographer [2]. Although shoulder sonography may be time consuming for the novice, with experience, a better understanding of the sonographic anatomy, and the use of a standardized protocol, the examination can be performed quickly [3]. In addition to its short acquisition time, shoulder sonography has a marketable advantage of being inexpensive when compared to MRI. However, the most distinct advantage is the ability to assess for pathology in real time both at static and dynamic states. Provocative maneuvers can be performed to assess for pathology amenable to be accentuated by positional maneuvers, for example, impingement syndromes [4]. In addition to grayscale imaging the use of color and/or power Doppler imaging can be utilized to detect hyperemia during the examination, which has been associated with symptomatic tendinopathy, inflammation, and repair states. In this chapter we discuss the approach to performing shoulder sonography, relevant anatomy, and relevant interpretation pitfalls.

A. Yemin (✉)
Envision Physician Services—Radiology Associates of Hollywood, Memorial Healthcare System, Hollywood, FL, USA
e-mail: avner.yemin@shcr.com

R. S. Adler
Department of Radiology, NYU Langone Health, New York, NY, USA
e-mail: Ronald.Adler@nyulangone.org

3.2 Sonographic Shoulder Anatomy

There are four muscles and tendons, which make up the rotator cuff: the supraspinatus, the infraspinatus, the subscapularis, and the teres minor. Normal muscle on sonography appears as a structure made up of a hypoechoic background with superimposition of multiple curvilinear and sometimes punctate echogenic areas corresponding to the perimysial connective tissue (Figs. 3.1 and 3.2).

The four tendons of the rotator cuff each has unique bony attachments, which are used as landmarks to assist in identification of each tendon. The supraspinatus tendon inserts onto the superior facet and superior half of the middle facet of the greater tuberosity. The infraspinatus tendon also inserts along the middle facet of the greater tuberosity, just posterior to the supraspinatus tendon and with some overlap of the fibers in a junctional zone. The teres minor

J. T. Bencardino (ed.), *The Shoulder*, https://doi.org/10.1007/978-3-030-06240-8_3

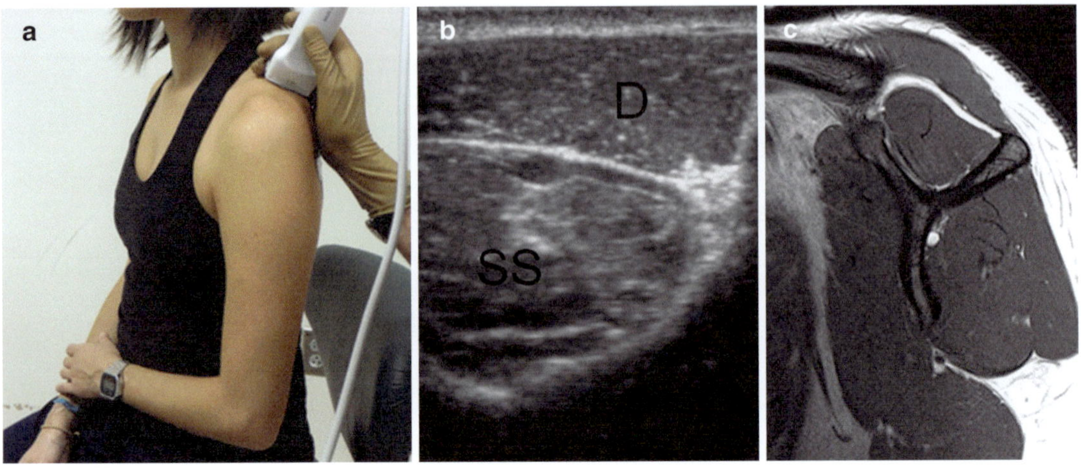

Fig. 3.1 Muscle imaging—supraspinatus patient positioning (**a**); short-axis sonographic image (**b**); MRI correlate (**c**); supraspinatus (SS); deltoid (D)

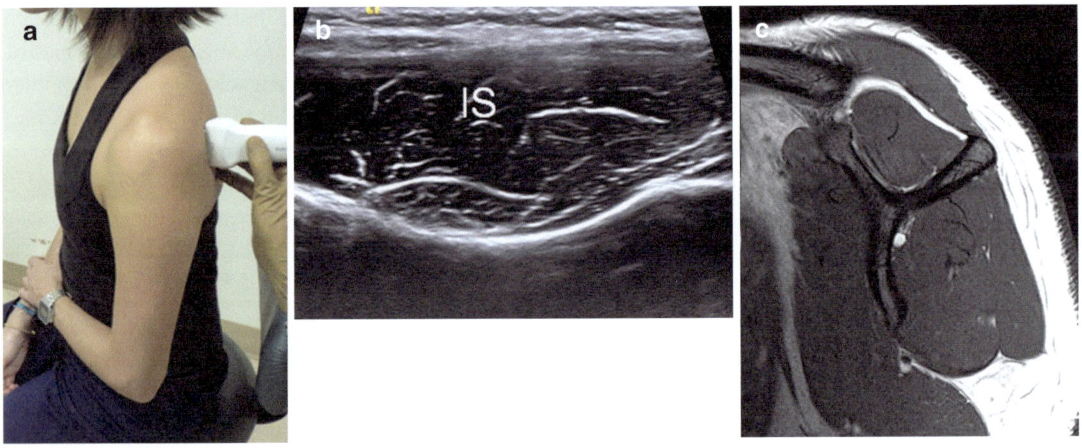

Fig. 3.2 Muscle imaging—infraspinatus patient positioning (**a**); short-axis sonographic image (**b**); MRI correlate (**c**); infraspinatus (IS)

tendon is positioned inferior to the infraspinatus tendon and thus inserts along the inferior facet of the greater tuberosity [5]. The subscapularis tendon inserts onto the lesser tuberosity of the humerus.

As demonstrated in Fig. 3.3, deep to the subdeltoid bursa is the supraspinatus tendon, which is a convex echogenic structure with well-demarcated convex margin that tapers distally as it inserts on the footprint. It is crucial to be able to distinguish the thin hypoechoic area, which is often seen as the tendon fiber insert, from a partial-thickness tear or tendinosis.

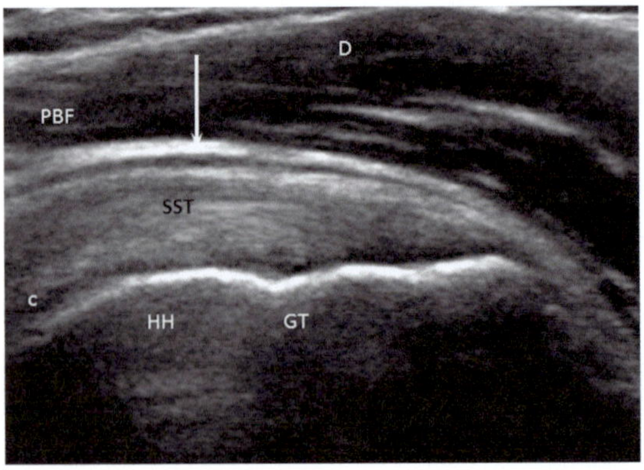

Fig. 3.3 Supraspinatus long-axis view—supraspinatus tendon (SST): deltoid (D); peri-bursal fat (PBF); subdeltoid bursa (arrow); convex tendon (c); greater tuberosity (GT); humeral head (HH)

The long head of the biceps tendon has both intra- and extra-articular components. It

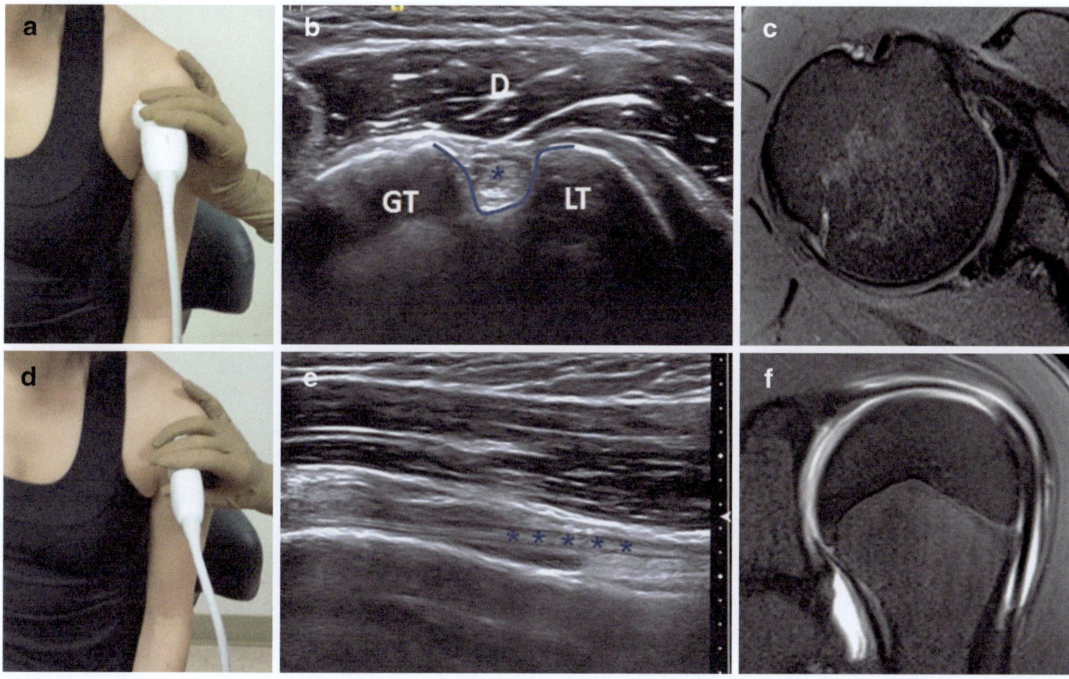

Fig. 3.4 Biceps tendon—short-axis patient positioning (**a**); short-axis sonographic image (**b**); MR correlate of short axis (**c**); long-axis patient positioning (**d**); long-axis sonographic image (**e**); MR correlate of long axis (**f**); biceps tendon (*) Greater tuberosity (GT); lesser tuberosity (LT); Biceps groove (curved line)

originates from the superior margin of the glenoid and courses anterolaterally through the rotator interval and extends inferiorly between the greater and lesser tuberosities in the bicipital groove (a.k.a. intertubercular groove), where it is considered extra-articular (Fig. 3.4).

The subacromial-subdeltoid bursa is a synovial lined space that lies deep to the deltoid and acromion. As demonstrated in Fig. 3.3, there is a distinct peri-bursal fat stripe deep to the deltoid. The subdeltoid bursa is interposed between the fat stripe and the superficial margin of the tendon and is generally seen as a thin hypoechoic line, usually less than 2 mm in thickness in normal individuals [3]. This can be distended in the setting of subacromial/subdeltoid bursitis.

3.3 Nomenclature

When performing ultrasound the orientation of the transducer is positioned in multiple different planes as we attempt to best view the tendons. Additionally certain positions are used to optimally view the different tendons creating oblique views. Therefore utilizing the standard anatomic planes for sonography can create confusion. As such it is convenient to discuss tendons in terms of long axis or short axis. The long-axis view assesses the tendon in length as it attaches on the footprint and the short-axis view is perpendicular to that (Fig. 3.5).

3.4 Anisotropy

The difficulty with scanning the shoulder in particular is that the structures are curvilinear which leads to issues with anisotropy so that when you are scanning initially the most echogenic portion is going to be that portion of the tendon which is perpendicular to the transducer scan plane. However, if the adjacent tendon fibers are angled, and not perpendicular to the transducer, the tendon will appear progressively hypoechoic due to anisotropy, which can easily be mistaken for tendinosis or tear. This problem

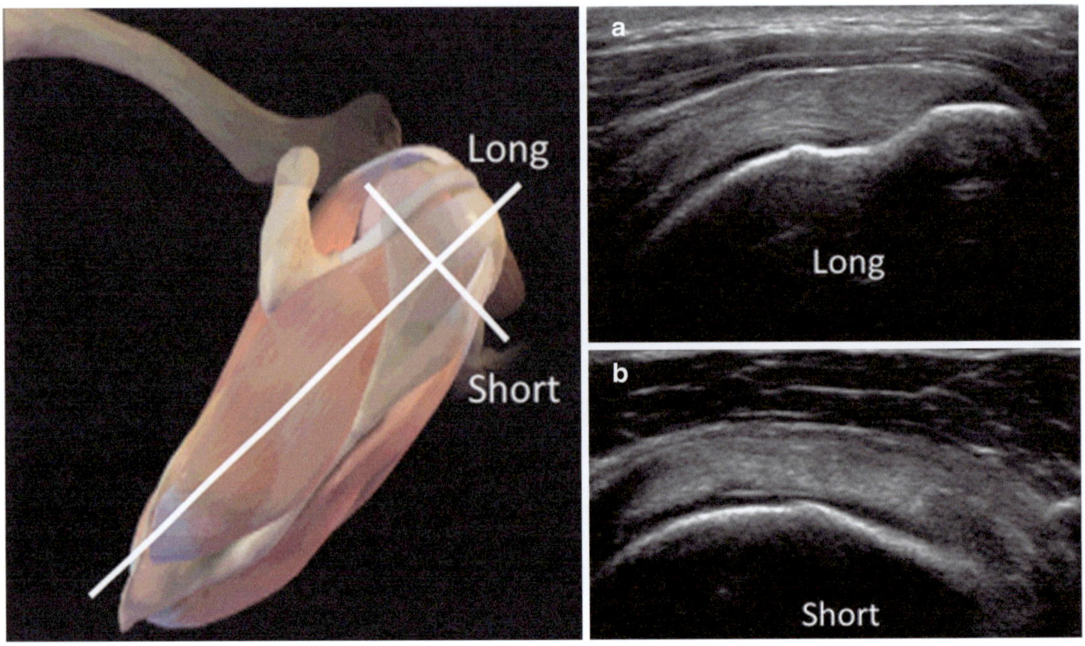

Fig. 3.5 Tendon orientation—long-axis (**a**) and short-axis (**b**) views

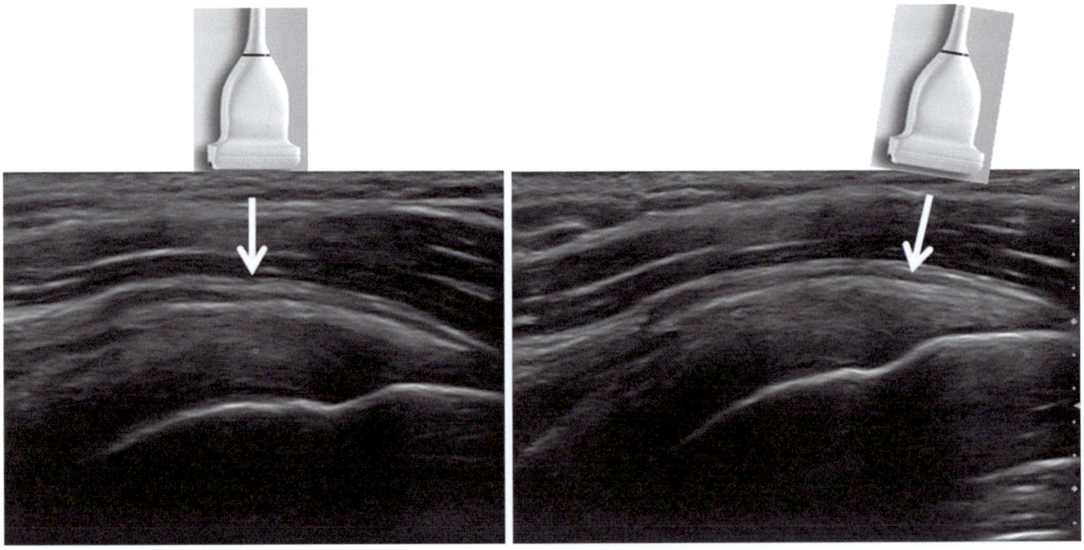

Fig. 3.6 Rocking the transducer to eliminate anisotropic effect at footprint

is very common, as an angle of as little as 2–3° has been shown to produce anisotropy [6]. Hence, when scanning, it is critical to reorient the transducer so that it is perpendicular to the tendon fibers being evaluated to exclude anisotropy for the hypoechoic nature of the tendon. This anisotropy is commonly seen at the tendon footprint where the tendon fibers are curvilinear as they attach to bone. Rocking of the transducer back and forth along the long axis can be used to show if there is a true tear or just anisotropy (Fig. 3.6).

Table 3.1 Standardized shoulder sonography protocol

Biceps	Short axis—3 images → proximal to distal	Long axis—2 images → proximal and distal
AC joint	1 image across joint	
Subscapularis	Short axis—3 images → near coracoid, mid, and distal	Long axis—2 images → proximal and distal
Muscle – Infraspinatus – Teres minor – Supraspinatus	Short axis only 1 image each	
Supraspinatus/infraspinatus (Crass or modified Crass)	Short axis—3 images → proximal to distal	Long axis—3 images → lateral (infraspinatus), mid (junctional zone), medial (near rotator interval)

3.5 Technique

Several different guidelines have been established for performance of shoulder sonography, some of which advocate that the sonographer is positioned in front of the patient and others advocate scanning from behind the patient [6–8]. We have found approaching the patient from the front to be most convenient and for the purposes of the chapter will be describing this technique. We advise having the patient sitting down on a chair, which can revolve to ease the transitions between steps. In addition patient positioning should be optimized to allow for the most ergonomically comfortable scanning position for the examiner.

The two most important aspect of shoulder sonography is to maintain a standardized protocol with a systematic approach and second is to properly position the arm to optimally look at all the shoulder structures (Table 3.1). We advise looking at the anterior structures first followed by posterior structures and lastly evaluating the supraspinatus tendon, as the positioning is usually the most uncomfortable for the patient, thus leaving the worst for last.

3.6 Step-by-Step Guideline

3.6.1 Step 1: Evaluating the Long Head of the Biceps Tendon (Fig. 3.4; Table 3.2)

The patient should be seated with the arm at their side with the elbow in 90-degree flexion and the forearm supinated. This position places the bicipital groove anteriorly. In short axis you should see the long head of the biceps tendon within the bicipital groove. By turning the transducer 90° you can assess the length of the long head of the biceps tendon as an echogenic fibrillar structure. In certain situations you may need to rock the transducer back and forth in order to make the transducer as parallel to the biceps tendon as possible.

Table 3.2 Biceps tendon guidelines

	Technique	Findings
Short axis first	– One image above groove – At least 2 below	– Tendon is an echogenic ellipse in the bicipital groove – Demonstrates fluid/synovitis
Long axis	– Turn transducer 90° – To avoid anisotropy tilt transducer to maximize echogenicity	Tendon is linear and fibrillar

3.6.2 Step 2: Evaluating the Acromioclavicular Joint (Fig. 3.7)

Start by palpating the acromioclavicular joint and placing the transducer in long axis along the top of the joint. You will be able to see the distal clavicle and acromion and the interposed joint capsule/fibrocartilage disc. When assessing the acromioclavicular joint look for joint capsular distension, osseous irregularities, joint widening, or a step-off between the clavicle and acromial process. If there is suspicion for a widened joint

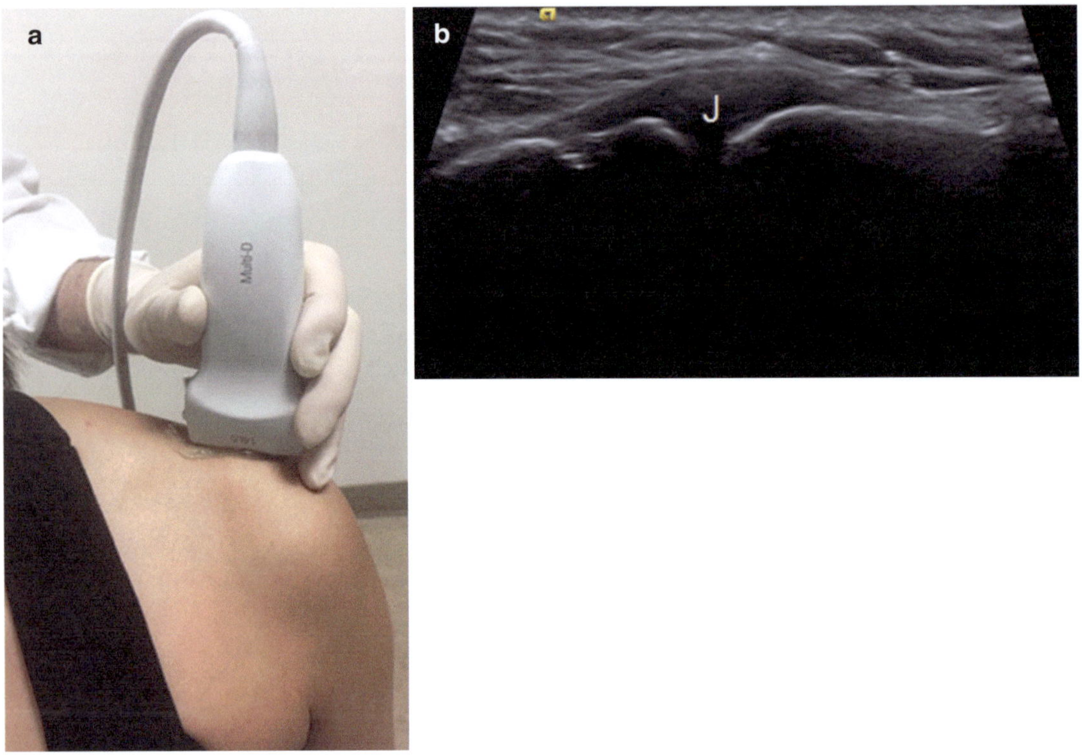

Fig. 3.7 Acromioclavicular joint imaging—patient positioning (**a**); sonographic image (**b**); joint capsule (J)

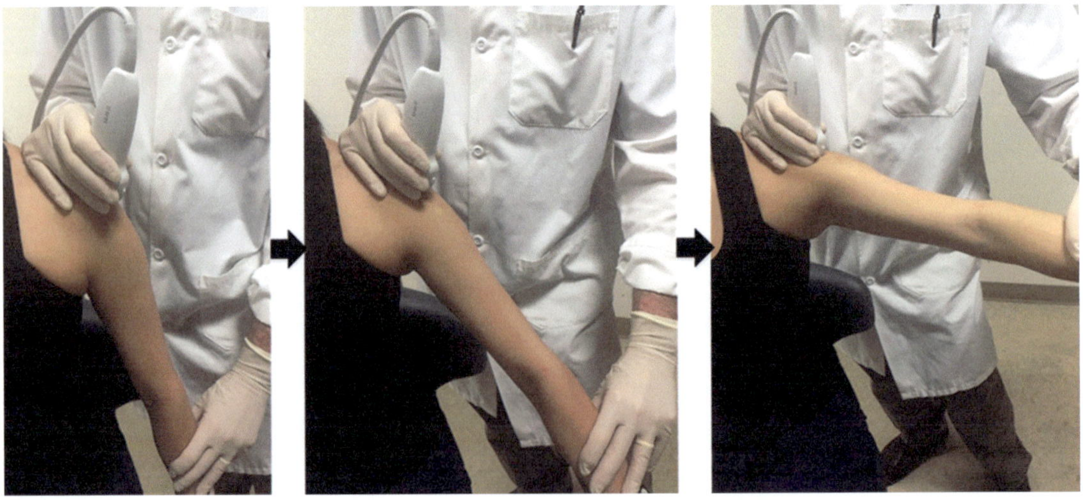

Fig. 3.8 Subacromial impingement dynamic imaging—patient positioning with progressive increase of arm abduction while imaging

or articular step-off dynamic maneuvers such as internally and externally rotating the patient's arm actively can be utilized.

Additionally dynamic maneuvers can be performed to assess for subacromial impingement (Fig. 3.8). This is done by placing the transducer just lateral to the acromial process and moving the patient's arm through a range of abduction and adduction while imaging. Findings of subacromial impingement include

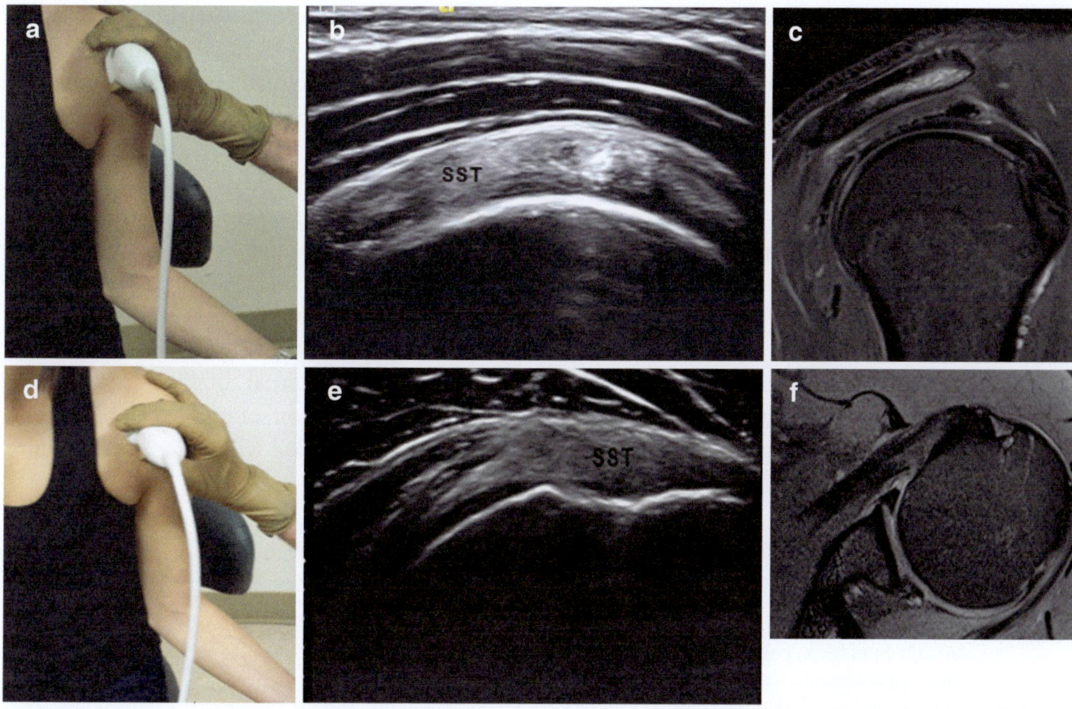

Fig. 3.9 Subscapularis tendon—short-axis patient positioning (**a**); short-axis sonographic image (**b**); MR correlate of short axis—multipennate (**c**); long-axis patient positioning (**d**); long-axis sonographic image (**e**); MR correlate of long axis (**f**); supraspinatus tendon (SST)

snapping of the bursal tissue and abnormal upward migration of the humeral head with respect to the acromion [8].

3.6.3 Step 3: Subscapularis Tendon (Fig. 3.9; Table 3.3)

The patient's arm should be placed in external rotation in order to bring the subscapularis away from the coracoid process which otherwise would partially impede visualization due to dense shadowing. External rotation will therefore expose the subscapularis tendon and place it in some degree of hyperextension. The footprint of the subscapularis tendon will be seen as a curvilinear structure tapering down to the bony attachment. Assessment of the subscapularis footprint is achieved by looking at the anatomic neck and the beginning of the humeral head articular cartilage (black line). As discussed in the nomenclature section, the long-axis view is in respect to the tendon length and is noted to be with the transducer in what would conventionally be a transverse orientation (anatomic axial plane). Hence, by turning the transducer 90° (transducer in the sagittal plane), we will be assessing the tendon in short axis. In this plane, the long head of the biceps tendon may appear as a separate round hyperechoic structure just superior to the subscapularis tendon. Given the multipennate structural arrangement of the subscapularis tendon, multiple round echogenic areas may be

Table 3.3 Subscapularis tendon

	Technique	Findings
Long-axis image first	Externally rotate forearm with transducer in fixed position	– Tendon footprint is a curvilinear structure tapering down to the bony attachment – Look for humeral anatomic neck and beginning of articular cartilage
Short axis	Turn transducer 90°	Tendon is multipennate

seen. This is a key concept, as we do not want to misinterpret these multiple tendon slips that eventually come together to form the single conjoined tendon as it inserts on the lesser tuberosity, for a tear.

3.6.4 Step 4: Supraspinatus/Infraspinatus Tendons and Rotator Interval (Table 3.4)

There are two different ways of looking at the supraspinatus tendon, each with relative advantages. The first provides for greater hyperextension in the Crass position [9] (Fig. 3.10). The Crass position entails placing the arm behind the back with the palm pointed out. In short axis you will see the biceps tendon medially, and the supraspinatus laterally. Reorienting the transducer 90° will demonstrate the supraspinatus tendon in long axis as a convex echogenic tendon with tapering as it extends to the footprint. The second approach is a modified Crass with the difference being that the hand is placed as if it was in the back pocket [10] (Fig. 3.11). The advantage of this is less external rotation which allows for better visualization of the rotator interval. Again the biceps tendon will be located medially

Table 3.4 Supraspinatus and infraspinatus tendon imaging

	Technique	Findings
Crass	– Internal rotation, hyperextension – Arm behind back, palm out, fingers toward scapula	**Short axis:** biceps tendon medially and the supraspinatus laterally **Long axis:** supraspinatus tendon in long axis → convex echogenic tendon with tapering as it extends to the footprint
Modified Crass	Arm behind back with hand in "back pocket"	**Short axis:** biceps tendon medially, then the rotator interval, then the supraspinatus laterally **Long axis:** supraspinatus tendon in long axis → may see less of the tendon

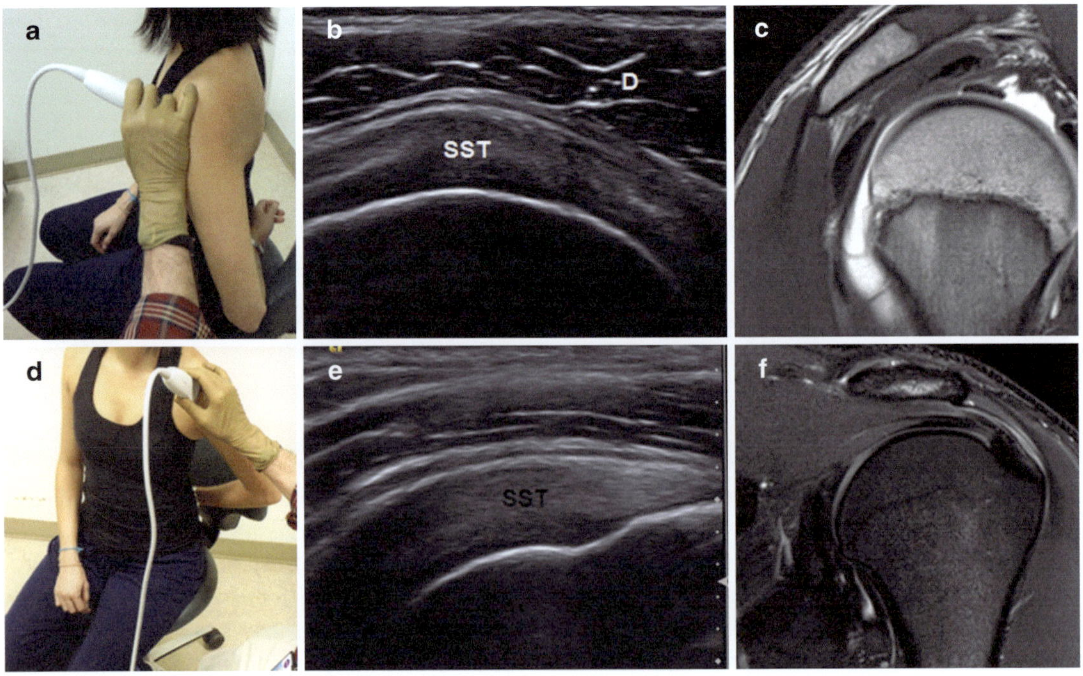

Fig. 3.10 Crass position: supraspinatus/infraspinatus and rotator interval—short-axis patient positioning (**a**); short-axis sonographic image (**b**); MR correlate of short axis (**c**); long-axis patient positioning (**d**); long-axis sonographic image (**e**); MR correlate of long axis (**f**); supraspinatus tendon (SST); deltoid (D)

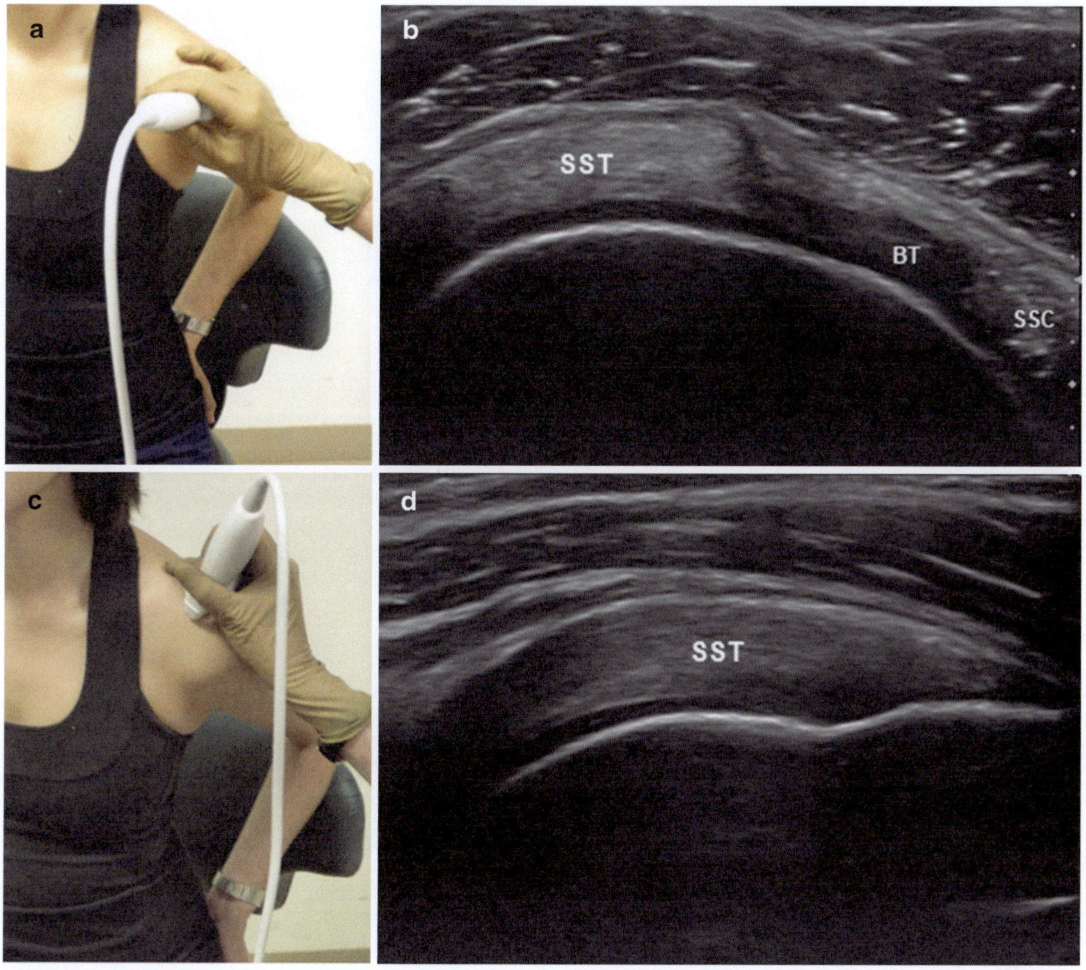

Fig. 3.11 Modified Crass supraspinatus/infraspinatus and rotator interval— short-axis patient positioning (**a**); short-axis sonographic image (**c**); long-axis patient positioning (**b**); long-axis sonographic image (**d**); supraspinatus (SST); biceps tendon (BT); subscapularis (SSC)

and the rotator interval and supraspinatus tendon laterally. The disadvantage is that you tend to not see as much of the tendon while the arm is in hyperextension. However, studies demonstrate no significant difference in the overall accuracy when comparing the two techniques [11]. If the patient can tolerate both positions we believe that there is added value in performing both with optimal visualization of both the supraspinatus tendon and the rotator interval in the modified Crass and Crass, respectively. Of note the modified Crass may be more comfortable for certain patients, especially in cases of adhesive capsulitis.

It is important to note, particularly when scanning the rotator cuff in short axis, that there is a transitional zone where there is a blending of both infraspinatus and supraspinatus fibers (Fig. 3.12). As a rule of thumb from the level of the rotator interval approximately 2 cm from its anterior margin will be supraspinatus tendon, then there is a junctional zone with mixed supraspinatus and infraspinatus fibers, and more posteriorly there will be the infraspinatus tendon.

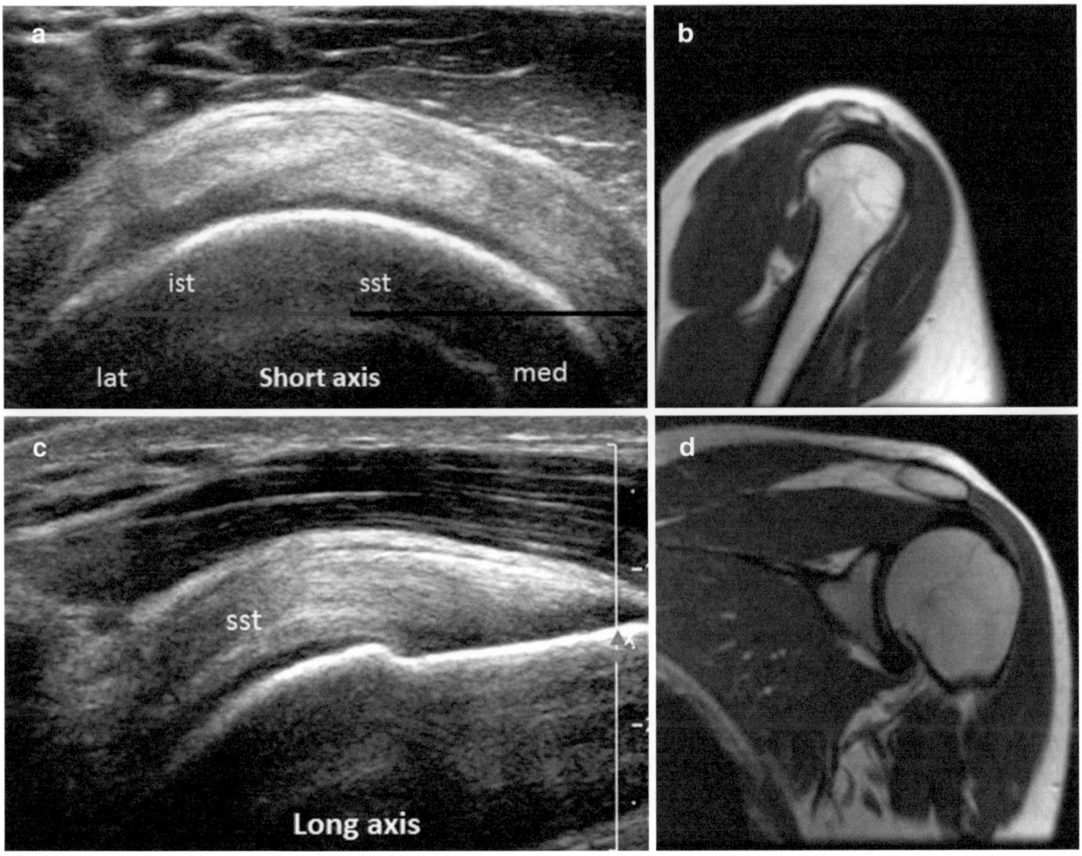

Fig. 3.12 Rotator cuff—short-axis sonographic image (**a**); short-axis MRI correlate (**b**); long-axis sonographic image (**c**); long-axis MRI correlate (**d**); supraspinatus tendon (SST); infraspinatus tendon (IST): In short axis generally 2 cm lateral to the rotator interval will be the supraspinatus tendon

3.6.5 Step 5: Muscle Evaluation—Supraspinatus (Fig. 3.1)

Muscle evaluation is crucial as atrophy and fatty infiltration have been shown to be associated with failed rotator cuff repairs and poor clinical outcomes [12]. Evaluation of the muscle is a fairly simple portion of the exam. Initially place the transducer in a sagittal orientation superior to the spine of the scapula to evaluate the supraspinatus muscle in the suprascapular fossa with the trapezius muscle overlying it. Again note that normal muscle is hypoechoic and within that hypoechoic background curvilinear echogenic areas are seen, corresponding to the perimysial connective tissue.

3.6.6 Step 6: Muscle Evaluation—Infraspinatus and Teres Minor (Fig. 3.2)

Position the transducer more posteriorly and caudally below the level of the scapular spine you will find the infraspinatus muscle in the infraspinatus fossa. Moving the transducer slightly caudally you will see the teres minor muscle.

Evaluation of the subscapularis muscle is limited due to the lack of a proper acoustic window, as the muscle lies deep to the pectoralis and thorax anteriorly, and the scapula posteriorly. Accounting for these limitations the muscle tissue interposed between the tendon fascicles can be imaged along the course of the multipennate tendon insertional fibers and, as described earlier, they should not be mistaken for a tendon tear.

3.7 Conclusion

Shoulder sonography has been proven to be a sensitive and specific diagnostic tool in assessing shoulder pathology. With the implementation of a standardized protocol, such as the one outlined in this chapter, accompanied by appropriate knowledge of the sonographic shoulder anatomy we believe that it can be utilized as a powerful addition to the radiologist's armamentarium.

References

1. De Jesus JO, Parker L, Frangos AJ, Nazarian LN. Accuracy of MRI, MR arthrography, and ultrasound in the diagnosis of rotator cuff tears: a meta-analysis. AJR Am J Roentgenol. 2009;192(6):1701–7.
2. Le Corroller T, Cohen M, Aswad R, Pauly V, Champsaur P. Sonography of the painful shoulder: role of the operator's experience. Skelet Radiol. 2008;37(11):979–86.
3. Jacobson JA. Shoulder US: anatomy, technique, and scanning pitfalls. Radiology. 2011;260(1):6–16.
4. Minagawa H, Itoi E, Konno N, Kido T, Sano A, Uramaya M, et al. Humeral attachment of the supraspinatus and infraspinatus tendons: an anatomic study. Arthroscopy. 1998;14(3):302–6.
5. Crass JR, van de Vegte GL, Harkavy LA. Tendon echogenicity: ex vivo study. Radiology. 1988;167(2):499–501.
6. Finnoff JT, Smith J, Peck ER. Ultrasonography of the shoulder. Phys Med Rehabil Clin N Am. 2010;21:481–507.
7. Moosikasuwan JB, Miller TT, Burke BJ. Rotator cuff tears: clinical, radiographic, and US findings. Radiographics. 2005;25:1591–607.
8. Bureau NJ, Beauchamp M, Cardinal E, Brassard P. Dynamic sonography evaluation of shoulder impingement syndrome. AJR Am J Roentgenol. 2006;187(1):216–20.
9. Crass JR, Craig EV, Feinberg SB. The hyperextended internal rotation view in rotator cuff ultrasonography. J Clin Ultrasound. 1987;15(6):416–20.
10. Ferri M, Finlay K, Popowich T, Stamp G, Schuringa P, Friedman L. Sonography of full-thickness supraspinatus tears: comparison of patient positioning technique with surgical correlation. AJR Am J Roentgenol. 2005;184(1):180–4.
11. Shah NP, Miller TT, Stock H, Adler RS. Sonography of supraspinatus tendon abnormalities in the neutral versus crass and modified crass positions a prospective study. J Ultrasound Med. 2012;31(8):1203–8.
12. Kuzel BR, Grindel S, Papandrea R, Ziegler D. Fatty infiltration and rotator cuff atrophy. J Am Acad Orthop Surg. 2013;21(10):613–23.

Image-Guided Procedures of the Shoulder

4

Ogonna Kenechi Nwawka, Shefali Kothary, and Theodore T. Miller

4.1 Introduction

Shoulder pain is a common complaint in the adult patient population, caused by a wide variety of conditions affecting the osseous and soft-tissue structures in the shoulder. Image-guided shoulder interventions are important for both diagnosis and treatment of conditions that affect the shoulder. Image-guided interventions can be performed with different imaging modalities including ultrasound (US), fluoroscopy, computed tomography (CT), and magnetic resonance imaging (MRI), depending on the anatomy, disease process, and type of intervention. This chapter provides technical guidelines for performing image-guided shoulder interventions, concentrating on sonographic guidance.

4.2 General Considerations

4.2.1 Imaging Techniques

Image-guided shoulder interventions are most commonly performed under US or fluoroscopy. The real-time nature of US imaging and lack of ionizing radiation are advantageous, and thus image guidance via US is recommended when available, especially in teenagers and young adults [1]. Multiple studies have demonstrated US as effective in image guidance for shoulder MR arthrography [2–4], with similar success rates when compared to fluoroscopic guidance [5, 6]. When performing US-guided procedures, a high-resolution, high-frequency transducer should be used. Typically at our institution, we use a 12–15 MHz linear transducer for procedures around the shoulder.

Fluoroscopy is also commonly used to guide therapeutic injections, and during joint aspiration and instillation of intra-articular contrast for arthrography. The glenohumeral joint is easily accessed under fluoroscopic guidance, with well-established technique [7]. Although CT and MRI are typically reserved for performing biopsies around the shoulder, there is literature supporting their use in guidance for arthrography [8–10], particularly when sonographic or fluoroscopic guidance is not available.

4.2.2 Procedure

As part of the pre-procedure preparation, the site of needle puncture should be marked with indelible ink under image guidance.

The needle gauge and length are selected based on the procedure to be performed and the patient's body habitus. In an average-size person, all injections around the shoulder can be performed with 22–25-gauge 1.5–3.5 in. needles.

O. K. Nwawka · S. Kothary · T. T. Miller (✉)
Division of Ultrasound, Department of Radiology and Imaging, Hospital for Special Surgery, Weill Medical College of Cornell University, New York, NY, USA
e-mail: nwawkao@hss.edu; millertt@hss.edu

J. T. Bencardino (ed.), *The Shoulder*, https://doi.org/10.1007/978-3-030-06240-8_4

Aspirations are usually performed with an 18-gauge 1.5 or 3.5 in. needle depending on patient's body habitus and depth of the target. For optimal needle visualization during US procedures, the needle should be oriented as close to perpendicular to the orientation of the US beam as possible. The needle may be advanced in plane (i.e., longitudinal) or out of plane (i.e., short axis) to the transducer (Fig. 4.1). When inserting the needle in plane, it is important to visualize the entire length of the needle at all times and to visualize the needle bevel in order to avoid crosscutting error and misplacement of the needle tip [11] (Figs. 4.2 and 4.3). Rotating or gently agitating the needle may help in visualization of the needle tip.

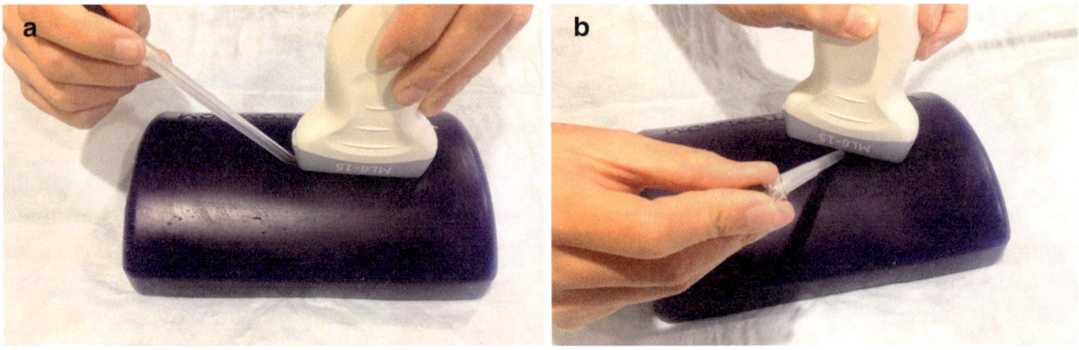

Fig. 4.1 Needle placement in plane (**a**) and out of plane (**b**) to the transducer

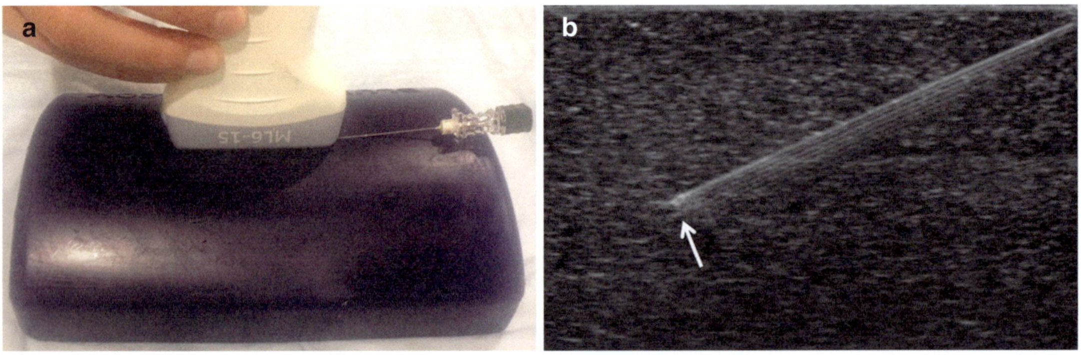

Fig. 4.2 In-plane needle placement with correct technique. The needle is in line with the transducer (**a**), and the entire length of the needle is seen on the US image, including the echogenic tip (**b**, arrow)

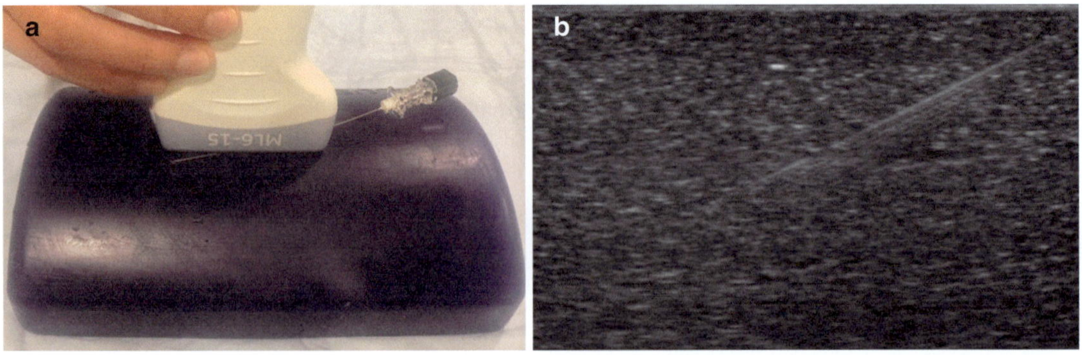

Fig. 4.3 In-plane needle placement with crosscutting error. The needle is not in line with the transducer (**a**), and the entire length of the needle is not visualized (**b**). This can result in misplacement of the needle tip

To maintain sterile technique during the procedure, the transducer should be prepped or covered with a sterile sheath, following manufacturer recommendations.

4.3 Glenohumeral Joint

4.3.1 Ultrasound

An anterior or posterior approach can be used, though the injection is typically performed via a posterior approach [11], with the patient in a lateral decubitus position and with the arm extended at the shoulder and bent at the elbow (Fig. 4.4). A 25-gauge 1.5 in. needle or a 22-gauge 3.5 in. needle should be used for the injection, depending on the patient's body habitus. The needle is inserted in plane to the transducer via a lateral-to-medial approach (Fig. 4.4). The target for the injection should be the articular cartilage over the humeral head or the posterior recess of the glenohumeral joint (Fig. 4.5a). If present, a joint effusion within the posterior recess of the glenohumeral joint is a good target. Once the needle contacts the humeral head articular cartilage or the fluid within the joint space, the needle should be within the joint. You may perform a test injection with anesthetic, e.g., 1% lidocaine to confirm intra-articular positioning of the needle tip. The test injectate should freely flow into the joint space without resistance; if not, the needle tip may be buried within the articular cartilage or in an extra-articular position and should be repositioned until intra-articular flow is confirmed. Subsequently, upon injection of the desired mixture, fluid should smoothly distend the posterior glenohumeral recess (Fig. 4.5b).

For the anterior US approach, the patient is placed supine with the arm by the side in external rotation. The injection is performed at the level of the coracoid, inserting the needle in a lateral-to-medial or medial-to lateral approach [4, 5]. As with the posterior approach, the target is the humeral head cartilage or fluid within the joint space (Fig. 4.6).

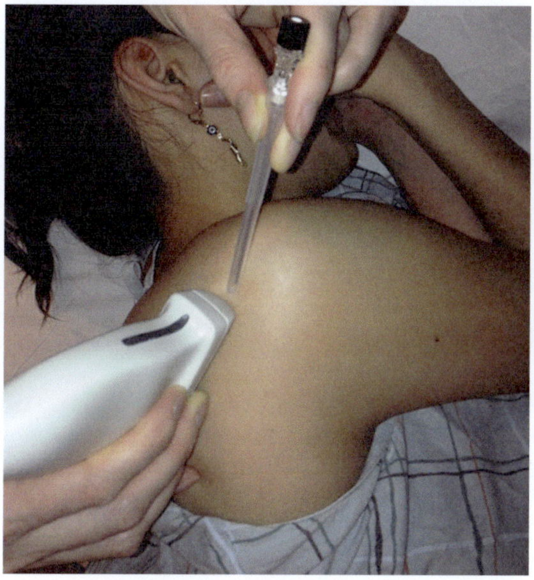

Fig. 4.4 Glenohumeral joint injection: Patient positioning and needle placement for posterior approach

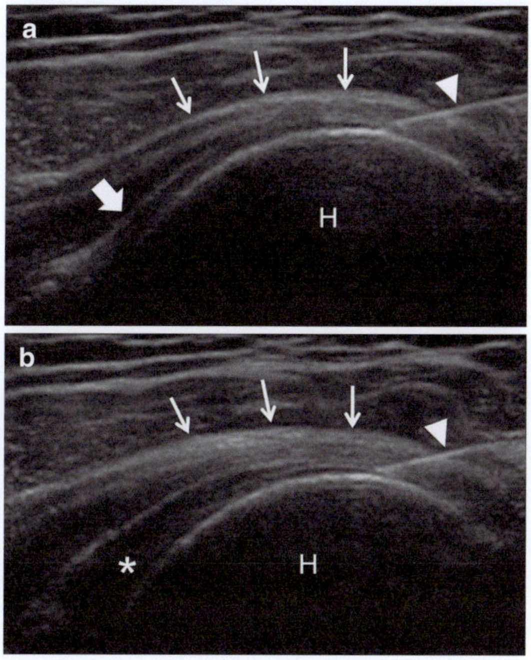

Fig. 4.5 (**a** and **b**) US images demonstrate needle placement (arrowhead) within the posterior glenohumeral joint prior to injection. Posteriorly, the glenohumeral joint is located deep to the infraspinatus tendon (arrows). Prior to injection, the posterior glenohumeral joint recess is collapsed (**a**, block arrow). During injection, there is distention of the posterior glenohumeral recess with injectate (asterisk). *H* humeral head

4.3.2 Fluoroscopy

When performing a glenohumeral joint injection under fluoroscopic guidance, an anterior approach is typically used. The patient is placed on the fluoroscopy table in a supine position, with the arm externally rotated and the forearm and wrist in supination (Fig. 4.7). A sand bag may be used to assure proper arm positioning during the procedure. The goal is for the humeral head to overlap the posterior glenoid rim, producing an ellipse (Fig. 4.8). The image intensifier (II) can also be slightly obliqued to obtain this appearance. The recommended target for glenohumeral joint injection varies, with some advocating the upper third of the ellipse and others advocating the middle or lower third [7, 12, 13]. All of these recommended positions fall just lateral to the medial cortex of the humeral head. A 22-gauge 3.5 in. needle is typically used for injection, though a 25-gauge 1.5 in. needle may also be sufficient depending on the patient's body

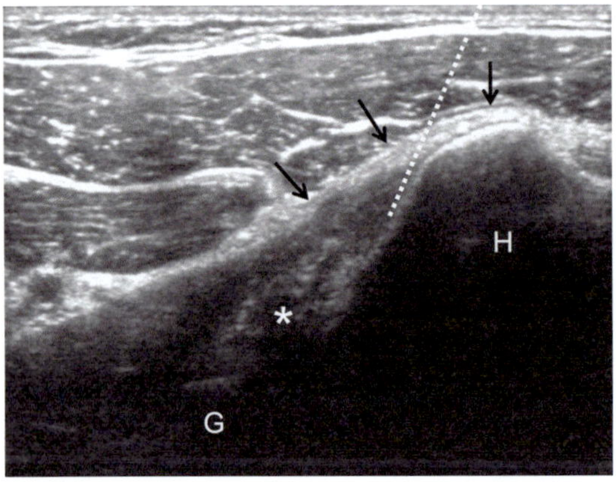

Fig. 4.6 Anterior approach for glenohumeral injection under US. Simulated needle trajectory for an anterior glenohumeral injection (dotted line). *H* humeral head, *G* Glenoid, * Anterior joint recess. Arrows—subscapularis tendon

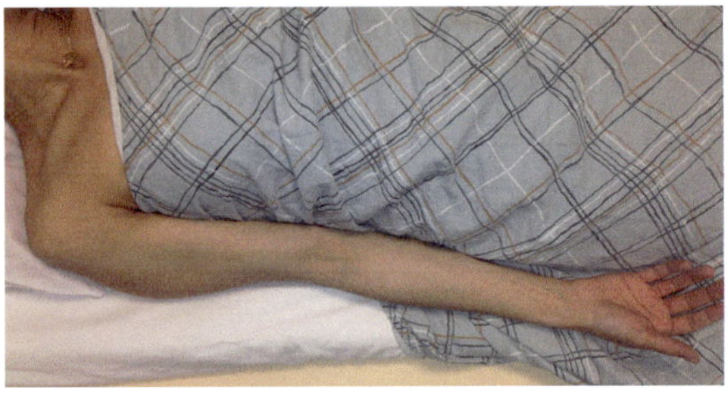

Fig. 4.7 Glenohumeral joint injection: Patient positioning

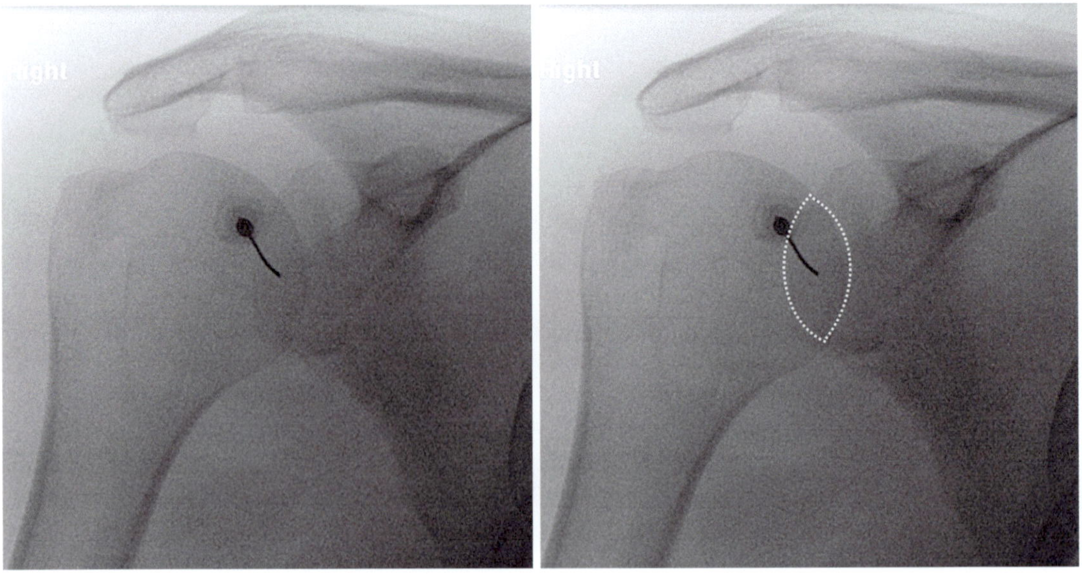

Fig. 4.8 Needle placement is recommended just lateral to the medial cortex of the humeral head, within the ellipse formed by the overlap of the glenoid and humeral head

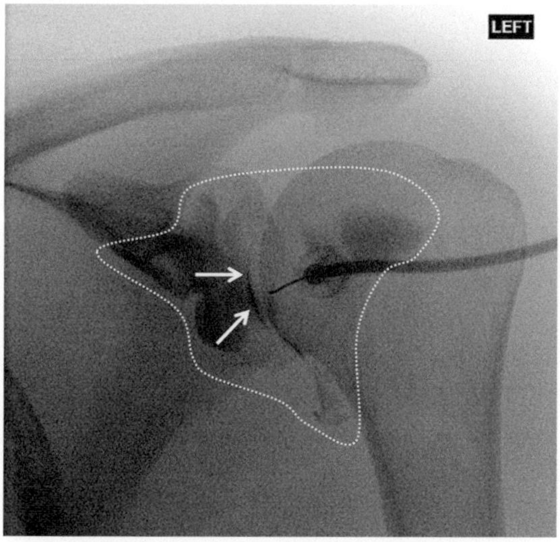

Fig. 4.9 Fluoroscopic image after intra-articular injection of contrast demonstrates contrast material in the joint space (arrows) and within the expected confines of the joint capsule (dotted line)

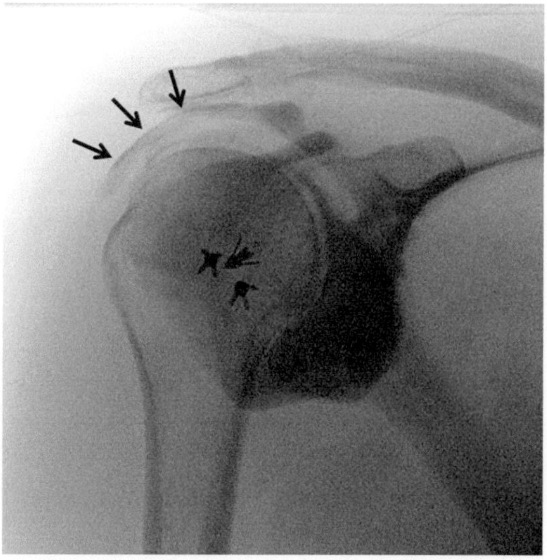

Fig. 4.10 Fluoroscopic image after intra-articular injection of contrast reveals contrast within the joint capsule and also extravasating into the subacromial-subdeltoid bursa (arrows), diagnostic of a rotator cuff tear. Suture anchors from prior rotator cuff repair are noted

habitus. Under intermittent fluoroscopy to check needle positioning, the needle should be advanced until contact is made with the bony surface of the humeral head. If the needle is advanced into the glenohumeral joint space, any further manipulation should be gentle in order to avoid damage to the articular cartilage and labrum [14]. Once the needle appears to be in a good position, a test injection should be performed with a low osmolar contrast material to confirm intra-articular positioning of the needle. An intra-articular injection should demonstrate contrast flowing freely away from the needle into the glenohumeral joint or within the expected confines of the joint capsule (Fig. 4.9). Lack of contrast spread may suggest injection into overlying muscle or tendon. Once the appropriate needle position is confirmed, the desired intra-articular medium may be instilled. During arthrography, the presence of a rotator cuff tear may be diagnosed by extra-articular extension of contrast into the overlying subacromial-subdeltoid bursa (Fig. 4.10).

Glenohumeral joint injections can also be performed under fluoroscopic guidance using a posterior approach. The positioning is advocated in patients with suspected anterior labral pathology or instability, as inadvertent extra-articular contrast extravasation posteriorly will not confound anterior pathology [14, 15]. The patient should be placed on the fluoroscopy table in a prone position, with a foam pad placed under the ipsilateral shoulder and thorax to oblique the shoulder and provide an en face view of the glenohumeral joint. The patient's arm should be in a neutral or internally rotated position. The needle target is just lateral to the medial cortex of the humeral head, similar to the anterior approach.

4.4 Glenohumeral Joint Aspiration

Glenohumeral joint aspiration is usually performed to obtain a sample of joint fluid for analysis when infection is suspected, usually in the prosthetic shoulder. The technique employed for an US-guided glenohumeral joint aspiration is similar to that used in injection, and either an anterior or a posterior approach may be used. The patient positioning is the same, and joint fluid is the desired target. Different from a joint injection, no test injection with anesthetic should be

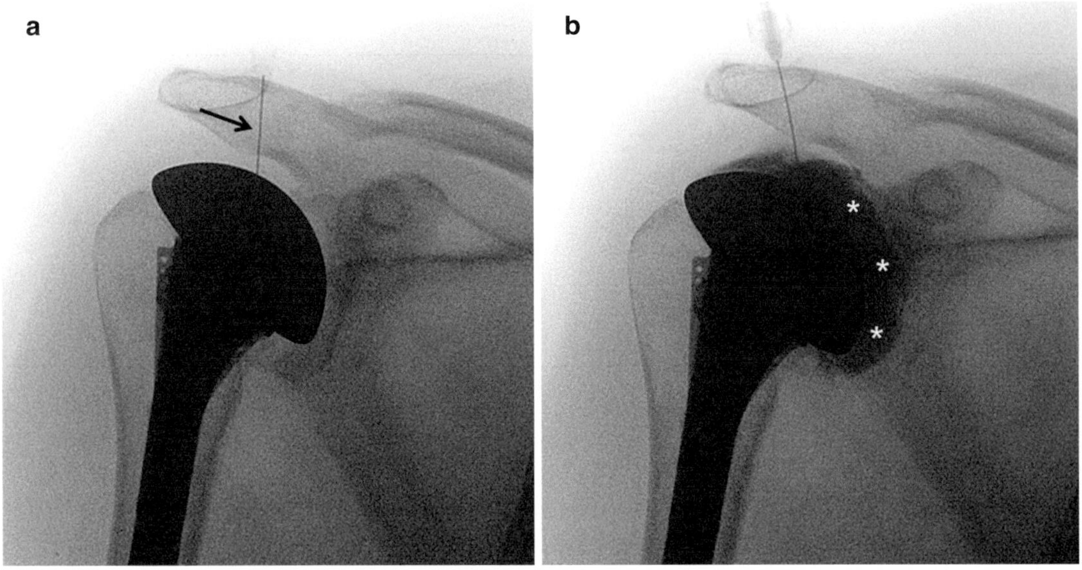

Fig. 4.11 (a) Fluoroscopic image demonstrate oblique needle trajectory (arrow) for glenohumeral joint aspiration/injection in a patient with a shoulder implant. When possible, the target should be the metallic humeral head component. During contrast injection (**b**), there is opacification of the joint pseudocapsule (*)

performed prior to aspiration of native joint fluid to avoid inaccurate cell count analysis and potential bactericide. If there is no visible joint fluid or no fluid can be aspirated on initial attempt, a lavage may be performed by injecting and re-aspirating sterile non-bacteriostatic and preservative-free saline to obtain a fluid sample for analysis. A large-bore needle (e.g., 18-gauge) is typically used for aspiration.

Glenohumeral joint aspiration under fluoroscopy is also similar to the technique used in injection. If aspiration is being performed in a prosthetic joint, the target should be the humeral head component. An oblique needle trajectory is recommended for better needle visualization over a metallic target like a prosthetic humeral component (Fig. 4.11). As with US, aspiration of native joint fluid should be attempted first before the instillation of intra-articular contrast.

4.5 Subacromial-Subdeltoid Bursa

The subacromial-subdeltoid (SASD) bursa is located deep to the acromioclavicular joint and extends like a saddle superficially over the rotator cuff. The bursa runs both anteroposteriorly and mediolaterally, and extends beyond the rotator cuff insertion. Therefore, the SASD bursa can be accessed via an anterior, lateral, or posterior approach [16] with the patient in a supine, lateral decubitus, or seated position.

A 25-gauge 1.5 in. needle or a 22-gauge 3.5 in. needle can be used for injection, depending on the patient's body habitus. 2–3 mL of an anesthetic and cortisone mixture is typically used for a therapeutic injection [16], although up to 10 mL can comfortably be injected into the bursa. For a lateral approach, the needle should be inserted in plane to the transducer via a lateral-to-medial approach (Fig. 4.12). The hypoechoic bursa between the echogenic peribursal fat should be targeted (Fig. 4.13a). Of note, fluid within the bursa is an excellent target if present. When holding the transducer, it is important not to use too much pressure as this can efface fluid within the SASD bursa. Once the needle appears to be in a good position, perform a test injection with anesthetic to confirm that the needle tip is within the bursa. If there is no visible fluid within the bursa, insert the needle between the peribursal fat stripes and inject anesthetic to create a visible plane. There should be smooth linear distention of the

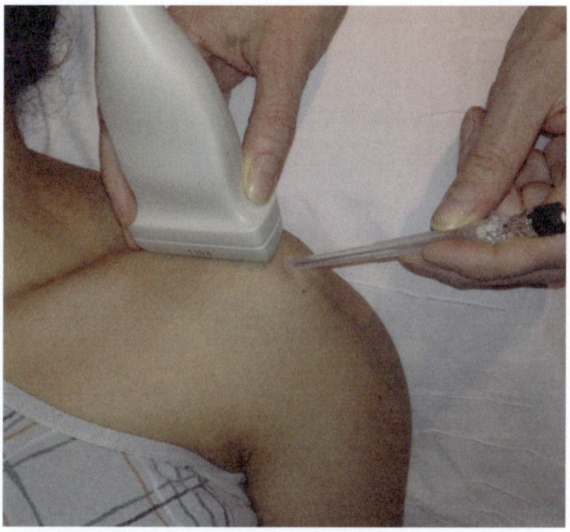

Fig. 4.12 Patient positioning and needle placement for SASD bursal injection

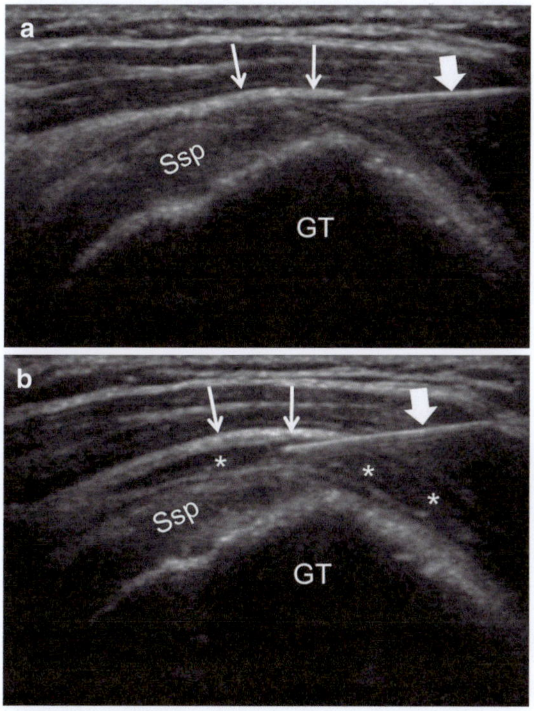

Fig. 4.13 Ultrasound images (**a** and **b**) demonstrate needle placement, for SASD bursal injection, with the tip of the needle (block arrow) within the echogenic peribursal fat (thin arrows). Postinjection, there is smooth distention of the SASD bursal with injectate (*, **b**). Note that the bursa extends lateral to the rotator cuff insertion. *Ssp* supraspinatus, *GT* greater tuberosity

SASD over the rotator cuff tendon, and fluid will extend lateral to the rotator cuff insertion (Fig. 4.13b).

An 18- or 20-gauge needle can be used for aspiration of the SASD bursa. The technique is the same as described above, with fluid as the target. If no fluid is present, a lavage can be performed to obtain a bursal fluid sample, using sterile saline.

4.6 Biceps Tendon Sheath

The long head of the biceps tendon (LHBT) originates at the supraglenoid tubercle of the scapula within the glenohumeral joint, extends through the rotator interval, and courses distally within the bicipital groove between the greater and lesser tuberosities of the humerus. The extra-articular LHBT sits within a tendon sheath, composed of a synovial membrane, as it travels within the bicipital groove. The tendon sheath, which communicates with the glenohumeral joint, can contain a small amount of physiologic fluid even in the absence of pathology. The proximal biceps is well seen with US at and distal to the bicipital groove, and US is the preferred method for image-guided injection.

The patient is positioned supine with the arm by the side in external rotation (Fig. 4.14). This will position the bicipital groove at the 12:00 position, allowing direct access to the biceps tendon sheath within the bicipital groove. A

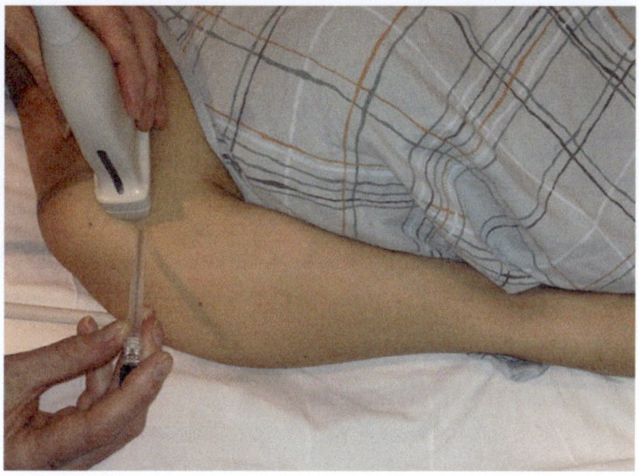

Fig. 4.14 Patient positioning and needle placement for LHBT US-guided injection

25-gauge 1.5 in.needle or a 22-gauge 3.5 in. needle may be used for injection, depending on the patient's body habitus. 3–4 mL of an anesthetic and cortisone mixture is typically injected for therapeutic purposes. The transducer is placed transversely over the bicipital groove, providing a short-axis view of the LHBT. The needle should be inserted into the tendon sheath at the level of the bicipital groove in plane to the transducer via a lateral-to-medial approach (Fig. 4.14). Fluid within the tendon sheath is an excellent target, if present. Rocking the transducer will help to distinguish anisotropy of the LHBT, which is normally echogenic, from fluid within the tendon sheath. Doppler imaging should also be used to identify and avoid the anterior humeral circumflex artery, which is often seen just lateral to the LHBT.

The needle should be advanced into the tendon sheath so that the tip sits adjacent to the superficial or deep aspect of the LHBT (Fig. 4.15a). Once the needle appears to be in a satisfactory position, a test injection with anesthetic should be performed to confirm appropriate needle positioning. The lidocaine should smoothly distend the biceps tendon sheath (Fig. 4.15b). Subsequently, the therapeutic mixture can be injected, and the injectate should circumferentially coat the LHBT. Distention of the biceps tendon sheath can also be confirmed by scanning the LHBT in long axis, which should demonstrate distal spread of injectate. Ultrasound-guided injection of the LHBT has shown to significantly reduce needle misplacement as compared with the blinded method (86% vs. 26%, respectively) [17].

4.7 Acromioclavicular Joint

The acromioclavicular (AC) joint is well seen under US and can be found by scanning laterally along the superior aspect of the clavicle. For US-guided injection, the patient is positioned supine, with the arm by the side in a neutral position. The injection can be easily performed with a 25-gauge 1.5 in. needle. With an intact joint capsule, usually not more than 1 mL can be injected into the AC joint. With advanced AC joint arthrosis, injectate may decompress into the SASD bursa.

The AC joint can be injected via an in-plane or out-of-plane approach. With an out-of-plane approach, the AC joint should be scanned in long axis with the transducer placed longitudinally over the AC joint and the needle advanced out of plane (i.e., short axis) to the transducer (Fig. 4.16a). Using this approach, both the acromion and clavicle are visualized

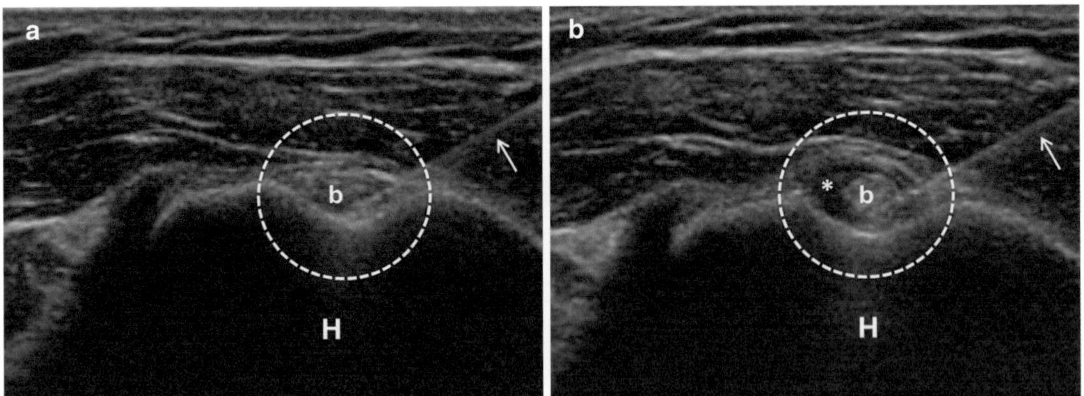

Fig. 4.15 Ultrasound images (**a**, **b**) demonstrate needle placement (arrow) within the LHBT sheath (circle). During injection, there is circumferential distention of the LHBT sheath with the injectate (**b**,*). *H* humeral head, *b* biceps tendon

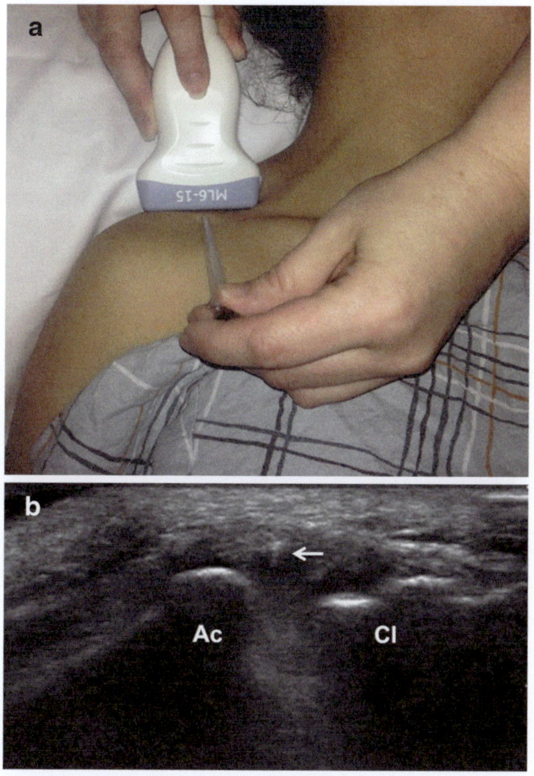

Fig. 4.16 (**a**) Patient positioning and needle placement for out-of-plane AC joint injection. (**b**) The echogenic tip of the needle (arrow) is seen within the acromioclavicular joint. *Ac* acromion, *Cl* clavicle

on the same image, and the tip of the needle will be seen en face as an echogenic dot (Fig. 4.16b).

For an in-plane approach, the transducer is placed transversely over the AC joint and the needle is advanced in plane to the transducer. The joint space can be found by scanning laterally from the clavicle or medially from the acromion. The hypoechoic space between the clavicle and acromion is the joint space (Fig. 4.17). Neither the clavicle nor the acromion will be seen on the sonographic image during this in-plane injection; only the joint space will be visualized. The needle shaft and tip should be visualized as the tip is inserted into the joint space (Fig. 4.18).

Once the needle appears to be within the joint space, a test injection should be performed to confirm intra-articular needle positioning with smooth distention of the joint space. Subsequently, the therapeutic mixture can be injected. A recent report has shown that ultrasound-guided AC joint injections have better outcome as compared with blinded injections due to the improved accuracy [18].

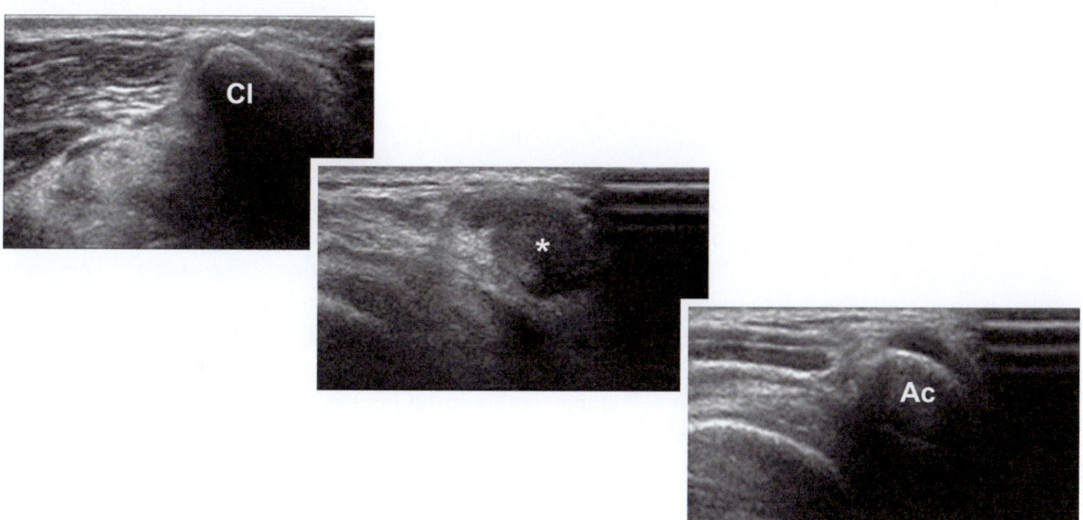

Fig. 4.17 Ultrasound images demonstrate the appearance of the acromioclavicular joint via an in-plane approach. The joint space (asterisk) is located between the clavicle (Cl), which is lateral, and the acromion (Ac), which is medial

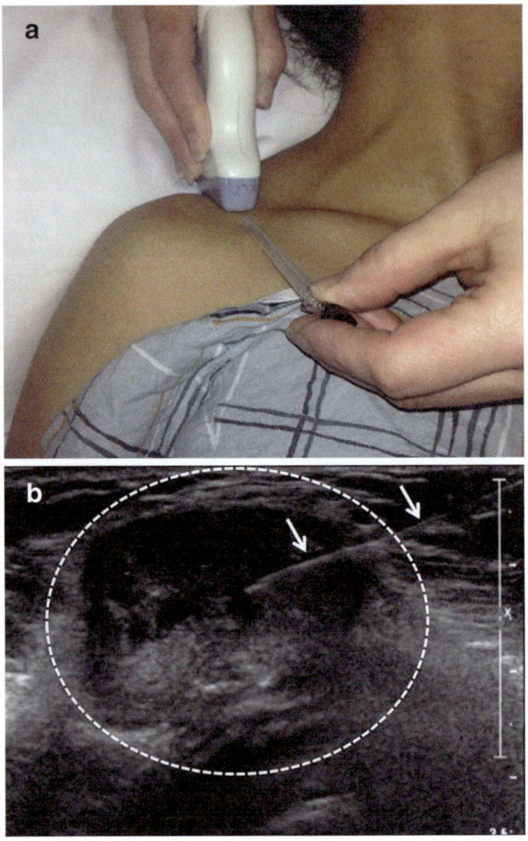

Fig. 4.18 (**a**) Patient positioning and needle placement for in-plane AC joint injection. (**b**) The entire length of the needle (arrows) is seen as it is advanced into the joint space (circle)

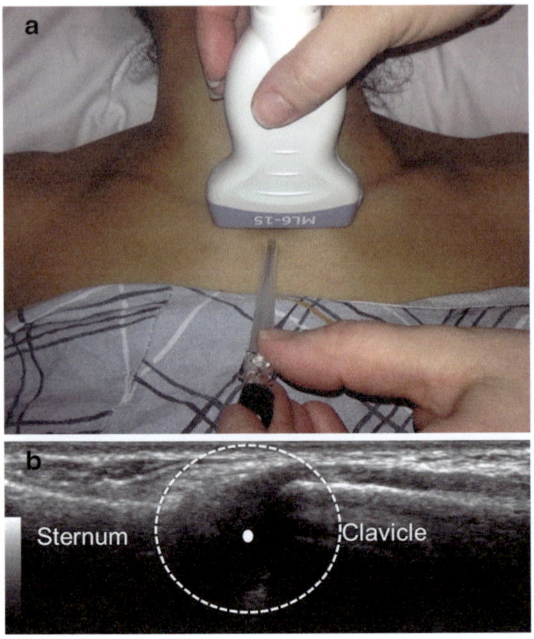

Fig. 4.19 (**a**) Patient positioning and needle placement for out-of-plane SC joint injection. (**b**) Simulated echogenic needle tip (round dot) within the SC joint (circle)

4.8 Sternoclavicular Joint

Similar to the AC joint, the sternoclavicular (SC) joint is superficial and well seen on US. The patient should be supine, with the arm by the side in a neutral position. The injection is easily performed with a 25-gauge 1.5 in. needle. A therapeutic volume of 1–2 mL of an anesthetic and cortisone mixture is recommended. The SC joint can be found by scanning longitudinally along the anterior aspect of the clavicle and moving medially over the clavicular head until the lateral border of the manubrium is visualized.

The injection technique is similar to that of the AC joint. With an out-of-plane approach, the SC joint should be scanned in long axis with the transducer placed longitudinally over the SC joint and the needle advanced straight down, out of plane to the transducer (Fig. 4.19a). Using this approach, both the sternum and clavicle are visualized on the same image, and the tip of the needle will be seen as an echogenic dot (Fig. 4.19b). With this technique, the operator must be aware of the depth of the needle tip at all times to avoid inadvertent injury to critical structures deep to the SC joint.

For an in-plane approach, the transducer is placed transversely over the SC joint and the needle is advanced in an oblique cranial direction, in plane to the transducer (Fig. 4.20a). The joint space can be found by scanning laterally from the clavicle or medially from the sternum. The hypoechoic space between the clavicle and acromion is the joint space. As with the AC joint, the needle shaft and tip should be seen as the tip is inserted into the SC joint space (Fig. 4.20b).

An alternative SC joint in-plane injection is performed with the transducer placed over the sternoclavicular joint in long axis, with the needle inserted in either a medial-to-lateral or a lateral-to-medial direction, using the

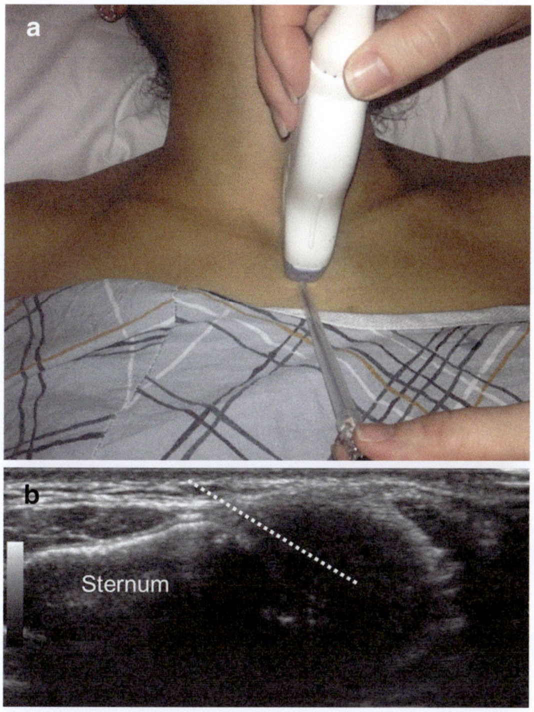

Fig. 4.20 (**a**) Patient positioning and needle placement for in-plane SC joint injection. (**b**) Simulated needle trajectory (dotted line) to target the SC joint

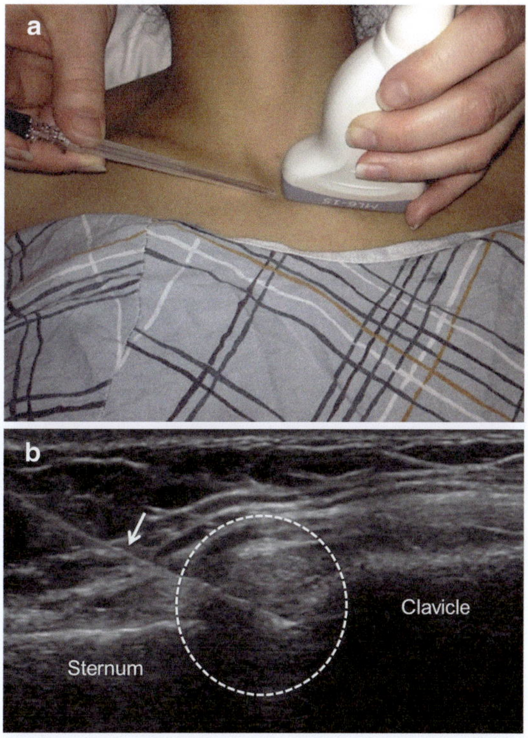

Fig. 4.21 (**a**) Patient positioning and needle placement for alternate in-plane SC joint injection. (**b**) The entire length of the needle is seen (arrow), with the needle tip within the SC joint (circle) and the clavicular head acting as a backstop. *Cl* clavicular head, *St* sternum

manubrium or clavicular head as a backstop for the needle tip, respectively (Fig. 4.21). This in-plane approach also allows for constant visualization of the needle tip and prevents inadvertent injury to critical structures deep to the SC joint. Once the needle appears to be within the joint space, a test injection with anesthetic can be performed to confirm intra-articular needle positioning and should result in capsular distention. Once confirmed, the therapeutic mixture may be injected.

4.9 Scapulothoracic Bursa

The scapulothoracic bursa is located deep to the scapula and superficial to the ribs (Fig. 4.22). Scapulothoracic bursal injection can easily and safely be performed under US guidance. A distended bursa is almost never visible on US, and so the injection should be performed at the site of the patient's maximum discomfort. The patient should be placed in a prone or prone oblique position, with the arm by the side (Fig. 4.23a). A 25-gauge 1.5 in. needle is typically used for this injection, although a 22-gauge 3.5 in. needle can also be used if required, depending on the patient's body habitus. The dose should consist of 2–3 mL of an anesthetic and cortisone mixture.

The space between the medial border of the scapula and rib should be targeted using a horizontal, medial-to-lateral needle approach (Fig. 4.23a). An in-plane approach is used for injection, with the transducer placed transversely over the scapulothoracic bursa medial border of the scapula. The injection should be performed at the level of a rib in order to provide a backstop, and the needle shaft should always be visualized as it is advanced deep to

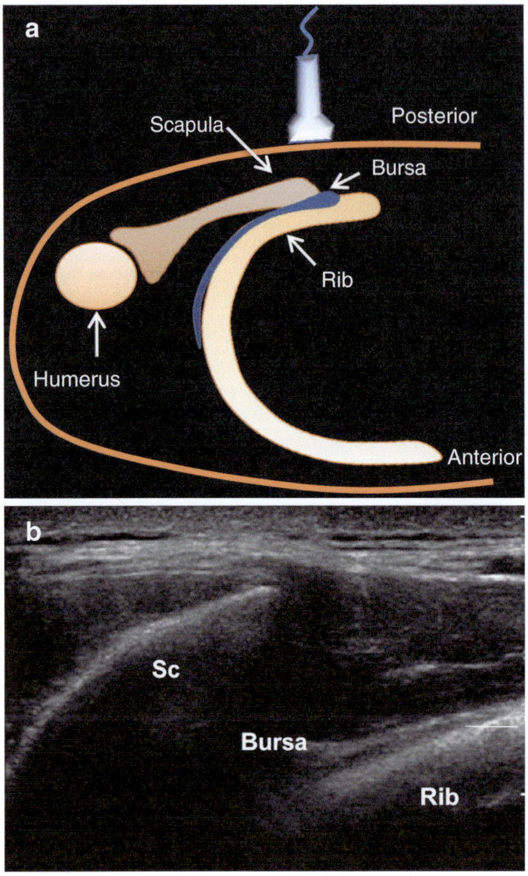

Fig. 4.22 Illustration (**a**) and ultrasound image (**b**) of the region of the scapulothoracic bursa. The bursa is not seen on US but is located between the scapular blade (Sc) and the rib

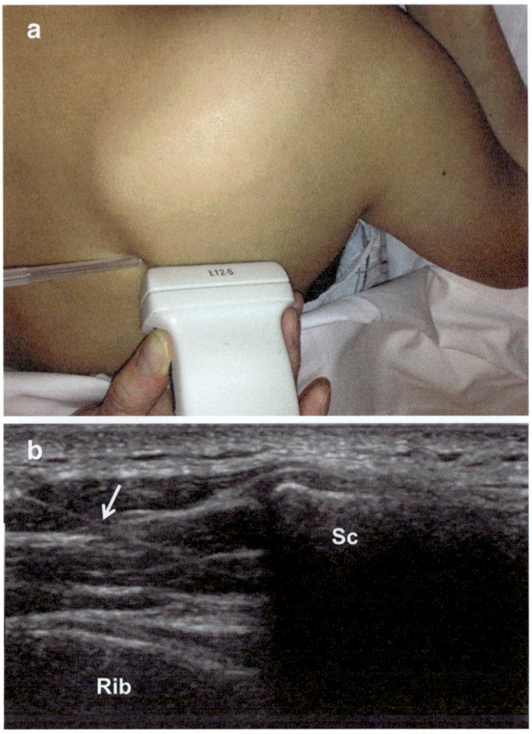

Fig. 4.23 (**a**) Patient positioning and needle placement. (**b**) Ultrasound image demonstrates needle placement (arrow) targeting the scapulothoracic bursa. *Sc* scapula

the scapula (Fig. 4.23b). It is imperative to stay superficial to the ribs in order to prevent a pneumothorax.

4.10 Calcific Tendinosis Lavage and Aspiration

Hydroxyapatite crystal deposition in the shoulder most commonly involves the rotator cuff tendons (calcific tendinosis) and/or the SASD bursa (calcific bursitis). Lavage and aspiration of the calcific deposits under US guidance is an effective method for treatment of calcific tendinosis, and it has been shown to give longer lasting relief than corticosteroid injection into the SASD bursa alone [19–21].

A diagnostic US should first be performed to identify the location and size of the calcific deposits (Fig. 4.24). If multiple calcific deposits are present, the largest deposits should be targeted. Echogenic calcific deposits may or may not demonstrate associated shadowing, and some will reveal associated hyperemia with Doppler evaluation [12, 22, 23].

Patient positioning will depend on the location of the calcific deposits to be targeted. However, the procedure will typically be performed with the patient in a supine or lateral decubitus position. An 18-gauge needle should be used, and the needle length can be 1.5 or 3.5 in., depending on the patient's body habitus. One- and two-needle aspiration techniques have been reported [20, 23, 24]. The lavage medium may consist of sterile saline alone, lidocaine alone, or saline with lidocaine in a 50–50 admixture. Some advocate the use of warmed saline in calcific tendinosis lavage, reporting improved

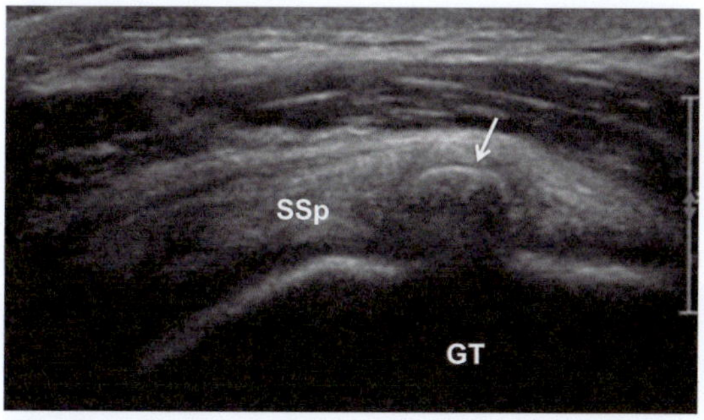

Fig. 4.24 Ultrasound image demonstrates an echogenic, shadowing focus of calcification (arrow) within the supraspinatus tendon, reflecting calcific tendinosis. *Ssp* supraspinatus tendon, *GT* greater tuberosity

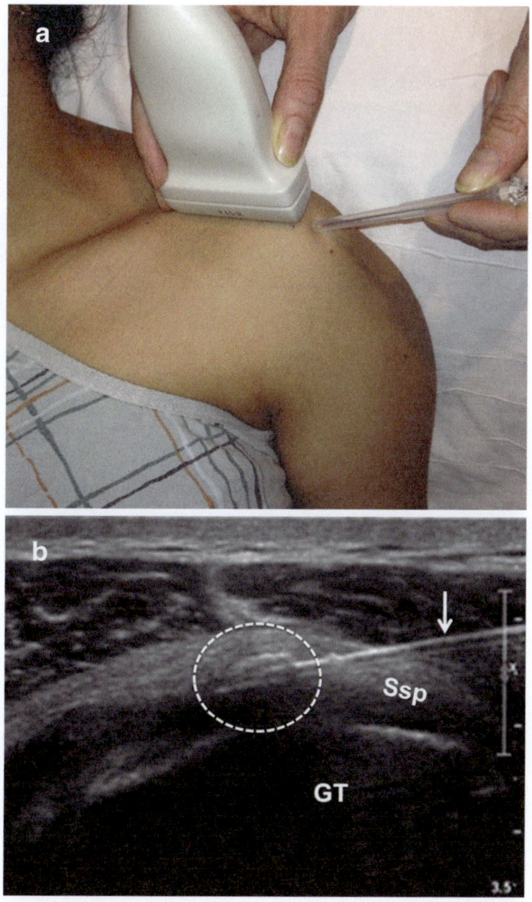

Fig. 4.25 (**a**) Patient positioning and needle placement. (**b**) Ultrasound image demonstrates optimal needle placement (arrow) with the needle tip at the center of the calcific deposit (circle). *Ssp* supraspinatus tendon, *GT* greater tuberosity

calcium dissolution and lower incidence of post-procedural bursitis [25]. Our technique is to use multiple aliquots of the lavage mixture, preferably in 5 or 10 mL syringes, and a one-needle aspiration technique. The needle should be directed into the center of the calcific deposit via an in-plane approach and the tip should be positioned in the center of the calcific deposit (Fig. 4.25). It is important to accurately puncture the calcific deposit in one pass, as this will help maintain pressure within the deposit during lavage. The saline syringe should be attached to the needle once it is in proper position and pulsed lavage should begin by applying repeated compression on the plunger of the syringe. Initial breakdown of the calcific deposit may occur with a palpable pop. Repeated plunger compression will cause further breakdown of the calcific deposit and calcific particles will be seen to waft back into the syringe each time the plunger is released (Fig. 4.26).

As lavage is performed, a hypoechoic, fluid-filled cavity will be created within the center of the calcific deposit. As fluid is pushed into the calcific deposit, the cavity will expand, and as it is withdrawn the cavity will collapse (Fig. 4.27). This is indicative of an effective lavage, and has been likened to a "fishmouth" appearance. Once the fluid in the syringe is cloudy and filled with calcium, the syringe should be replaced with a fresh saline syringe. Lavage should be performed

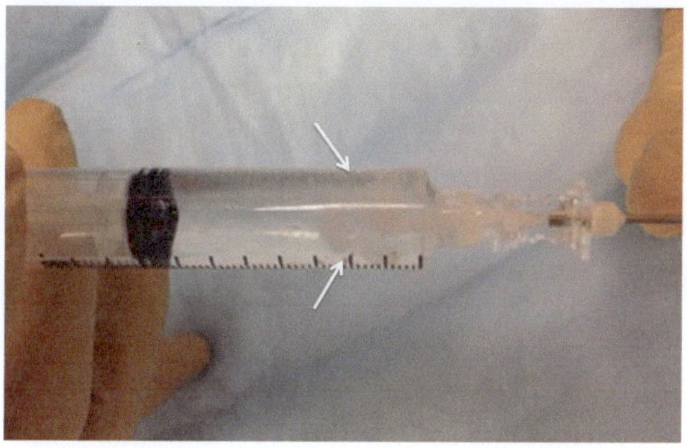

Fig. 4.26 Photograph depicts calcium (arrows) wafting into a syringe of saline during calcific tendinosis lavage

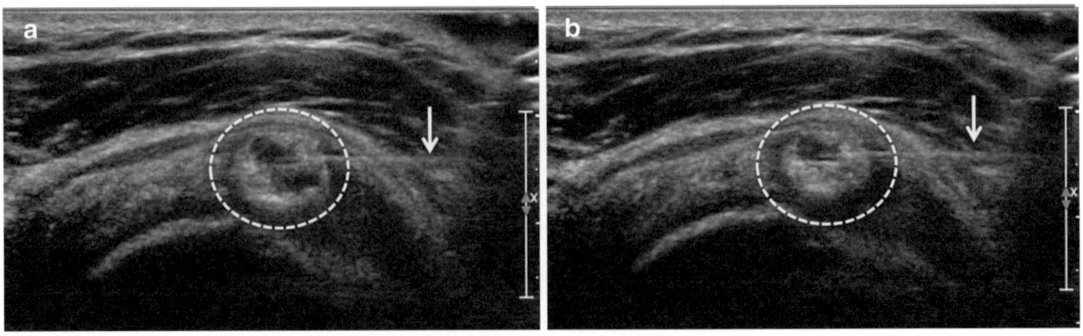

Fig. 4.27 (**a** and **b**) Ultrasound images demonstrate distention (**a**) and decompression (**b**) of the cavity (circle) within the calcific deposit during lavage and aspiration, producing a "fishmouth" appearance in real time. Arrow—needle

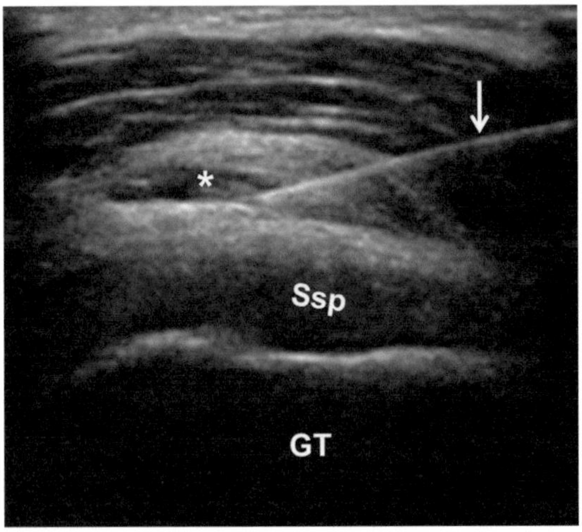

Fig. 4.28 Following lavage and aspiration of calcium, the needle (arrow) can be redirected into the overlying SASD bursa (asterisk) for cortisone injection. *Ssp* supraspinatus tendon, *GT* greater tuberosity

until calcium is no longer visualized entering the syringe. As the lavage of the calcium progresses, fluid injected into the calcific nidus may be seen to decompress into the overlying SASD.

Following calcium lavage and aspiration, the needle can be redirected into the overlying SASD bursa, and bursal injection with anesthetic and cortisone mixture should be performed using the same technique as described above in the SASD bursa section (Fig. 4.28). Performing this injection will help to prevent or minimize symptoms associated with painful calcific bursitis after the procedure is completed.

4.11 Ganglion/Paralabral Cyst Aspiration

Paralabral cysts are thought to occur due to injury of the capsulolabral complex, and indicate the presence of a labral tear. Synovial fluid can leak from the joint, through the tear, and into the para-articular soft tissues, resulting in the development of a paralabral cyst. In the shoulder, these cysts are most commonly seen in the spinoglenoid notch and may extend into the suprascapular notch. US can detect paralabral cysts about the shoulder, particularly within the spinoglenoid notch [26] (Fig. 4.29), and can be used for guidance of aspiration and fenestration of these cysts.

Spinoglenoid or suprascapular notch paralabral cyst aspiration can be performed in a prone, prone oblique, or lateral decubitus position, depending on the cyst location. An 18-gauge needle is recommended, as the contents are usually viscous, and the length of the needle will vary depending on the depth of the cyst. The cyst may be targeted with the needle in plane to the transducer via a medial-to-lateral or lateral-to medial approach (Fig. 4.30). Before and while advancing the needle, it is important to look for the suprascapular neurovascular bundle which is located in the region of the spinoglenoid notch. Color or power Doppler imaging can be useful for identification. Once the needle tip is inserted into the center of the paralabral cyst, the fluid within the cyst should be aspirated, with the aim

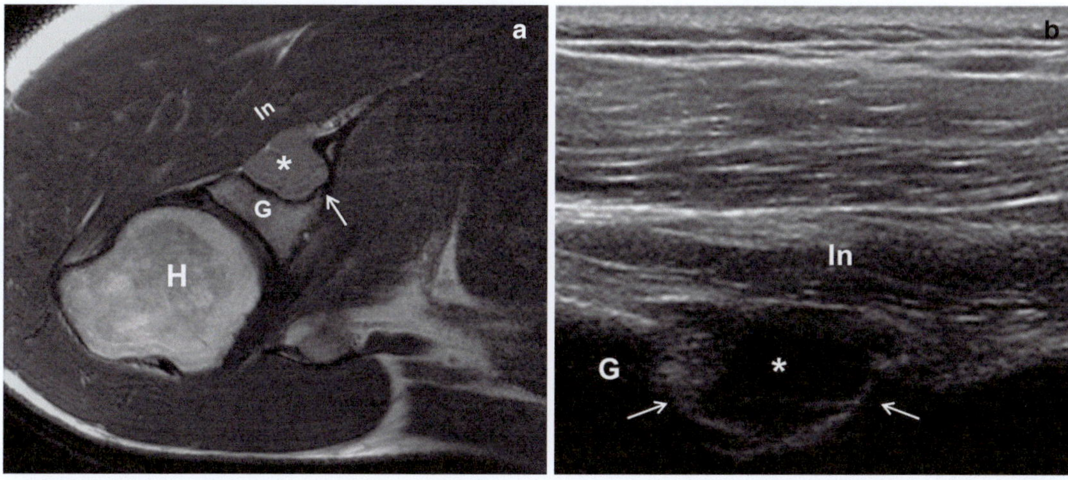

Fig. 4.29 Axial T1-weighted MR image (**a**) and corresponding ultrasound image (**b**) demonstrate a paralabral cyst (asterisk) within the spinoglenoid notch (arrows). The spinoglenoid notch is located deep to the infraspinatus. *In* infraspinatus muscle, *G* glenoid

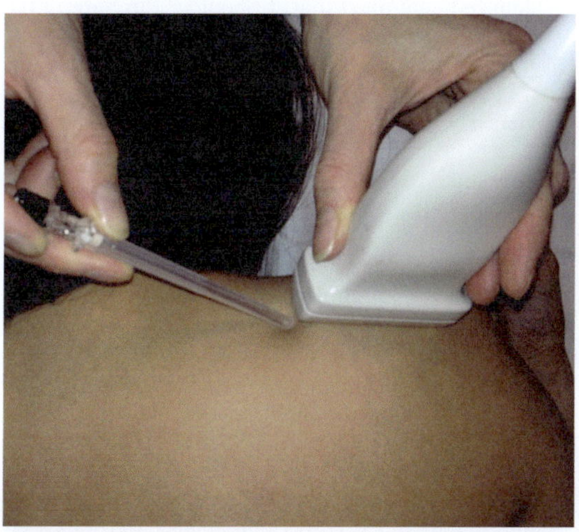

Fig. 4.30 Patient positioning and needle placement for aspiration of a spinoglenoid cyst

of complete decompression of the cyst (Fig. 4.31). Lavage by injection of anesthetic and re-aspiration may aid in complete decompression. Subsequently, the cyst wall should be fenestrated with multiple needle passes. Following paralabral cyst aspiration and fenestration, a mixture of 1–2 mL of anesthetic and cortisone can be injected into the region of the decompressed cyst, with care taken not to re-distend the cyst. Alternatively, the anesthetic-cortisone mixture

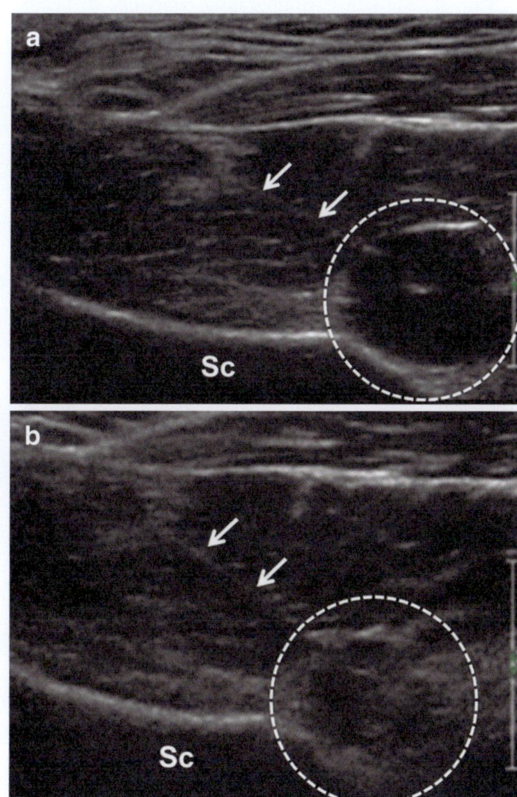

Fig. 4.31 Ultrasound images (**a**, **b**) demonstrating a needle (arrows) within the spinoglenoid notch cyst (circles). Post-aspiration (**b**), there is decompression of the spinoglenoid notch cyst

may be used to lavage the cyst cavity during fenestration, and any excess of the mixture is re-aspirated to avoid leaving the cyst distended. Although evidence is sparse, cortisone injection is thought to diminish inflammation which is proposed as a pain generator and a causative factor in cyst formation [26, 27]. Corticosteroid injection in the region of the cyst may also help decrease inflammation of the suprascapular nerve, which is commonly entrapped in patients with symptomatic paralabral cysts in the shoulder [26, 28, 29].

References

1. Otjen J, Parnell SE, Menashe S, Thapa MM. Ultrasound-guided joint injections for MR arthrography in pediatric patients: how we do it. Pediatr Radiol. 2015;45:308–16.. quiz 305-7
2. Valls R, Melloni P. Sonographic guidance of needle position for MR arthrography of the shoulder. AJR Am J Roentgenol. 1997;169:845–7.
3. Gokalp G, Dusak A, Yazici Z. Efficacy of ultrasonography-guided shoulder MR arthrography using a posterior approach. Skelet Radiol. 2010;39:575–9.
4. Ogul H, Bayraktutan U, Ozgokce M, et al. Ultrasound-guided shoulder MR arthrography: comparison of rotator interval and posterior approach. Clin Imaging. 2014;38:11–7.
5. Ng AW, Hung EH, Griffith JF, Tong CS, Cho CC. Comparison of ultrasound versus fluoroscopic guided rotator cuff interval approach for MR arthrography. Clin Imaging. 2013;37:548–53.
6. Rutten MJ, Collins JM, Maresch BJ, et al. Glenohumeral joint injection: a comparative study of ultrasound and fluoroscopically guided techniques before MR arthrography. Eur Radiol. 2009;19:722–30.
7. Schneider R, Ghelman B, Kaye JJ. A simplified injection technique for shoulder arthrography. Radiology. 1975;114:738–9.
8. Mulligan ME. CT-guided shoulder arthrography at the rotator cuff interval. AJR Am J Roentgenol. 2008;191:W58–61.
9. Soh E, Bearcroft PW, Graves MJ, Black R, Lomas DJ. MR-guided direct arthrography of the glenohumeral joint. Clin Radiol. 2008;63:1336–41.. discussion 1342-3
10. Hilfiker PR, Weishaupt D, Schmid M, Dubno B, Hodler J, Debatin JF. Real-time MR-guided joint puncture and arthrography: preliminary results. Eur Radiol. 1999;9:201–4.
11. Jacobson JA. Fundamentals of musculoskeletal ultrasound. Philadelphia, PA: Saunders/Elsevier; 2007. p. 345.
12. Jacobson JA, Lin J, Jamadar DA, Hayes CW. Aids to successful shoulder arthrography performed with a fluoroscopically guided anterior approach. Radiographics. 2003;23:373–8.. discussion 379
13. Miller TT. MR arthrography of the shoulder and hip after fluoroscopic landmarking. Skelet Radiol. 2000;29:81–4.
14. Chung CB, Dwek JR, Feng S, Resnick D. MR arthrography of the glenohumeral joint: a tailored approach. AJR Am J Roentgenol. 2001;177:217–9.
15. Farmer KD, Hughes PM. MR arthrography of the shoulder: fluoroscopically guided technique using a posterior approach. AJR Am J Roentgenol. 2002;178:433–4.
16. Molini L, Mariacher S, Bianchi S. US guided corticosteroid injection into the subacromial-subdeltoid bursa: technique and approach. J Ultrasound. 2012;15:61–8.
17. T H, Sakurai G, Morimoto M, Komei T, Takakura Y, Tanaka Y. Accuracy of the biceps tendon sheath injection: ultrasound-guided or unguided injection? A randomized controlled trial. J Shoulder Elb Surg. 2011 Oct;20(7):1069–73.
18. Park KD, Kim TK, Lee J, Lee WY, Ahn JK, Park Y. Palpation versus ultrasound-guided acromioclavicular joint intra-articular corticosteroid injections: a retrospective comparative clinical study. Pain Physician. 2015;18(4):333–41.
19. de Witte PB, Selten JW, Navas A, et al. Calcific tendinitis of the rotator cuff: a randomized controlled trial of ultrasound-guided needling and lavage versus subacromial corticosteroids. Am J Sports Med. 2013;41:1665–73.
20. del Cura JL, Torre I, Zabala R, Legorburu A. Sonographically guided percutaneous needle lavage in calcific tendinitis of the shoulder: short- and long-term results. AJR Am J Roentgenol. 2007;189:W128–34.
21. Levy O. Ultrasound-guided barbotage in addition to ultrasound-guided corticosteroid injection improved outcomes in calcific tendinitis of the rotator cuff. J Bone Joint Surg Am. 2014;96:335.
22. Le Goff B, Berthelot JM, Guillot P, Glemarec J, Maugars Y. Assessment of calcific tendonitis of rotator cuff by ultrasonography: comparison between symptomatic and asymptomatic shoulders. Joint Bone Spine. 2010;77:258–63.
23. Saboeiro GR. Sonography in the treatment of calcific tendinitis of the rotator cuff. J Ultrasound Med. 2012;31:1513–8.
24. Sconfienza LM, Vigano S, Martini C, et al. Double-needle ultrasound-guided percutaneous treatment of rotator cuff calcific tendinitis: tips & tricks. Skelet Radiol. 2013;42:19–24.

25. Sconfienza LM, Bandirali M, Serafini G, et al. Rotator cuff calcific tendinitis: does warm saline solution improve the short-term outcome of double-needle US-guided treatment? Radiology. 2012;262:560–6.
26. Hashimoto BE, Hayes AS, Ager JD. Sonographic diagnosis and treatment of ganglion cysts causing suprascapular nerve entrapment. J Ultrasound Med. 1994;13:671–4.
27. Breidahl WH, Adler RS. Ultrasound-guided injection of ganglia with corticosteroids. Skelet Radiol. 1996;25:635–8.
28. Biedert RM. Atrophy of the infraspinatus muscle caused by a suprascapular ganglion. Clin J Sport Med. 1996;6:262–3.. discussion 264
29. Neviaser TJ, Ain BR, Neviaser RJ. Suprascapular nerve denervation secondary to attenuation by a ganglionic cyst. J Bone Joint Surg Am. 1986;68:627–8.

Part II

Rotator Cuff, Biceps and Rotator Interval

Imaging Diagnosis of Rotator Cuff Pathology and Impingement Syndromes

5

Eric Y. Chang and Christine B. Chung

5.1 Introduction

Rotator cuff disease, which includes tendinopathy and tearing, is incredibly common. A systematic review in 2014 has shown that the prevalence of rotator cuff disease increases with age, from approximately 10% in patients under 20 years of age to approximately 60% in patients greater than 80 years of age [1]. There are a number of controversies that exist when discussing the rotator cuff, including symptomatology and pathoetiology. Although it is clear that cuff disease can be symptomatic and necessitate treatment, the determination of which abnormalities are symptomatic or which are best treated with surgical intervention remains a challenge [2–6].

The etiology of rotator cuff disease is multifactorial with intrinsic and extrinsic contributions [7, 8]. Intrinsic mechanisms are associated with the tendon itself and the *degenerative-microtrauma model* is likely to be critical to the development of cuff disease in many patients [9]. This model supposes that age-related tendon damage [10, 11] compounded by chronic, repetitive microtrauma results in adverse cellular changes, release of inflammatory mediators, and apoptosis [12, 13]. Extrinsic mechanisms include anatomic variables external to the tendon, such as the various impingement syndromes.

In most patients, it is generally favored that intrinsic mechanisms play a greater role in cuff disease compared with extrinsic factors [14–18]. This is referred to as the *intrinsic theory* of cuff disease, which states that cuff dysfunction is the causal abnormality, leading to decentering of the humeral lead and resultant formation of enthesophytes and tuberosity lesions [19]. Although biologically engineered scaffolds [20], exogenous growth factors [21], and cellular therapies [22] targeting intrinsic mechanisms are increasing, surgical therapy of cuff disease and treatment of associated extrinsic lesions remain the most widely available nonconservative treatment options. Therefore, it is critical for the radiologist and surgeon to identify the lesions that can be associated with shoulder pain and cases which may be amenable to available treatment.

The diagnosis of impingement syndromes requires all available information, including history, physical examination, and imaging. A practical and commonly used classification scheme of the various shoulder impingement syndromes is to divide based on those where the pathogenesis resides outside the glenohumeral joint capsule (termed *external* impingement) and those residing inside the glenohumeral joint capsule (termed *internal* impingement). External impingement syndromes include *subacromial impingement* and *subcoracoid impingement*. Internal impingement syndromes include *posterosuperior*

E. Y. Chang (✉) · C. B. Chung
Department of Radiology, VA San Diego Healthcare System, San Diego, CA, USA

Department of Radiology, University of California, San Diego Medical Center, San Diego, CA, USA

J. T. Bencardino (ed.), *The Shoulder*, https://doi.org/10.1007/978-3-030-06240-8_5

impingement, which belongs in the spectrum of abnormalities leading to the disabled throwing shoulder, and *anterosuperior impingement*. Each impingement syndrome is a distinct entity, predominantly affecting different demographics of patients, but more than one type of impingement syndrome may be seen in an individual.

This chapter reviews (1) the imaging anatomy of the structures related to impingement, including the rotator cuff and biceps pulley; (2) the multi-modality imaging manifestations of rotator cuff disease and the various shoulder impingement syndromes; and (3) the expected and abnormal appearances after surgical therapy.

5.2 Imaging Anatomy

The supraspinatus, infraspinatus, teres minor, and subscapularis contribute to the rotator cuff. The rotator cuff is composed of approximately 75% water and the dry weight composition is approximately 67% type I collagen [23] and 1–5% proteoglycan/glycosaminoglycan [24]. The rotator cuff ultrastructure is complex, with up to five distinct layers that are visible with histological evaluation [25] or MR imaging [26, 27].

An important component of the rotator cuff is the *rotator cable* [28]. Of note, the term *rotator cable* is most commonly utilized in the radiological literature; however the same structure has been described under different names, including the *ligamentum semicirculare humeri* [29, 30], the *transverse band* [25], and the *circular fiber system* [31]. The rotator cable has been described to be an extension of fibrous tissue extending through the rotator interval, which has been termed the coracohumeral ligament (CHL) [25, 32] or the coracoglenohumeral ligament (CGHL) [30] (Fig. 5.1a). The differences in terminology reflect the different perspectives of the dense connective tissue in the rotator interval. While some consider the CHL and superior glenohumeral ligament (SGHL) as separate structures, others have suggested that these structures be considered a single functional unit, called either the CHL (with the SGHL representing a limited portion of this structure) [32] or the CGHL [30].

Burkhart et al. outlined the function of the rotator cable-crescent complex in 1993 [28]. Much like a suspension bridge, the rotator cuff and cable have anterior and posterior supporting limbs, represented by the anterior attachment of the supraspinatus tendon and the posterior attachment of the infraspinatus tendon, respectively. Tears that occur in the thinner, crescentic portion of the cuff between the two intact limbs are felt to be stress-shielded by the cable, explaining why some cuff tears may be less biomechanically significant [28]. In contrast, tears of the rotator cable itself or of the supporting limbs can have dire biomechanical consequences and should be considered for early repair [33–36]. While the rotator cable is consistently identified on anatomic dissections and at surgery [28, 37, 38], it can be seen frequently but not invariably on imaging [37–40]. This may be due to the less conspicuous appearance on imaging (Fig. 5.1b).

The deepest layer of the rotator cuff is the glenohumeral joint capsule [25]. Although previously thought to be only 1–2 mm thick [25], Nimura et al. found a much more substantial contribution of the capsule to the rotator cuff, representing more than half the total tendon width at some locations. According to Nimura et al., the minimum capsular width was 3.5 mm, located near the posterior portion of the supraspinatus footprint, and this was suspected to represent the *crescent* [41]. The joint capsule was found to be thickest at the anterior margin of the greater tuberosity and posterior margin of the infraspinatus tendon, measuring 5.6 and 9.1 mm on average, respectively [42]. These are believed to represent the greater tuberosity attachment sites of the rotator cable [41].

Our understanding of anatomy pertinent to each rotator cuff muscle and tendon continues to evolve. Classic descriptions in standard anatomical textbooks [43, 44] are now known to be inaccurate or incomplete since significant contributions to the literature have occurred within the last decade. Each cuff component has unique anatomical considerations that are important to biomechanical function. This is particularly relevant to the radiologist for diagnosis and to the orthopedic surgeon for anatomic

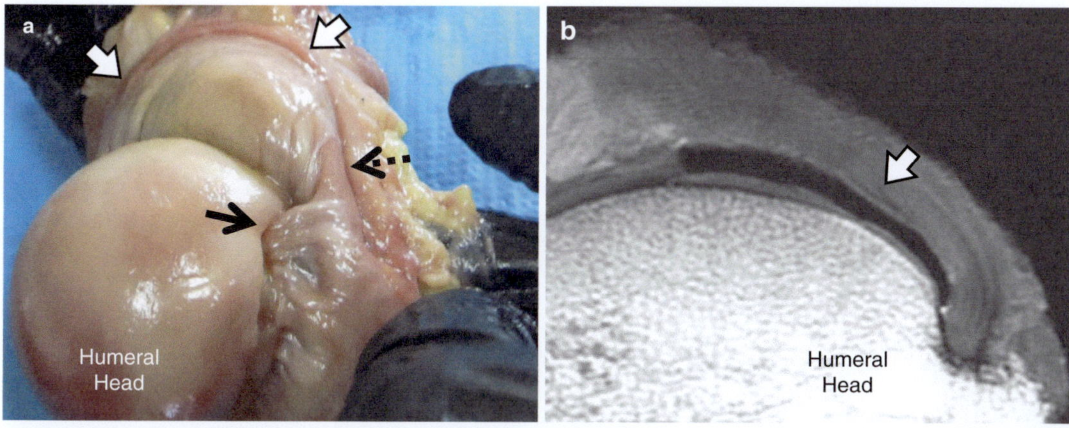

Fig. 5.1 Left shoulder of a cadaveric specimen (94-year-old man). (**a**) Photograph of dissection, viewed from anterosuperior, after reflection of the rotator cuff and capsule shows a distinct rotator cable (thick arrows), which is a continuation of the coracohumeral ligament (black dashed arrow). The superior glenohumeral ligament (black arrow) inserts onto the fovea capitis of the humerus. Diffuse chondrosis is present over the humeral head. (**b**) Coronal oblique intermediate-weighted MR image of the same specimen shows the rotator cable as a thickening of the deep surface of the supraspinatus tendon (thick white arrow), which is less apparent compared with the gross image. Dissected specimen is imaged in air, which appears black in the image

restoration. Pertinent soft tissue and osseous anatomy for each component is further described below.

5.2.1 Supraspinatus

The supraspinatus muscle originates from supraspinous fossa as well as the superior surface of the scapular spine and is composed of distinct anterior and posterior muscle bellies. The anterior muscle belly is approximately 3–6 times larger and also demonstrates a larger variation of pennation angles compared with the posterior belly [45, 46]. The greater force generation and different contraction forces present within the anterior belly may explain the higher incidence of anterior tendon tears [45, 47].

The anterior belly gives rise to a longer, cord-like tendon whereas the posterior belly gives rise to a shorter, quadrangular shaped tendon [45] (Fig. 5.2). The humeral attachment of the rotator cuff tendon is frequently referred to as the *footprint*, a term coined by Tierney et al. in 1999 [48]. The footprint of the supraspinatus was first delineated by Minagawa et al. [49], but has subsequently been redefined and refined several times. Our current knowledge of the supraspinatus footprint is that it predominantly occupies the anteromedial portion of the superior facet (or highest impression) of the greater tuberosity and is triangular or trapezoidal in shape [50, 51]. The lateral-most attachment extends over the lip of the greater tuberosity [48]. Anatomic studies have shown that in approximately a quarter of specimens, fibers from the anterior tendon of the supraspinatus cover the bicipital groove and attach to the lesser tuberosity [50, 51]. Moser et al. described an "aponeurotic expansion" of the anterior supraspinatus tendon, coursing anterior and lateral to the long head of the biceps tendon, inserting distally onto the pectoralis major tendon and evident in approximately half of their cadaveric shoulders and clinical cases [52, 53]. According to Moser et al., this same structure has been previously mistermed a *fourth head of the pectoralis major* [54] and an *accessory biceps tendon* [55–57]. Precise delineation of the anatomy in the anterosuperior aspect of the shoulder requires reconciliation of the rapidly evolving anatomical, surgical, and imaging literature.

The dimensions of the cuff footprint are clinically relevant since partial-thickness tears should be graded as low, moderate, or high grade based

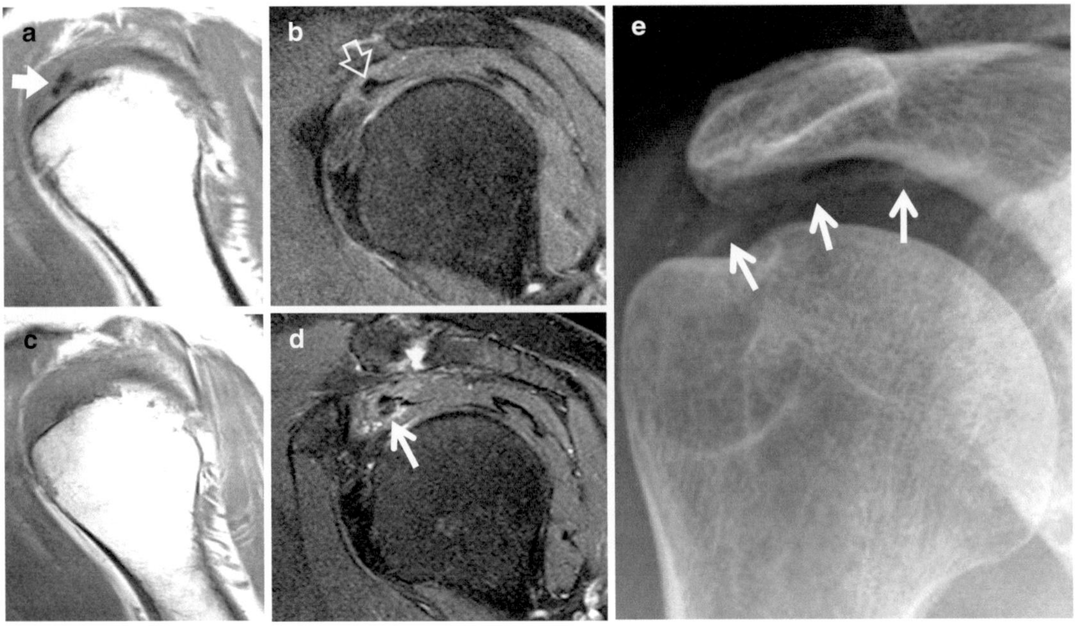

Fig. 5.2 Anatomy and pathology of the anterior muscle belly of the supraspinatus in a 50-year-old man. (**a** and **b**) Sagittal oblique T1-weighted and T2-weighted fat-suppressed MR images, respectively, show calcium hydroxyapatite deposition in the supraspinatus tendon near the footprint (thick arrow). More medially, cordlike tendon of anterior belly is evident (open arrow). Mild subacromial-subdeltoid bursitis was present (not shown). (**c** and **d**) 4 years later, calcium hydroxyapatite had migrated towards the myotendinous junction of the anterior belly with surrounding edema (thin arrow) which separates the tendons of the anterior and posterior muscle bellies of the supraspinatus. (**e**) Concurrent radiograph confirms intra-tendinous migration of crystals (thin arrows)

on depth [58] and anatomic restoration in the setting of repair requires knowledge of the footprint. Unfortunately, reported cuff footprint dimensions have varied widely in the literature, likely due to a combination of variables, including the precise delineation of the boundaries of the footprint, differences in degrees of capsular dissection from the tendon [42], as well as individual variation such as age, gender, patient size, and race. For instance, Curtis et al. described that the supraspinatus tendon extends over the lateral lip of the greater tuberosity [48]; however it is likely that the authors were measuring a portion of the infraspinatus footprint onto what is now called the *lateral facet* [59] (discussed in further detail below). On cadaveric studies, mean supraspinatus footprint width (medial-lateral dimension) has been reported to vary considerably, ranging from 6.7 to 16 mm [42, 46, 48, 50, 51, 60, 61]. Based on the current concept that the supraspinatus footprint is not as large as previously described, mean length (anterior-posterior dimension) measures approximately 20.9–32 mm medially and 1.3–6.4 mm laterally [50, 51]. In contrast to gross measurements, there is a paucity of imaging-based tendon measurements, which some may argue would be the most useful for clinical practice. Karthiekeyan et al. [62] performed ultrasound-based measurements in 120 young healthy shoulders and found mean supraspinatus footprint widths of 14.9 mm in men and 13.5 mm in women. In the same study, mean supraspinatus tendon thickness was 5.6 mm in men and 4.9 mm in women.

5.2.2 Infraspinatus

The infraspinatus muscle originates from the infraspinous fossa as well as the inferior surface of the scapular spine and is composed of two distinct portions. The *oblique* (or inferior) portion is approximately four to five times larger than the *transverse* (or superior) portion [63, 64]. The infraspinatus tendon attaches to the greater tuberosity and, similar to the supraspinatus, the footprint has also been redefined and refined several times in recent years. Kato et al. demonstrated that the footprint is entirely composed of the tendon arising from the oblique portion and that the tendon of the transverse portion is membrane-like and attaches to the posterior surface of the tendinous portion of the oblique part [63, 64].

The greater tuberosity footprint of the oblique portion is larger than what has been historically described. Standard anatomical textbooks recognize three facets (or impressions) of the greater tuberosity: superior (or horizontal), middle (or oblique), and inferior (or vertical) [43, 44]. More recent studies have suggested that the infraspinatus footprint occupies the entire middle facet and approximately half of the superior facet [50, 51]. However, in 2015, Nozaki et al. proposed a fourth facet (or impression) of the greater tuberosity, which they termed the *lateral* facet (Fig. 5.3) [59]. The lateral facet is triangular in shape, variable in size, located posterolateral to the superior facet, and was recognized in all 87 specimens of their study. The authors demonstrated that the anterior extent of the infraspinatus footprint is onto the lateral facet. The orientation of the facets of the humeral tuberosities is related to rotator cuff muscle function and may represent an anatomical factor involved in pathogenesis of rotator cuff tears [65, 66]. Le Corroller et al. demonstrated that a decrease in dorsal orientation of the middle facet in the sagittal plane was associated with higher likelihood of cuff tearing [65].

Similar to the supraspinatus tendon, the reported infraspinatus footprint dimensions have varied widely in the literature. On cadaveric studies, mean infraspinatus footprint width (medial-lateral dimension) has been reported to range from 6.9 to 15.1 mm [42, 48, 50, 51, 60]. Based on the current concept that the footprint of the infraspinatus occupies the entire middle facet and approximately half of the superior facet (or lateral facet), the mean length (anterior-posterior dimension) measures 22.9 mm medially and 25.6–32.7 mm laterally [50, 51]. Of note, Mochizuki et al. found a far anterolateral extent of the infraspinatus footprint, with mean distance between the most anterior edge of the footprint and the bicipital groove measuring 1.3 mm [51]. Lumsdaine et al. found a greater mean distance between the most anterior edge of the infraspinatus footprint and the bicipital groove, measuring 6.4 mm [50]. The differences may be due to ethnic variation since Mochizuki et al. used 128 shoulders from Japanese donors whereas Lumsdaine et al. used 54 shoulders from Australian Caucasoid donors. Using ultrasound on young healthy shoulders, Karthiekeyan et al. [62] found that the mean thickness of the infraspinatus tendon measures 4.9 mm in men and 4.4 mm in women. Michelin et al. measured a mean infraspinatus tendon thickness of 2.2 mm on MRI [67] and 2.4 mm on ultrasound [68].

5.2.3 Teres Minor

The teres minor muscle originates from the middle portion of the lateral edge of the scapula and a variable dense fascia of the infraspinatus muscle [69]. At the myotendinous junction, the teres minor appears as superior and inferior bundles [70]. The superior bundle originates from the lateral edge of the scapula and inserts onto the inferior facet as an oval footprint. The inferior bundle originates from both the lateral edge of the scapula and a dense fascial septum between the infraspinatus and teres minor muscles, and attaches as a band to the surgical neck of the humerus. Saji et al. dissected seven shoulders and found that the dense fascia was aplastic in one case. In the setting of an absent fascia, the teres muscle extends to cover the infraspinatus and the borders between

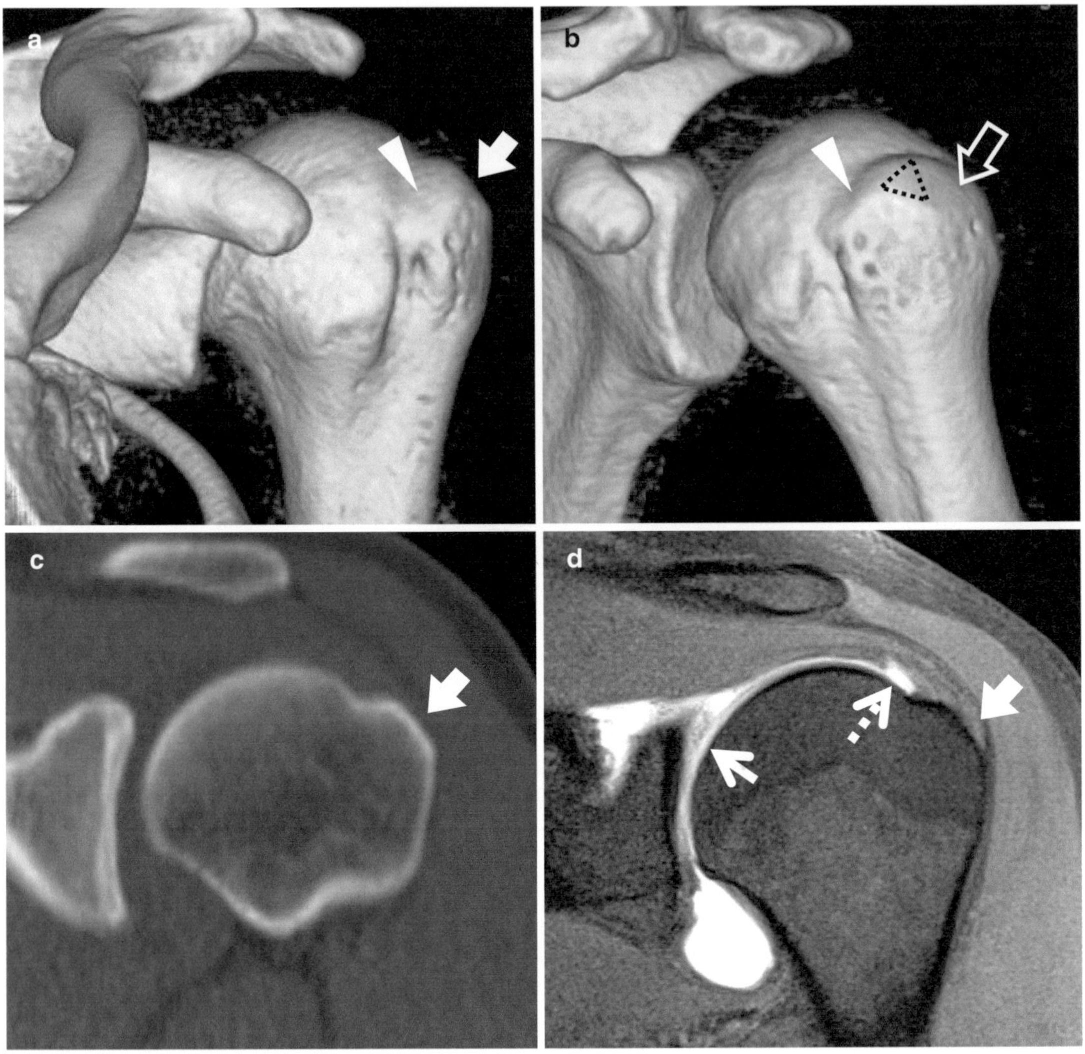

Fig. 5.3 30-Year-old man with a large lateral facet of the greater tuberosity as described by Nozaki et al. (**a** and **b**) Volume-rendered CT images shows the lateral facet in profile (**a**, thick arrow) and en face (**b**, dashed outline). Superior (arrowhead) and middle (open arrow) facets are marked. (**c** and **d**) Coronal oblique CT and T1-weighted fat-suppressed MR arthrogram images show the large lateral facet (thick arrows), which is located posterolateral to the superior facet and represents the anterior infraspinatus footprint and the bursal side of the cuff at this location. Also evident is moderate-grade partial-thickness articular sided tearing of the supraspinatus tendon (dashed arrow) and posterosuperior labral tearing with adjacent chondral damage (thin arrow)

the infraspinatus and teres minor muscles can be difficult to identify on MR imaging [71] (Fig. 5.4).

Similar to the rest of the cuff, reported mean dimensions of the footprint vary widely in the literature. On cadaveric studies, mean width (medial-lateral dimension) ranges from 11.4 to 21 mm and mean length (superior-inferior dimension) ranges from 20.7 to 29 mm [48, 60].

5.2.4 Subscapularis

The subscapularis muscle originates from the medial two-thirds of the anterior surface of the scapula [72]. The superior two-thirds of the subscapularis muscle transitions to tendon at the level of the glenoid and blends with joint capsule fibers before inserting onto the lesser tuberosity [73, 74]. The inferior one-third is the so-called

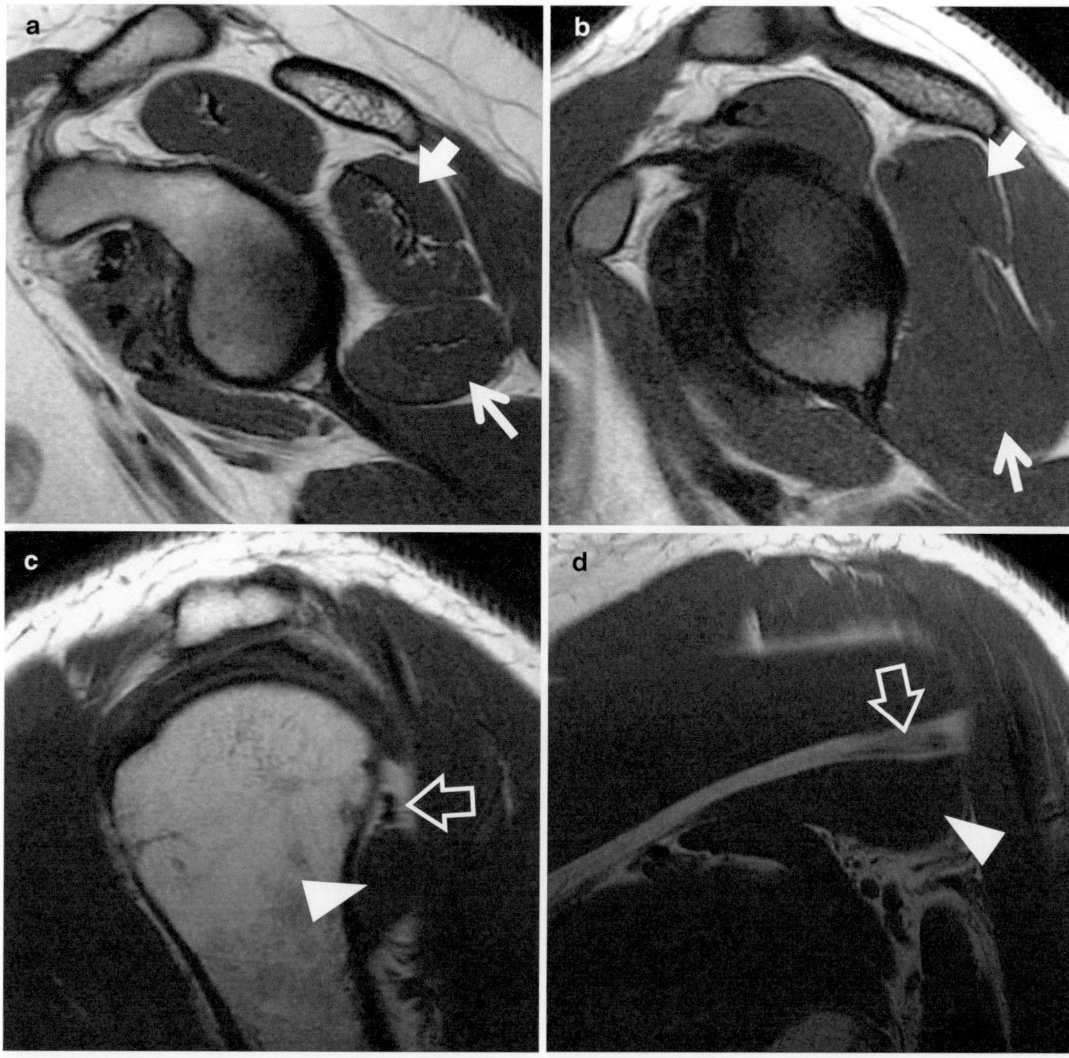

Fig. 5.4 Anatomic variations and pathology of the teres minor muscle. (**a**) Sagittal oblique T1-weighted image of a 21-year-old woman with well-delineated infraspinatus (thick arrow) and teres minor (thin arrow) muscles. (**b**) Sagittal oblique T1-weighted image of a 23-year-old woman with an indistinct boundary between the infraspinatus (thick arrow) and teres minor (thin arrow) muscles, indicating a hypoplastic fascial septum. (**c** and **d**) Sagittal and coronal oblique T1-weighted images in a 53-year-old man with selective atrophy of the superior bundle of the teres minor muscle. An oval-shaped tendon arises from the atrophic superior muscle bundle (open arrow) and attaches onto the inferior facet of the greater tuberosity. The normal inferior bundle attaches onto the posterior aspect of the surgical neck of the humerus (arrowhead)

muscular insertion, attaching onto the surgical neck of the humerus via a thin, membranous structure [66, 73, 74].

Similar to the rest of the cuff, our knowledge of the subscapularis tendon and footprint continues to evolve. The subscapularis tendon is composed of several smaller intramuscular tendons and the superior-most insertion is a thin slip, which attaches to the fovea capitis of the humerus [70, 73] (Fig. 5.5). Many authors have found that the superior glenohumeral ligament also attaches to the fovea capitis [75–77], although some have

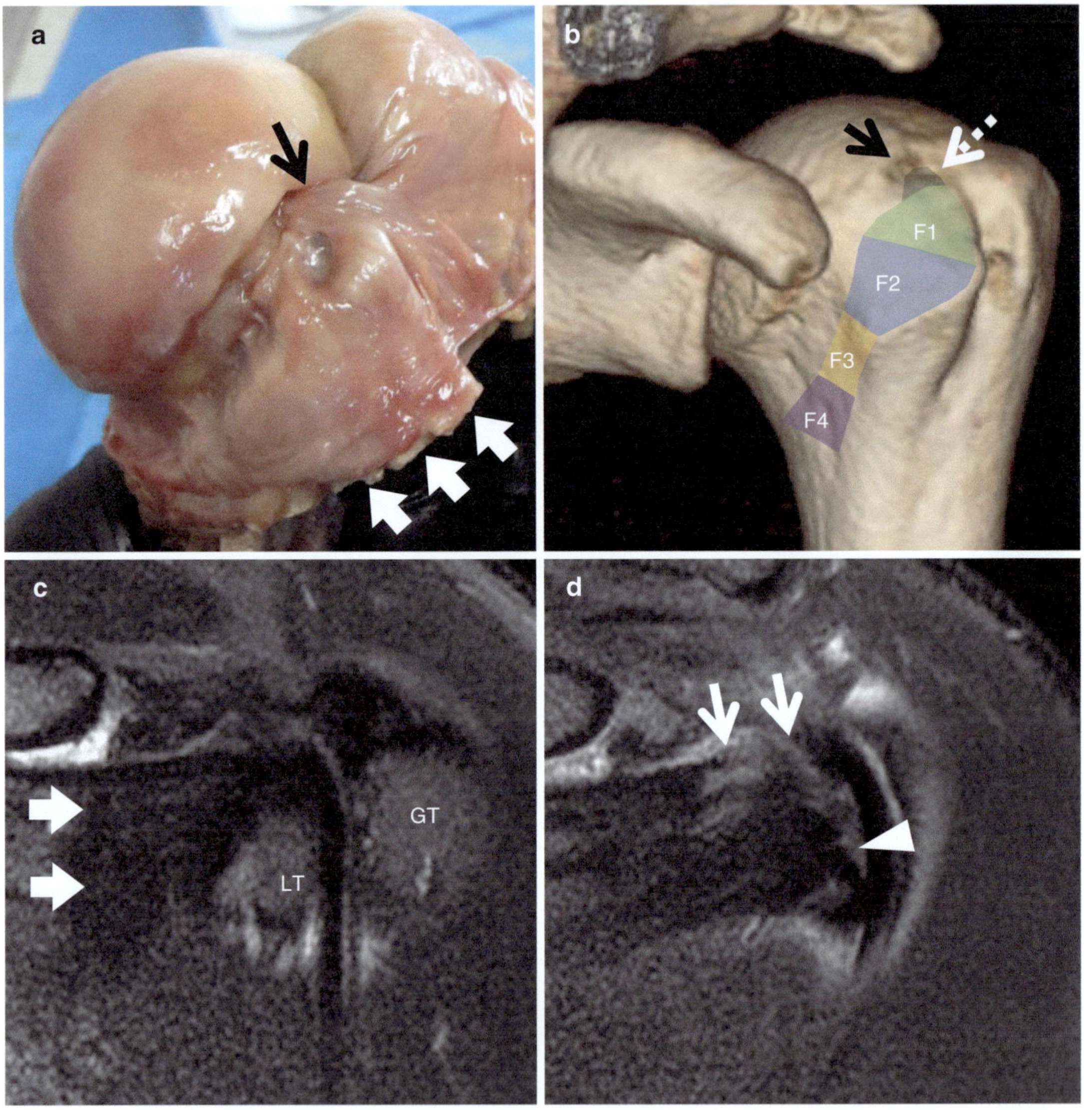

Fig. 5.5 Subscapularis anatomy and pathology. (**a**) Left cadaveric shoulder specimen (same specimen shown in Fig. 5.1, viewed from anterosuperior), after the subscapularis tendon was cut and reflected (thick arrows), shows the articular side of the tendon. Both the superior glenohumeral ligament and superior-most subscapularis tendon insert onto the fovea capitis of the humerus (black arrow). The rotator cable is less apparent than in Fig. 5.1 due to the far reflection of the superior cuff. (**b**) Volume-rendered CT image of the left shoulder of a 34-year-old man demonstrates the four facets of the subscapularis footprint (F1-F4) as described by Yoo et al. [66] as well as superior-most tendon fibers which insert onto the fovea capitis as described by Arai et al. [73] (dashed arrow). (**c**) Coronal oblique T2-weighted fat-suppressed MR image of a 24-year-old man shows an intact subscapularis tendon (thick arrows) inserting onto the top two facets of the lesser tuberosity (LT). Greater tuberosity (GT) is marked. (**d**) Coronal oblique T2-weighted fat-suppressed MR image of a 46-year-old man shows a tear of subscapularis tendon, which involves the superior-most tendon fibers and first two facet attachments. Tear is of full thickness at the first facet (disrupted from articular side through lateral hood, thin arrows) and partial thickness at the second facet (arrowhead)

suggested that the superior glenohumeral ligament attaches to the tendinous slip of the subscapularis instead [78].

Although prior authors have described the footprint of the subscapularis to be shaped as a comma [48, 79] or the state of Nevada [74], a study in 2015 [66] has found that the footprint is best evaluated from a three-dimensional perspective. In a cadaveric and clinical study, Yoo et al. described the three-dimensional footprint anatomy, which consists of four bony facets [66]. The superior-most facet consists of approximately one-third of the entire footprint and the top two facets consist of 60% of the entire footprint. The third and fourth facets represent the so-called *muscular* insertion onto the surgical neck of the humerus (Fig. 5.5b).

Similar to the rest of the cuff, reported mean dimensions of the footprint vary; however, based on cadaveric studies, the mean width (medial-lateral dimension) ranges from 15 to 26 mm and mean length (superior-inferior dimension) ranges from 18 to 24 mm [48, 60, 74, 79]. Yoo et al. [66] found a mean width of 13.5 mm and a combined mean length of 51.5 mm; however their measurements were oblique relative to the standard imaging planes used with imaging, and therefore cannot be directly compared using CT or MRI. Based on studies that have evaluated the mean widths of both supraspinatus and subscapularis tendon footprints [48, 60, 66], a practical guideline is that the superior aspect of the subscapularis footprint should be approximately 25–40% greater than the supraspinatus footprint. Using ultrasound, mean subscapularis tendon thickness has been described to be 4.4 mm in men and 3.8 mm in women [62].

5.2.5 Biceps Pulley

The biceps pulley (or reflection pulley) [32, 78, 80] is an important part of the rotator interval, serving to maintain the position of the long head of the biceps tendon, and the detailed anatomy is covered in Chap. 13. In brief, the pulley system is a tendoligamentous sling, consisting of the coracohumeral ligament (CHL), superior glenohumeral ligament (SGHL), and fibers of the supraspinatus and subscapularis tendons (Fig. 5.6). As described above, the precise delineation of the CHL and SGHL is debatable and some experts advocate for the consideration of these ligaments as a single ligamentous structure with variable parts rather than separate ligaments [30, 32]. However, many other experts describe each structure individually.

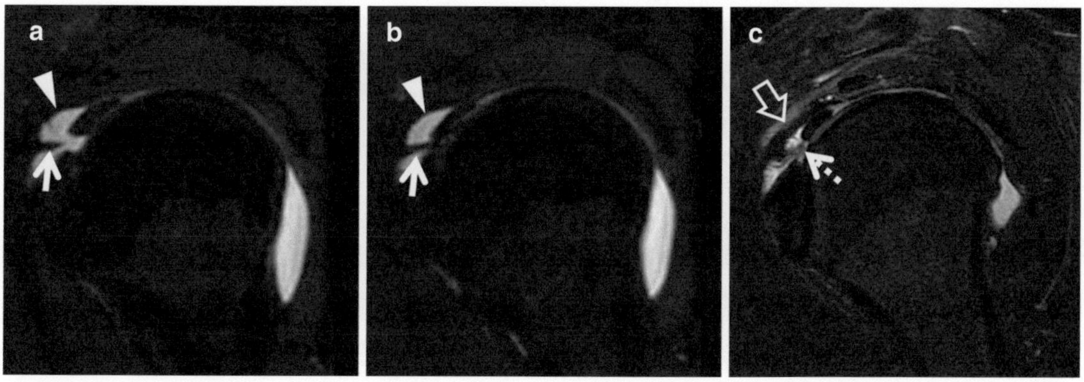

Fig. 5.6 Normal and abnormal biceps pulleys. (**a** and **b**) Reformatted sagittal-oblique MR arthrogram image from a T1-weighted fat-suppressed 3D-FSE acquisition shows a normal biceps pulley, including a normal superior glenohumeral ligament (white arrows) and coracohumeral ligament (arrowheads). (**c**) Sagittal-oblique T2-weighted fat-suppressed image shows a thick coracohumeral ligament (open arrow) with partial tearing of the superior glenohumeral ligament (dashed arrow), consistent with chronic injury. Improved visualization of these structures is made possible due to the presence of a joint effusion and synovial proliferation in the subacromial-subdeltoid bursa

5.3 Pathologic Conditions

This section describes the external (subacromial and subcoracoid) and internal (posterosuperior and anterosuperior) impingement syndromes as well as their imaging manifestations. Subacromial, subcoracoid, and anterosuperior impingement syndromes can affect adults of all ages while posterosuperior impingement is more common in young and middle-aged individuals involved in repetitive overhead motions. By far the most common impingement syndrome is subacromial impingement. For this chapter, rotator cuff disease is discussed together with subacromial impingement, although some degree of cuff disease is typically present in all of the impingement syndromes.

5.3.1 Rotator Cuff Disease and Subacromial Impingement

5.3.1.1 Rotator Cuff Disease: Definition and Characterization

Rotator cuff disease is an umbrella term that can include calcific tendinitis, muscle tearing, or disorders involving the glenohumeral joint capsule (adhesive capsulitis) or subacromial-subdeltoid bursa (tendinobursitis). However, in this chapter we use the term *rotator cuff disease* to refer to tendinopathy and tendon tearing. At the histologic level, tendinosis is characterized by microscopic collagen fiber disruption, a decrease in type I collagen, glycosaminoglycan accumulation, and an increase in water content [81–83].

Tendon tears are macroscopically evident, either by gross inspection or by imaging. Partial-thickness tears can be classified into articular sided, bursal sided, or intra-substance tears (also referred to as interstitial, intratendinous, or concealed tears). It is generally agreed upon that articular sided tears are at least twice as common as bursal sided tears [58, 84] and both have been associated with shoulder impingement syndromes [8]. Cadaveric studies have shown pure intra-substance tears to be twice as common as articular sided tears [85]; however this has not been confirmed in patients at surgery or on imaging, which may be due to inherent limitations with what is considered the reference standard. Partial-thickness tears typically begin 13–15 mm posterior to the biceps tendon, near the junction of the supraspinatus and infraspinatus tendons [86].

The typical site of initiation in the medial-lateral dimension may vary depending on the type of partial-thickness tear. In a study of 12 en bloc surgical specimens with bursal sided tears, Fukuda et al.. found all the tears developing within 1 cm of the insertion, with nine beginning slightly farther away from the insertion [87]. In a similar study of 17 specimens with intra-substance tears, Fukuda et al. found 11 (65%) of the specimens with tears that extended into the enthesis (insertion) [88]. To our knowledge, a histological study documenting the frequencies of articular sided tear initiation sites in the medial-lateral dimension has not been performed, but most authors consider these tears to begin at [86] or near [89] the humeral insertion.

The most commonly used classification of partial-thickness tears is the Ellman classification, which characterizes the cuff based on the assumption that an average intact cuff thickness is 10–12 mm [58]. Partial-thickness tears can be classified as low grade (grade 1, <3 mm deep), moderate grade (grade 2, 3–6 mm deep), or high grade (grade 3, >6 mm deep). The natural history of partial-thickness cuff tears is not well understood and some authors have found low rates of tear progression; however there is biomechanical evidence to support repair of tears involving greater than 50% of the tendon [90]. Based on available data, tears that involve less than 50% of the tendon can be debrided with good results [91].

Full-thickness tendon tears allow communication between the glenohumeral joint and subacromial-subdeltoid bursa. A full-thickness tear can be pinhole in size or involve an entire tendon (which is referred to as a full-thickness, full-width tendon tear). Compared with partial-thickness tears, full-thickness tears are associated with more synovial inflammation and tendon degeneration

[92]. Full-thickness tears of the supraspinatus and infraspinatus tendons can be classified based on shape at the time of surgery [93] or on preoperative MRI [94], although one study found limited concordance for L-shaped tears [95]. A practical method of reporting is to describe the tendons involved and to measure the anterior-posterior and medial-lateral (retraction) dimensions of the tear [96]. Some authors define *massive* cuff tears as full-thickness tears that are greater than 5 cm in the largest dimension and involve two or more rotator cuff tendons [97, 98]. Of note, measurement precision can be limited in the setting of markedly degenerated tissue edges, even at surgery [99]. Delamination of the cuff, defined as intratendinous horizontal splitting between the articular and bursal layers, is common and estimated to be approximately 56% on non-contrast MRI exams [100]. The presence of delamination should be detected on imaging since it can be missed during routine arthroscopy and result in lower healing rates if untreated [101].

Changes in muscle volume can be seen in rotator cuff disease, particularly with chronic tendon tears, likely due to a combination of mechanical unloading [102] and denervation [103]. Although part of the same process, fatty infiltration and muscle atrophy have been shown to be independent predictors of functional outcome after repair [104]. Fatty infiltration and muscle atrophy can be readily detected on CT, ultrasound, and MRI. Both of these processes are important [105, 106], but a complete discussion of muscle disease is beyond the scope of this chapter.

5.3.1.2 External Subacromial Impingement Syndrome: Definition and Associations

The term *impingement syndrome* can be defined as a painful, localized compression of the rotator cuff tendon [107]. The most common subtype of the shoulder impingement syndromes is *external subacromial impingement*, which refers to compression of the rotator cuff by the coracoacromial arch above and the humerus below. There exist so many different uses of the term *subacromial impingement syndrome* in the literature that several authors have proposed abandoning the term altogether and instead using the term *subacromial pain syndrome* [108] or *rotator cuff disease* [109], or simply describing tendinosis or tears of the rotator cuff [110]. However, the term *impingement syndrome* remains commonly used in practice and is recognized as a disease in the tenth revision of the International Statistical Classification of Diseases and Related Health Problems (ICD) published by the World Health Organization.

Much of the controversy behind the term stems from authors who differ in their belief of the relative importance of the factors involved in rotator cuff disease. In 1972, Charles Neer introduced the concept of *impingement syndrome* in his landmark article which included 100 cadaveric scapulae and 46 patients [111]. He suggested that rotator cuff disease resulted from impingement from the anterior one-third of the acromion, coracoacromial ligament, and acromioclavicular joint on the supraspinatus tendon, sometimes extending onto the anterior infraspinatus tendon and long head of the biceps tendon. The belief that extrinsic compression was the primary cause of rotator cuff tendon disease led to the use of the term *impingement syndrome* to be synonymous with *rotator cuff disease* in general [109]. However, we now know that rotator cuff disease can be asymptomatic and therefore labeling all tendon abnormalities as *impingement syndrome* would be inappropriate. In addition, using dynamic ultrasound and MRI, authors have shown that asymptomatic contact can occur between the intact rotator cuff and the acromion, coracoacromial ligament, and acromioclavicular joint, which is felt to be physiologic [112, 113]. Contact alone cannot be labeled as *impingement syndrome* since, by a common definition, pain must be present.

It is now widely recognized that the pathophysiologic cause of rotator cuff disease is multifactorial, although the relative importance of each component remains debated. Regardless of whether or not contact between the cuff and extrinsic structures is causative (primary) or secondarily involved, after the rotator cuff tendon becomes diseased, nociceptive units in tendon, bursa, and subchondral bone become sensitized [114, 115] and physiologic contact forces can induce pain. This is supported by a study from Gellhorn et al. in 2015, who utilized intense focused ultrasound and were not able to elicit sensation in a control group, but in patients with rotator cuff disease sensations were elicited in the cuff, subacromial bursa, and subchondral bone at intensities less than half of what was used in the control group [116].

An abundance of literature has demonstrated many associations between rotator cuff disease and extrinsic structures, including congenital and developmental variants in bone and soft-tissue shape, acquired and often degenerative bone production, as well as os acromiale. The reader should be aware that statistically significant association is insufficient to establish causality without evidence of direction of influence. However, despite the continued controversy of causation, most practitioners would agree that it is important to be aware of lesions that have been associated with rotator cuff disease.

Neer described *proliferative spurs* which were frequently present in cases of impingement, and when anterolateral acromioplasty and coracoacromial ligament release were performed, patient satisfaction and relief of pain were achieved [111]. Subsequent literature has shown that the proliferative spurs described by Neer represent coracoacromial enthesophytes [88, 117, 118] (Fig. 5.7). Coracoacromial enthesophytes as well as lateral deltoid enthesophytes have been associated with full-thickness cuff tears in symptomatic patients [119].

Bigliani et al. [120] proposed a classification of acromial morphology: type I, flat; type II, curved; and type III, hooked. Classification of acromial morphology is controversial with several investigators showing poor reliability using radiographs [121–127]. This may arise from differences in projection angle or confusion in terminology and misclassification of type I and II acromions with subacromial enthesophytes as type III acromions [128]. These differences may explain the vastly conflicting results of some studies. For instance, Nicholson et al. found that acromial morphology is an age-independent, primary anatomic characteristic [129], whereas others have found it to be an age-dependent acquired characteristic [130, 131]. Many authors have found associations of Bigliani type III acromion morphology with cuff degeneration and tearing [122, 123, 132–137]. In addition some authors have found associations of cuff disease with acromial slope in the sagittal [138, 139] or coronal planes [18, 139, 140], whereas others have not [17]. Previous reports have suggested that scapular dyskinesia was involved in the pathogenesis of impingement syndrome [141]; however a systematic review by Ratcliffe et al. in 2014 demonstrated that there is insufficient evidence to support this [142].

Inferiorly directed osteophytes from the acromioclavicular joint have also been associated with rotator cuff tears [143–145]. Many studies have advocated for arthroscopic distal clavicular resection in the presence of rotator cuff pathologies, although nearly all were level IV evidence [146–153]. Randomized, controlled trials (level I evidence) published in 2014 [154] and 2015 [155] found that arthroscopic distal clavicular resection did not result in better clinical or structural outcomes compared with rotator cuff repair alone. In addition, distal clavicular resection can lead to symptomatic acromioclavicular joint instability [154]. However, arthroscopic distal clavicular resection is still frequently performed and therefore radiologists should make note of large osteophytes when present.

Anatomic studies have also focused on the coracoacromial ligament and its role in impingement. The CAL can have a variety of shapes including a Y-, V-, quadrangular, broad band, and multi-banded configurations [156, 157]. Subacromial enthesophytes preferentially form at the anterolateral aspect of the CAL [158]. Additionally, CAL morphologies that demonstrate more than one band have been associated with rotator cuff degeneration [156]. Although some authors have advocated for coracoacromial ligament release, either alone or in combination with other procedures [159–162], biomechanical studies have suggested that the ligament is an important restraint to superior subluxation of the humeral head [163].

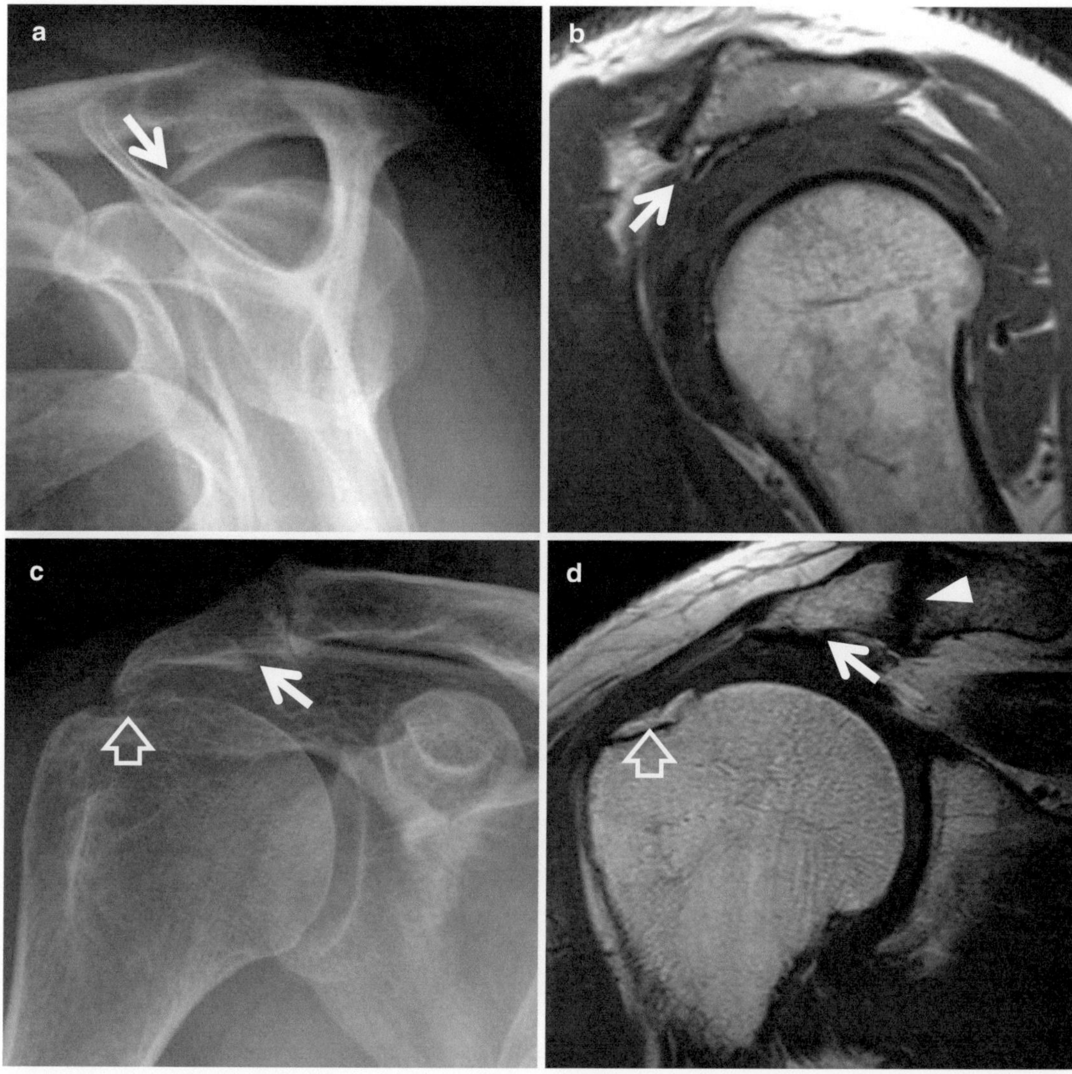

Fig. 5.7 Subacromial enthesophytes associated with rotator cuff disease and external subacromial impingement in a 62-year-old man (**a** and **b**) and a 60-year-old man (**c** and **d**). (**a** and **b**) Supraspinatus outlet radiograph and sagittal-oblique T1-weighted MR image show a large subacromial enthesophyte (thin arrows), which was associated with a full-thickness full-width tear of the supraspinatus and partial-thickness tearing of the biceps tendon (not shown). (**c** and **d**) AP radiograph and coronal oblique T1-weighted MR image show subacromial (thin arrows) and greater tuberosity (open arrows) enthesophytes, which were associated with rotator cuff and biceps tendon disease (not shown). Acromioclavicular joint osteoarthrosis is present (arrowhead)

Os acromiale results from failure of fusion of the anterior acromion during development and has been associated with impingement syndromes and rotator cuff disease [164, 165]. A meta-analysis in 2014 pooled data from 26 articles reported a 7% crude prevalence of os acromiale [166]. The acromial apophysis is composed of four ossification centers: basi-acromion, meta-acromion, meso-acromion, and pre-acromion. The type of os acromiale is defined by the unfused segment immediately anterior to the site of nonunion (Fig. 5.8). The os meso-acromiale subtype is most common (failed fusion between the meta-acromial and meso-acromial ossification centers) (Fig. 5.8a, b) [129, 164, 167]. Pain can arise from the nonunion site itself or from dynamic impinge-

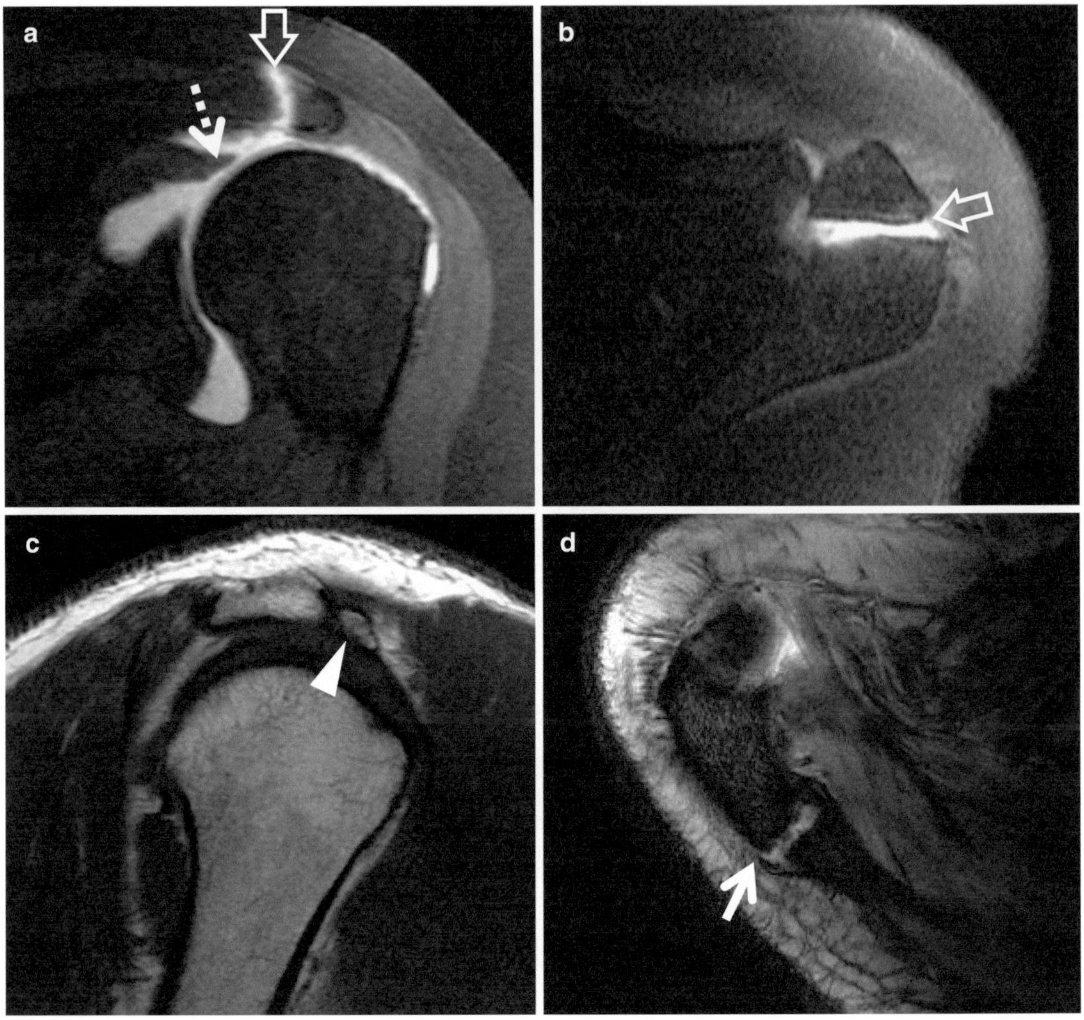

Fig. 5.8 Os acromiale variants in three different patients. (**a** and **b**) Coronal oblique and axial T1-weighted fat-suppressed MR images after contrast injection into the glenohumeral joint show communication with the subacromial-subdeltoid bursa through a retracted, full-thickness supraspinatus tendon tear (dashed arrow). In addition, there is superior subluxation of the humerus with contrast extending into an unstable os meso-acromiale (open arrow). (**c**) Sagittal-oblique T1-weighted MR image shows an os pre-acromiale (arrowhead). (**d**) Axial gradient fat-suppressed MR image shows an os meta-acromiale with degenerative changes (arrow)

ment, whereby deltoid contraction during arm elevation narrows the cuff outlet [168].

5.3.1.3 Radiographic and CT Findings

Radiography is the most appropriate initial imaging modality for evaluation of shoulder pain of any etiology [169]. Calcium hydroxyapatite deposition, fractures, acromioclavicular osteoarthrosis, and glenohumeral osteoarthrosis can be readily diagnosed with radiographs. Local radiographic protocols vary, but all radiographic shoulder studies should include a frontal radiograph, which can either be an anteroposterior (AP) projection with the humerus in neutral, internal, or external rotation or be a Grashey projection, which is in the plane of the scapula.

Although radiographs cannot directly visualize the rotator cuff, the acromiohumeral distance has been used to indirectly evaluate the tendon. A systematic review in 2015 has questioned the reliability of this measurement on radiographs, particularly using non-standardized techniques [170]. Despite this, the acromiohumeral distance continues to be used in general practice. A measurement of less than 6–7 mm has been reported to be a specific sign of a full-thickness cuff tear [171] and the amount of reduced distance is correlated with the size of the tear [172, 173]. More recently, Goutallier et al. suggested that an AHD of less than 6 mm almost systematically involves a full-thickness, full-width, or near-full-width tear of the infraspinatus tendon with advanced fatty degeneration, and is not amenable to surgical repair [174].

Osseous changes near the tuberosities of the humerus have also been reported to be associated with cuff disease. Most but not all [175] studies have found an association between intraosseous cystic changes near the superior facet of the greater tuberosity and cuff disease [176–180]. Similarly, most but not all [178] studies have found the same association for cysts near the lesser tuberosity [181–183]. However, more posteriorly located cysts near the bare area generally have not shown an association with cuff disease [176, 177, 184] and have been considered a normal variant by some authors [185].

The association of enthesophytes, cortical thickening, and subcortical sclerosis at the tuberosities and cuff disease is less well established. There are conflicting results in the literature with some authors finding an association between enthesophyte formation/subcortical sclerosis at the greater tuberosity, and rotator cuff disease (Fig. 5.7c, d) [175, 186] whereas others have found no association [187]. Koh et al. reported that the Grashey view is more sensitive than conventional AP view for the detection of greater tuberosity enthesophytes, cysts, and sclerosis [186].

A subacromial enthesophyte is a highly specific but late radiographic finding of external subacromial impingement (Fig. 5.7) [188–190]. To improve detection of a subacromial enthesophyte, the AP projection can be modified with 30-degree caudal angulation of the beam [189, 191]. The supraspinatus outlet view (also known as the modified trans-scapular lateral or Y- views) is obtained at 5–10° of caudal angulation and can also demonstrate acromial morphology and subacromial enthesophytes (Fig. 5.7a) [191]. Fluoroscopy has a limited role in the evaluation of patients with cuff disease, but may help identify subacromial enthesophytes [192] and may be useful for directing injections.

An os acromiale can be detected on radiographs, with a higher sensitivity using the axillary radiograph compared with the AP view or the supraspinatus outlet view (73.5%) [193]. Familiarity with the appearance of the overlapping shadows of the os acromiale and remaining acromion on the AP and supraspinatus outlet views can facilitate detection [193]. Despite this, a meta-analysis in 2014 demonstrated that crude radiological prevalence (4.2%) was less than half of the true anatomical prevalence (9.6%), confirming the suboptimal sensitivity of radiographs [166].

Computed tomography (CT) arthrography has also been used for evaluation of the rotator cuff, particularly when MR imaging is contraindicated. For evaluation of full-thickness tears of the supraspinatus and infraspinatus tendons, sensitivity and specificity of CT arthrography have been reported to be similar to those of MR arthrography [194, 195]. However, sensitivity for subscapularis tendon tear detection has been shown to be lower compared with the other cuff tendons when evaluated with CT arthrography [194, 196, 197]. In addition, CT arthrography with intra-articular contrast is less sensitive than MRI for partial-thickness tears, especially bursal sided tears [194, 195].

5.3.1.4 Ultrasound Findings

Ultrasound technique and findings of the normal and abnormal rotator cuff are covered in *the Sonographic Evaluation of the Shoulder* chapter. A meta-analysis by Roy et al. in 2015 has found that ultrasound demonstrates comparable diagnostic accuracy to MRI and MR arthrography for the characterization of full-thickness cuff tears with overall sensitivity and specificity estimates greater than 90% [198]. As for the diagnosis of partial tears and tendinopathy on ultrasound, estimates for specificity were high (94%), but sensitivity was lower (68% for partial tears and 79%

for tendinopathy). When considering accuracy, cost, and safety, the authors concluded that ultrasound was the best option [198]. When greater tuberosity irregularities are detected on ultrasound, the operator should have a high index of suspicion for rotator cuff tearing since this finding has been shown to be a reliable indicator [199].

Dynamic assessment of the rotator cuff and surrounding structures can also be performed with ultrasound. Dynamic imaging signs that have been associated with subacromial impingement include increased thickness (also referred as *gathering* or *bunching*) of the subacromial-subdeltoid bursa [200, 201] or supraspinatus tendon [201] lateral to the coracoacromial arch during arm abduction. Less commonly, upward migration of the humeral head during active elevation of the arm prevents passage of the greater tuberosity and cuff beneath the acromion [201]. Other authors have found that thickening of the bursa during abduction is a less useful sign for impingement since it may be seen to a similar degree in healthy volunteers [202] and may be negative in approximately 20% of patients with impingement [203]. Patient pain during dynamic maneuvers should be noted since diagnostic accuracy for impingement is increased when both objective ultrasound signs and subjective pain are simultaneously present [204, 205].

5.3.1.5 MR Findings

There are limited studies evaluating the accuracy of diagnosing tendinosis on MRI. This is largely due to the complex structure as well as the orientation of the rotator cuff. On MRI, tendinosis of cylindrical tendons such as the Achilles is diagnosed by the presence of increased signal intensity [206]. However, unlike the Achilles tendon which demonstrates parallel orientation to the main magnetic field (B_0) through its course, the superior rotator cuff tendon makes a near-90-degree turn as it originates from the muscle and inserts onto the greater tuberosity. It is well known that as collagen fiber orientation approaches 54.7° relative to the main magnetic field, frequency changes from dipolar interactions are minimized and signal intensity is maximum [207]. This is known as the *magic angle effect* [208] and up to a sixfold change in signal intensity has been shown in histologically normal regions of the rotator cuff tendon at 3 T depending on orientation [27]. Furthermore, the rotator cuff is composed of distinct tendons that course in different orientations. For instance, at the superior facet of the greater tuberosity, the predominant orientation of the supraspinatus is medial to lateral whereas the predominant orientation of the anterior infraspinatus tendon fibers is anterior to posterior. This can result in different signal intensities of the individual contributions to the cuff [26, 27, 67].

However, not all increases in intratendinous signal are artifactual and MRI-histology correlation studies have shown that signal increases and increased thickness of the cuff tendon can correlate with histologically determined tendinosis [209, 210]. A practical approach for the diagnosis of tendinosis is to rely on the combined findings of increased signal intensity within the cuff without extension to the articular or bursal surfaces as well as swelling, or increased thickness of the tendon [211]. The signal intensity abnormality should be less than that of fluid. Additionally, in the setting of increased signal without tendon caliber change, recognizing the usual location of the magic angle effect in the adducted shoulder (downsloping region) can prevent false-positive diagnoses [211]. Sein et al. found excellent intra-observer reliability for the grading of MRI-determined supraspinatus tendinosis at 1.5 T (intraclass correlation coefficient, ICC, 0.85), but only fair to good inter-observer reliability (ICC, 0.55). At 3 T, Bauer et al. found excellent intra-observer reliability (kappa, 0.84–0.93) and moderate-to-good inter-observer reliability (kappa, 0.55–0.74) [212].

Partial-thickness tears of the rotator cuff can be diagnosed when there is signal abnormality extending to a surface of the cuff, approaching the intensity of fluid. Increased linear fluid-signal intensity that extends along the long axis of the tendon can represent a partial-thickness intrasubstance tear [34] or delamination when there is communication with the bursal or articular surfaces. The accuracy of MRI for partial-thickness cuff tears is lower than that for full-thickness cuff tears, and meta-analyses have found standard MRI to demonstrate 64–67% sensitivity and 92–94% specificity and direct MR arthrography to demonstrate 83–86% sensitivity and 93–96% specificity [198, 213]. Pitfalls for the diagnosis of a partial-thickness tear include volume averaging for small tears due to a low ratio between tear size and voxel size as well as fibrovascular tissue residing in the tear, both of which will cause signal intensity to be less than that of fluid. A unique partial-thickness bursal sided tear involves the transverse head of the infraspinatus tendon, which can be avulsed and retracted from the oblique portion [26, 63].

Full-thickness tears of the rotator cuff typically demonstrate a fluid signal intensity defect [214]. MRI is very accurate for full-thickness cuff tears with meta-analyses showing 90–92% sensitivity and 93% specificity for standard MRI and 90–95% sensitivity and 95–99% specificity with direct MR arthrography [198, 213]. For the diagnosis of partial- or full-thickness tendon tears using indirect MR arthrography, studies have shown comparable sensitivity, specificity, and accuracy with direct MR arthrography [215, 216]. In addition, a study in 2014 has suggested that a single 3D T1-weighted FSE sequence is comparable to conventional 2D sequences [217].

5.3.2 External Subcoracoid Impingement

5.3.2.1 Definition

External subcoracoid impingement (also known as coracoid impingement) is an uncommon cause of anterior shoulder pain, resulting from impingement of the subscapularis or biceps tendon between the coracoid process and lesser tuberosity [218–221]. Unfortunately a literature review by Martetschlager et al. [222] in 2011 found that our knowledge of subcoracoid impingement is not supported by rigorous scientific studies, especially with regard to diagnosis, physical examination, imaging, treatment options, and expected outcomes. In fact, there have been no prospective randomized trials or comparative studies published to date. However, the concept of subcoracoid impingement has been recognized for over a century [223].

External subcoracoid impingement may be due to idiopathic, iatrogenic, or traumatic causes. Idiopathic causes include anatomic variations, such as a long coracoid process, protuberant lesser tuberosity, or space-occupying lesions including ganglion cysts and heterotopic ossification [220, 222, 224–228]. Iatrogenic causes include surgical procedures such as coracoid transfer, posterior glenoid osteotomy, or acromionectomy [220]. Posttraumatic causes can be due to fractures of the scapula, including the coracoid process, glenoid or neck, or proximal humerus [220]. Furthermore, anterior glenohumeral instability can also cause narrowing of the coracohumeral distance [229, 230].

The diagnosis of subcoracoid impingement is challenging. Symptoms are described as dull, anterior shoulder pain aggravated by forward flexion and internal rotation [220]. The most common findings reported on imaging include subscapularis tendon disease (either bursal sided or articular sided [8]) and/or narrowing of the coracohumeral interval, which is the space between the coracoid process and anterior humerus.

5.3.2.2 Radiographic and CT Findings

Radiographs may demonstrate a far laterally projecting or a chevron-shaped coracoid process on the AP or supraspinatus outlet views, respectively [231, 232]. Axillary views have not been reported to be helpful for diagnosis [233]. Cystic changes near the lesser tuberosity may be present [233]. The coracoid index was first described on CT, defined as the lateral projection of the coracoid process beyond the glenoid joint line [233]. Dines et al. reported a mean value of 8.2 mm (range—2.5 to 25 mm) in healthy shoulders and an index of 23.5 mm in one of their patients [233]. The coracohumeral interval has also been measured on CT. In healthy shoulders, Gerber et al. reported a mean value of 8.7 mm for an adducted arm and 6.8 mm for the arm in flexion and internal rotation, concluding that subcoracoid impingement was more likely during forward flexion of a shoulder

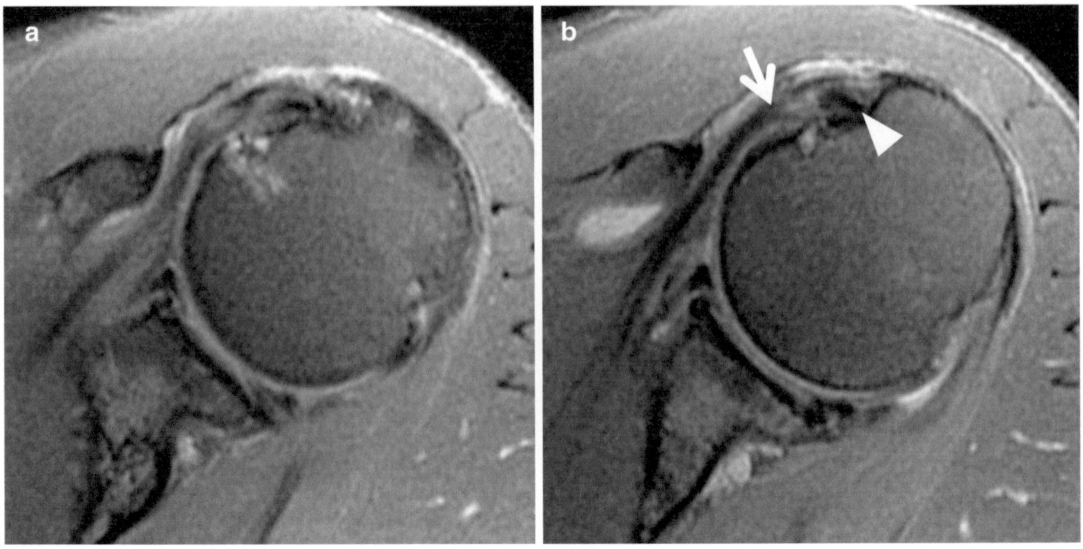

Fig. 5.9 67-year-old man with left shoulder pain. (**a** and **b**) Axial intermediate-weighted MR images show a high-grade partial-thickness tear of the subscapularis tendon involving the articular side and lateral hood (arrow). The biceps tendon is also partially torn and medially subluxed (arrowhead). There is a narrowed coracohumeral interval, measuring 5 mm, with cystic changes within the lesser tuberosity. Subcoracoid and subacromial-subdeltoid bursitis is present. Subcoracoid impingement was raised which was clinically confirmed

with a far laterally projecting coracoid tip close to the scapular neck [234]. Masala et al. also found that CT was useful for the measurement of the coracohumeral interval and was sensitive to even slight bone changes [235]. Abnormal coracohumeral interval values have been described on MRI and subsequently adopted to CT, although to date there are no studies correlating measurements made between the two modalities.

5.3.2.3 Ultrasound Findings

Tracy et al. performed sonography on asymptomatic volunteers and patients with the clinical diagnosis of subcoracoid impingement. Using a linear array transducer with the arm adducted across the chest, mean coracohumeral distance was 12.2 mm (range 7.8–17.5 mm) for the volunteers and 7.9 mm (range 5.9–9.6 mm) for the patients. In addition, in patients with subcoracoid impingement, bursal thickening in the subcoracoid region can be seen which can cause an anterior snapping sensation visible on dynamic sonography [236, 237]. As described above, ultrasound is also useful for the diagnosis of subscapularis tendon disease, including tendinosis.

5.3.2.4 MR Findings

Several investigators have reported on coracohumeral intervals as measured on MRI [8, 238–245] (Fig. 5.9). Although previous authors have found statistically significant differences in mean values between individuals with and without subcoracoid impingement, no ideal cutoff value exists with high sensitivity and specificity [241]. However, in patients clinically suspected to have subcoracoid impingement, a value of 6 mm or less has been used to be consistent with the disease [8, 241–244].

Associated subscapularis tendon disease can be diagnosed on MRI. Partial-thickness tendon tears can be articular sided, bursal sided (involving the anterior surface), or intra-substance (also called *interstitial delamination* [246] or a *concealed lesion* [66]). Full-thickness tears demonstrate a focus of complete tendon discontinuity [247], which can either extend from the articular side to the bursal side or extend from the articular side to the lateral edge of the tendon (also termed the *lateral hood* or *lateral end* [66]) when involving the footprint (Fig. 5.5d). Several classifications of subscapularis tendon tears exist, including the LaFosse [248], Fox and Romeo [249], and the Yoo classifications [66]. However, similar to the superior cuff, a practical method is to describe partial- or full-thickness involvement and the location of the tear, and provide measurements in the superior-inferior and medial-lateral (retraction) directions. Involvement of the inferior, extra-articular portion of the tendon (so-called muscular attachment) or tears of the myotendinous portions should be described since these may influence the decision for an open rather than arthroscopic approach for repair [250].

Combined full-thickness tears that involve the subscapularis and supraspinatus tendons are referred to as anterosuperior rotator cuff tears [251], and have been associated with combined subcoracoid and subacromial impingement [242]. The retracted edges of the two tendons can be connected by a bridge of connective tissue which has been described to represent the coracohumeral ligament [25, 32, 252]. This tissue has been called the "comma sign" [253] at surgery or the "bridging sign" on MRI [254] and may be thickened to various degrees. Recognition of this sign is useful to avoid misdiagnosing an intact subscapularis tendon [254] or a medially dislocated long head of the biceps tendon.

5.3.3 Internal Posterosuperior Impingement

5.3.3.1 Definition

The term *posterosuperior impingement* is typically, but not always, used in association with the throwing shoulder [255, 256]. Similar to external subacromial impingement, the term and concept of *posterosuperior impingement* are controversial. It is generally accepted that there is physiologic contact of the undersurface of the cuff against the edge of the glenoid in the abducted, externally rotated position [257, 258]. Furthermore, it is generally accepted that posterosuperior impingement can cause articular sided tears of the superior rotator cuff in throwing athletes. However, there are two different views of posterosuperior impingement in the literature with regard to throwing athletes: those who believe that it explains the mechanism of most articular sided tears of the superior rotator cuff and those who believe that it explains only a minority of them.

In 1992, Walch et al. proposed that repetitive, forceful contact leads to cuff tearing in throwing athletes [255, 259]. Subsequent authors supported this view for several years, although there was disagreement about the anterior capsuloligamentous structures in the disabled throwing shoulder [256, 257]. Some believed that the presence of anterior instability worsened internal impingement [256, 260, 261], whereas others believed that instability was not a typical part of the pathology in the throwing shoulder [257]. Burkhart et al., in a series of articles published in 2003, summarized the literature and proposed a pathologic cascade in the throwing shoulder, beginning with acquired posteroinferior capsular contracture [262]. This results in a posterosuperior shift of the glenohumeral contact point during the late cocking phase, allowing hyper-external rotation of the humerus due to reduced camming effect, but causing peel-back forces which could lead to a SLAP lesion. Burkhart theorized that cuff failure in throwing athletes was typically due to repetitive tensile and torsional loading rather than impingement, although cuff tearing due to internal impingement could be seen in pitchers who hyper-externally rotate their arms in excess of 130° during the late cocking phase [262, 263].

Unfortunately, there is no consensus of the causative pathophysiologic process of the disabled throwing shoulder. In the literature, there are several imaging findings that have been associated with *posterosuperior impingement* and the disabled throwing shoulder. However, it should be emphasized that the use of the term *posterosuperior impingement* differs between individual physicians and practices. The radiologist is urged to reconcile their nomenclature with their referring physicians.

5.3.3.2 Radiographic and CT Findings

In patients diagnosed with posterosuperior internal impingement, cystic changes of the greater tuberosity may be seen on radiographs in approximately half [264], although similar findings have also been reported in 39% of asymptomatic professional baseball pitchers [265]. Remodeling of the posterior glenoid rim can also be seen radiographically, although cross-sectional imaging would optimally evaluate this region [264].

Bennett lesions, which are described as mineralization near the posteroinferior glenoid rim, have been defined exclusively in baseball pitchers, although they are seen in approximately 22% of asymptomatic major league baseball pitchers [265–267]. Bennett lesions are theorized to be caused by traction on the posterior band of the inferior glenohumeral ligament and may also be identified on CT [268, 269].

5.3.3.3 Ultrasound Findings

As described above, ultrasound is sensitive for partial-thickness articular sided tears of the rotator cuff. In patients diagnosed with posterosuperior internal impingement, ultrasound may demonstrate cortical irregularity of the posterolateral humeral head region [270]. In addition, posterosuperior labral detachment or tears may be seen, characterized as an anechoic or hypoechoic cleft between the labrum and glenoid or within the labral substance, respectively. This may be emphasized with dynamic ultrasound and may be associated with paralabral ganglion cysts [270]. Posterior capsular thickening may be associated with the diagnosis of internal impingement and can be measured with ultrasound [271].

5.3.3.4 MR Findings

Direct MR arthrography is most useful for evaluation of the constellation of imaging findings associated with posterosuperior internal impingement, which includes cystic changes near the posterolateral humeral head, partial-thickness articular sided tears of the infraspinatus and posterior supraspinatus tendons, and posterosuperior labral lesions [272–274] (Fig. 5.10). For partial-thickness cuff tears, meta-analyses have found that direct MR arthrography is slightly superior to standard MRI with a higher range of sensitivity (83–86% vs. 64–67%, respectively), but comparable specificity (93–96% vs. 92–94%, respectively) [198, 213]. For labral tears, meta-analyses have found that direct MR arthrography appears marginally superior to standard MRI with higher sensitivity (83 vs. 79%, respectively) and specificity (93 vs. 87%) [275, 276]. In pitchers with glenohumeral internal rotation deficits, posterior capsular fibrosis may be evident on MR arthrography [277]. Tuite et al. found a tendency for a thicker posteroinferior labrum and shallower capsular recess in overhead throwing athletes with internal impingement and internal rotation deficit compared with controls using the standard, adducted MRI position [278].

The abducted and externally rotated (ABER) position may be helpful to detect delamination of the rotator cuff tendon (Fig. 5.10d) and for increased accuracy for diagnosis of labral lesions [279–281], although it adds an extra 5–10 min to the examination due to necessary patient repositioning and coil changes. As described above, physiologic contact between the undersurface of the rotator cuff and posterosuperior glenoid in the ABER position is considered physiologic [257].

5.3.4 Internal Anterosuperior Impingement

5.3.4.1 Definition

Anterosuperior impingement is less well defined compared with the previously discussed entities. This entity was first described in 2000 by Gerber and Sebesta in 16 patients, nearly all of whom were involved with regular overhead activity, most during their profession as manual laborers [282]. The authors postulated that repetitive contact of the superior subscapularis tendon and biceps pulley against the anterosuperior glenoid rim caused damage to these structures since pain could be reproduced when the arm was horizontally adducted, internally rotated, and positioned with various degrees of anterior elevation [282].

In 2002, Struhl reported on ten nonathletic patients who demonstrated partial-thickness articular sided tears of the supraspinatus tendon which appeared to be compressed between the humeral head and the anterosuperior labrum [283]. Struhl

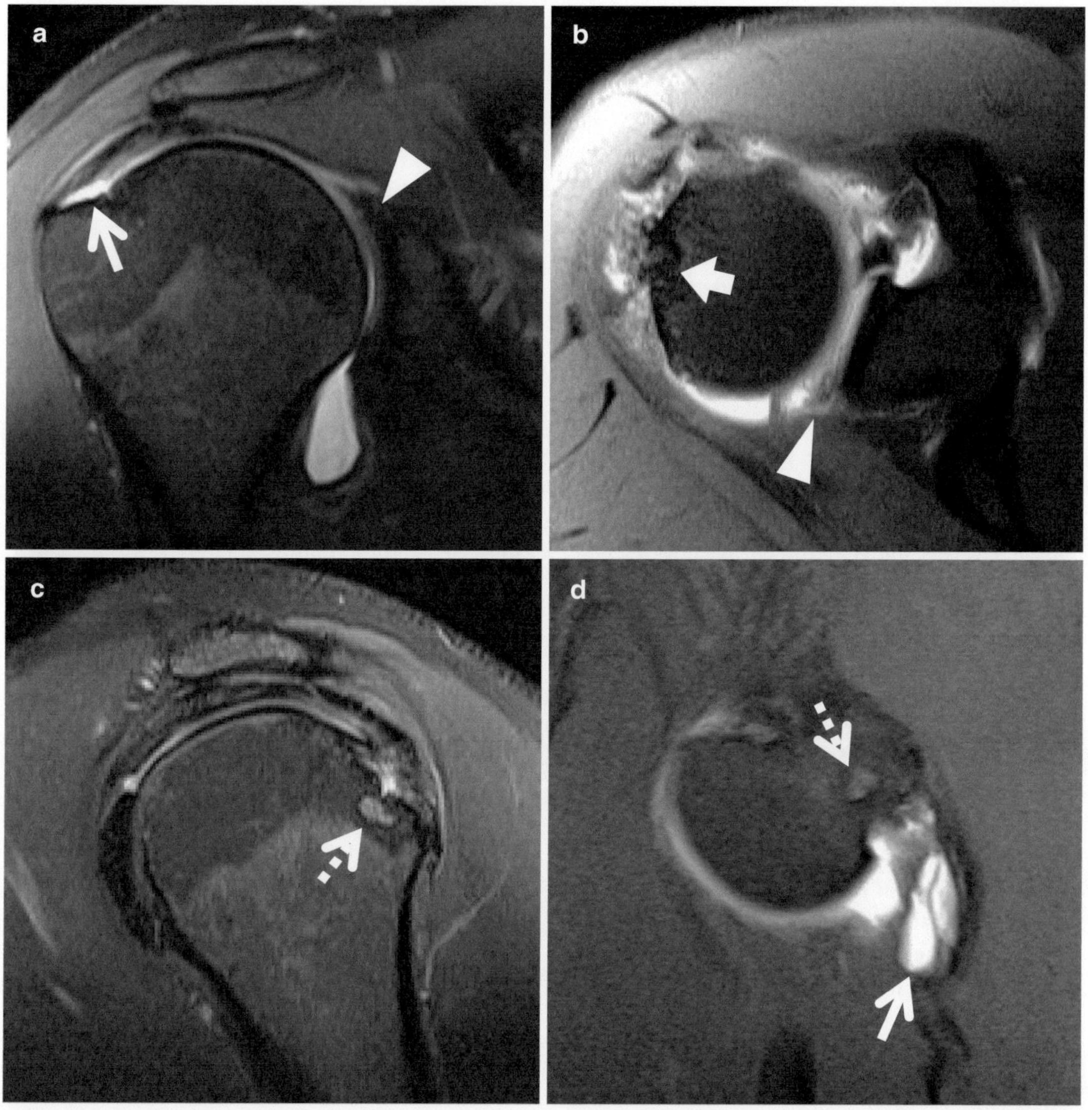

Fig. 5.10 MR arthrogram images of a 30-year-old major league baseball pitcher with shoulder pain. (**a**) Coronal intermediate-weighted fat-suppressed image shows a high-grade, partial-thickness, articular sided tear at the footprint of the supraspinatus-infraspinatus tendon junction (arrow). A posterosuperior labral tear is present (arrowhead). (**b**) Axial T1-weighted fat-suppressed image confirms labral tear (arrowhead) and shows marked irregularity at the greater tuberosity (thick arrow). (**c**) Sagittal intermediate-weighted fat-suppressed image confirms cystic changes near the posterosuperior aspect of the humeral head with adjacent articular sided tearing of the infraspinatus tendon. (**d**) ABER view improves delineation of the extent of medial delamination (arrow). The same posterosuperior humeral head cyst is seen (dashed arrow)

stated that contact of the cuff and superior labrum was normal in the intact shoulder, but abnormal in the setting of cuff tears. Nearly all his patients had identical clinical presentations to subacromial impingement, but the arthroscopic findings were consistent with the entity of *anterior internal impingement*. Subsequent authors have interpreted his study to refer to anterosuperior internal impingement [284, 285]. Notably, Struhl did not diagnose biceps pulley lesions in any of his patients and in only two of the ten cases was a subscapularis tendon tear present [283].

In 2004, Habermeyer defined *anterosuperior impingement* as the presence of an anterosuperior labral lesion and positive impingement of the subscapularis tendon between the lesser tuberosity and anterosuperior glenoid rim in the flexed, horizontally adducted, and internally rotated position during arthroscopy [284]. He included 89 patients, none of whom performed regular overhead activity, but all with surgically confirmed pulley lesions. Notably he excluded patients with complete tears of the supraspinatus or subscapularis tendons. He found that the presence of anterosuperior impingement increased when a partial-thickness articular sided tear of the subscapularis tendon was present. Habermeyer proposed a classification scheme and outlined the pathologic cascade, which begins with a degenerative or traumatic tear of the biceps pulley [284]. During the anterosuperior impingement position, the long head of the biceps tendon medially subluxates and causes a tear of the subscapularis tendon. Due to a lack of dynamic soft-tissue restraints, the humeral head migrates anterosuperiorly, impinging against the glenoid rim and causing the entity of anterosuperior impingement [284].

The diagnosis of anterosuperior impingement is very challenging and there are only a handful of scientific articles from which to draw conclusions. First, there is no patient population that is typically affected. Anterosuperior impingement has been diagnosed in young and elderly patients [282, 284]. Additionally, patients may be regularly engaged in overhead activities [282] or not [284], or may even be wheelchair bound [272, 286]. Second, clinical tests have not been reported to be sensitive or specific for this entity [283, 285]. Third, the existing literature does not support a mandatory lesion. The pulley system was surgically intact in 3 of the 16 patients in Gerber and Sebesta's study [282] and in presumably most of the patients in Struhl's study [283]. Furthermore, anterosuperior impingement has been diagnosed in many patients without subscapularis tendon lesions [283, 284]. Fourth, although used as a criterion in Habermeyer's study [284], subsequent cadaveric and in vivo MRI studies have shown that contact between the subscapularis tendon and glenoid rim typically occurs during the Hawkins position (90-degree forward elevation and maximal internal rotation) [287, 288]. Finally, authors have noted that anterosuperior impingement tests may be negative in patients with pulley lesions, suggesting that anterosuperior impingement is not the only pathomechanism for pulley lesions [289].

5.3.4.2 Imaging Findings

As described above, there are no pathognomonic lesions for the diagnosis of anterosuperior impingement. However, several articles have focused on the biceps pulley, and in particular the superior glenohumeral ligament [284, 290]. Habermeyer [284] described a surgical classification scheme for intra-articular lesions associated with anterosuperior impingement which has been adopted to MR arthrography: group 1 lesions involve the superior glenohumeral ligament (SGHL), group 2 lesions involve the SGHL with partial-thickness articular sided supraspinatus tendon tears, group 3 lesions involve the SGHL with partial-thickness articular sided subscapularis tendon tears, and group 4 lesions involve the SGHL with both partial-thickness articular sided supraspinatus and subscapularis tendon tears.

Diagnosis of SGHL abnormalities can be readily made with MR arthrography [77, 291], or in the presence of a joint effusion (Figs. 5.6c and 5.11a). The biceps tendon may be subluxed, dislocated, and torn to various degrees [284]. Subscapularis tendon tears are usually visible to some degree in all three standard imaging planes, including coronal oblique (Fig. 5.5), sagittal oblique [290], and axial (Fig. 5.9) [292] planes and all three should be used for complete evaluation. According to Habermeyer's theory, an unstable biceps tendon causes the subscapularis tendon to tear, and these would invariably involve the superior-most fibers (Fig. 5.11). However, it should be reinforced that full-thickness tears of the subscapularis tendon are excluded in Habermeyer's classification Scheme [284], although they may be seen in later stages of the disease.

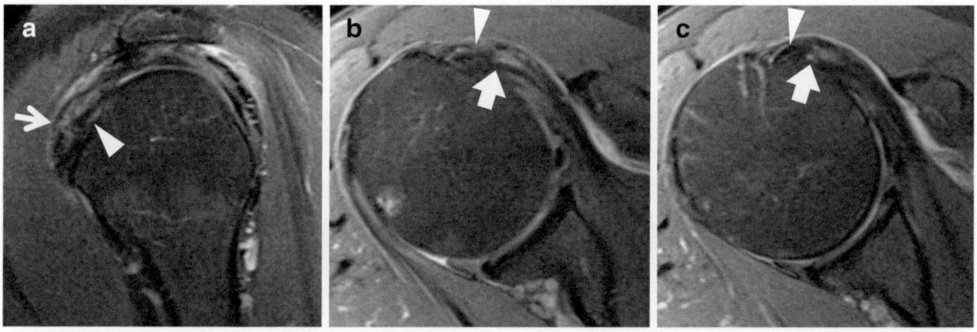

Fig. 5.11 53-year-old woman with shoulder pain during elevation and internal rotation of the arm. (**a**) Sagittal-oblique intermediate-weighted fat-suppressed image shows a tear of the superior glenohumeral ligament (arrow) and partial tearing of the long head of the biceps tendon (arrowhead). Subacromial-subdeltoid and subcoracoid bursitis is present. (**b** and **c**) Axial intermediate-weighted fat-suppressed images including at the level of the superior edge of the subscapularis tendon (**b**) show tendon tearing involving the superior-most fibers of the subscapularis at the lateral hood with delamination (thick arrow). The partially torn long head of the biceps tendon is medially subluxed (arrowhead). Anterosuperior impingement was suggested based on imaging, and confirmed by the orthopedic surgeon

5.4 Postoperative Imaging

Surgical therapy for the impingement syndromes is primarily directed at the rotator cuff, which includes debridement or repair. Although many surgeons routinely perform partial acromioplasty and coracoacromial ligament release, existing level I and level II studies do not support their routine use [293]. Incidence of rotator cuff repairs is increasing, particularly with arthroscopic techniques [294], which have become favored over open or mini-open techniques. In general, arthroscopic repair of full-thickness rotator cuff tears leads to good clinical outcomes [295, 296]. Structural failure after cuff repair is common, although counterintuitively a number of studies with high levels of evidence have shown a lack of correlation between recurrent tear and clinical or functional outcomes [295, 297]. This was confirmed in a systemic review and meta-analysis published in 2015 covering over 30 years of studies [296]. The reasons behind this are unclear and this remains an area of intense study.

5.4.1 Techniques

For appropriate interpretation of postoperative images, familiarity with the common techniques used for repair is necessary. High-grade partial-thickness tendon tears can be repaired through an arthroscopic trans-tendon repair technique where a single row of suture anchors are placed at the medial margin of the rotator cuff footprint [298, 299] or surgical completion of the tear and subsequent full-thickness cuff repair [300]. A meta-analysis published in 2015 found that the existing evidence supports the trans-tendon technique rather than tear conversion followed by repair for partial-thickness articular sided tears involving more than 50% of the thickness [301]. Full-thickness tendon tears can be repaired in a number of different ways, which depend on surgeon preference and many patient variables. The goal of surgical treatment of full-thickness tendon tears is to recreate the native anatomy. However, full-thickness tears that have a large medial-lateral component with poor mobility of the retracted tendon edge result in fewer choices for the orthopedic surgeon. Side-to-side suturing of the tendon edges can be performed to close the defect, either without (Fig. 5.12) [302] or with fixation of the converged tendon margin to bone [303].

Torn rotator cuff tendons that can be reduced to the greater tuberosity without undue tension are transfixed with sutures that pass through bone tunnels or through a suture anchor. These anchors can be made of metal alloy or biocomposite material, which may be partially or entirely bioresorbable [304]. Traditionally, arthroscopic rotator cuff repair used a single row of suture

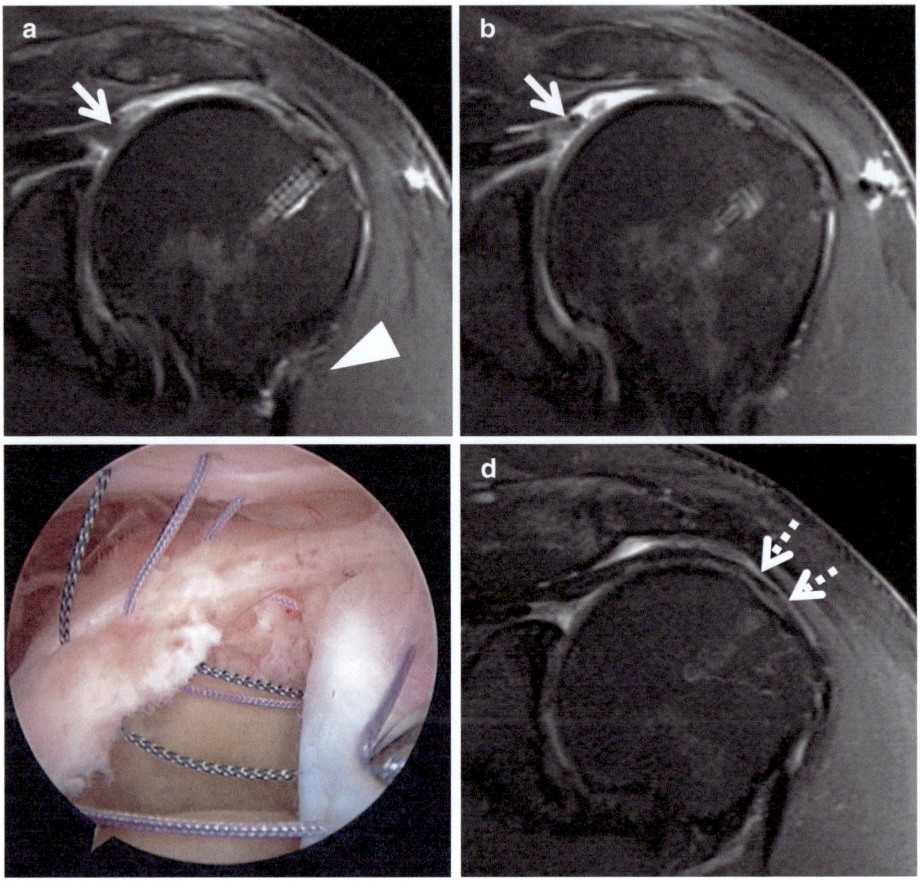

Fig. 5.12 54-year-old man with previous cuff repair 1 year prior, now with worsening shoulder pain and U-shaped tear. (**a** and **b**) Coronal oblique intermediate-weighted fat-suppressed MR images show a full-thickness retear of the supraspinatus tendon with differential retraction to the glenoid margin. Superior migration of the humeral head is evident. (**c**) Arthroscopic image during revision surgery with scope in subacromial-subdeltoid bursa through posterior portal shows side-to-side tendon repair. Sutures extend across U-shaped tear. (**d**) Coronal oblique intermediate-weighted fat-suppressed MR image 3 years after revision surgery shows an attenuated but intact repair (dashed arrows). Subacromial-subdeltoid bursitis was present, but no full-thickness tear was visualized

anchors placed in the greater tuberosity in a linear anterior-to-posterior configuration, which could either be medial or lateral. However, this has been shown to only restore approximately 67% of the original cuff footprint [305], and the double-row repair was devised in an attempt to create more surface contact between the healing tendon and bone. The double-row repair was initially described with a medial row of anchors with sutures in a mattress configuration and a lateral row of anchors with sutures in a simple configuration, but subsequent studies showed limited contact pressures between tendon and bone compared with newer double-row techniques [306, 307]. One double-row technique that has gained popularity is the transosseous equivalent, otherwise known as the suture bridge technique. This was developed in 2006 by Park et al. [308] to optimize footprint contact area, pressure, and pullout strength. The transosseous equivalent technique uses a medial row of suture anchors and a lateral row of knotless anchors. The double-row techniques, including the transosseous equivalent technique, are significantly stronger than single-row repairs in time-zero cadaveric studies and several studies have suggested higher rates of healing [295, 297, 309]. True arthroscopic transosseous (anchorless) fixation has also been described [310], although biomechanical studies have shown superior results with transosseous equivalent techniques [311].

5.4.2 Imaging

In patients with persistent or new shoulder pain after surgical therapy, imaging may be indicated. First-line imaging modalities of the postoperative cuff include ultrasound, MRI, or MR arthrography. Prickett et al. used ultrasound to evaluate postoperative rotator cuff integrity and reported the sensitivity, specificity, and accuracy to be 91, 86, and 89%, respectively [312]. However, Lee et al. found that accuracy of ultrasound for the postoperative cuff was 78% when compared to MR arthrography [313]. They found that ultrasound accuracy increased to 93% with the use of intra-articular contrast (arthrosonography) [313]. MRI without or with intra-articular contrast can be used to evaluate the status of the repaired rotator cuff [300, 314–316] (Fig. 5.13). The appearance of the repaired rotator cuff on

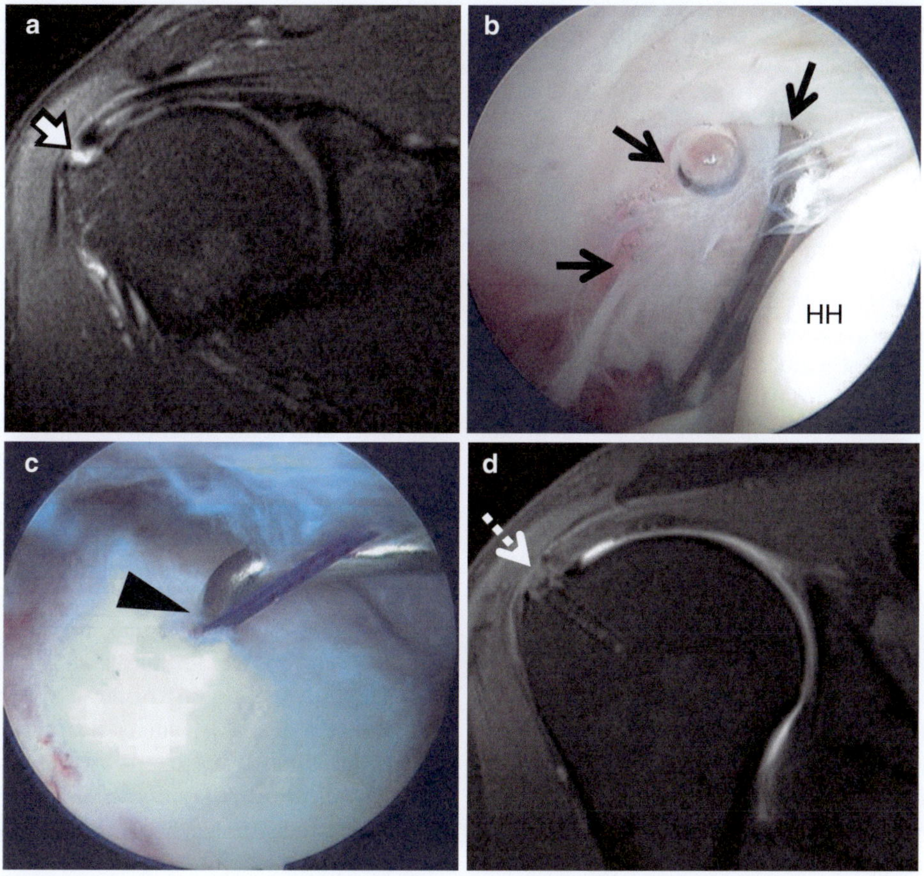

Fig. 5.13 52-year-old man with repair of full-thickness supraspinatus tendon tear. (**a**) Coronal oblique intermediate-weighted MR image shows a focal full-thickness tear of the supraspinatus tendon at the footprint (thick arrow) with delamination. (**b**) Arthroscopic image in glenohumeral joint through posterior portal confirms articular sided supraspinatus tendon tear (black arrows). Humeral head (HH) is marked. (**c**) Arthroscopic image in subacromial-subdeltoid bursa through posterior portal after purple marking suture was placed through articular side. Probe easily extended through bursal surface, confirming the focal full-thickness tear (black arrowhead). (**d**) Coronal oblique T1-weighted fat-suppressed image 2 years after repair shows well-healed footprint after single-row repair (dashed arrow)

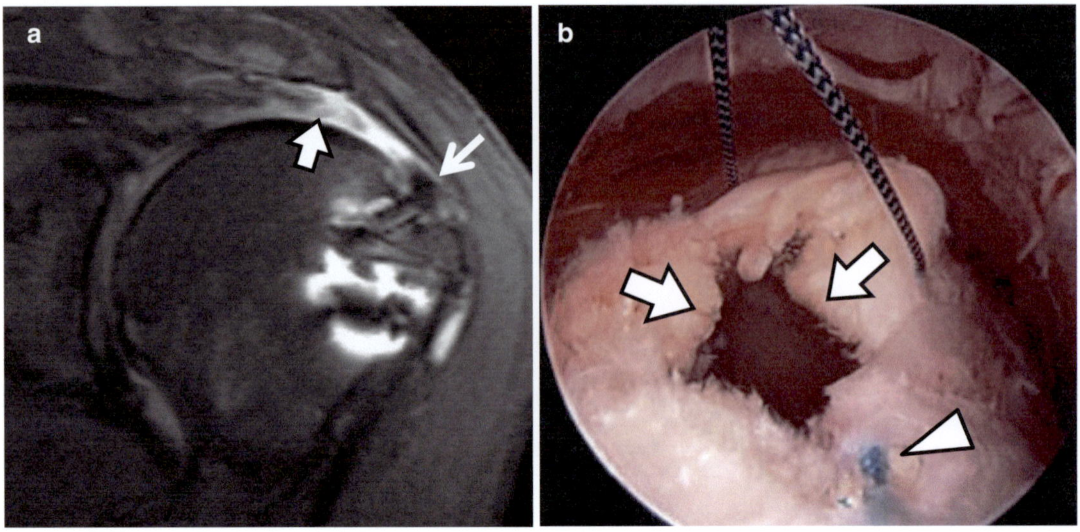

Fig. 5.14 65-Year-old woman status post-rotator cuff repair 4 months prior with worsening shoulder pain and characteristic failure location after double-row repair. (**a**) Coronal oblique intermediate-weighted fat-suppressed MR image shows a full-thickness retear of the distal supraspinatus tendon with retraction (thick arrow). Small amount of tendon remains visible at the footprint (thin arrow). (**b**) Arthroscopic image during revision surgery with scope in subacromial-subdeltoid bursa through posterior portal confirms full-thickness retear (thick arrows). Tear is centered medial to the medial row (arrowhead marks medial row suture from initial repair)

MRI varies depending on the time of imaging. Within the first 3 months, there can be increased signal within the repaired cuff and the appearance of poor footprint coverage, which can improve by the first postoperative year [317]. In a group of 15 asymptomatic patients 1.5–5 years after rotator cuff repair, Spielmann et al. found that only 10% of tendons demonstrated normal low signal intensity [318].

If there is unequivocal full-thickness fluid signal traversing the entire repaired tendon at any time point, a retear can be diagnosed [317, 319]. Structural failure, as determined with imaging, is common after both single-row and double-row repair techniques. Multiple studies with high levels of evidence show conflicting results regarding retear rates after each technique, suggesting that there may not be a true difference between these techniques [320, 321]. However, studies have suggested characteristic tear patterns which are dependent on technique. Cho et al. found that in a single-row repair group, 74% of retearing occurred at the insertion site of the cuff, whereas in a transosseous equivalent group, 74% of retearing occurred in the tendon near the medial row [322]. Similar to the transosseous equivalent technique, the failure pattern in the double-row suture anchor method tends to involve the tendon near the medial row rather than at the insertion [323] (Fig. 5.14).

In 2015, Saccomanno et al. performed a systematic review of MRI criteria for the assessment of rotator cuff repair and identified 26 different criteria that have been previously used [324]. This included structural integrity, footprint coverage, tendon thickness, signal intensity, partial retearing, and muscle atrophy and fatty infiltration. The principal finding of the study was that, with the data available, only structural integrity showed good intra- and inter-observer reliability [324]. Specifically, reliability was highest when a binary classification scheme was used (dichotomization of cuffs into intact versus retear groups).

5.5 Conclusion

In summary, rotator cuff disease is common and the diagnosis of impingement syndromes requires all available information, including history, physical examination, and imaging. Our knowledge of the anatomy involving the rotator cuff is rapidly evolving, and this has many clinical implications. The etiology of rotator cuff disease is multifactorial with intrinsic and extrinsic contributions and knowledge of both mechanisms is required for targeted therapy. Evaluation of the rotator cuff after surgery is challenging, but imaging plays an important role and familiarity with the different repair techniques as well as expected and abnormal postoperative appearances will aid the radiologist in making an accurate diagnosis.

References

1. Teunis T, Lubberts B, Reilly BT, Ring D. A systematic review and pooled analysis of the prevalence of rotator cuff disease with increasing age. J Shoulder Elb Surg. 2014;23(12):1913–21. https://doi.org/10.1016/j.jse.2014.08.001.
2. Chakravarty K, Webley M. Shoulder joint movement and its relationship to disability in the elderly. J Rheumatol. 1993;20(8):1359–61.
3. Chard MD, Hazleman BL. Shoulder disorders in the elderly (a hospital study). Ann Rheum Dis. 1987;46(9):684–7.
4. Chard MD, Hazleman R, Hazleman BL, King RH, Reiss BB. Shoulder disorders in the elderly: a community survey. Arthritis Rheum. 1991;34(6):766–9.
5. van der Windt DA, Koes BW, de Jong BA, Bouter LM. Shoulder disorders in general practice: incidence, patient characteristics, and management. Ann Rheum Dis. 1995;54(12):959–64.
6. Dunn WR, Kuhn JE, Sanders R, An Q, Baumgarten KM, Bishop JY, Brophy RH, Carey JL, Holloway GB, Jones GL, Ma CB, Marx RG, McCarty EC, Poddar SK, Smith MV, Spencer EE, Vidal AF, Wolf BR, Wright RW. Symptoms of pain do not correlate with rotator cuff tear severity: a cross-sectional study of 393 patients with a symptomatic atraumatic full-thickness rotator cuff tear. J Bone Joint Surg Am. 2014;96:793. https://doi.org/10.2106/jbjs.l.01304.
7. Factor D, Dale B. Current concepts of rotator cuff tendinopathy. Int J Sports Phys Ther. 2014;9(2):274–88.
8. Lo IK, Burkhart SS. The etiology and assessment of subscapularis tendon tears: a case for subcoracoid impingement, the roller-wringer effect, and TUFF lesions of the subscapularis. Arthroscopy. 2003;19(10):1142–50. https://doi.org/10.1016/j.arthro.2003.10.024.
9. Nho SJ, Yadav H, Shindle MK, Macgillivray JD. Rotator cuff degeneration: etiology and pathogenesis. Am J Sports Med. 2008;36(5):987–93. https://doi.org/10.1177/0363546508317344.
10. Milgrom C, Schaffler M, Gilbert S, van Holsbeeck M. Rotator-cuff changes in asymptomatic adults. The effect of age, hand dominance and gender. J Bone Joint Surg. 1995;77(2):296–8.
11. Tempelhof S, Rupp S, Seil R. Age-related prevalence of rotator cuff tears in asymptomatic shoulders. J Shoulder Elb Surg. 1999;8(4):296–9.
12. Yuan J, Murrell GA, Wei AQ, Wang MX. Apoptosis in rotator cuff tendonopathy. J Orthop Res. 2002;20(6):1372–9. https://doi.org/10.1016/S0736-0266(02)00075-X.
13. Perry SM, McIlhenny SE, Hoffman MC, Soslowsky LJ. Inflammatory and angiogenic mRNA levels are altered in a supraspinatus tendon overuse animal model. J Shoulder Elb Surg. 2005;14(1 Suppl S):79S–83S. https://doi.org/10.1016/j.jse.2004.09.020.
14. Jia XF, Ji JH, Pannirselvam V, Petersen SA, McFarland EG. Does a positive neer impingement sign reflect rotator cuff contact with the acromion? Clin Orthop Relat Res. 2011;469(3):813–8. https://doi.org/10.1007/s11999-010-1590-3.
15. Hyvonen P, Paivansalo M, Lehtiniemi H, Leppilahti J, Jalovaara P. Supraspinatus outlet view in the diagnosis of stages II and III impingement syndrome. Acta Radiol. 2001;42(5):441–6. https://doi.org/10.1080/028418501127347151.
16. Chang EY, Moses DA, Babb JS, Schweitzer ME. Shoulder impingement: objective 3D shape analysis of acromial morphologic features. Radiology. 2006;239(2):497–505. https://doi.org/10.1148/radiol.2392050324.
17. Moses DA, Chang EY, Schweitzer ME. The scapuloacromial angle: a 3D analysis of acromial slope and its relationship with shoulder impingement. J Magn Reson Imaging. 2006;24(6):1371–7. https://doi.org/10.1002/jmri.20763.
18. Banas MP, Miller RJ, Totterman S. Relationship between the lateral acromion angle and rotator cuff disease. J Shoulder Elb Surg. 1995;4(6):454–61.
19. Harrison AK, Flatow EL. Subacromial impingement syndrome. J Am Acad Orthop Surg. 2011;19(11):701–8.
20. Ricchetti ET, Aurora A, Iannotti JP, Derwin KA. Scaffold devices for rotator cuff repair. J Shoulder Elb Surg. 2012;21(2):251–65. https://doi.org/10.1016/j.jse.2011.10.003.
21. Gulotta LV, Rodeo SA. Growth factors for rotator cuff repair. Clin Sports Med. 2009;28(1):13. https://doi.org/10.1016/j.csm.2008.09.002.
22. Obaid H, Connell D. Cell therapy in tendon disorders what is the current evidence? Am J Sport Med. 2010;38(10):2123–32. https://doi.org/10.1177/0363546510373574.
23. Riley GP, Harrall RL, Constant CR, Chard MD, Cawston TE, Hazleman BL. Tendon degeneration and chronic shoulder pain: changes in the collagen composition of the human rotator cuff tendons in rotator cuff tendinitis. Ann Rheum Dis. 1994;53(6):359–66.

24. Matuszewski PE, Chen YL, Szczesny SE, Lake SP, Elliott DM, Soslowsky LJ, Dodge GR. Regional variation in human supraspinatus tendon proteoglycans: decorin, biglycan, and aggrecan. Connect Tissue Res. 2012;53(5):343–8. https://doi.org/10.3109/03008207.2012.654866.
25. Clark JM, Harryman DT 2nd. Tendons, ligaments, and capsule of the rotator cuff. Gross and microscopic anatomy. J Bone Joint Surg Am. 1992;74(5):713–25.
26. Chang EY, Chung CB. Current concepts on imaging diagnosis of rotator cuff disease. Semin Musculoskelet Radiol. 2014;18(4):412–24. https://doi.org/10.1055/s-0034-1384830.
27. Chang EY, Szeverenyi NM, Statum S, Chung CB. Rotator cuff tendon ultrastructure assessment with reduced-orientation dipolar anisotropy fiber imaging. Am J Roentgenol. 2014;202(4):W376–8.
28. Burkhart SS, Esch JC, Jolson RS. The rotator crescent and rotator cable: an anatomic description of the shoulder's "suspension bridge". Arthroscopy. 1993;9(6):611–6.
29. Kolts I, Busch LC, Tomusk H, Arend A, Eller A, Merila M, Russlies M. Anatomy of the coracohumeral and coracoglenoidal ligaments. Ann Anat. 2000;182(6):563–6. https://doi.org/10.1016/S0940-9602(00)80105-3.
30. Pouliart N, Somers K, Eid S, Gagey O. Variations in the superior capsuloligamentous complex and description of a new ligament. J Shoulder Elb Surg. 2007;16(6):821–36. https://doi.org/10.1016/j.jse.2007.02.138.
31. Gohlke F, Essigkrug B, Schmitz F. The pattern of the collagen fiber bundles of the capsule of the glenohumeral joint. J Shoulder Elb Surg. 1994;3(3):111–28. https://doi.org/10.1016/S1058-2746(09)80090-6.
32. Arai R, Nimura A, Yamaguchi K, Yoshimura H, Sugaya H, Saji T, Matsuda S, Akita K. The anatomy of the coracohumeral ligament and its relation to the subscapularis muscle. J Shoulder Elb Surg. 2014;23(10):1575–81. https://doi.org/10.1016/j.jse.2014.02.009.
33. Nguyen ML, Quigley RJ, Galle SE, McGarry MH, Jun BJ, Gupta R, Burkhart SS, Lee TQ. Margin convergence anchorage to bone for reconstruction of the anterior attachment of the rotator cable. Arthroscopy. 2012;28(9):1237–45. https://doi.org/10.1016/j.arthro.2012.02.016.
34. Mesiha MM, Derwin KA, Sibole SC, Erdemir A, McCarron JA. The biomechanical relevance of anterior rotator cuff cable tears in a cadaveric shoulder model. J Bone Joint Surg. 2013;95(20):1817–24. https://doi.org/10.2106/JBJS.L.00784.
35. Araki D, Miller RM, Fujimaki Y, Hoshino Y, Musahl V, Debski RE. Effect of tear location on propagation of isolated supraspinatus tendon tears during increasing levels of cyclic loading. J Bone Joint Surg. 2015;97(4):273–8. https://doi.org/10.2106/JBJS.N.00062.
36. Namdari S, Donegan RP, Dahiya N, Galatz LM, Yamaguchi K, Keener JD. Characteristics of small to medium-sized rotator cuff tears with and without disruption of the anterior supraspinatus tendon. J Shoulder Elb Surg. 2014;23(1):20–7. https://doi.org/10.1016/j.jse.2013.05.015.
37. Morag Y, Jamadar DA, Boon TA, Bedi A, Caoili EM, Jacobson JA. Ultrasound of the rotator cable: prevalence and morphology in asymptomatic shoulders. AJR Am J Roentgenol. 2012;198(1):W27–30. https://doi.org/10.2214/AJR.10.5796.
38. Gyftopoulos S, Bencardino J, Nevsky G, Hall G, Soofi Y, Desai P, Jazrawi L, Recht MP. Rotator cable: MRI study of its appearance in the intact rotator cuff with anatomic and histologic correlation. AJR Am J Roentgenol. 2013;200(5):1101–5. https://doi.org/10.2214/AJR.12.9312.
39. Morag Y, Jacobson JA, Lucas D, Miller B, Brigido MK, Jamadar DA. US appearance of the rotator cable with histologic correlation: preliminary results. Radiology. 2006;241(2):485–91. https://doi.org/10.1148/radiol.2412050800.
40. Sheah K, Bredella MA, Warner JJP, Halpern EF, Palmer WE. Transverse thickening along the articular surface of the rotator cuff consistent with the rotator cable: identification with MR arthrography and relevance in rotator cuff evaluation. AJR Am J Roentgenol. 2009;193(3):679–86.
41. Nimura A, Akita K. Reply to: "The superior capsule of the shoulder joint complements the insertion of the rotator cuff". J Shoulder Elb Surg. 2013;22(2):e20–1. https://doi.org/10.1016/j.jse.2012.11.018.
42. Nimura A, Kato A, Yamaguchi K, Mochizuki T, Okawa A, Sugaya H, Akita K. The superior capsule of the shoulder joint complements the insertion of the rotator cuff. J Shoulder Elb Surg. 2012;21(7):867–72. https://doi.org/10.1016/j.jse.2011.04.034.
43. Cunningham DJ, Romanes GJ. Cunningham's manual of practical anatomy. Oxford medical publications. 15th ed. New York: Oxford University Press; 1986.
44. Gray H, Standring S, Ellis H, Berkovitz BKB. Gray's anatomy: the anatomical basis of clinical practice. 39th ed. New York: Elsevier Churchill Livingstone; 2005.
45. Kim SY, Boynton EL, Ravichandiran K, Fung LY, Bleakney R, Agur AM. Three-dimensional study of the musculotendinous architecture of supraspinatus and its functional correlations. Clin Anat. 2007;20(6):648–55. https://doi.org/10.1002/ca.20469.
46. Roh MS, Wang VM, April EW, Pollock RG, Bigliani LU, Flatow EL. Anterior and posterior musculotendinous anatomy of the supraspinatus. J Shoulder Elb Surg. 2000;9(5):436–40. https://doi.org/10.1067/mse.2000.108387.
47. Huang CY, Wang VM, Pawluk RJ, Bucchieri JS, Levine WN, Bigliani LU, Mow VC, Flatow EL. Inhomogeneous mechanical behavior of the human supraspinatus tendon under uniaxial loading. J Orthop Res. 2005;23(4):924–30. https://doi.org/10.1016/j.orthres.2004.02.016.

48. Curtis AS, Burbank KM, Tierney JJ, Scheller AD, Curran AR. The insertional footprint of the rotator cuff: an anatomic study. Arthroscopy. 2006;22(6):609 e601. https://doi.org/10.1016/j.arthro.2006.04.001.
49. Minagawa H, Itoi E, Konno N, Kido T, Sano A, Urayama M, Sato K. Humeral attachment of the supraspinatus and infraspinatus tendons: an anatomic study. Arthroscopy. 1998;14(3):302–6.
50. Lumsdaine W, Smith A, Walker RG, Benz D, Mohammed KD, Stewart F. Morphology of the humeral insertion of the supraspinatus and infraspinatus tendons: application to rotator cuff repair. Clin Anat. 2015;28(6):767–73. https://doi.org/10.1002/ca.22548.
51. Mochizuki T, Sugaya H, Uomizu M, Maeda K, Matsuki K, Sekiya I, Muneta T, Akita K. Humeral insertion of the supraspinatus and infraspinatus. New anatomical findings regarding the footprint of the rotator cuff. J Bone Joint Surg Am. 2008;90(5):962–9. https://doi.org/10.2106/JBJS.G.00427.
52. Moser TP, Cardinal E, Bureau NJ, Guillin R, Lanneville P, Grabs D. The aponeurotic expansion of the supraspinatus tendon: anatomy and prevalence in a series of 150 shoulder MRIs. Skelet Radiol. 2015;44(2):223–31. https://doi.org/10.1007/s00256-014-1993-4.
53. Brodie CG. Note on the transverse-humeral, coraco-acromial, and coraco-humeral ligaments, &c. J Anat Physiol. 1890;24(Pt 2):247–52.
54. Hammad RB, Mohamed A. Unilateral four-headed pectoralis muscle major. Mcgill J Med. 2006;9(1):28–30.
55. Gheno R, Zoner CS, Buck FM, Nico MA, Haghighi P, Trudell DJ, Resnick D. Accessory head of biceps brachii muscle: anatomy, histology, and MRI in cadavers. AJR Am J Roentgenol. 2010;194(1):W80–3. https://doi.org/10.2214/AJR.09.3158.
56. Lutterbach-Penna RA, Brigido MK, Robertson B, Kim SM, Jacobson JA, Fessell DP. Sonography of the accessory head of the biceps brachii. J Ultrasound Med. 2014;33(10):1851–4. https://doi.org/10.7863/ultra.33.10.1851.
57. Moser TP, Bureau NJ, Grabs D, Cardinal E. Accessory head of the biceps tendon versus aponeurotic expansion of the supraspinatus tendon. J Ultrasound Med. 2015;34(1):173–4. https://doi.org/10.7863/ultra.34.1.173.
58. Ellman H. Diagnosis and treatment of incomplete rotator cuff tears. Clin Orthop Relat Res. 1990;254:64–74.
59. Nozaki T, Nimura A, Fujishiro H, Mochizuki T, Yamaguchi K, Kato R, Sugaya H, Akita K. The anatomic relationship between the morphology of the greater tubercle of the humerus and the insertion of the infraspinatus tendon. J Shoulder Elb Surg. 2015;24(4):555–60. https://doi.org/10.1016/j.jse.2014.09.038.
60. Dugas JR, Campbell DA, Warren RF, Robie BH, Millett PJ. Anatomy and dimensions of rotator cuff insertions. J Shoulder Elb Surg. 2002;11(5):498–503.
61. Ruotolo C, Fow JE, Nottage WM. The supraspinatus footprint: an anatomic study of the supraspinatus insertion. Arthroscopy. 2004;20(3):246–9. https://doi.org/10.1016/j.arthro.2004.01.002.
62. Karthikeyan S, Rai SB, Parsons H, Drew S, Smith CD, Griffin DR. Ultrasound dimensions of the rotator cuff in young healthy adults. J Shoulder Elb Surg. 2014;23(8):1107–12. https://doi.org/10.1016/j.jse.2013.11.012.
63. Kato A, Nimura A, Yamaguchi K, Mochizuki T, Sugaya H, Akita K. An anatomical study of the transverse part of the infraspinatus muscle that is closely related with the supraspinatus muscle. Surg Radiol Anat. 2012;34(3):257–65. https://doi.org/10.1007/s00276-011-0872-0.
64. Seo JB, Yoo JS, Jang HS, Kim JS. Correlation of clinical symptoms and function with fatty degeneration of infraspinatus in rotator cuff tear. Knee Surg Sports Traumatol Arthrosc. 2015;23(5):1481–8. https://doi.org/10.1007/s00167-014-2857-0.
65. Le Corroller T, Aswad R, Pauly V, Champsaur P. Orientation of the rotator cuff insertion facets on the humerus: comparison between individuals with intact and torn rotator cuffs. Ann Anat. 2009;191(2):218–24. https://doi.org/10.1016/j.aanat.2008.10.003.
66. Yoo JC, Rhee YG, Shin SJ, Park YB, McGarry MH, Jun BJ, Lee TQ. Subscapularis tendon tear classification based on 3-dimensional anatomic footprint: a cadaveric and prospective clinical observational study. Arthroscopy. 2015;31(1):19–28. https://doi.org/10.1016/j.arthro.2014.08.015.
67. Michelin P, Trintignac A, Dacher JN, Carvalhana G, Lefebvre V, Duparc F. Magnetic resonance anatomy of the superior part of the rotator cuff in normal shoulders, assessment and practical implication. Surg Radiol Anat. 2014;36(10):993–1000. https://doi.org/10.1007/s00276-014-1331-5.
68. Michelin P, Kasprzak K, Dacher J, Lefebvre V, Duparc F. Ultrasound and anatomical assessment of the infraspinatus tendon through anterosuperolateral approach. Eur Radiol. 2015;25:1–6. https://doi.org/10.1007/s00330-015-3614-6.
69. Resnick D, Kang HS, Pretterklieber ML. Internal derangements of joints. 2nd ed. Philadelphia: Saunders/Elsevier; 2007.
70. Nimura A, Akita K, Sugaya H. Rotator cuff. In: Bain GI, Itoi E, Di Giacomo G, Sugaya H, editors. Normal and pathological anatomy of the shoulder. Berlin Heidelberg: Springer; 2015. p. 199–205. https://doi.org/10.1007/978-3-662-45719-1_20.
71. Saji T, Arai R, Harada H, Tsukiyama H, Miura T, Matsuda S Anatomical study on the origin and the insertion of the teres minor muscle. In: ISAKOS, Toronto, Canada; 2013. p. 2013.
72. Gray H, Clemente CD. Anatomy of the human body. 30th ed. Philadelphia: Lea & Febiger; 1985.
73. Arai R, Sugaya H, Mochizuki T, Nimura A, Moriishi J, Akita K. Subscapularis tendon tear: an anatomic and clinical investigation. Arthroscopy.

2008;24(9):997–1004. https://doi.org/10.1016/j.arthro.2008.04.076.
74. Richards DP, Burkhart SS, Tehrany AM, Wirth MA. The subscapularis footprint: an anatomic description of its insertion site. Arthroscopy. 2007;23(3):251–4. https://doi.org/10.1016/j.arthro.2006.11.023.
75. DePalma AF. Surgery of the shoulder. 3rd ed. Philadelphia: Lippincott; 1983.
76. Di Giacomo G (2008) Atlas of functional shoulder anatomy.
77. Pouliart N, Boulet C, Maeseneer MD, Shahabpour M. Advanced imaging of the glenohumeral ligaments. Semin Musculoskelet Radiol. 2014;18(4):374–97. https://doi.org/10.1055/s-0034-1384827.
78. Arai R, Mochizuki T, Yamaguchi K, Sugaya H, Kobayashi M, Nakamura T, Akita K. Functional anatomy of the superior glenohumeral and coracohumeral ligaments and the subscapularis tendon in view of stabilization of the long head of the biceps tendon. J Shoulder Elb Surg. 2010;19(1):58–64. https://doi.org/10.1016/j.jse.2009.04.001.
79. D'Addesi LL, Anbari A, Reish MW, Brahmabhatt S, Kelly JD. The subscapularis footprint: an anatomic study of the subscapularis tendon insertion. Arthroscopy. 2006;22(9):937–40. https://doi.org/10.1016/j.arthro.2006.04.101.
80. Werner A, Mueller T, Boehm D, Gohlke F. The stabilizing sling for the long head of the biceps tendon in the rotator cuff interval. A histoanatomic study. Am J Sports Med. 2000;28(1):28–31.
81. Chard MD, Cawston TE, Riley GP, Gresham GA, Hazleman BL. Rotator cuff degeneration and lateral epicondylitis: a comparative histological study. Ann Rheum Dis. 1994;53(1):30–4.
82. Jarvinen M, Jozsa L, Kannus P, Jarvinen TL, Kvist M, Leadbetter W. Histopathological findings in chronic tendon disorders. Scand J Med Sci Sports. 1997;7(2):86–95.
83. Berenson MC, Blevins FT, Plaas AH, Vogel KG. Proteoglycans of human rotator cuff tendons. J Orthop Res. 1996;14(4):518–25. https://doi.org/10.1002/jor.1100140404.
84. Weber SC. Arthroscopic debridement and acromioplasty versus mini-open repair in the treatment of significant partial-thickness rotator cuff tears. Arthroscopy. 1999;15(2):126–31. https://doi.org/10.1053/ar.1999.v15.0150121.
85. Fukuda H. The management of partial-thickness tears of the rotator cuff. J Bone Joint Surg. 2003;85(1):3–11.
86. Kim HM, Dahiya N, Teefey SA, Middleton WD, Stobbs G, Steger-May K, Yamaguchi K, Keener JD. Location and initiation of degenerative rotator cuff tears: an analysis of three hundred and sixty shoulders. J Bone Joint Surg Am. 2010;92(5):1088–96. https://doi.org/10.2106/JBJS.I.00686.
87. Fukuda H, Hamada K, Yamanaka K. Pathology and pathogenesis of bursal-side rotator cuff tears viewed from en bloc histologic sections. Clin Orthop Relat Res. 1990;254:75–80.
88. Fukuda H, Hamada K, Nakajima T, Tomonaga A. Pathology and pathogenesis of the intratendinous tearing of the rotator cuff viewed from en bloc histologic sections. Clin Orthop Relat Res. 1994;304:60–7.
89. Codman EA, Akerson IB. The pathology associated with rupture of the supraspinatus tendon. Ann Surg. 1931;93(1):348–59.
90. Mazzocca AD, Rincon LM, O'Connor RW, Obopilwe E, Andersen M, Geaney L, Arciero RA. Intra-articular partial-thickness rotator cuff tears: analysis of injured and repaired strain behavior. Am J Sports Med. 2008;36(1):110–6. https://doi.org/10.1177/0363546507307502.
91. Strauss EJ, Salata MJ, Kercher J, Barker JU, McGill K, Bach BR Jr, Romeo AA, Verma NN. Multimedia article. The arthroscopic management of partial-thickness rotator cuff tears: a systematic review of the literature. Arthroscopy. 2011;27(4):568–80.
92. Shindle MK, Chen CCT, Robertson C, DiTullio AE, Paulus MC, Clinton CM, Cordasco FA, Rodeo SA, Warren RF. Full-thickness supraspinatus tears are associated with more synovial inflammation and tissue degeneration than partial-thickness tears. J Shoulder Elb Surg. 2011;20(6):917–27. https://doi.org/10.1016/j.jse.2011.02.015.
93. Lo IK, Burkhart SS. Current concepts in arthroscopic rotator cuff repair. Am J Sports Med. 2003;31(2):308–24.
94. Sela Y, Eshed I, Shapira S, Oran A, Vogel G, Herman A, Perry M. Rotator cuff tears: correlation between geometric tear patterns on MRI and arthroscopy and pre- and postoperative clinical findings. Acta Radiol. 2015;56(2):182–9. https://doi.org/10.1177/0284185114520861.
95. Lee YH, Kim AH, Suh JS. Magnetic resonance visualization of surgical classification of rotator cuff tear: comparison with three-dimensional shoulder magnetic resonance arthrography at 3.0 T. Clin Imag. 2014;38(6):858–63. https://doi.org/10.1016/j.clinimag.2014.07.003.
96. Tauro JC. Arthroscopic repair of large rotator cuff tears using the interval slide technique. Arthroscopy. 2004;20(1):13–21.
97. Cofield RH. Subscapular muscle transposition for repair of chronic rotator cuff tears. Surg Gynecol Obstet. 1982;154(5):667–72.
98. Pill SG, Phillips J, Kissenberth MJ, Hawkins RJ. Decision making in massive rotator cuff tears. Instr Course Lect. 2012;61:97–111.
99. Delaney RA, Lin A, Warner JJ. Nonarthroplasty options for the management of massive and irreparable rotator cuff tears. Clin Sports Med. 2012;31(4):727–48. https://doi.org/10.1016/j.csm.2012.07.008.
100. Choo HJ, Lee SJ, Kim JH, Kim DW, Park YM, Kim OH, Kim SJ. Delaminated tears of the rotator cuff: prevalence, characteristics, and diagnostic accuracy using indirect MR arthrography. AJR Am J Roentgenol. 2015;204(2):360–6. https://doi.org/10.2214/AJR.14.12555.

101. Han Y, Shin JH, Seok CW, Lee CH, Kim SH. Is posterior delamination in arthroscopic rotator cuff repair hidden to the posterior viewing portal? Arthroscopy. 2013;29(11):1740–7. https://doi.org/10.1016/j.arthro.2013.08.021.
102. Meyer DC, Hoppeler H, von Rechenberg B, Gerber C. A pathomechanical concept explains muscle loss and fatty muscular changes following surgical tendon release. J Orthop Res. 2004;22(5):1004–7.
103. Albritton MJ, Graham RD, Richards RS 2nd, Basamania CJ. An anatomic study of the effects on the suprascapular nerve due to retraction of the supraspinatus muscle after a rotator cuff tear. J Shoulder Elb Surg. 2003;12(5):497–500.
104. Gladstone JN, Bishop JY, Lo IK, Flatow EL. Fatty infiltration and atrophy of the rotator cuff do not improve after rotator cuff repair and correlate with poor functional outcome. Am J Sports Med. 2007;35(5):719–28. https://doi.org/10.1177/0363546506297539.
105. Kuzel BR, Grindel S, Papandrea R, Ziegler D. Fatty infiltration and rotator cuff atrophy. J Am Acad Orthop Surg. 2013;21(10):613–23. https://doi.org/10.5435/JAAOS-21-10-613.
106. Chaudhury S, Dines JS, Delos D, Warren RF, Voigt C, Rodeo SA. Role of fatty infiltration in the pathophysiology and outcomes of rotator cuff tears. Arthritis Care Res. 2012;64(1):76–82. https://doi.org/10.1002/acr.20552.
107. Sarkar K, Taine W, Uhthoff HK. The ultrastructure of the coracoacromial ligament in patients with chronic impingement syndrome. Clin Orthop Relat Res. 1990;254:49–54.
108. Diercks R, Bron C, Dorrestijn O, Meskers C, Naber R, de Ruiter T, Willems J, Winters J, van der Woude HJ, Dutch Orthopaedic A. Guideline for diagnosis and treatment of subacromial pain syndrome: a multidisciplinary review by the Dutch Orthopaedic Association. Acta Orthop. 2014;85(3):314–22. https://doi.org/10.3109/17453674.2014.920991.
109. McFarland EG, Maffulli N, Del Buono A, Murrell GA, Garzon-Muvdi J, Petersen SA. Impingement is not impingement: the case for calling it "Rotator Cuff Disease". Muscles Ligaments Tendons J. 2013;3(3):196–200.
110. Papadonikolakis A, McKenna M, Warme W, Martin BI, Matsen FA 3rd. Published evidence relevant to the diagnosis of impingement syndrome of the shoulder. J Bone Joint Surg Am. 2011;93(19):1827–32. https://doi.org/10.2106/JBJS.J.01748.
111. Neer CS 2nd. Anterior acromioplasty for the chronic impingement syndrome in the shoulder: a preliminary report. Muscles Ligaments Tendons J. 1972;54(1):41–50.
112. Yamamoto N, Muraki T, Sperling JW, Steinmann SP, Itoi E, Cofield RH, An KN. Contact between the coracoacromial arch and the rotator cuff tendons in nonpathologic situations: a cadaveric study. J Shoulder Elb Surg. 2010;19(5):681–7. https://doi.org/10.1016/j.jse.2009.12.006.
113. Tasaki A, Nimura A, Nozaki T, Yamakawa A, Niitsu M, Morita W, Hoshikawa Y, Akita K. Quantitative and qualitative analyses of subacromial impingement by kinematic open MRI. Knee Surg Sport Tr A. 2015;23(5):1489–97. https://doi.org/10.1007/s00167-014-2876-x.
114. Alfredson H, Forsgren S, Thorsen K, Lorentzon R. In vivo microdialysis and immunohistochemical analyses of tendon tissue demonstrated high amounts of free glutamate and glutamate NMDAR1 receptors, but no signs of inflammation, in Jumper's knee. J Orthopaed Res. 2001;19(5):881–6. https://doi.org/10.1016/S0736-0266(01)00016-X.
115. Alfredson H, Lorentzon R. Chronic tendon pain: no signs of chemical inflammation but high concentrations of the neurotransmitter glutamate. Implications for treatment? Curr Drug Targets. 2002;3(1):43–54. https://doi.org/10.2174/1389450023348028.
116. Gellhorn AC, Gillenwater C, Mourad PD. Intense focused ultrasound stimulation of the rotator cuff: evaluation of the source of pain in rotator cuff tears and tendinopathy. Ultrasound Med Biol. 2015;41(9):2412–9. https://doi.org/10.1016/j.ultrasmedbio.2015.05.005.
117. Ozaki J, Fujimoto S, Nakagawa Y, Masuhara K, Tamai S. Tears of the rotator cuff of the shoulder associated with pathological changes in the acromion. A study in cadavera. Muscles Ligaments Tendons J. 1988;70(8):1224–30.
118. Getz JD, Recht MP, Piraino DW, Schils JP, Latimer BM, Jellema LM, Obuchowski NA. Acromial morphology: relation to sex, age, symmetry, and subacromial enthesophytes. Radiology. 1996;199(3):737–42. https://doi.org/10.1148/radiology.199.3.8637998.
119. Fujisawa Y, Mihata T, Murase T, Sugamoto K, Neo M. Three-dimensional analysis of acromial morphologic characteristics in patients with and without rotator cuff tears using a reconstructed computed tomography model. Am J Sport Med. 2014;42(11):2621–6. https://doi.org/10.1177/0363546514544683.
120. Bigliani LU, Morrison DS, April EW. The morphology of the acromion and its relationship to rotator cuff tears. Orthop Trans. 1986;10:216.
121. Zuckerman JD, Kummer FJ, Cuomo F, Greller M. Interobserver reliability of acromial morphology classification: an anatomic study. J Shoulder Elb Surg. 1997;6(3):286–7.
122. Peh WC, Farmer TH, Totty WG. Acromial arch shape: assessment with MR imaging. Radiology. 1995;195(2):501–5. https://doi.org/10.1148/radiology.195.2.7724774.
123. Epstein RE, Schweitzer ME, Frieman BG, Fenlin JM Jr, Mitchell DG. Hooked acromion: prevalence on MR images of painful shoulders. Radiology. 1993;187(2):479–81. https://doi.org/10.1148/radiology.187.2.8475294.
124. Mayerhoefer ME, Breitenseher MJ, Roposch A, Treitl C, Wurnig C. Comparison of MRI and conven-

tional radiography for assessment of acromial shape. AJR Am J Roentgenol. 2005;184(2):671–5. https://doi.org/10.2214/ajr.184.2.01840671.
125. Haygood TM, Langlotz CP, Kneeland JB, Iannotti JP, Williams GR Jr, Dalinka MK. Categorization of acromial shape: interobserver variability with MR imaging and conventional radiography. AJR Am J Roentgenol. 1994;162(6):1377–82. https://doi.org/10.2214/ajr.162.6.8192003.
126. Bright AS, Torpey B, Magid D, Codd T, McFarland EG. Reliability of radiographic evaluation for acromial morphology. Skelet Radiol. 1997;26(12):718–21.
127. Jacobson SR, Speer KP, Moor JT, Janda DH, Saddemi SR, MacDonald PB, Mallon WJ. Reliability of radiographic assessment of acromial morphology. J Shoulder Elb Surg. 1995;4(6):449–53.
128. Chambler AF, Emery RJ. Acromial morphology: the enigma of terminology. Knee Surg Sports Traumatol Arthrosc. 1997;5(4):268–72. https://doi.org/10.1007/s001670050062.
129. Nicholson GP, Goodman DA, Flatow EL, Bigliani LU. The acromion: morphologic condition and age-related changes. A study of 420 scapulas. J Shoulder Elb Surg. 1996;5:1):1–11.
130. Shah NN, Bayliss NC, Malcolm A. Shape of the acromion: congenital or acquired--a macroscopic, radiographic, and microscopic study of acromion. J Shoulder Elb Surg. 2001;10(4):309–16. https://doi.org/10.1067/mse.2001.114681.
131. Speer KP, Osbahr DC, Montella BJ, Apple AS, Mair SD. Acromial morphotype in the young asymptomatic athletic shoulder. J Shoulder Elb Surg. 2001;10(5):434–7. https://doi.org/10.1067/mse.2001.117124.
132. Toivonen DA, Tuite MJ, Orwin JF. Acromial structure and tears of the rotator cuff. J Shoulder Elb Surg. 1995;4(5):376–83.
133. Tuite MJ, Toivonen DA, Orwin JF, Wright DH. Acromial angle on radiographs of the shoulder: correlation with the impingement syndrome and rotator cuff tears. AJR Am J Roentgenol. 1995;165(3):609–13. https://doi.org/10.2214/ajr.165.3.7645479.
134. Farley TE, Neumann CH, Steinbach LS, Petersen SA. The coracoacromial arch: MR evaluation and correlation with rotator cuff pathology. Skelet Radiol. 1994;23(8):641–5.
135. Wang JC, Horner G, Brown ED, Shapiro MS. The relationship between acromial morphology and conservative treatment of patients with impingement syndrome. Orthopedics. 2000;23(6):557–9.
136. Tasu JP, Miquel A, Rocher L, Molina V, Gagey O, Blery M. MR evaluation of factors predicting the development of rotator cuff tears. J Comput Assist Tomogr. 2001;25(2):159–63.
137. Panni AS, Milano G, Lucania L, Fabbriciani C, Logroscino CA. Histological analysis of the coracoacromial arch: Correlation between age-related changes and rotator cuff tears. Arthroscopy. 1996;12(5):531–40. https://doi.org/10.1016/S0749-8063(96)90190-5.
138. Zuckerman JD, Kummer FJ, Cuomo F, Simon J, Rosenblum S, Katz N. The influence of coracoacromial arch anatomy on rotator cuff tears. J Shoulder Elb Surg. 1992;1(1):4–14. https://doi.org/10.1016/S1058-2746(09)80010-4.
139. Balke M, Liem D, Greshake O, Hoeher J, Bouillon B, Banerjee M. Differences in acromial morphology of shoulders in patients with degenerative and traumatic supraspinatus tendon tears. Knee Surg Sports Traumatol Arthrosc. 2014;24(7):2200–5. https://doi.org/10.1007/s00167-014-3499-y.
140. MacGillivray JD, Fealy S, Potter HG, O'Brien SJ. Multiplanar analysis of acromion morphology. Am J Sports Med. 1998;26(6):836–40.
141. Kibler WB. Scapular involvement in impingement: signs and symptoms. Instr Course Lect. 2006;55:35–43.
142. Ratcliffe E, Pickering S, McLean S, Lewis J. Is there a relationship between subacromial impingement syndrome and scapular orientation? A systematic review. Brit J Sport Med. 2014;48(16):1251–U1282. https://doi.org/10.1136/bjsports-2013-092389.
143. Petersson CJ, Gentz CF. Ruptures of the supraspinatus tendon. The significance of distally pointing acromioclavicular osteophytes. Clin Orthop Relat Res. 1983;174:143–8.
144. Cuomo F, Kummer FJ, Zuckerman JD, Lyon T, Blair B, Olsen T. The influence of acromioclavicular joint morphology on rotator cuff tears. J Shoulder Elb Surg. 1998;7(6):555–9.
145. de Abreu MR, Chung CB, Wesselly M, Jin-Kim H, Resnick D. Acromioclavicular joint osteoarthritis: comparison of findings derived from MR imaging and conventional radiography. Clin Imaging. 2005;29(4):273–7. https://doi.org/10.1016/j.clinimag.2004.11.021.
146. Blasiak A, Mojzesz M, Brzoska R, Solecki W, Binkowska A. Results of arthroscopic treatment of rotator cuff tear with the resection of symptomatic acromioclavicular joint with degenerative changes. Pol Orthop Traumatol. 2013;78:229–34.
147. Daluga DJ, Dobozi W. The influence of distal clavicle resection and rotator cuff repair on the effectiveness of anterior acromioplasty. Clin Orthop Relat Res. 1989;247:117–23.
148. Kay SP, Dragoo JL, Lee R. Long-term results of arthroscopic resection of the distal clavicle with concomitant subacromial decompression. Arthroscopy. 2003;19(8):805–9.
149. Kim J, Chung J, Ok H. Asymptomatic acromioclavicular joint arthritis in arthroscopic rotator cuff tendon repair: a prospective randomized comparison study. Arch Orthop Trauma Surg. 2011;131(3):363–9. https://doi.org/10.1007/s00402-010-1216-y.
150. Levine WN, Soong M, Ahmad CS, Blaine TA, Bigliani LU. Arthroscopic distal clavicle resec-

tion: a comparison of bursal and direct approaches. Arthroscopy. 2006;22(5):516–20. https://doi.org/10.1016/j.arthro.2006.01.013.
151. Lozman PR, Hechtman KS, Uribe JW. Combined arthroscopic management of impingement syndrome and acromioclavicular joint arthritis. J South Orthop Assoc. 1995;4(3):177–81.
152. Snyder SJ, Banas MP, Karzel RP. The arthroscopic Mumford procedure: an analysis of results. Arthroscopy. 1995;11(2):157–64.
153. Razmjou H, ElMaraghy A, Dwyer T, Fournier-Gosselin S, Devereaux M, Holtby R. Outcome of distal clavicle resection in patients with acromioclavicular joint osteoarthritis and full-thickness rotator cuff tear. Knee surgery, sports traumatology. Arthroscopy. 2015;23(2):585–90. https://doi.org/10.1007/s00167-014-3114-2.
154. Oh JH, Kim JY, Choi JH, Park S-M. Is arthroscopic distal clavicle resection necessary for patients with radiological acromioclavicular joint arthritis and rotator cuff tears? A prospective randomized comparative study. Am J Sports Med. 2014;42(11):2567–73. https://doi.org/10.1177/0363546514547254.
155. Park YB, Koh KH, Shon MS, Park YE, Yoo JC. Arthroscopic distal clavicle resection in symptomatic acromioclavicular joint arthritis combined with rotator cuff tear: a prospective randomized trial. Am J Sports Med. 2015;43(4):985–90. https://doi.org/10.1177/0363546514563911.
156. Kesmezacar H, Akgun I, Ogut T, Gokay S, Uzun I. The coracoacromial ligament: the morphology and relation to rotator cuff pathology. J Shoulder Elb Surg. 2008;17(1):182–8. https://doi.org/10.1016/j.jse.2007.05.015.
157. Holt EM, Allibone RO. Anatomic variants of the coracoacromial ligament. J Shoulder Elb Surg. 1995;4(5):370–5.
158. Fealy S, April EW, Khazzam M, Armengol-Barallat J, Bigliani LU. The coracoacromial ligament: morphology and study of acromial enthesopathy. J Shoulder Elb Surg. 2005;14(5):542–8. https://doi.org/10.1016/j.jse.2005.02.006.
159. Abrams GD, Gupta AK, Hussey KE, Tetteh ES, Karas V, Bach BR Jr, Cole BJ, Romeo AA, Verma NN. Arthroscopic repair of full-thickness rotator cuff tears with and without acromioplasty: randomized prospective trial with 2-year follow-up. Am J Sports Med. 2014;42(6):1296–303. https://doi.org/10.1177/0363546514529091.
160. Gartsman GM, O'Connor DP. Arthroscopic rotator cuff repair with and without arthroscopic subacromial decompression: a prospective, randomized study of one-year outcomes. J Shoulder Elb Surg. 2004;13(4):424–6. https://doi.org/10.1016/S1058274604000527.
161. MacDonald P, McRae S, Leiter J, Mascarenhas R, Lapner P. Arthroscopic rotator cuff repair with and without acromioplasty in the treatment of full-thickness rotator cuff tears: a multicenter, randomized controlled trial. J Bone Joint Surg Am. 2011;93(21):1953–60. https://doi.org/10.2106/JBJS.K.00488.
162. Milano G, Grasso A, Salvatore M, Zarelli D, Deriu L, Fabbriciani C. Arthroscopic rotator cuff repair with and without subacromial decompression: a prospective randomized study. Arthroscopy. 2007;23(1):81–8. https://doi.org/10.1016/j.arthro.2006.10.011.
163. Moorman CT, Warren RF, Deng XH, Wickiewicz TL, Torzilli PA. Role of coracoacromial ligament and related structures in glenohumeral stability: a cadaveric study. J Surg Orthop Adv. 2012;21(4):210–7.
164. Edelson JG, Zuckerman J, Hershkovitz I. Os acromiale: anatomy and surgical implications. J Bone Joint Surg. 1993;75(4):551–5.
165. Mudge MK, Wood VE, Frykman GK. Rotator cuff tears associated with os acromiale. Muscles Ligaments Tendons J. 1984;66(3):427–9.
166. Yammine K. The prevalence of os acromiale: A systematic review and meta-analysis. Clin Anat. 2014;27(4):610–21. https://doi.org/10.1002/ca.22343.
167. Sammarco VJ. Os acromiale: frequency, anatomy, and clinical implications. J Bone Joint Surg Am. 2000;82(3):394–400.
168. Kurtz CA, Humble BJ, Rodosky MW, Sekiya JK. Symptomatic os acromiale. J Am Acad Orthop Surg. 2006;14(1):12–9.
169. Wise JN, Daffner RH, Weissman BN, Bancroft L, Bennett DL, Blebea JS, Bruno MA, Fries IB, Jacobson JA, Luchs JS, Morrison WB, Resnik CS, Roberts CC, Schweitzer ME, Seeger LL, Stoller DW, Taljanovic MS. ACR Appropriateness Criteria(R) on acute shoulder pain. J Am Coll Radiol. 2011;8(9):602–9. https://doi.org/10.1016/j.jacr.2011.05.008.
170. McCreesh KM, Crotty JM, Lewis JS. Acromiohumeral distance measurement in rotator cuff tendinopathy: is there a reliable, clinically applicable method? A systematic review. Brit J Sport Med. 2015;49(5):298–305. https://doi.org/10.1136/bjsports-2012-092063.
171. Petersson CJ, Redlund-Johnell I. The subacromial space in normal shoulder radiographs. Acta Orthop Scand. 1984;55(1):57–8.
172. Saupe N, Pfirrmann CWA, Schmid MR, Jost B, Werner CML, Zanetti M. Association between rotator cuff abnormalities and reduced acromiohumeral distance. Am J Roentgenol. 2006;187(2):376–82. https://doi.org/10.2214/Ajr.05.0435.
173. Nove-Josserand L, Levigne C, Noel E, Walch G. The acromio-humeral interval. A study of the factors influencing its height. Rev Chir Orthop Reparatrice Appar Mot. 1996;82(5):379–85.
174. Goutallier D, Le Guilloux P, Postel JM, Radier C, Bernageau J, Zilber S. Acromio humeral distance less than six millimeter: Its meaning in full-thickness rotator cuff tear. Orthop Traumatol Sur. 2011;97(3):246–51. https://doi.org/10.1016/j.otsr.2011.01.010.

175. Huang LF, Rubin DA, Britton CA. Greater tuberosity changes as revealed by radiography: lack of clinical usefulness in patients with rotator cuff disease. Am J Roentgenol. 1999;172(5):1381–8.
176. Fritz LB, Ouellette HA, O'Hanley TA, Kassarjian A, Palmer WE. Cystic changes at supraspinatus and infraspinatus tendon insertion sites: Association with age and rotator cuff disorders in 238 patients. Radiology. 2007;244(1):239–48. https://doi.org/10.1148/radiol.2441050029.
177. Sano A, Itoi E, Konno N, Kido T, Urayama M, Sato K. Cystic changes of the humeral head on MR imaging - Relation to age and cuff-tears. Acta Orthop Scand. 1998;69(4):397–400. https://doi.org/10.3109/17453679808999054.
178. Suluova F, Kanatli U, Ozturk BY, Esen E, Bolukbasi S. Humeral head cysts: association with rotator cuff tears and age. Eur J Orthop Surg Traumatol. 2014;24(5):733–9. https://doi.org/10.1007/s00590-013-1247-5.
179. Studler U, Pfirrmann CW, Jost B, Rousson V, Hodler J, Zanetti M. Abnormalities of the lesser tuberosity on radiography and MRI: association with subscapularis tendon lesions. AJR Am J Roentgenol. 2008;191(1):100–6. https://doi.org/10.2214/AJR.07.3056.
180. Pan Y-W, Mok D, Tsiouri C, Chidambaram R. The association between radiographic greater tuberosity cystic change and rotator cuff tears: a study of 105 consecutive cases. Shoulder Elbow. 2011;3(4):205–9. https://doi.org/10.1111/j.1758-5740.2011.00143.x.
181. Wissman RD, Ingalls J, Hendry D, Gorman D, Kenter K. Cysts within and adjacent to the lesser tuberosity: correlation with shoulder arthroscopy. Skelet Radiol. 2012;41(9):1105–10. https://doi.org/10.1007/s00256-012-1366-9.
182. Wissman R, Hendry D, Gorman D, Kapur S, Ingalls J, Ying J, Kenter K. Cysts within and adjacent to the lesser tuberosity: correlation with shoulder arthroscopy. Am J Roentgenol. 2010;194(5):1105.
183. Celikyay F, Yuksekkaya R, Deniz C, Inal S, Gokce E, Acu B. Locations of lesser tuberosity cysts and their association with subscapularis, supraspinatus, and long head of the biceps tendon disorders. Acta Radiol. 2014;56(12):1494–500. https://doi.org/10.1177/0284185114561821.
184. Williams M, Lambert RG, Jhangri GS, Grace M, Zelazo J, Wong B, Dhillon SS. Humeral head cysts and rotator cuff tears: an MR arthrographic study. Skelet Radiol. 2006;35(12):909–14. https://doi.org/10.1007/s00256-006-0157-6.
185. Jin W, Ryu KN, Park YK, Lee WK, Ko SH, Yang DM. Cystic lesions in the posterosuperior portion of the humeral head on MR arthrography: correlations with gross and histologic findings in cadavers. AJR Am J Roentgenol. 2005;184(4):1211–5. https://doi.org/10.2214/ajr.184.4.01841211.
186. Koh KH, Han KY, Yoon YC, Lee SW, Yoo JC. True anteroposterior (Grashey) view as a screening radiograph for further imaging study in rotator cuff tear. J Shoulder Elb Surg. 2013;22(7):901–7. https://doi.org/10.1016/j.jse.2012.09.015.
187. Pearsall AW, Bonsell S, Heitman RJ, Helms CA, Osbahr D, Speer KP. Radiographic findings associated with symptomatic rotator cuff tears. J Shoulder Elb Surg. 2003;12(2):122–7. https://doi.org/10.1067/mse.2003.19.
188. Berens DL, Lockie LM. Ossification of the coracoacromial ligament. Radiology. 1960;74:802–5. https://doi.org/10.1148/74.5.802.
189. Cone RO 3rd, Resnick D, Danzig L. Shoulder impingement syndrome: radiographic evaluation. Radiology. 1984;150(1):29–33. https://doi.org/10.1148/radiology.150.1.6689783.
190. Kieft GJ, Bloem JL, Rozing PM, Obermann WR. Rotator cuff impingement syndrome: MR imaging. Radiology. 1988;166(1 Pt 1):211–4. https://doi.org/10.1148/radiology.166.1.3336681.
191. Kilcoyne RF, Reddy PK, Lyons F, Rockwood CA. Optimal plain film imaging of the shoulder impingement syndrome. Am J Roentgenol. 1989;153(4):795–7.
192. Newhouse KE, el-Khoury GY, Nepola JV, Montgomery WJ. The shoulder impingement view: a fluoroscopic technique for the detection of subacromial spurs. AJR Am J Roentgenol. 1988;151(3):539–41. https://doi.org/10.2214/ajr.151.3.539.
193. Lee DH, Lee KH, Lopez-Ben R, Bradley EL. The double-density sign: a radiographic finding suggestive of an os acromiale. J Bone Joint Surg Am. 2004;86-A(12):2666–70.
194. Omoumi P, Bafort AC, Dubuc JE, Malghem J, Vande Berg BC, Lecouvet FE. Evaluation of rotator cuff tendon tears: comparison of multidetector CT arthrography and 1.5-T MR arthrography. Radiology. 2012;264(3):812–22. https://doi.org/10.1148/radiol.12112062.
195. Mahmoud MK, Badran YM, Zaki HG, Ali AH. One-shot MR and MDCT arthrography of shoulder lesions with arthroscopic correlation. Egypt J Radiol Nucl Med. 2013;44(2):273–81. https://doi.org/10.1016/j.ejrnm.2013.01.002.
196. Szymanski C, Staquet V, Deladerriere JY, Vervoort T, Audebert S, Maynou C. Reproducibility and reliability of subscapularis tendon assessment using CT-arthrography. Orthop Traumatol-Sur. 2013;99(1):2–9. https://doi.org/10.1016/j.otsr.2012.07.014.
197. Charousset C, Bellaiche L, Duranthon LD, Grimberg J. Accuracy of CT arthrography in the assessment of tears of the rotator cuff. J Bone Joint Surg. 2005;87b(6):824–8. https://doi.org/10.1302/0301-620x.87b6.15836.
198. Roy JS, Braen C, Leblond J, Desmeules F, Dionne CE, MacDermid JC, Bureau NJ, Fremont P. Diagnostic accuracy of ultrasonography, MRI and MR arthrography in the characterisation of rotator cuff disorders: a meta-analysis. Br J Sports Med. 2015;49(20):1316–28. https://doi.org/10.1136/bjsports-2014-094148.

199. Wohlwend JR, van Holsbeeck M, Craig J, Shirazi K, Habra G, Jacobsen G, Bouffard JA. The association between irregular greater tuberosities and rotator cuff tears: a sonographic study. Am J Roentgenol. 1998;171(1):229–33.
200. Farin PU, Jaroma H, Harju A, Soimakallio S. Shoulder impingement syndrome: sonographic evaluation. Radiology. 1990;176(3):845–9. https://doi.org/10.1148/radiology.176.3.2202014.
201. Bureau NJ, Beauchamp M, Cardinal E, Brassard P. Dynamic sonography evaluation of shoulder impingement syndrome. AJR Am J Roentgenol. 2006;187(1):216–20. https://doi.org/10.2214/AJR.05.0528.
202. Daghir AA, Sookur PA, Shah S, Watson M. Dynamic ultrasound of the subacromial-subdeltoid bursa in patients with shoulder impingement: a comparison with normal volunteers. Skelet Radiol. 2012;41(9):1047–53. https://doi.org/10.1007/s00256-011-1295-z.
203. Read JW, Perko M. Shoulder ultrasound: diagnostic accuracy for impingement syndrome, rotator cuff tear, and biceps tendon pathology. J Shoulder Elb Surg. 1998;7(3):264–71.
204. Read JW, Perko M. Ultrasound diagnosis of subacromial impingement for lesions of the rotator cuff. Australas J Ultrasound Med. 2010;13(2):11–5.
205. Khoury V, Cardinal E, Bureau NJ. Musculoskeletal sonography: a dynamic tool for usual and unusual disorders. AJR Am J Roentgenol. 2007;188(1):W63–73. https://doi.org/10.2214/AJR.06.0579.
206. Karjalainen PT, Soila K, Aronen HJ, Pihlajamaki HK, Tynninen O, Paavonen T, Tirman PF. MR imaging of overuse injuries of the Achilles tendon. AJR Am J Roentgenol. 2000;175(1):251–60. https://doi.org/10.2214/ajr.175.1.1750251.
207. Krasnosselskaia LV, Fullerton GD, Dodd SJ, Cameron IL. Water in tendon: orientational analysis of the free induction decay. Magn Reson Med. 2005;54(2):280–8. https://doi.org/10.1002/mrm.20540.
208. Berendsen HJC. Nuclear magnetic resonance study of collagen HYDRATION. J Chem Phys. 1962;36(12):3297. https://doi.org/10.1063/1.1732460.
209. Gagey N, Quillard J, Gagey O, Meduri G, Bittoun J, Lassau JP. Tendon of the normal supraspinatus muscle: correlations between MR imaging and histology. Surg Radiol Anat. 1995;17(4):329–34.
210. Kjellin I, Ho CP, Cervilla V, Haghighi P, Kerr R, Vangness CT, Friedman RJ, Trudell D, Resnick D. Alterations in the supraspinatus tendon at MR imaging: correlation with histopathologic findings in cadavers. Radiology. 1991;181(3):837–41. https://doi.org/10.1148/radiology.181.3.1947107.
211. Tuite MJ. Magnetic resonance imaging of rotator cuff disease and external impingement. Magn Reson Imaging Clin N Am. 2012;20(2):187–200, ix. https://doi.org/10.1016/j.mric.2012.01.011.
212. Bauer S, Wang A, Butler R, Fallon M, Nairn R, Budgeon C, Breidahl W, Zheng MH. Reliability of a 3 T MRI protocol for objective grading of supraspinatus tendonosis and partial thickness tears. J Orthop Surg Res. 2014;9:128. https://doi.org/10.1186/s13018-014-0128-x.
213. de Jesus JO, Parker L, Frangos AJ, Nazarian LN. Accuracy of MRI, MR arthrography, and ultrasound in the diagnosis of rotator cuff tears: a meta-analysis. AJR Am J Roentgenol. 2009;192(6):1701–7. https://doi.org/10.2214/AJR.08.1241.
214. Farley TE, Neumann CH, Steinbach LS, Jahnke AJ, Petersen SS. Full-thickness tears of the rotator cuff of the shoulder: diagnosis with MR imaging. AJR Am J Roentgenol. 1992;158(2):347–51. https://doi.org/10.2214/ajr.158.2.1729796.
215. Lee JH, Yoon YC, Jee S. Diagnostic performance of indirect MR arthrography for the diagnosis of rotator cuff tears at 3.0T. Acta Radiol. 2014;56(6):720–6. https://doi.org/10.1177/0284185114537817.
216. Jung JY, Yoon YC, Yi SK, Yoo J, Choe BK. Comparison study of indirect MR arthrography and direct MR arthrography of the shoulder. Skelet Radiol. 2009;38(7):659–67. https://doi.org/10.1007/s00256-009-0660-7.
217. Lee JH, Yoon YC, Jee S, Kwon JW, Cha JG, Yoo JC. Comparison of three-dimensional isotropic and two-dimensional conventional indirect MR arthrography for the diagnosis of rotator cuff tears. Korean J Radiol. 2014;15(6):771–80. https://doi.org/10.3348/kjr.2014.15.6.771.
218. Dumontier C, Sautet A, Gagey O, Apoil A. Rotator interval lesions and their relation to coracoid impingement syndrome. J Shoulder Elb Surg. 1999;8(2):130–5. https://doi.org/10.1016/S1058-2746(99)90005-8.
219. Ferrick MR. Coracoid impingement - A case report and review of the literature. Am J Sport Med. 2000;28(1):117–9.
220. Gerber C, Terrier F, Ganz R. The role of the coracoid process in the chronic impingement syndrome. J Bone Joint Surg. 1985;67(5):703–8.
221. Paulson MM, Watnik NF, Dines DM. Coracoid impingement syndrome, rotator interval reconstruction, and biceps tenodesis in the overhead athlete (Reprinted from Operative Techniques in Sports Medicine, October, 2000). Orthop Clin N Am. 2001;32(3):485. https://doi.org/10.1016/S0030-5898(05)70217-0.
222. Martetschlager F, Rios D, Boykin RE, Giphart JE, de Waha A, Millett PJ. Coracoid impingement: current concepts. Knee surgery, sports traumatology. Arthroscopy. 2012;20(11):2148–55. https://doi.org/10.1007/s00167-012-2013-7.
223. Goldthwait JE. An anatomic and mechanical study of the shoulder-joint, explaining many of the cases of painful shoulder, many of the recurrent dislocations, and many of the cases of brachial neuralgias or neuritis. J Bone Joint Surg. 1909;s2-6(4):579.

224. Arrigoni P, Brady PC, Burkhart SS. Calcific tendonitis of the subscapularis tendon causing subcoracoid stenosis and coracoid impingement. Arthroscopy. 2006;22(10):1139 e1131–3. https://doi.org/10.1016/j.arthro.2005.06.028.
225. Franceschi F, Longo UG, Ruzzini L, Rizzello G, Denaro V. Arthroscopic management of calcific tendinitis of the subscapularis tendon. Knee Surg Sports Traumatol Arthrosc. 2007;15(12):1482–5. https://doi.org/10.1007/s00167-007-0340-x.
226. Ko JY, Shih CH, Chen WJ, Yamamoto R. Coracoid impingement caused by a ganglion from the subscapularis tendon. A case report. J Bone Joint Surg. 1994;76(11):1709–11.
227. Peidro L, Serra A, Suso S. Subcoracoid impingement after ossification of the subscapularis tendon. J Shoulder Elb Surg. 1999;8(2):170–1.
228. Terabayashi N, Fukuta M, Ito Y, Takigami I, Nishimoto Y, Shimizu K. Shoulder impingement syndrome due to a ganglion cyst below the coracoacromial ligament: a case report. J Bone Joint Surg. 2011;93(8):e36. https://doi.org/10.2106/JBJS.J.00810.
229. Patte D. The subcoracoid impingement. Clin Orthop Relat Res. 1990;254:55–9.
230. Radas CB, Pieper HG. The coracoid impingement of the subscapularis tendon: a cadaver study. J Shoulder Elb Surg. 2004;13(2):154–9. https://doi.org/10.1016/S1058274603003124.
231. Kragh JF Jr, Doukas WC, Basamania CJ. Primary coracoid impingement syndrome. Am J Orthop (Belle Mead NJ). 2004;33(5):229–32.. discussion 232
232. Okoro T, Reddy VR, Pimpelnarkar A. Coracoid impingement syndrome: a literature review. Curr Rev Musculoskelet Med. 2009;2(1):51–5. https://doi.org/10.1007/s12178-009-9044-9.
233. Dines DM, Warren RF, Inglis AE, Pavlov H. The coracoid impingement syndrome. J Bone Joint Surg. 1990;72(2):314–6.
234. Gerber C, Terrier F, Zehnder R, Ganz R. The subcoracoid space. An anatomic study. Clin Orthop Relat Res. 1987;215:132–8.
235. Masala S, Fanucci E, Maiotti M, Nardocci M, Gaudioso C, Apruzzese A, Di Mario M, Simonetti G. Impingement syndrome of the shoulder. Clinical data and radiologic findings. Radiol Med. 1995;89(1–2):18–21.
236. Finnoff JT, Thompson JM, Collins M, Dahm D. Subcoracoid bursitis as an unusual cause of painful anterior shoulder snapping in a weight lifter. Am J Sports Med. 2010;38(8):1687–92. https://doi.org/10.1177/0363546510369546.
237. Drakes S, Thomas S, Kim S, Guerrero L, Lee SW. Ultrasonography of subcoracoid bursal impingement syndrome. Pm&R. 2015;7(3):329–33. https://doi.org/10.1016/j.pmrj.2014.09.015.
238. Bonutti PM, Norfray JF, Friedman RJ, Genez BM. Kinematic Mri of the Shoulder. J Comput Assist Tomogr. 1993;17(4):666–9.
239. Richards DP, Burkhart SS, Campbell SE. Relation between narrowed coracohumeral distance and subscapularis tears. Arthroscopy. 2005;21(10):1223–8. https://doi.org/10.1016/j.arthro.2005.06.015.
240. Friedman RJ, Bonutti PM, Genez B. Cine magnetic resonance imaging of the subcoracoid region. Orthopedics. 1998;21(5):545–8.
241. Giaroli EL, Major NM, Lemley DE, Lee J. Coracohumeral interval imaging in subcoracoid impingement syndrome on MRI. AJR Am J Roentgenol. 2006;186(1):242–6. https://doi.org/10.2214/AJR.04.0830.
242. Lo IK, Parten PM, Burkhart SS. Combined subcoracoid and subacromial impingement in association with anterosuperior rotator cuff tears: An arthroscopic approach. Arthroscopy. 2003;19(10):1068–78. https://doi.org/10.1016/j.arthro.2003.10.016.
243. Nove-Josserand L, Boulahia A, Levigne C, Noel E, Walch G. Coraco-humeral space and rotator cuff tears. Rev Chir Orthop Reparatrice Appar Mot. 1999;85(7):677–83.
244. Lo IKY, Burkhart SS. Arthroscopic coracoplasty through the rotator interval. Arthroscopy. 2003;19(6):667–71. https://doi.org/10.1016/S0749-8063(03)00219-6.
245. Nove-Josserand L, Edwards TB, O'Connor DP, Walch G. The acromiohumeral and coracohumeral intervals are abnormal in rotator cuff tears with muscular fatty degeneration. Clin Orthop Relat Res. 2005;433:90–6.
246. Walz DM, Miller TT, Chen S, Hofman J. MR imaging of delamination tears of the rotator cuff tendons. Skelet Radiol. 2007;36(5):411–6. https://doi.org/10.1007/s00256-006-0265-3.
247. Deutsch A, Altchek DW, Veltri DM, Potter HG, Warren RF. Traumatic tears of the subscapularis tendon. Clinical diagnosis, magnetic resonance imaging findings, and operative treatment. Am J Sports Med. 1997;25(1):13–22.
248. Lafosse L, Jost B, Reiland Y, Audebert S, Toussaint B, Gobezie R. Structural integrity and clinical outcomes after arthroscopic repair of isolated subscapularis tears. J Bone Joint Surg. 2007;89(6):1184–93. https://doi.org/10.2106/JBJS.F.00007.
249. Fox J, Romeo AA Arthroscopic subscapularis repair. In: Annual Meeting of the American Academy of Orthopaedic Surgeons, New Orleans, LA, 2003.
250. Osti L, Soldati F, Buono AD, Buda M. Arthroscopic repair of the subscapularis tendon: indications, limits and technical features. Muscles Ligaments Tendons J. 2013;3(3):213–9.
251. Kim SJ, Jung M, Lee JH, Kim C, Chun YM. Arthroscopic repair of anterosuperior rotator cuff tears: in-continuity technique vs. disruption of subscapularis-supraspinatus tear margin: comparison of clinical outcomes and structural integrity between the two techniques. J Bone Joint Surg Am. 2014;96(24):2056–61. https://doi.org/10.2106/JBJS.N.00293.

252. Visona E, Cerciello S, Godeneche A, Neyton L, Fessy MH, Nove-Josserand L. The "comma sign": an anatomical investigation (dissection of the rotator interval in 14 cadaveric shoulders). Surgical Radiol Anatomy. 2015;37(7):793–8. https://doi.org/10.1007/s00276-015-1420-0.
253. Lo IK, Burkhart SS. The comma sign: An arthroscopic guide to the torn subscapularis tendon. Arthroscopy. 2003;19(3):334–7. https://doi.org/10.1053/jars.2003.50080.
254. Jung JY, Yoon YC, Cha DI, Yoo JC, Jung JY. The "bridging sign": a MR finding for combined full-thickness tears of the subscapularis tendon and the supraspinatus tendon. Acta Radiol. 2013;54(1):83–8. https://doi.org/10.1258/ar.2012.120353.
255. Walch G, Boileau P, Noel E, Donell ST. Impingement of the deep surface of the supraspinatus tendon on the posterosuperior glenoid rim: An arthroscopic study. J Shoulder Elb Surg. 1992;1(5):238–45. https://doi.org/10.1016/S1058-2746(09)80065-7.
256. Jobe CM. Posterior superior glenoid impingement: expanded spectrum. Arthroscopy. 1995;11(5):530–6.
257. Halbrecht JL, Tirman P, Atkin D. Internal impingement of the shoulder: comparison of findings between the throwing and nonthrowing shoulders of college baseball players. Arthroscopy. 1999;15(3):253–8. https://doi.org/10.1016/S0749-8063(99)70030-7.
258. McFarland EG, Hsu CY, Neira C, O'Neil O. Internal impingement of the shoulder: a clinical and arthroscopic analysis. J Shoulder Elb Surg. 1999;8(5):458–60. https://doi.org/10.1016/S1058-2746(99)90076-9.
259. Walch G, Liotard JP, Boileau P, Noel E. Posterosuperior glenoid impingement. Another impingement of the shoulder. J Radiol. 1993;74(1):47–50.
260. Jobe FW, Giangarra CE, Kvitne RS, Glousman RE. Anterior capsulolabral reconstruction of the shoulder in athletes in overhand sports. Am J Sports Med. 1991;19(5):428–34. https://doi.org/10.1177/036354659101900502.
261. Mihata T, McGarry MH, Neo M, Ohue M, Lee TQ. Effect of anterior capsular laxity on horizontal abduction and forceful internal impingement in a cadaveric model of the throwing shoulder. Am J Sports Med. 2015;43(7):1758–63. https://doi.org/10.1177/0363546515582025.
262. Burkhart SS, Morgan CD, Kibler WB. The disabled throwing shoulder: spectrum of pathology Part I: pathoanatomy and biomechanics. Arthroscopy. 2003;19(4):404–20. https://doi.org/10.1053/jars.2003.50128.
263. Levitz CL, Dugas J, Andrews JR. The use of arthroscopic thermal capsulorrhaphy to treat internal impingement in baseball players. Arthroscopy. 2001;17(6):573–7. https://doi.org/10.1053/jars.2001.24853.
264. Mithöfer K, Fealy S, Altchek DW. Arthroscopic Treatment of Internal Impingement of the Shoulder. Tech Should Elbow Surg. 2004;5(2):66–75.
265. Wright RW, Steger-May K, Klein SE. Radiographic findings in the shoulder and elbow of major league baseball pitchers. Am J Sport Med. 2007;35(11):1839–43. https://doi.org/10.1177/0363546507304493.
266. Bennett GE. Shoulder and elbow lesions distinctive of baseball players. Ann Surg. 1947;126(1):107–10.
267. Wright RW, Paletta GA Jr. Prevalence of the Bennett lesion of the shoulder in major league pitchers. Am J Sports Med. 2004;32(1):121–4.
268. Nakagawa S, Yoneda M, Hayashida K, Mizuno N, Yamada S. Posterior shoulder pain in throwing athletes with a Bennett lesion: Factors that influence throwing pain. J Shoulder Elb Surg. 2006;15(1):72–7. https://doi.org/10.1016/j.jse.2005.05.010.
269. Ferrari JD, Ferrari DA, Coumas J, Pappas AM. Posterior ossification of the shoulder - the bennett lesion - etiology, diagnosis, and treatment. Am J Sport Med. 1994;22(2):171–6. https://doi.org/10.1177/036354659402200204.
270. Yablon CM, Bedi A, Morag Y, Jacobson JA. Ultrasonography of the shoulder with arthroscopic correlation. Clin Sports Med. 2013;32(3):391–408. https://doi.org/10.1016/j.csm.2013.03.001.
271. Thomas SJ, Swanik CB, Higginson JS, Kaminski TW, Swanik KA, Bartolozzi AR, Abboud JA, Nazarian LN. A bilateral comparison of posterior capsule thickness and its correlation with glenohumeral range of motion and scapular upward rotation in collegiate baseball players. J Shoulder Elb Surg. 2011;20(5):708–16. https://doi.org/10.1016/j.jse.2010.08.031.
272. Kirchhoff C, Imhoff AB. Posterosuperior and anterosuperior impingement of the shoulder in overhead athletes-evolving concepts. Int Orthop. 2010;34(7):1049–58. https://doi.org/10.1007/s00264-010-1038-0.
273. Giaroli EL, Major NM, Higgins LD. MRI of internal impingement of the shoulder. AJR Am J Roentgenol. 2005;185(4):925–9. https://doi.org/10.2214/AJR.04.0971.
274. Tirman PFJ, Bost FW, Garvin GJ, Peterfy CG, Mall JC, Steinbach LS, Feller JF, Crues JV. Posterosuperior glenoid impingement of the shoulder - findings at Mr-imaging and Mr arthrography with Arthroscopic correlation. Radiology. 1994;193(2):431–6.
275. Smith TO, Drew BT, Toms AP. A meta-analysis of the diagnostic test accuracy of MRA and MRI for the detection of glenoid labral injury. Arch Orthop Trauma Surg. 2012;132(7):905–19. https://doi.org/10.1007/s00402-012-1493-8.
276. Chang EY, Fliszar E, Chung CB. Superior labrum anterior and posterior lesions and microinstability. Magn Reson Imaging Clin N Am. 2012;20(2):277–94., x-xi. https://doi.org/10.1016/j.mric.2012.01.002.
277. Tehranzadeh AD, Fronek J, Resnick D. Posterior capsular fibrosis in professional baseball pitchers: case series of MR arthrographic findings in six patients with glenohumeral internal rotational

deficit. Clin Imaging. 2007;31(5):343–8. https://doi.org/10.1016/j.clinimag.2007.05.005.
278. Tuite MJ, Petersen BD, Wise SM, Fine JP, Kaplan LD, Orwin JF. Shoulder MR arthrography of the posterior labrocapsular complex in overhead throwers with pathologic internal impingement and internal rotation deficit. Skelet Radiol. 2007;36(6):495–502. https://doi.org/10.1007/s00256-007-0278-6.
279. Jung JY, Ha DH, Lee SM, Blacksin MF, Kim KA, Kim JW. Displaceability of SLAP lesion on shoulder MR arthrography with external rotation position. Skelet Radiol. 2011;40(8):1047–55. https://doi.org/10.1007/s00256-011-1134-2.
280. Saleem AM, Lee JK, Novak LM. Usefulness of the abduction and external rotation views in shoulder MR arthrography. AJR Am J Roentgenol. 2008;191(4):1024–30. https://doi.org/10.2214/AJR.07.3962.
281. Mulyadi E, Harish S, O'Neill J, Rebello R. MRI of impingement syndromes of the shoulder. Clin Radiol. 2009;64(3):307–18. https://doi.org/10.1016/j.crad.2008.08.013.
282. Gerber C, Sebesta A. Impingement of the deep surface of the subscapularis tendon and the reflection pulley on the anterosuperior glenoid rim: a preliminary report. J Shoulder Elb Surg. 2000;9(6):483–90. https://doi.org/10.1067/mse.2000.109322.
283. Struhl S. Anterior internal impingement: an arthroscopic observation. Arthroscopy. 2002;18(1):2–7.
284. Habermeyer P, Magosch P, Pritsch M, Scheibel MT, Lichtenberg S. Anterosuperior impingement of the shoulder as a result of pulley lesions: a prospective arthroscopic study. J Shoulder Elb Surg. 2004;13(1):5–12. https://doi.org/10.1016/j.jse.2003.09.013.
285. Garofalo R, Karlsson J, Nordenson U, Cesari E, Conti M, Castagna A. Anterior-superior internal impingement of the shoulder: an evidence-based review. Knee Surg Sports Traumatol Arthrosc. 2010;18(12):1688–93. https://doi.org/10.1007/s00167-010-1232-z.
286. Krzycki J, Tischer T, Imhoff AB. The para-shoulder: lesions of the anterior-superior complex (Labrum, SGHL, SSC) and their arthroscopic treatment. Z Orthop Ihre Grenzgeb. 2006;144(5):446–8. https://doi.org/10.1055/s-2006-954403.
287. Valadie AL, Jobe CM, Pink MM, Ekman EF, Jobe FW. Anatomy of provocative tests for impingement syndrome of the shoulder. J Shoulder Elb Surg. 2000;9(1):36–46. https://doi.org/10.1016/S1058-2746(00)90008-9.
288. Pappas GP, Blemker SS, Beaulieu CF, McAdams TR, Whalen ST, Gold GE. In vivo anatomy of the Neer and Hawkins sign positions for shoulder impingement. J Shoulder Elb Surg. 2006;15(1):40–9. https://doi.org/10.1016/j.jse.2005.04.007.
289. Baumann B, Genning K, Bohm D, Rolf O, Gohlke F. Arthroscopic prevalence of pulley lesions in 1007 consecutive patients. J Shoulder Elb Surg. 2008;17(1):14–20. https://doi.org/10.1016/j.jse.2007.04.011.
290. Barile A, Lanni G, Conti L, Mariani S, Calvisi V, Castagna A, Rossi F, Masciocchi C. Lesions of the biceps pulley as cause of anterosuperior impingement of the shoulder in the athlete: potentials and limits of MR arthrography compared with arthroscopy. Radiol Med. 2013;118(1):112–22. https://doi.org/10.1007/s11547-012-0838-2.
291. Chandnani VP, Gagliardi JA, Murnane TG, Bradley YC, DeBerardino TA, Spaeth J, Hansen MF. Glenohumeral ligaments and shoulder capsular mechanism: evaluation with MR arthrography. Radiology. 1995;196(1):27–32. https://doi.org/10.1148/radiology.196.1.7784579.
292. Nakata W, Katou S, Fujita A, Nakata M, Lefor AT, Sugimoto H. Biceps pulley: normal anatomy and associated lesions at MR arthrography. Radiographics. 2011;31(3):791–810. https://doi.org/10.1148/rg.313105507.
293. Familiari F, Gonzalez-Zapata A, Iannò B, Galasso O, Gasparini G, McFarland E. Is acromioplasty necessary in the setting of full-thickness rotator cuff tears? A systematic review. J Orthopaed Traumatol. 2015;16:1–8. https://doi.org/10.1007/s10195-015-0353-z.
294. Ensor KL, Kwon YW, Dibeneditto MR, Zuckerman JD, Rokito AS. The rising incidence of rotator cuff repairs. J Shoulder Elb Surg. 2013;22(12):1628–32. https://doi.org/10.1016/j.jse.2013.01.006.
295. Chen M, Xu W, Dong Q, Huang Q, Xie Z, Mao Y. Outcomes of single-row versus double-row arthroscopic rotator cuff repair: a systematic review and meta-analysis of current evidence. Arthroscopy. 2013;29(8):1437–49. https://doi.org/10.1016/j.arthro.2013.03.076.
296. McElvany MD, McGoldrick E, Gee AO, Neradilek MB, Matsen FA 3rd. Rotator cuff repair: published evidence on factors associated with repair integrity and clinical outcome. Am J Sports Med. 2015;43(2):491–500. https://doi.org/10.1177/0363546514529644.
297. Millett PJ, Warth RJ, Dornan GJ, Lee JT, Spiegl UJ. Clinical and structural outcomes after arthroscopic single-row versus double-row rotator cuff repair: a systematic review and meta-analysis of level I randomized clinical trials. J Shoulder Elb Surg. 2014;23(4):586–97. https://doi.org/10.1016/j.jse.2013.10.006.
298. Ide J, Maeda S, Takagi K. Arthroscopic transtendon repair of partial-thickness articular-side tears of the rotator cuff: anatomical and clinical study. Am J Sports Med. 2005;33(11):1672–9. https://doi.org/10.1177/0363546505277141.
299. Lo IK, Burkhart SS. Transtendon arthroscopic repair of partial-thickness, articular surface tears of the rotator cuff. Arthroscopy. 2004;20(2):214–20. https://doi.org/10.1016/j.arthro.2003.11.042.
300. Iyengar JJ, Porat S, Burnett KR, Marrero-Perez L, Hernandez VH, Nottage WM. Magnetic resonance imaging tendon integrity assessment after arthroscopic partial-thickness rotator cuff repair. Arthroscopy. 2011;27(3):306–13. https://doi.org/10.1016/j.arthro.2010.08.017.

301. Sun L, Zhang Q, Ge H, Sun Y, Cheng B. Which is the best repair of articular-sided rotator cuff tears: a meta-analysis. J Orthop Surg Res. 2015;10(1):84. https://doi.org/10.1186/s13018-015-0224-6.
302. Wolf EM, Pennington WT, Agrawal V. Arthroscopic side-to-side rotator cuff repair. Arthroscopy. 2005;21(7):881–7. https://doi.org/10.1016/j.arthro.2005.03.014.
303. Burkhart SS. The principle of margin convergence in rotator cuff repair as a means of strain reduction at the tear margin. Ann Biomed Eng. 2004;32(1):166–70.
304. Suchenski M, McCarthy MB, Chowaniec D, Hansen D, McKinnon W, Apostolakos J, Arciero R, Mazzocca AD. Material properties and composition of soft-tissue fixation. Arthroscopy. 2010;26(6):821–31. https://doi.org/10.1016/j.arthro.2009.12.026.
305. Apreleva M, Ozbaydar M, Fitzgibbons PG, Warner JJ. Rotator cuff tears: the effect of the reconstruction method on three-dimensional repair site area. Arthroscopy. 2002;18(5):519–26. https://doi.org/10.1053/jars.2002.32930.
306. Park MC, ElAttrache NS, Tibone JE, Ahmad CS, Jun BJ, Lee TQ. Part I: footprint contact characteristics for a transosseous-equivalent rotator cuff repair technique compared with a double-row repair technique. J Shoulder Elb Surg. 2007;16(4):461–8. https://doi.org/10.1016/j.jse.2006.09.010.
307. Denard PJ, Burkhart SS. The evolution of suture anchors in arthroscopic rotator cuff repair. Arthroscopy. 2013;29(9):1589–95. https://doi.org/10.1016/j.arthro.2013.05.011.
308. Park MC, Elattrache NS, Ahmad CS, Tibone JE. "Transosseous-equivalent" rotator cuff repair technique. Arthroscopy. 2006;22(12):1360 e1361–5. https://doi.org/10.1016/j.arthro.2006.07.017.
309. Voos JE, Barnthouse CD, Scott AR. Arthroscopic rotator cuff repair: techniques in 2012. Clin Sports Med. 2012;31(4):633–44. https://doi.org/10.1016/j.csm.2012.07.002.
310. Garofalo R, Castagna A, Borroni M, Krishnan SG. Arthroscopic transosseous (anchorless) rotator cuff repair. Knee Surg Sports Traumatol Arthrosc. 2012;20(6):1031–5. https://doi.org/10.1007/s00167-011-1725-4.
311. Salata MJ, Sherman SL, Lin EC, Sershon RA, Gupta A, Shewman E, Wang VM, Cole BJ, Romeo AA, Verma NN. Biomechanical evaluation of transosseous rotator cuff repair: do anchors really matter? Am J Sports Med. 2013;41(2):283–90. https://doi.org/10.1177/0363546512469092.
312. Prickett WD, Teefey SA, Galatz LM, Calfee RP, Middleton WD, Yamaguchi K. Accuracy of ultrasound imaging of the rotator cuff in shoulders that are painful postoperatively. J Bone Joint Surg Am. 2003;85-A(6):1084–9.
313. Lee KW, Yang DS, Chun TJ, Bae KW, Choy WS, Park HJ. A comparison of conventional ultrasonography and arthrosonography in the assessment of cuff integrity after rotator cuff repair. Clin Orthop Surg. 2014;6(3):336–42. https://doi.org/10.4055/cios.2014.6.3.336.
314. Duc SR, Mengiardi B, Pfirrmann CW, Jost B, Hodler J, Zanetti M. Diagnostic performance of MR arthrography after rotator cuff repair. AJR Am J Roentgenol. 2006;186(1):237–41. https://doi.org/10.2214/AJR.04.1818.
315. Kim S-J, Kim S-H, Lim S-H, Chun Y-M. Use of magnetic resonance arthrography to compare clinical features and structural integrity after arthroscopic repair of bursal versus articular side partial-thickness rotator cuff tears. Am J Sports Med. 2013;41(9):2041–7.
316. Tudisco C, Bisicchia S, Savarese E, Fiori R, Bartolucci DA, Masala S, Simonetti G. Single-row vs. double-row arthroscopic rotator cuff repair: clinical and 3 Tesla MR arthrography results. BMC Musculoskelet Disord. 2013;14:43. https://doi.org/10.1186/1471-2474-14-43.
317. Crim J, Burks R, Manaster BJ, Hanrahan C, Hung M, Greis P. Temporal evolution of MRI findings after arthroscopic rotator cuff repair. AJR Am J Roentgenol. 2010;195(6):1361–6. https://doi.org/10.2214/AJR.10.4436.
318. Spielmann AL, Forster BB, Kokan P, Hawkins RH, Janzen DL. Shoulder after rotator cuff repair: MR imaging findings in asymptomatic individuals--initial experience. Radiology. 1999;213(3):705–8. https://doi.org/10.1148/radiology.213.3.r99dc09705.
319. Owen RS, Iannotti JP, Kneeland JB, Dalinka MK, Deren JA, Oleaga L. Shoulder after surgery: MR imaging with surgical validation. Radiology. 1993;186(2):443–7. https://doi.org/10.1148/radiology.186.2.8421748.
320. Koh KH, Kang KC, Lim TK, Shon MS, Yoo JC. Prospective randomized clinical trial of single- versus double-row suture anchor repair in 2- to 4-cm rotator cuff tears: clinical and magnetic resonance imaging results. Arthroscopy. 2011;27(4):453–62. https://doi.org/10.1016/j.arthro.2010.11.059.
321. Franceschi F, Ruzzini L, Longo UG, Martina FM, Zobel BB, Maffulli N, Denaro V. Equivalent clinical results of arthroscopic single-row and double-row suture anchor repair for rotator cuff tears: a randomized controlled trial. Am J Sports Med. 2007;35(8):1254–60. https://doi.org/10.1177/0363546507302218.
322. Cho NS, Yi JW, Lee BG, Rhee YG. Retear patterns after arthroscopic rotator cuff repair: single-row versus suture bridge technique. Am J Sports Med. 2010;38(4):664–71. https://doi.org/10.1177/0363546509350081.
323. Hayashida K, Tanaka M, Koizumi K, Kakiuchi M. Characteristic retear patterns assessed by magnetic resonance imaging after arthroscopic double-row rotator cuff repair. Arthroscopy. 2012;28(4):458–64. https://doi.org/10.1016/j.arthro.2011.09.006.
324. Saccomanno MF, Cazzato G, Fodale M, Sircana G, Milano G. Magnetic resonance imaging criteria for the assessment of the rotator cuff after repair: a systematic review. Knee Surg Sports Traumatol Arthrosc. 2015;23(2):423–42. https://doi.org/10.1007/s00167-014-3486-3.

Imaging Diagnosis of Biceps Tendon and Rotator Interval Pathology

6

Luis S. Beltran, Eric Ledermann, Sana Ali, and Javier Beltran

6.1 Introduction

Rotator interval pathology is associated with biceps instability, glenohumeral instability, and adhesive capsulitis, all of which can be challenging to clinically diagnose and treat. The complex anatomy and orientation of the structures in this region within a relatively small space can make it difficult to evaluate by imaging; however, improvements in MR technology have better allowed detection of disease in this region. Furthermore, it is important to realize that the rotator interval is not routinely evaluated upon arthroscopic investigation unless the clinical examination or imaging points to pathology at this level. Imaging, therefore, plays a critical role in helping the clinician make the diagnosis and initiate appropriate treatment.

6.2 Normal Anatomy of the Rotator Interval

A triangular space, the rotator cuff interval, resides in the anterior-superior aspect of the shoulder bounded by the anterior fibers of the supraspinatus tendon superiorly, the cranial fibers of the subscapularis tendon inferiorly, and the coracoid process at its base (Fig. 6.1).

The rotator interval capsule (RIC), the most anterior-superior portion of the glenohumeral joint capsule, traverses the rotator interval and is reinforced by two ligaments, one internally by the superior glenohumeral ligament (SGHL) and the other externally by the coracohumeral ligament (CHL). Distally, the RIC joins the CHL and SGHL along the medial and lateral aspects of the bicipital groove maintaining the long head of the biceps tendon (LHBT) in normal anatomical location.

The CHL is a relatively constant structure only found to be hypoplastic or absent in 6% (4 of 63) of shoulder dissections [1, 2]. It originates along the lateral aspect of the base of the coracoid process of the scapula just abutting the external surface of the glenohumeral joint. The CHL is formed by two bands: a smaller band, medially, and a larger band, laterally, which are not always seen with clear distinction [1]. The medial band of the CHL (MCHL) merges distally with the SGHL to form a ligament (SGHL-MCHL) complex. The complex then surrounds the medial and inferior aspects of the intra-articular portion of LHBT forming a sling-like structure that cradles the biceps tendon, before inserting on the lesser tuberosity. At the lesser tuberosity insertion it then merges with the RIC along with the superior fibers of the subscapularis tendon. The lateral band of the CHL (LCHL) surrounds the superior and lateral aspects of the intra-articular LHBT before inserting on the greater tuberosity. At that

L. S. Beltran (✉)
Department of Radiology, Brigham and Women's Hospital, Harvard Medical School, Boston, MA, USA
e-mail: lbeltran@bwh.harvard.edu

E. Ledermann · S. Ali · J. Beltran
Department of Radiology, Maimonides Medical Center, Brooklyn, NY, USA

J. T. Bencardino (ed.), *The Shoulder*, https://doi.org/10.1007/978-3-030-06240-8_6

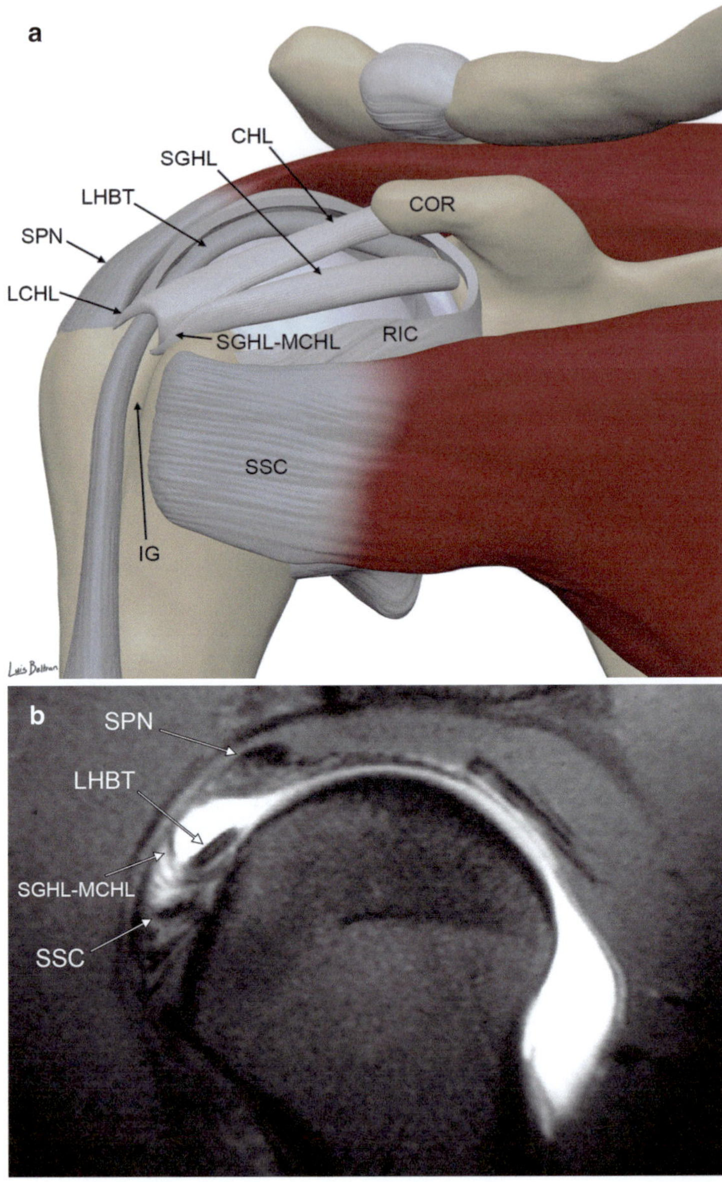

Fig. 6.1 Normal anatomy of rotator interval. (**a**) Illustration and (**b**) sagittal fat-saturated T1-weighted MR arthrogram image demonstrate rotator interval structures including long head of the biceps tendon (LHBT), coracohumeral ligament (CHL), superior glenohumeral ligament (SGHL), subscapularis tendon (SSC), supraspinatus tendon (SPN), and rotator interval capsule (RIC). In the illustration, RIC, SGHL, CHL, SSC, and SPN are partially resected to visualize underlying structures. COR, coracoid process; IG, intertubercular groove; SGHLMCHL, superior glenohumeral ligament-medial coracohumeral ligament complex. Illustration and MR image reprinted with permission from Beltran LS, Beltran J. Biceps and rotator interval: imaging update. Semin Musculoskelet Radiol. Thieme Medical Publishers; 2014;18:425–35

point, it merges with the anterior margin of the supraspinatus tendon. The coracohumeral ligament remains lax and unengaged with the arm in internal rotation and adduction.

The SGHL, like the CHL, is rarely absent, only reported unseen in 3% of patients at arthroscopy [3]. Its origin is the supraglenoid tubercle which resides just anterior to the origin of the LHBT; however variable origins do include the superior labrum, LHBT, and middle glenohumeral ligament [3]. The SGHL courses anterior and inferior to, and maintains close approximation to, the LHBT within the rotator interval forming a ligament (SGHL-MCHL) complex with the CHL. This complex surrounds and cradles the biceps tendon and maintains its position. Distally, the SGHL inserts into the fovea capitis of the humerus, a small depression above the lesser tuberosity, further contributing to the stability of the LHBT.

The intra-articular portion of the LHBT originates from either the supraglenoid tubercle of the glenoid osseous rim, the posterosuperior labrum, or a combination of both [4]. Variant anatomy of the distal biceps brachii muscle is common, with the literature reporting 9–23% variance in multiple supernumerary heads [5, 6]. Proximal anomalies are quite rare with respect to the intra-articular LHBT6 (Fig. 6.2). The LHBT courses obliquely through the rotator interval making a 30- to 45-degree turn along the anterior surface of the humeral head before exiting the joint. It then resides with the space between the lesser and greater tuberosities at the intertubercular groove. The function and normal anatomical position of the LHBT depend greatly on the integrity of these surrounding support structures including the static stabilizers (RIC, CHL, SGHL) and the dynamic stabilizers (supraspinatus and subscapularis tendons). Together, these stabilizing structures comprise the complex commonly referred to as the biceps reflection pulley [1, 7]. The

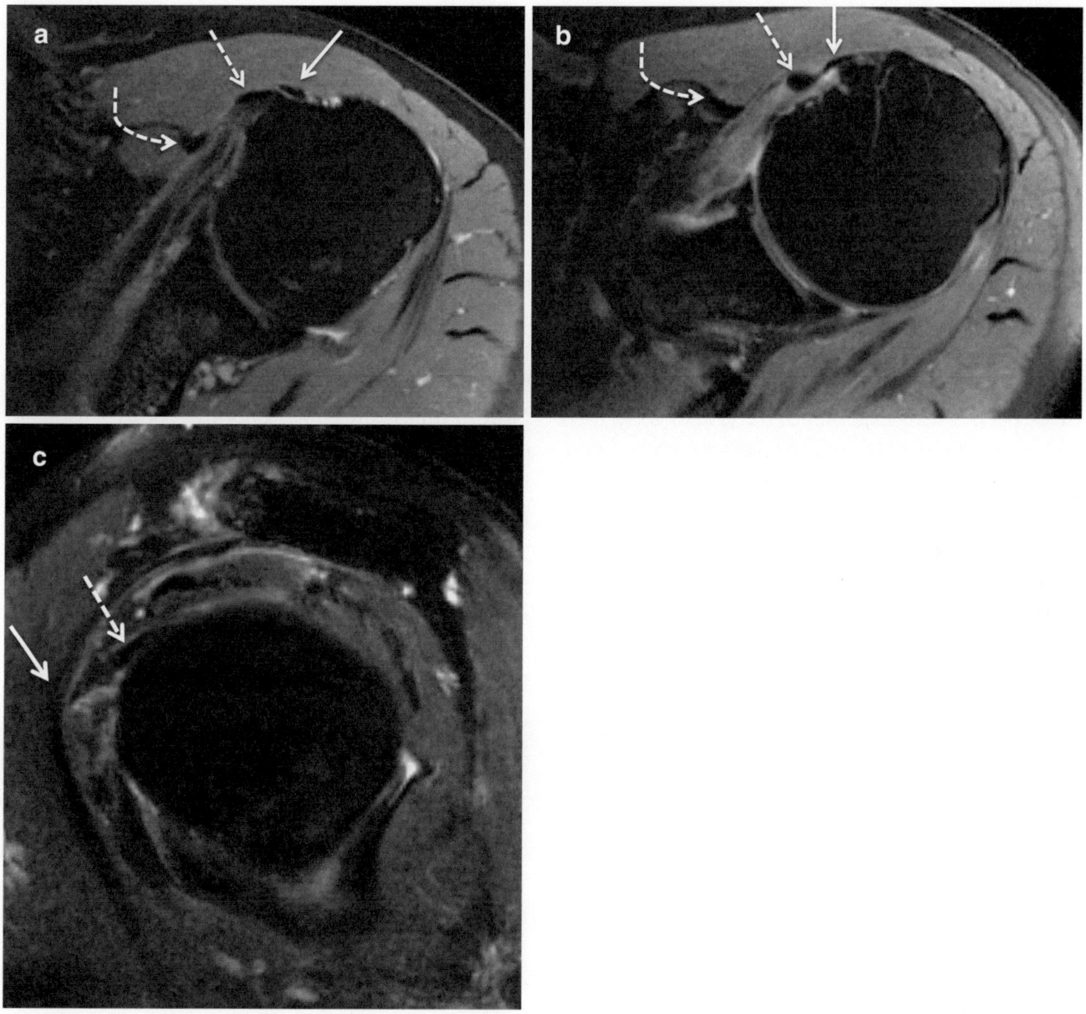

Fig. 6.2 Supernumerary tendons of biceps brachii muscle. (**a**, **b**) Axial fat-saturated and (**c**) sagittal fat-saturated T2 MR images demonstrate three distinct tendon slips of biceps brachii muscle in proximal arm including a supernumerary third tendon (solid arrow in **a** and **b**) located lateral to long head of biceps tendon (LHBT) (straight dashed arrow in **a** and **b**) and short head of biceps tendon (SHBT) (curved dashed arrow in **a** and **b**). The supernumerary tendon originates from superior aspect of rotator interval capsule, which is a variant anatomical origin (solid arrow in **c**). The other intra-articular LHBT originates from the supraglenoid tubercle of glenoid (dashed arrow in **c**), which is the most common anatomical origin

biceps reflection pulley is responsible for limiting medial subluxation of the LHBT when the arm is abducted and externally rotated. Injuries to any of the components, mentioned above, are referred to as "pulley lesions" [8, 9].

6.3 Pathology of the Rotator Interval

6.3.1 Biceps Tendon Pathology

Three categories of tendinopathy exist of the LHBT: impingement tendinopathy, tendinopathy with subluxation, and attrition tendinopathy [10]. Impingement tendinopathy of the proximal biceps tendon is commonly associated with rotator cuff pathology as a result of impingement between the head of the humerus, the acromion, and the coracohumeral ligament during elevation and external rotation of the arm [11, 12]. Tendinopathy with subluxation results from injury to the coracohumeral ligament and superior glenohumeral ligament [12]. Attrition tendinopathy, also described as primary tendinitis [10, 13], is the result of new local bone formation causing stenosis of the bicipital groove which may lead to adhesions. In a study of 122 complete rotator cuff tears by Chen et al. [11], the biceps long-head tendon was evaluated via arthroscopy or open surgery, showing that the incidence of biceps tendinitis was 41%, subluxation was 8%, dislocation was 10%, partial tear was 12%, and complete rupture was 5%. The typical clinical scenario of proximal biceps tendon injury is presentation with anterior shoulder pain and loss of forward arm flexion. When these symptoms are isolated, treatment is often conservative with options including nonsteroidal anti-inflammatory drugs (NSAIDS), physical therapy, and/or steroid injection near the biceps groove around the biceps tendon. Surgical treatment may be necessary when symptoms are over 3 months in duration, if conservative methods fail, or if there are other associated injuries to the rotator cuff or labrum [14]. In patients with impingement, surgical subacromial decompression is performed [12]. Direct therapy of the biceps tendon includes shaving of the tendon in mild or early disease and biceps tenotomy or tenodesis for more advanced disease [13] (Fig. 6.3). Biceps tenotomy includes the resection of the intra-articular portion of the biceps tendon, whereas biceps tenodesis involves resection of the intra-articular portion of the biceps tendon and reattachment of the distal tendon stump to the humeral neck or subpectoral proximal humeral shaft.

6.3.2 Biceps Reflection Pulley Injury

Position of the biceps tendon within the rotator interval and bicipital groove depends heavily on the stability of the biceps reflection pulley. The prevalence of biceps pulley lesions from arthroscopic data is 7%, representing a considerable source of morbidity [15]. Traumatic and nontraumatic causes can lead to biceps reflection pulley injury. Traumatic injuries usually result from a fall on the outstretched arm in combination with full external or internal rotation or a backward fall onto the hand or elbow [16]. Nontraumatic injury generally occurs due to chronic repetitive overhand activity typically seen with throwing sports [17] such as baseball, tennis, and volleyball. Injury to the biceps reflection pulley may also occur in association with rotator cuff tears. In particular, far-anterior supraspinatus tendon footprint insertion and superior subscapularis footprint insertion (also known as anterosuperior rotator cuff tears) tears may dissect to involve the CHL and SGHL, respectively [1]. Injury to this region of the cuff may result in instability of the biceps tendon resulting in biceps tendon subluxation or, worse, dislocation [17, 18].

Clinically, biceps pulley injury can be challenging to diagnose and is often referred to as "hidden lesion" because it can be missed during open and arthroscopic examination [19]. Two separate but similar classification systems of biceps pulley injuries have been described by Habermeyer et al. and Bennett, respectively, which are based on arthroscopic studies [7, 20]. Injury to the biceps reflection pulley can result in medial subluxation or dislocation of the biceps tendon toward the glenohumeral joint or take a

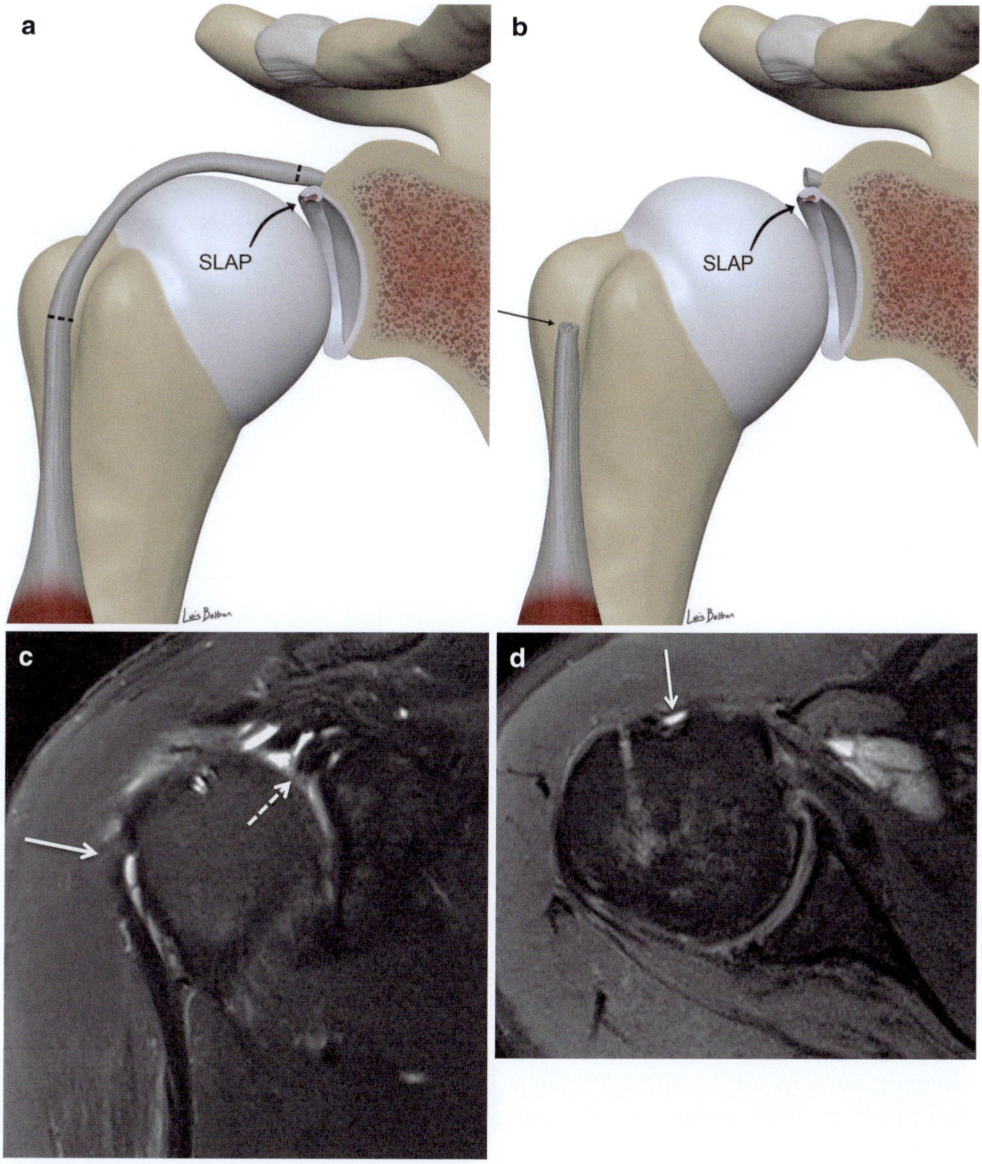

Fig. 6.3 Biceps tenotomy and tenodesis. (**a**) Preoperative illustration of incision sites for biceps tenotomy and tenodesis (dashed lines). Postoperative appearance of biceps tenotomy is demonstrated in (**b**) illustration and (**c**) coronal and (**d**) axial fat-suppressed T2 MR images demonstrating resection of the intra-articular biceps tendon at the level of the supraglenoid tubercle and humeral head (dashed lines in **a**). MRI normally shows a resected biceps tendon stump at the level of the humeral head (solid straight arrow in **b**, **c**), postoperative changes at the supraglenoid tubercle where the tendon insertion has been resected (dashed arrow in **c**), and non-visualization of the intra-articular portion of the long head of the biceps tendon with an empty bicipital groove (arrow in **d**). Biceps tenodesis is demonstrated in (**e**) illustration and (**f**) coronal proton density and (**g**) axial fat-suppressed proton density MR images. When a tenodesis is performed, the same incisions are made in the biceps tendon (dashed lines in **a**) coupled with fixation devices (screw, anchor, or sutures) at the attachment of the distal portion of the biceps tendon to the humeral head (arrows in **e**, **f**, and **g**) or more distally along the subpectoral proximal humeral shaft (not shown). Labral tears, specifically, superior labrum anterior and posterior (SLAP) tears (curved arrows in **a**, **b**, and **e**), are a form of concurrent injury leading to the need for performing biceps tenotomy/tenodesis in the treatment of biceps tendon pathology. Illustrations reprinted with permission from Beltran LS, Beltran J. Biceps and rotator interval: imaging update. Semin Musculoskelet Radiol. Thieme Medical Publishers; 2014;18:425–35

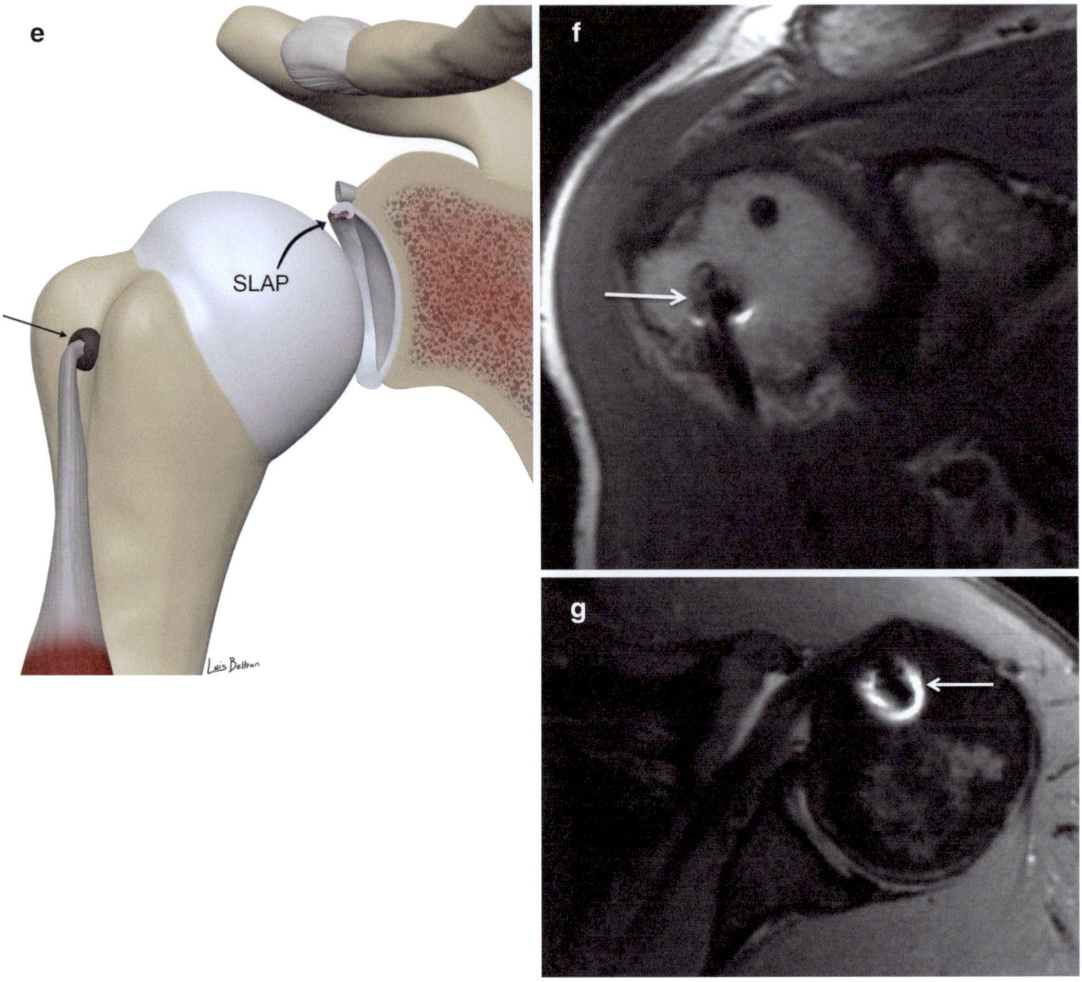

Fig. 6.3 (continued)

more anterior extra-articular course depending on which structures of the biceps reflection pulley are injured. Knowledge of the anatomy and classification systems of biceps pulley injuries can assist the clinician to ensure inspecting the appropriate regions during surgery to avoid pathology being missed [7, 20]. Choice of treatment of biceps pulley lesions varies. Some studies support surgical interventions and repair of the biceps pulley structures with the goal of restoring the stability of the biceps tendon [21, 22]. However, biceps tenodesis currently is most often performed in these patients [1].

6.3.3 Rotator Interval Laxity and Instability

The inferior glenohumeral ligament and the glenohumeral joint capsule are the most important static stabilizers of the glenohumeral joint [3]. The middle and superior glenohumeral ligaments play a more minor role because they are frequently hypoplastic or congenitally absent [23, 24]. The rotator cuff muscles are the major dynamic stabilizers of the glenohumeral joint which aid in balancing translational (destabilizing) forces with compressive (stabilizing) forces maintaining glenohumeral joint stability throughout its arc of motion [25–29]. This concavity-compression mechanism holds the glenohumeral joint at middle range of motion when the capsulolabral structures are unengaged and at terminal range of motion when rotator cuff muscle activity inhibits motion and decreases strain on the glenohumeral ligaments [30–33]. The biceps tendon also plays a key role in maintaining superior stability of the glenohumeral joint [24]. The glenoid labrum on the other hand acts as a conduit of stability by acting as an anchor site of ligamentous attachment and less significantly by providing increased depth to the glenoid fossa [3, 23].

Injury to the rotator interval capsule normally results in posterior and inferior glenohumeral joint instability [34]. Clinically this leads to excessive inferior translation with the shoulder in adduction and external rotation. Harryman et al. [35] demonstrated that resection of the rotator interval capsule in cadavers resulted in inferior and posterior translation of the adducted shoulder, and subsequent overlapping redundancy of the rotator interval capsule causes increased resistance to inferior and posterior translation. The role of the rotator interval capsule to glenohumeral joint stability is believed to be that it provides an anatomical negative-pressure seal to the anterior-superior joint capsule between the humeral head and glenoid fossa [20, 36, 37]. The CHL is also thought to be an important stabilizer providing additional structural support; however, its role is not as significant as the rotator interval capsule [9]. Ligamentous injury, particularly the SGHL and CHL, has been shown to result in inferior glenohumeral joint instability [37–39]. Furthermore, predisposition to glenohumeral instability is seen in individuals with developmental defects of the rotator interval [38, 40]. Preferred treatment of rotator interval laxity presenting with instability is imbrication of the rotator interval capsule, performed either arthroscopically or with an open approach [40–43].

6.3.4 Adhesive Capsulitis

Adhesive capsulitis, also known as frozen shoulder, was first described in 1934 by Codman [44] and has a prevalence of 2% in the general population [45]. The condition affects women more commonly than men and tends to occur between 40 and 60 years of age [45], but it can occur at any age. Clinically, affected patients present with shoulder pain symptoms which are most pronounced in the evening, shoulder stiffness lasting >1 month, and absence of other abnormalities explaining the symptoms [46]. Spontaneous resolution seems to occur in almost all patients; however, symptoms can persist for approximately 2 years [44]. There is a spectrum and temporal evolution of symptoms with varied clinical presentation and duration that consists of three phases [47]. Phase one is the "painful freezing phase" where the dominant symptom is pain along with shoulder stiffness lasting for 10–36 weeks. The second stage is the "adhesive phase" with near-complete loss of passive and active range of motion but gradual pain subsidence at 4–12 months. The third and final stage is the "resolution phase" during which normal range of motion returns to the shoulder spontaneously usually seen at 12–42 months.

In the literature, adhesive capsulitis is classified into a primary (idiopathic) type with no discoverable inciting event and a secondary type associated with specific injury or an underlying etiology [48]. The secondary type is further subcategorized by etiology into the intrinsic type in which rotator cuff injury or prolonged immobilization (e.g., sports injury) is the inciting event; the extrinsic type associated with a recent abnormality, such as ipsilateral breast surgery, cervical radiculopathy, or stroke; and the systemic type in which a systemic process triggers the onset as seen with diabetes, hypothyroidism, and hyperthyroidism.

The pathophysiologic mechanism in adhesive capsulitis includes a cascade of events that occur in the glenohumeral joint capsule, ligaments, and synovium beginning with an initial injury or underlying systemic disease that leads to thickening, contraction, and adhesion with decreased capsular compliance [49, 50]. Studies have shown immunocytochemical evidence of both proliferative fibroblasts and acute and chronic inflammatory cells [51–53].

Prompt diagnosis and treatment are critical in adhesive capsulitis because significant delays can lead to increased patient morbidity [54, 55]. Usually conservative treatment with physical therapy and intra-articular steroid injection into the glenohumeral joint is first-line therapy, which is associated with shortened duration of joint stiffness [55]. Surgical treatment is performed for refractory cases after at least 3–6 months of appropriate nonoperative treatment. Invasive therapy consists of manipulation under anesthesia to release adhesions or arthroscopic capsular release [54].

6.4 Imaging of the Rotator Interval

6.4.1 Imaging of the Biceps Tendon

Signs of tendon pathology in general throughout the body on MR include changes in caliber, contour irregularities, signal intensity abnormalities, partial or complete tears, and subluxation or dislocation [12, 56, 57]. However, evaluation of the biceps tendon may be complicated on MRI due to its curved course [58], relatively small diameter [56], normal size variability [59, 60], and magic-angle artifacts of the tendon [56].

Although MR arthrography has inherent advantages compared with standard MR imaging in the direct assessment of altered morphology of various joints, it has been shown that MR arthrography does not improve diagnostic accuracy compared with standard MR imaging when specifically analyzing the biceps tendon [12]. In the detection of biceps tendon pathology of the shoulder, the specificities of MR arthrography and computed tomography arthrography are high (94% and 95%, respectively); however, the sensitivities of both are low (27% and 31%, respectively) [57].

The proximal subacromial intra-articular portion of the LHBT from the biceps anchor to the rotator interval is best visualized on sagittal MR images [12]. The descending extra-articular portion within the intertubercular groove is better assessed on axial MR images [12]. The normal biceps tendon is homogeneously hypointense and round or ovoid on MR imaging with sizes ranging from 2 to 5 mm [12] (Fig. 6.4); however, flattening of the tendon, particularly at the entrance to the intertubercular groove, is commonly due to higher forces on the tendon at this level [12]. Increased MR signal and size of the tendon are consistent with tendinosis, which is also referred to as degeneration (Fig. 6.4) [12, 56, 57].

Disruption and attenuation of a portion of the tendon fibers indicate a partial tendon tear, usually longitudinal with split tearing of the tendon fibers and an appearance of two or more distinct tendon bands (Fig. 6.4). A complete tear manifests as non-visualization of the tendon (Fig. 6.4) [12]. Subluxation and dislocation manifest as visualization of the LHBT partially or completely (respectively) outside of the intertubercular groove (Fig. 6.4). Postoperative changes due to biceps tenotomy again show non-visualization of the intra-articular LHBT but now has accompanying postoperative changes at the supraglenoid tubercle where the tendon origin was resected, which should prompt query for a history of surgical resection (Fig. 6.3). Following biceps tenodesis, the previously mentioned MRI findings are also associated with a fixation device (screw, anchor, or sutures) appearing with a small foci of magnetic susceptibility artifact at the surgical reattachment of the distal portion of the resected biceps tendon stump to the humeral head or the proximal humeral shaft in a subpectoral location (Fig. 6.3). Radiographs if available should be correlated because they may show radiodense metal hardware in the proximal humerus; however, sometimes bioabsorbable screws are used, and these will be radiographically occult and a focal area of osseous rarefaction outlining the insertion of the bioabsorbable screw might be the only visible finding.

Entrapment of the LHBT refers to an internal impingement at the glenohumeral joint presenting with pain and locking of the shoulder on elevation of the arm. Typically this results from severe tendinosis and thickening of the biceps tendon leading to its impingement [61]. This pathology was first described by Boileau et al. in a study [62] in which they evaluated 21 patients who on physical examination had tenderness at the site of the bicipital groove associated with loss of passive motion in the final 10–20° of arm

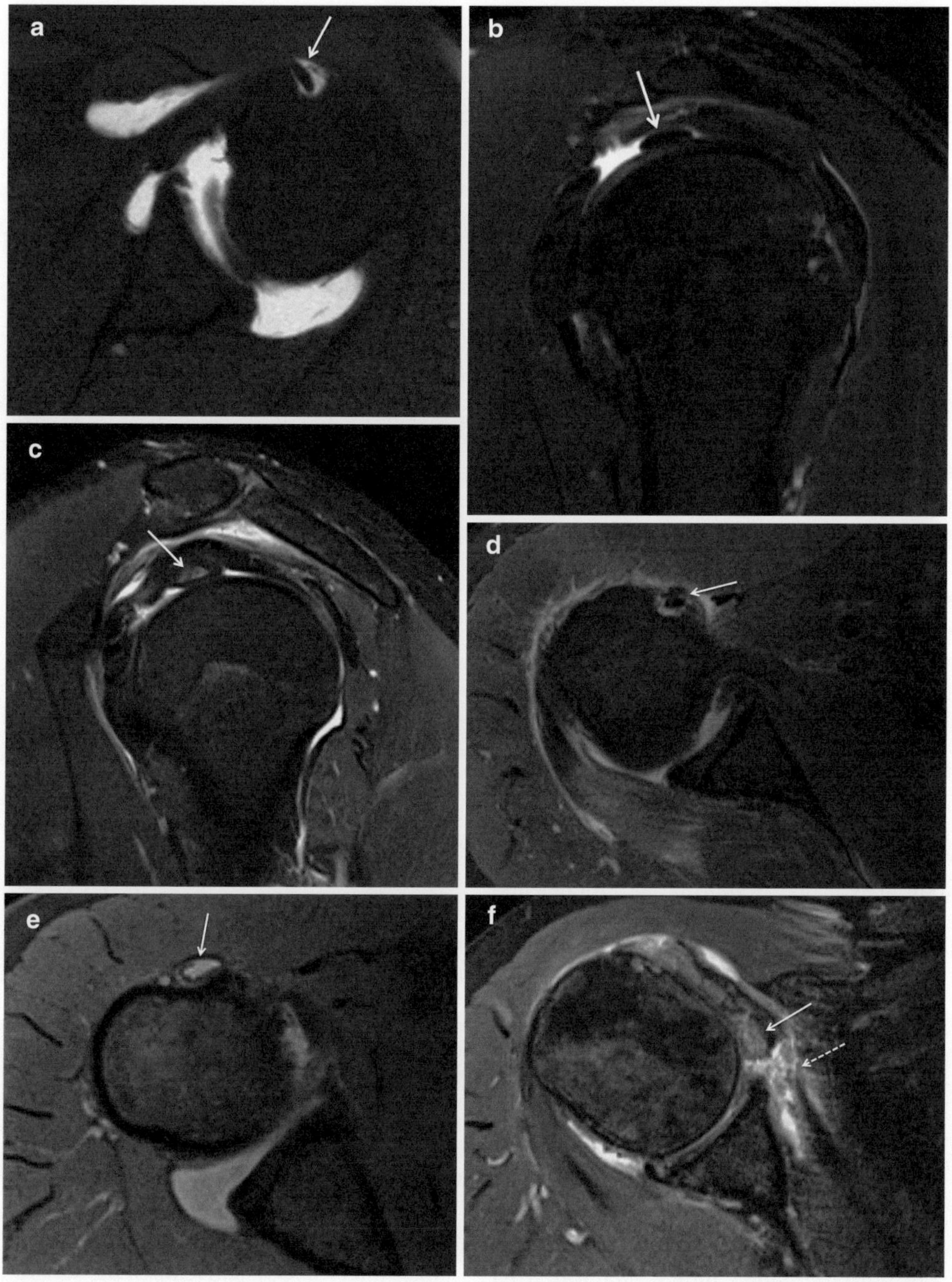

Fig. 6.4 Normal and pathologic appearance of long head of biceps tendon (LHBT) on MRI. (**a**) Axial fat-saturated T1 MR arthrogram image and (**b**) sagittal fat-saturated T2 MR image demonstrate normal LHBT (arrows in **a** and **b**) with normal diameter ranging from 2 to 5 mm and homogeneous hypointense signal. The normal extra-articular LHBT is located within the bicipital groove of humerus and best seen on axial images (**a**), and intra-articular LHBT is located in rotator interval best seen on sagittal images (**b**). (**c**) Sagittal T2 fat-saturated MR image demonstrates biceps tendinosis or degeneration with increased signal and thickening of tendon (arrow in **c**). (**d**) Axial fat-saturated proton density MR images demonstrate a partial tear of the biceps tendon with splitting of the tendon fibers (arrow in **d**), and (**e**) complete tear of biceps tendon with non-visualization of tendon within bicipital groove (arrow). (**f**) Axial fat-saturated proton density MR image demonstrates medial dislocation of the biceps tendon (solid arrow) from bicipital groove associated with a complete tear of the subscapularis tendon (dashed arrow)

elevation. On arthrography, every patient had a similar characteristic morphology of the LHBT related to hypertrophy of the intra-articular biceps tendon from tendinosis, which they referred to as the "hourglass biceps." During arthroscopic surgery, entrapment of the hypertrophic biceps tendon was demonstrated in every case with dynamic intraoperative maneuvering they called the "hourglass test," involving forward elevation of the arm with the elbow extended. During this test, they noticed a characteristic buckling of the tendon fibers, between the humeral head and the glenoid osseous margins creating an hourglass appearance, as it was pinched in its midportion. They deduced that the entrapment leads to the hypertrophy of the intra-articular portion of the tendon, which leads to a disproportion between the tendon size and the cross-sectional size of the bicipital groove, preventing normal sliding in the bicipital groove, resulting in entrapment or mechanical blockage. All cases showed restoration of complete normal arm elevation, symmetrical to the contralateral asymptomatic arm, following resection of the intra-articular portion of the biceps tendon via either biceps tenodesis or tenotomy. The diagnosis of the hourglass biceps is made primarily by the combination of the appropriate clinical history and surgical findings described; however, MRI and MR arthrography may suggest the diagnosis when there is this characteristic hypertrophic appearance of the intra-articular biceps tendon with hourglass morphology (Fig. 6.5).

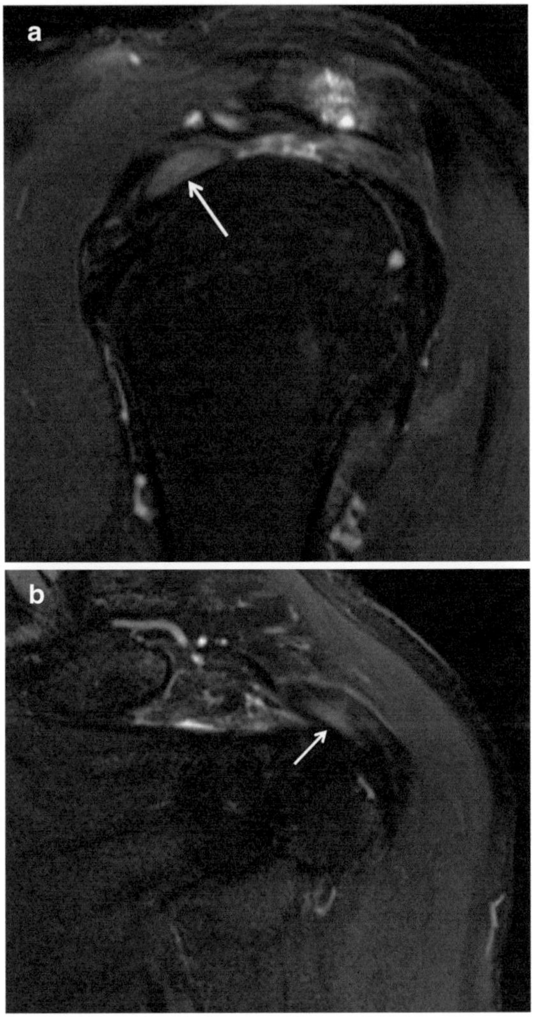

Fig. 6.5 Hourglass biceps morphology. (**a**) Sagittal and (**b**) coronal fat-saturated T2 MR images demonstrate severe tendinosis of intra-articular biceps tendon with marked thickening and increased signal at entry into bicipital groove resulting in an hourglass morphology (arrows), which can be associated with impingement of the tendon

6.4.2 Imaging of the Biceps Reflection Pulley

Clinical tests are often equivocal in the diagnosis of biceps reflection pulley injury; therefore MRI is often recommended for the diagnosis in order to avoid unnecessary diagnostic arthroscopy [15, 63, 64]. Diagnostic criteria of biceps pulley injury on MRI include dislocation or medial subluxation of the biceps tendon from the intertubercular groove (Figs. 6.4 and 6.6) [16, 20, 65, 66], tearing of the superior fibers of the subscapularis tendon (Figs. 6.4 and 6.6) and anterior fibers of the supraspinatus tendon (Fig. 6.6) around the rotator interval [66], and tears of the superior glenohumeral and coracohumeral ligaments (Fig. 6.6) [66].

Weishaupt el al. [66] demonstrated an overall high sensitivity of 86–93% and a high specificity of 80–100% in the detection of biceps reflection pulley lesions on MR arthrography using several criteria including tears of the coracohumeral and superior glenohumeral ligaments, abnormal position

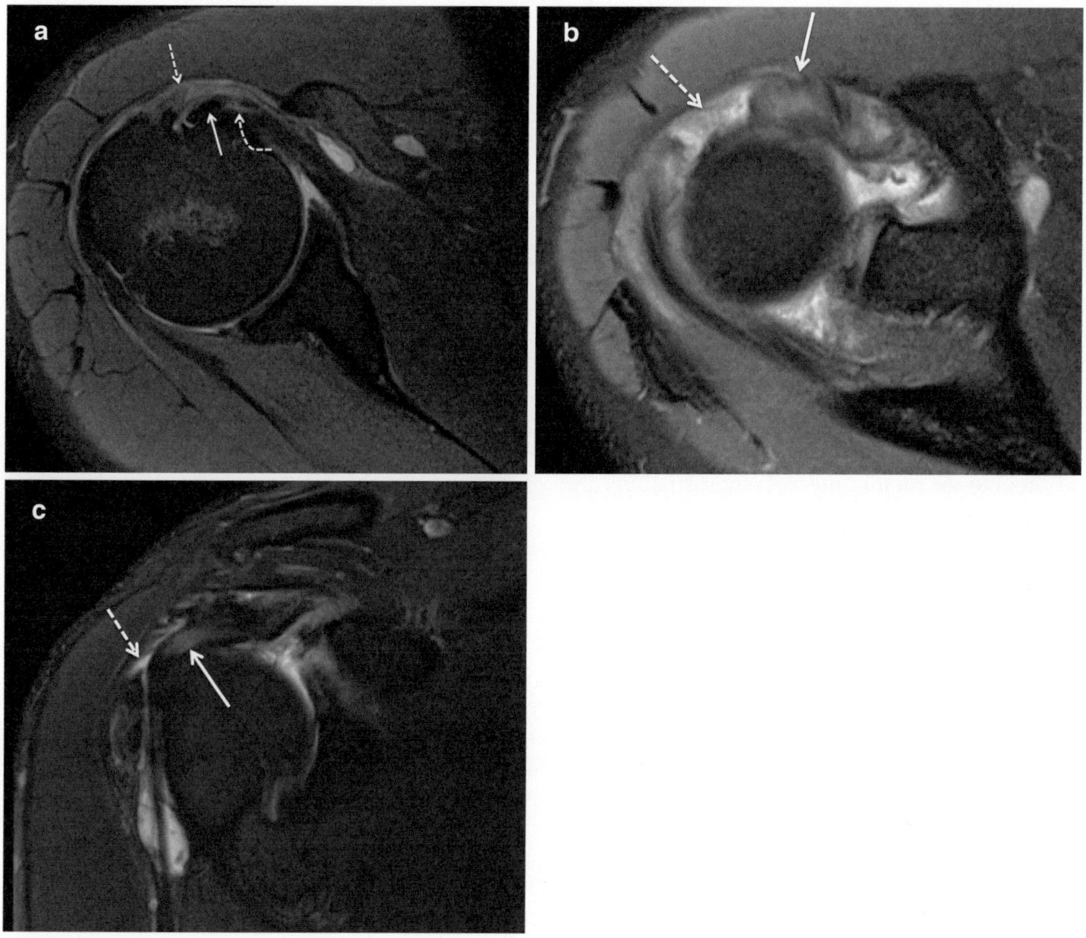

Fig. 6.6 Biceps reflection pulley injuries. (**a**) Axial fat-saturated proton density MR image demonstrates medial subluxation of biceps tendon from bicipital groove (solid arrow) associated with partial tear of subscapularis tendon (dashed curved arrow) and partial tear of coracohumeral ligament insertion (dashed straight arrow). (**b**) Axial and (**c**) coronal fat-saturated proton density MR images demonstrate medial subluxation and severe tendinosis of biceps tendon (solid arrow in **b**, **c**) associated with a full-thickness tear of anterior supraspinatus tendon insertion (dashed arrow in **b**, **c**)

and tearing of the biceps tendon, and tears of superior border of the subscapularis tendon. According to Weishaupt et al. [66], the most accurate criterion for the diagnosis of a pulley lesion was an abnormality of the superior border of the subscapularis tendon. This finding had a sensitivity of 86–100% and a specificity of 70–80%.

However, a more recent arthroscopic study by Braun et al. [67] prospectively evaluated 229 shoulders in consecutive patients who underwent shoulder arthroscopy and found that, with the shoulder in neutral position, the biceps tendon was located within the intertubercular groove in ~36 of 67 patients (54%) who had a biceps pulley tear. Additionally, the arthroscopic incidence of isolated pulley lesions is substantial, ranging from 29 to 74% [7, 15, 67]. Taking this additional arthroscopic data into consideration, Schaeffeler et al. [68] more recently suggested that many pulley lesions may be overlooked by following the more traditional MR imaging criteria of biceps tendon location and superior subscapularis integrity because the shoulder is usually examined in the neutral position during MR imaging and inference of an intact biceps pulley based on its anatomical location and/or unremarkable appearance of the superior subscapularis tendon can be inaccurate.

The study by Schaeffeler et al. [68] retrospectively evaluated 80 patients with arthroscopically proven intact or torn biceps pulley systems. They assessed for the presence of a biceps pulley lesion on MR arthrography using several specific criteria, including medial subluxation of the biceps tendon on transverse images, displacement of the biceps tendon relative to the subscapularis tendon on oblique sagittal images (displacement sign), presence of biceps tendinopathy, nonvisibility or discontinuity of the SGHL, and rotator cuff tears adjacent to the rotator interval (supraspinatus and subscapularis tendons). They reported high overall sensitivity of 82–89% and high specificity of 87–98% using these criteria, which was concordant with previous data from Weishaupt et al. [66]. They found that the displacement sign (sensitivity 75–86%, specificity 90–98%), nonvisibility or discontinuity of the SGHL (sensitivity 75–89%, specificity 75–83%), and tendinopathy of the biceps tendon (sensitivity 64–93%, specificity 81–96%) were the most accurate measures for the detection of pulley lesions. Subluxation of the biceps tendon was highly specific (96–100%) but insensitive (36–64%). Also tears of the subscapularis tendon around the rotator interval were highly specific (92–100%) but insensitive (54–86%). Conversely, tears of the supraspinatus tendon around the rotator interval were the least accurate with low sensitivities (58–87%) and low specificities (61–76%).

Studies performed by Weishaupt et al. [66] and Scaeffeler et al. [68] had similar overall sensitivities and specificities, but there were some significant differences in their results regarding the irregularity of the superior border of the subscapularis tendon, which was highly sensitive for pulley lesions in the study by Weishaupt et al. but insensitive in the study by Schaeffeler et al. Schaeffeler et al. postulated that their study population had a high number of patients with an unremarkable subscapularis tendon (Habermeyer group I and II lesions) [7], and they suggested that isolated pulley lesions with a normal subscapularis tendon were underrepresented in the study of Weishaupt et al.

As opposed to Schaeffeler et al., Weishaupt et al. observed that the tears of the SGHL were specific but insensitive. Schaeffeler et al. proposed that improvements in MR imaging techniques over the course of the 10 years between their two studies and a better understanding of the anatomy may have improved the better visualization of the SGHL in the latter series. The study by Schaeffeler et al. included both 1.5-T and 3-T MR studies between 2006 and 2010, whereas the earlier study by Weishaupt et al. was performed on a 1.0-T scanner between 1995 and 1997, which also supports this assumption. While review-type articles correlating biceps pulley lesions on MRI with arthroscopic classification have been previously published [1, 61], Schaeffeler et al. [68] note that Bennett's arthroscopic classification of pulley lesions is specifically not applicable for MR arthrography because the detailed anatomy at the apex of the rotator interval cannot be visualized on MRI with the same accuracy as arthroscopy.

6.4.3 Imaging of Rotator Interval Laxity

The diagnosis of rotator interval laxity is largely a clinical diagnosis based on history and physical examination demonstrating posterior and inferior glenohumeral joint instability. Imaging may play a supportive role in cases where clinical history and examination are inconclusive. MR arthrography is more accurate than conventional nonarthrographic MRI because arthrography can show extra-articular contrast material in the region of the rotator interval typically collecting in the subcoracoid space [69, 70]. This finding may suggest disruption of the rotator interval capsule, particularly if the rotator cuff is intact, in the appropriate clinical setting.

A study by Vinson et al. [71] demonstrated intra-articular contrast extending to the cortex of the undersurface of the coracoid in five patients with an arthroscopically proven lesion of the rotator interval who presented with signs of shoulder instability. Tears of the rotator interval capsule can also be seen directly on conventional and/or arthrographic MRI as irregularity, thinning, or focal discontinuity of the rotator interval capsule [72]. Patients with glenohumeral instability associated with rotator interval laxity may also have increased joint space volume and size in the rotator interval on MR arthrography [73]. A retrospective study of 120 shoulders by Kim et al. [73] separated subjects into groups with and without clinical glenohumeral instability. Kim et al. measured the size and calculated the volume of the rotator interval using MR arthrography and found statistically significant differences between the two groups, with larger rotator interval dimensions and volumes in those with clinical instability.

6.4.4 Imaging of Adhesive Capsulitis

Imaging with MRI or ultrasound has an important supportive diagnostic role in the diagnosis of adhesive capsulitis because symptoms may be misleading and clinical diagnosis can be challenging, particularly in the early stages of disease and when not all of the diagnostic criteria are met. Furthermore, imaging may also help identify other underlying conditions that can be masked by the clinical symptoms of adhesive capsulitis.

The CHL is considered to be the key structure of the rotator interval involved in the pathologic changes of adhesive capsulitis [2, 74–76] because this normally flexible structure becomes stiff and inelastic resulting in limited external rotation [1] (Fig. 6.7). Thickening of the CHL >4 mm was shown to have a specificity of 95% and a sensitivity of 59% on MR arthrography by Mengiardi et al. [77] (Fig. 6.7). This is best seen on sagittal images; however, coronal and axial images can occasionally be useful to confirm suspected thickening of this ligament. The SGHL is often also involved and thickened (Fig. 6.7); however, this has not been studied systematically to the best of our knowledge. Additional findings frequently associated with adhesive capsulitis on MR imaging included synovial hypertrophy within the rotator interval, which is seen as replacement of the normal fat signal in this region by edema secondary to granulation tissue or scar tissue [77] (Fig. 6.7). Ultrasound has also demonstrated these findings by showing edema and synovitis with increased vascularity on Doppler imaging of the rotator interval [78] (Fig. 6.7). Additionally, thickening and edema of the rotator interval capsule >7 mm on MR arthrography were shown to have a specificity of 86% and sensitivity of 64% by Mengiardi et al. [77].

Additional changes associated with adhesive capsulitis outside of the rotator interval can be seen on MR imaging. A study by Emig et al. [50] showed that thickening of the axillary recess joint capsule and inferior glenohumeral ligaments >4 mm has a specificity of 95% and sensitivity of 70% (Fig. 6.7). Additionally, Mengiardi et al. [77] demonstrated a significantly reduced axillary recess volume in patients with adhesive capsulitis on MR arthrography compared with control subjects (Fig. 6.7). However, the authors noted that this may not be a true abnormality of adhesive capsulitis but rather a manifestation of the reduced volume of contrast that can be injected in patients with adhesive capsulitis before there is early leakage of contrast material secondary to weakening in the joint capsule. It is also important to note that axillary recess volume showed no significant difference on conventional non-arthrographic MR imaging between patients with adhesive capsulitis and asymptomatic volunteers in a study by Emig et al. [50]. Thus, this measurement is not considered to be useful on conventional non-arthrographic MRI.

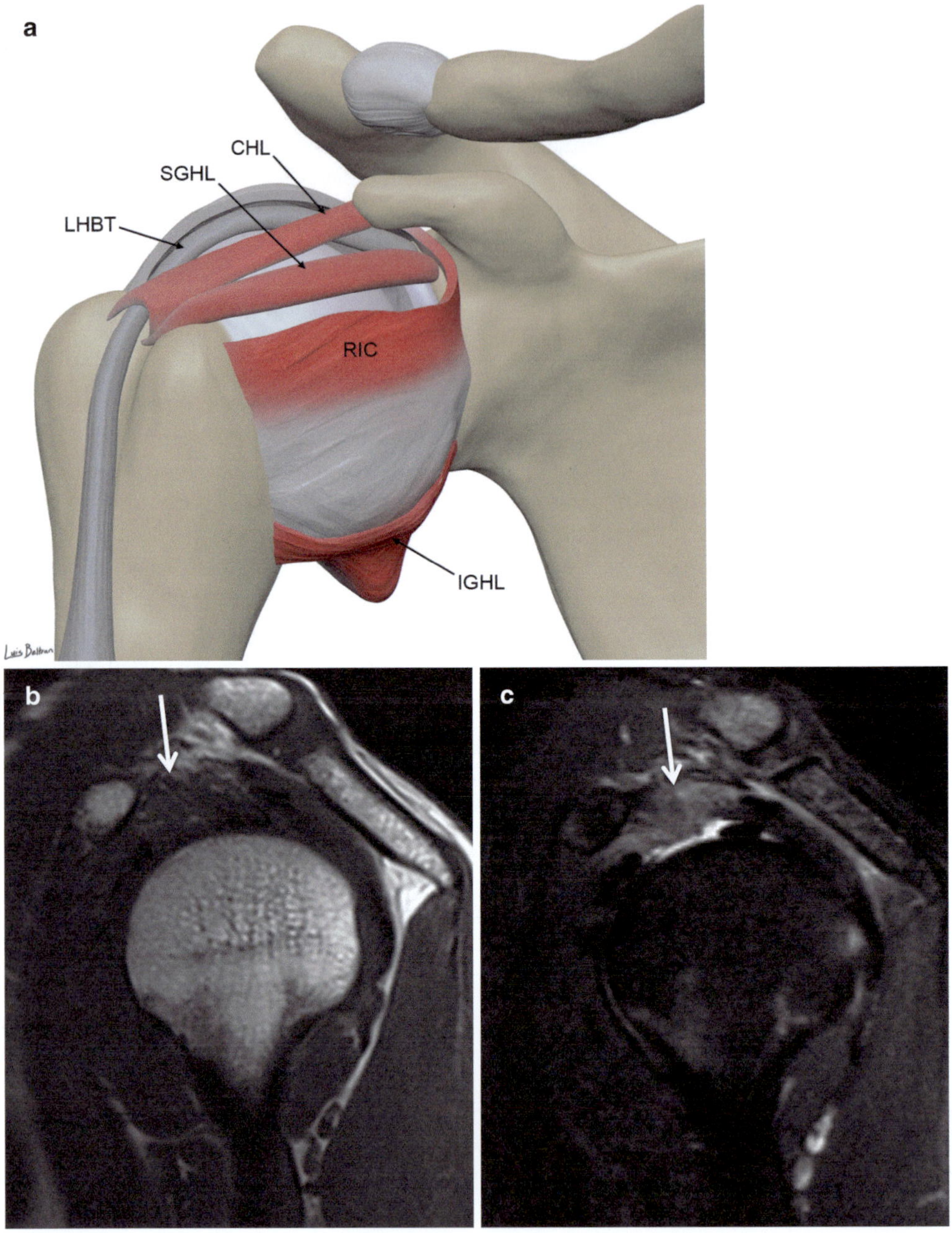

Fig. 6.7 Adhesive capsulitis. (**a**) Illustration of involved structures in adhesive capsulitis highlighted in red indicating adhesions and inflammation in rotator interval and thickening and inflammation of joint capsule. (**b**) Sagittal T1 and (**c**) sagittal fat-saturated T2 MR images demonstrate thickening and indistinct margin of coracohumeral ligament (CHL) (arrow in **b**) associated with edematous effacement of normal surrounding fat signal in rotator interval (arrow in **c**). (**d**) Transverse ultrasound image of the anterior shoulder shows increased vascularity in rotator interval on power Doppler (red foci) due to edema and synovitis. (**e**) Axial fat-saturated proton density MR image demonstrates thickening and increased signal of SGHL (arrow). (**f**) Coronal fat-saturated T2 MR image demonstrates thickening and increased signal due to edema in the axillary recess joint capsule and inferior glenohumeral ligaments (arrow). (**g**) Coronal fat-saturated T1 MR arthrogram image demonstrates reduced axillary recess volume following intra-articular injection of contrast (arrow). HUM, humeral head; IGHL, inferior glenohumeral ligament; LHBT, long head of the biceps tendon; RIC, rotator interval capsule; SGHL, superior glenohumeral ligament; COR, coracoid. Illustration reprinted with permission from Beltran LS, Beltran J. Biceps and rotator interval: imaging update. Semin Musculoskelet Radiol. Thieme Medical Publishers; 2014;18:425–35

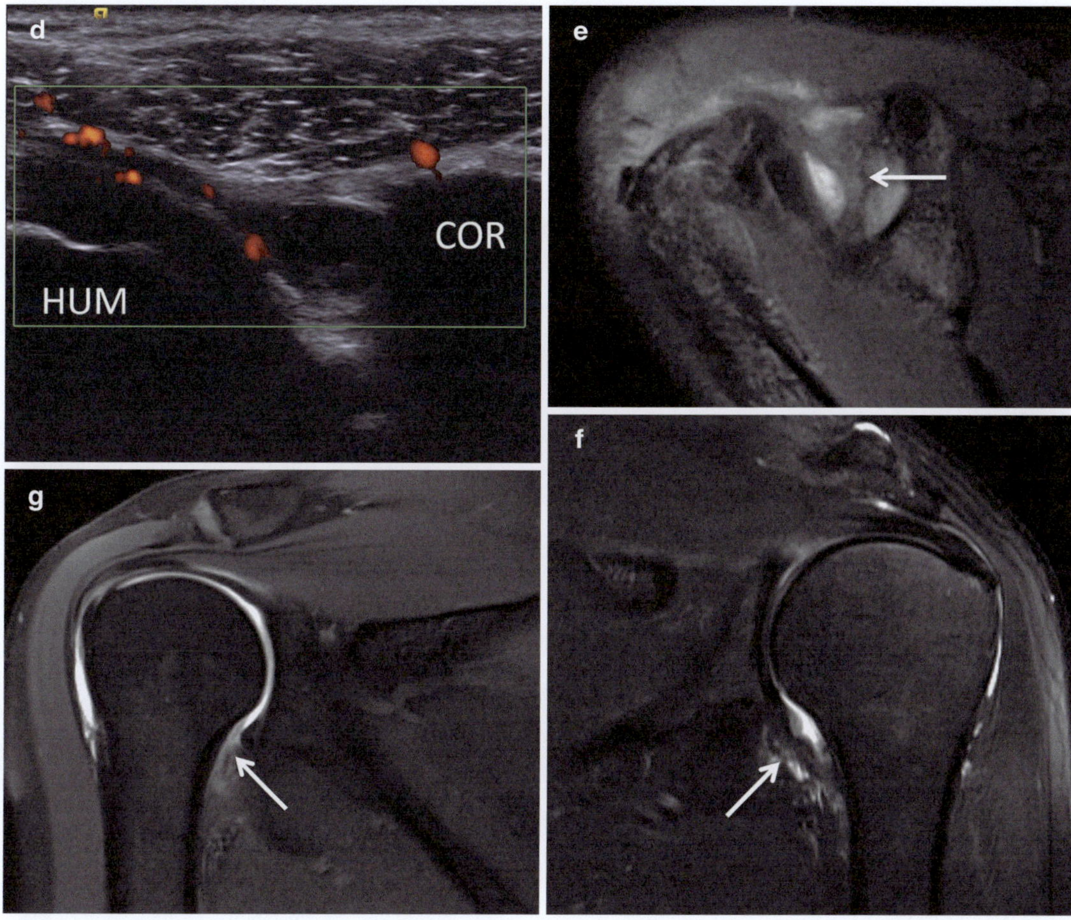

Fig. 6.7 (continued)

6.5 Conclusion

The rotator interval is a complex anatomical area containing many important structures that contribute to the stability and normal function of the shoulder joint. We discussed the normal anatomy, clinical and imaging appearances, and treatment options of pathology in the rotator interval and its structures. The complex anatomy of the rotator interval within a relatively small space makes it challenging to evaluate on MR imaging; however, improvements in MR technology as well as a better understanding of the anatomy have allowed improved detection of disease in this region. Additionally, diagnosis of pathology in this area can be clinically challenging, underscoring the important role of imaging in assisting the clinician to make the diagnosis and initiate appropriate treatment.

References

1. Petchprapa CN, Beltran LS, Jazrawi LM, Kwon YW, Babb JS, Recht MP. The rotator interval: a review of anatomy, function, and normal and abnormal MRI appearance. AJR Am J Roentgenol. 2010;195(3):567–76.
2. Neer CS II, Satterlee CC, Dalsey RM, Flatow EL. The anatomy and potential effects of contracture of the coracohumeral ligament. Clin Orthop Relat Res. 1992;280:182–5.
3. Shankman S, Bencardino J, Beltran J. Glenohumeral instability: evaluation using MR arthrography of the shoulder. Skelet Radiol. 1999;28(7):365–82.
4. Vangsness CT Jr, Jorgenson SS, Watson T, Johnson DL. The origin of the long head of the biceps from

the scapula and glenoid labrum. An anatomical study of 100 shoulders. J Bone Joint Surg Br. 1994;76(6):951–4.
5. Abu-Hijleh MFM. Three-headed biceps brachii muscle associated with duplicated musculocutaneous nerve. Clin Anat. 2005;18(5):376–9.
6. Gaskin CM, Golish SR, Blount KJ, Diduch DR. Anomalies of the long head of the biceps brachii tendon: clinical significance, MR arthrographic findings, and arthroscopic correlation in two patients. Skelet Radiol. 2007;36(8):785–9.
7. Habermeyer P, Magosch P, Pritsch M, Scheibel MT, Lichtenberg S. Anterosuperior impingement of the shoulder as a result of pulley lesions: a prospective arthroscopic study. J Shoulder Elb Surg. 2004;13(1):5–12.
8. Edelson JG, Taitz C, Grishkan A. The coracohumeral ligament. Anatomy of a substantial but neglected structure. J Bone Joint Surg Br. 1991;73(1):150–3.
9. Morag Y, Jacobson JA, Shields G, et al. MR arthrography of rotator interval, long head of the biceps brachii, and biceps pulley of the shoulder. Radiology. 2005;235(1):2130.
10. Burkhead WJ. The biceps tendon. In: Rockwood CJ, Matson FI, editors. The shoulder. Philadelphia: WB Saunders; 1990. p. 791–836.
11. Chen C-H, Hsu K-Y, Chen W-J, Shih C-H. Incidence and severity of biceps long head tendon lesion in patients with complete rotator cuff tears. J Trauma. 2005;58(6):1189–93.
12. Zanetti M, Weishaupt D, Gerber C, Hodler J. Tendinopathy and rupture of the tendon of the long head of the biceps brachii muscle: evaluation with MR arthrography. AJR Am J Roentgenol. 1998;170(6):1557–61.
13. Curtis AS, Snyder SJ. Evaluation and treatment of biceps tendon pathology. Orthop Clin North Am. 1993;24(1):33–43.
14. Hsu AR, Ghodadra NS, Provencher MT, Lewis PB, Bach BR. Biceps tenotomy versus tenodesis: a review of clinical outcomes and biomechanical results. J Shoulder Elbow Surg. 2011;20(2):326–32.
15. Baumann B, Genning K, Böhm D, Rolf O, Gohlke F. Arthroscopic prevalence of pulley lesions in 1007 consecutive patients. J Shoulder Elb Surg. 2008;17(1):14–20.
16. Walch G, Nové-Josserand L, Boileau P, Levigne C. Subluxations and dislocations of the tendon of the long head of the biceps. J Shoulder Elb Surg. 1998;7(2):100–8.
17. Gerber C, Sebesta A. Impingement of the deep surface of the subscapularis tendon and the reflection pulley on the anterosuperior glenoid rim: a preliminary report. J Shoulder Elb Surg. 2000;9(6):483–90.
18. Habermeyer P, Krieter C, Tang K-L, Lichtenberg S, Magosch P. A new arthroscopic classification of articular-sided supraspinatus footprint lesions: a prospective comparison with Snyder's and Ellman's classification. J Shoulder Elb Surg. 2008;17(6):909–13.
19. Hunt SA, Kwon YW, Zuckerman JD. The rotator interval: anatomy, pathology, and strategies for treatment. J Am Acad Orthop Surg. 2007;15(4):218–27.
20. Bennett WF. Subscapularis, medial, and lateral head coracohumeral ligament insertion anatomy. Arthroscopic appearance and incidence of "hidden" rotator interval lesions. Arthroscopy. 2001;17(2):173–80.
21. Stoller DW. Magnetic resonance imaging in orthopaedics and sports medicine. Philadelphia: Lippincott Williams & Wilkins; 2006.
22. Bennett WF. Arthroscopic repair of anterosuperior (supraspinatus/ subscapularis) rotator cuff tears: a prospective cohort with 2- to 4- year follow-up. Classification of biceps subluxation/instability. Arthroscopy. 2003;19(1):21–33.
23. O'Connell PW, Nuber GW, Mileski RA, Lautenschlager E. The contribution of the glenohumeral ligaments to anterior stability of the shoulder joint. Am J Sports Med. 1990;18(6):579–84.
24. Warner JJ, McMahon PJ. The role of the long head of the biceps brachii in superior stability of the glenohumeral joint. J Bone Joint Surg Am. 1995;77(3):366–72.
25. Lazarus MD, Sidles JA, Harryman DT II, Matsen FA III. Effect of a chondral-labral defect on glenoid concavity and glenohumeral stability. A cadaveric model. J Bone Joint Surg Am. 1996;78(1):94–102.
26. Lippitt SB, Vanderhooft JE, Harris SL, Sidles JA, Harryman DT II, Matsen FA III. Glenohumeral stability from concavity-compression: a quantitative analysis. J Shoulder Elb Surg. 1993;2(1):27–35.
27. Lippitt S, Matsen F. Mechanisms of glenohumeral joint stability. Clin Orthop Relat Res. 1993;291:20–8.
28. Matsen FA III, Harryman DT II, Sidles JA. Mechanics of glenohumeral instability. Clin Sports Med. 1991;10(4):783–8.
29. Porcellini G, Caranzano F, Campi F, Pellegrini A, Paladini P. Glenohumeral instability and rotator cuff tear. Sports Med Arthrosc. 2011;19(4):395–400.
30. Bigliani LUL, Kelkar R, Flatow ELE, Pollock RGR, Mow VCV. Glenohumeral stability. Biomechanical properties of passive and active stabilizers. Clin Orthop Relat Res. 1996;330:13–30.
31. Howell SM, Kraft TA. The role of the supraspinatus and infraspinatus muscles in glenohumeral kinematics of anterior should instability. Clin Orthop Relat Res. 1991;263:128–34.
32. Lee SB, Kim KJ, O'Driscoll SW, Morrey BF, An KN. Dynamic glenohumeral stability provided by the rotator cuff muscles in the mid-range and end-range of motion. A study in cadavera. J Bone Joint Surg Am. 2000;82(6):849–57.
33. Neviaser RJ, Neviaser TJ, Neviaser JS. Anterior dislocation of the shoulder and rotator cuff rupture. Clin Orthop Relat Res. 1993;291:103–6.
34. Steinbach LS. MRI of shoulder instability. Eur J Radiol. 2008;68(1):57–71.
35. Harryman DT II, Sidles JA, Harris SL, Matsen FA III. The role of the rotator interval capsule in passive

motion and stability of the shoulder. J Bone Joint Surg Am. 1992;74(1):53–66.
36. Jost B, Koch PP, Gerber C. Anatomy and functional aspects of the rotator interval. J Shoulder Elb Surg. 2000;9(4):336–41.
37. Itoi E, Berglund LJ, Grabowski JJ, Naggar L, Morrey BF, An KN. Superior-inferior stability of the shoulder: role of the coracohumeral ligament and the rotator interval capsule. Mayo Clin Proc. 1998;73(6):508–15.
38. Burkart AC, Debski RE. Anatomy and function of the glenohumeral ligaments in anterior shoulder instability. Clin Orthop Relat Res. 2002;400:32–9.
39. Warner JJJ, Deng XHX, Warren RFR, Torzilli PAP. Static capsuloligamentous restraints to superior-inferior translation of the glenohumeral joint. Am J Sports Med. 1992;20(6):675–85.
40. Field LD, Warren RF, O'Brien SJ, Altchek DW, Wickiewicz TL. Isolated closure of rotator interval defects for shoulder instability. Am J Sports Med. 1995;23(5):557–63.
41. Karas SG. Arthroscopic rotator interval repair and anterior portal closure: an alternative technique. Arthroscopy. 2002;18(4):436–9.
42. Gartsman GMG, Taverna E, Hammerman SMS. Arthroscopic rotator interval repair in glenohumeral instability: description of an operative technique. Arthroscopy. 1999;15(3):330–2.
43. Treacy SH, Field LD, Savoie FH. Rotator interval capsule closure: an arthroscopic technique. Arthroscopy. 1997;13(1):103–6.
44. Codman EA. Tendinitis of the short rotators. In: Codman EA, editor. Ruptures of the supraspinatus tendon and other lesions on or about the subacromial bursa. Boston: Thomas Todd Co; 1934. p. 91–9.
45. Hannafin JA, Chiaia TA. Adhesive capsulitis. A treatment approach. Clin Orthop Relat Res. 2000;372:95–109.
46. Manske RC, Prohaska D. Diagnosis and management of adhesive capsulitis. Curr Rev Musculoskelet Med. 2008;1(3–4):180–9.
47. Hazleman BL. Frozen shoulder. In: Rockwood CJ, Matsen FI, editors. The shoulder. 2nd ed. Philadelphia: WB Saunders; 1990. p. 623–77.
48. Sedeek S, Chye-Andrew TH. Adhesive capsulitis: is arthroscopic capsular release necessary? Current review. OA Orthopaedics. 2013;1(1):8.
49. Hulstyn MJ, Weiss AP. Adhesive capsulitis of the shoulder. Orthop Rev. 1993;22(4):425–33.
50. Emig EW, Schweitzer ME, Karasick D, Lubowitz J. Adhesive capsulitis of the shoulder: MR diagnosis. AJR Am J Roentgenol. 1995;164(6):1457–9.
51. Rodeo SA, Hannafin JA, Tom J, Warren RF, Wickiewicz TL. Immunolocalizationof cytokines and their receptors in adhesive capsulitis of the shoulder. J Orthop Res. 1997;15(3):427–36.
52. Simmonds FA. Shoulder pain with particular reference to the frozen shoulder. J Bone Joint Surg Br. 1949;31B(3):426–32.
53. Bunker TD, Anthony PP. The pathology of frozen shoulder. A Dupuytren-like disease. J Bone Joint Surg Br. 1995;77(5):677–83.
54. Tasto JP, Elias DW. Adhesive capsulitis. Sports Med Arthrosc. 2007;15(4):216–21.
55. Carette S, Moffet H, Tardif J, et al. Intra-articular corticosteroids, supervised physiotherapy, or a combination of the two in the treatment of adhesive capsulitis of the shoulder: a placebo-controlled trial. Arthritis Rheum. 2003;48(3):829–38.
56. Buck FM, Grehn H, Hilbe M, Pfirrmann CWA, Manzanell S, Hodler J. Degeneration of the long biceps tendon: comparison of MRI with gross anatomy and histology. AJR Am J Roentgenol. 2009;193(5):1367–75.
57. De Maeseneer M, Boulet C, Pouliart N, et al. Assessment of the long head of the biceps tendon of the shoulder with 3T magnetic resonance arthrography and CT arthrography. Eur J Radiol. 2012;81(5):934–9.
58. Erickson SJ, Fitzgerald SW, Quinn SF, Carrera GF, Black KP, Lawson TL. Long bicipital tendon of the shoulder: normal anatomy and pathologic findings on MR imaging. AJR Am J Roentgenol. 1992;158(5):1091–6.
59. Toshiaki A, Itoi E, Minagawa H, et al. Cross-sectional area of the tendon and the muscle of the biceps brachii in shoulders with rotator cuff tears: a study of 14 cadaveric shoulders. Acta Orthop. 2005;76(4):509–12.
60. Demondion X, Maynou C, Van Cortenbosch B, Klein K, Leroy X, Mestdagh H. Relationship between the tendon of the long head of the biceps brachii muscle and the glenoid labrum [in French]. Morphologie. 2001;85(269):5–8.
61. Beltran LS, Nikac V, Beltran J. Internal impingement syndromes. Magn Reson Imaging Clin N Am. 2012;20(2):201–11.. ix–x
62. Boileau P, Ahrens PM, Hatzidakis AM. Entrapment of the long head of the biceps tendon: the hourglass biceps—a cause of pain and locking of the shoulder. J Shoulder Elb Surg. 2004;13(3):249–57.
63. Bennett WF. Specificity of the Speed's test: arthroscopic technique for evaluating the biceps tendon at the level of the bicipital groove. Arthroscopy. 1998;14(8):789–96.
64. Chung CB, Dwek JR, Cho GJ, Lektrakul N, Trudell D, Resnick D. Rotator cuff interval: evaluation with MR imaging and MR arthrography of the shoulder in 32 cadavers. J Comput Assist Tomogr. 2000;24(5):738–43.
65. Walch G, Nove-Josserand L, Levigne C, Renaud E. Tears of the supraspinatus tendon associated with "hidden" lesions of the rotator interval. J Shoulder Elb Surg. 1994;3(6):353–60.
66. Weishaupt D, Zanetti M, Tanner A, Gerber C, Hodler J. Lesions of the reflection pulley of the long biceps tendon. MR arthrographic findings. Investig Radiol. 1999;34(7):463–9.
67. Braun S, Horan MP, Elser F, Millett PJ. Lesions of the biceps pulley. Am J Sports Med. 2011;39(4):790–5.
68. Schaeffeler C, Waldt S, Holzapfel K, et al. Lesions of the biceps pulley: diagnostic accuracy of MR arthrography of the shoulder and evaluation of previously described and new diagnostic signs. Radiology. 2012;264(2):504–13.

69. Grainger AJ, Tirman PF, Elliott JM, Kingzett-Taylor A, Steinbach LS, Genant HK. MR anatomy of the subcoracoid bursa and the association of subcoracoid effusion with tears of the anterior rotator cuff and the rotator interval. AJR Am J Roentgenol. 2000;174(5):1377–80.
70. Le Huec JC, Schaeverbeke T, Moinard M, et al. Traumatic tear of the rotator interval. J Shoulder Elb Surg. 1996;5(1):41–6.
71. Vinson EN, Major NM, Higgins LD. Magnetic resonance imaging findings associated with surgically proven rotator interval lesions. Skelet Radiol. 2007;36(5):405–10.
72. Bigoni BJ, Chung CB. MR imaging of the rotator cuff interval. Radiol Clin N Am. 2006;44(4):525–36.. viii
73. Kim K-C, Rhee K-J, Shin H-D, Kim Y-M. Estimating the dimensions of the rotator interval with use of magnetic resonance arthrography. J Bone Joint Surg Am. 2007;89(11):2450–5.
74. Omari A, Bunker TD. Open surgical release for frozen shoulder: surgical findings and results of the release. J Shoulder Elb Surg. 2001;10(4):353–7.
75. Ozaki J, Nakagawa Y, Sakurai G, Tamai S. Recalcitrant chronic adhesive capsulitis of the shoulder. Role of contracture of the coracohumeral ligament and rotator interval in pathogenesis and treatment. J Bone Joint Surg Am. 1989;71(10):1511–5.
76. Warner JJ, Allen A, Marks PH, Wong P. Arthroscopic release for chronic, refractory adhesive capsulitis of the shoulder. J Bone Joint Surg Am. 1996;78(12):1808–16.
77. Mengiardi B, Pfirrmann CWA, Gerber C, Hodler J, Zanetti M. Frozen shoulder: MR arthrographic findings. Radiology. 2004;233(2):486–92.
78. Lee JC, Sykes C, Saifuddin A, Connell D. Adhesive capsulitis: sonographic changes in the rotator cuff interval with arthroscopic correlation. Skelet Radiol. 2005;34(9):522–7.

Part III

The Labrum

Imaging Diagnosis of Glenohumeral Instability with Clinical Implications

7

Luis S. Beltran, Monica Tafur, and Jenny T. Bencardino

Learning Objectives
- Discuss the imaging techniques to evaluate the shoulder for glenohumeral instability with an emphasis on MRI
- Describe the normal anatomical structures of the shoulder that pertain to glenohumeral stability
- Cover the imaging findings and clinical implications of glenohumeral instability

7.1 Epidemiology

The prevalence of shoulder dislocation is approximately 1–2% [1–5] in the general population; however recurrent shoulder dislocation can be as high as 92% in young athletic patients after a first-time anterior shoulder dislocation which does not undergo operative treatment [6, 7]. Predictors of recurrent dislocation after an initial dislocation include patient age, gender, and athletic involvement or physical activity [8]. The age of initial dislocation is the most common predisposing factor for recurrent dislocation [9–16], and the rate of recurrent dislocation decreases based on patient age alone [17]. In one study by Te Slaa et al., patients younger than 18 years of age had a 71% recurrence rate at 5-year follow-up compared to the overall group of 16–39-year-old patients who demonstrated a recurrence rate of 55% [16]. Shoulder dislocation is three times more likely to occur in men compared to women [5]. In addition to seeing a higher prevalence of shoulder dislocation in athletes, other specific populations in which there is greater physical activity, such as military personnel, also demonstrate increased rates of shoulder dislocation compared to the general population [18, 19].

7.2 Imaging Technique

Imaging of the shoulder to evaluate for glenohumeral instability is often first performed with radiography to evaluate the osseous structures for glenohumeral joint dislocation and/or fracture. This includes AP views with the humerus in internal and external rotation, scapular Y, and axillary views of the affected shoulder. Occasionally, additional views are requested by the orthopedic surgeon including a Stryker notch view to assess for a humeral head fracture and/or a West Point view to evaluate the anteroinferior glenoid [8]. If initial radiographic evaluation

L. S. Beltran (✉)
Brigham and Women's Hospital, Department of Radiology, Harvard Medical School, Boston, MA, USA
e-mail: lbeltran@bwh.harvard.edu

M. Tafur
Department of Radiology, Michael's Hospital, University of Toronto, Toronto, ON, Canada

J. T. Bencardino
Department of Radiology, New York University Langone Health, New York, NY, USA

Penn Medicine, Department of Radiology, Perelman School of Medicine at the University of Pennsylvania, Philadelphia, PA, USA

J. T. Bencardino (ed.), *The Shoulder*, https://doi.org/10.1007/978-3-030-06240-8_7

demonstrates evidence of bone loss along the humeral head or glenoid and/or if the patient has a history of multiple prior dislocation events, then cross-sectional imaging with CT or MRI is ordered for further evaluation.

Typically, for a routine shoulder MRI, the patient is in the supine position within the MRI scanner and the arm is supinated with the thumb facing laterally. To maintain the hand in this position, a sandbag is placed on the hand if the patient can tolerate this. A phased-array shoulder coil is placed on the shoulder to optimize signal in the joint; however if the shoulder coil is too small for the patient secondary to large body habitus, a body-phased array coil can be used instead. A typical MRI protocol of the shoulder will often include a combination of fluid-sensitive fat-suppressed images to detect pathology and nonfat-suppressed images to evaluate anatomic detail. This is often in the form of coronal oblique proton density (PD), coronal oblique fat-saturated T2 (FST2), sagittal T1, sagittal FST2, and axial fat-saturated proton density sequences (FSPD). If the patient has metal orthopedic hardware, the protocol can be modified to reduce metal artifact by increasing the turbo factor and bandwidth, increasing the number of excitations (NEX), and decreasing the slice thickness. Additionally, frequency-selective fat saturation should be avoided and instead short tau inversion recovery (STIR) sequences should be used to suppress fat since STIR is less susceptible to metal artifact compared to frequency-selective fat saturation techniques.

Injection of contrast material into the glenohumeral joint for MR arthrography is usually performed to evaluate for abnormal extension of contrast material into the labrum indicating a labral tear which is a frequent finding in glenohumeral instability, and it can also help to evaluate for injury to the joint capsule and rotator cuff. An injection of dilute gadolinium contrast is performed into the glenohumeral joint and the patient is shortly thereafter placed in the MR scanner for imaging. The contrast mixture is prepared by mixing 0.1 mL of gadolinium with 20 cc syringe of normal saline, which can be injected under ultrasound or fluoroscopic guidance immediately before the MRI study is performed. Approximately 12–15 mL of contrast material is sufficient to optimally distend the joint. The MRI sequences may vary from institution to institution but typically a coronal oblique fat-saturated T1, coronal oblique fat-saturated T2, sagittal T1, axial fat-saturated T1, and oblique axial fat-saturated T1 MR sequences with the arm in abduction and external rotation (ABER) are performed. To position the shoulder in the ABER position, the patient is instructed to place the hand of the affected extremity with the palm up behind the head of the patient with the elbow flexed. This position produces traction of the anterior-inferior glenohumeral joint capsule over the labrum which optimizes evaluation of this region for extension of contrast material into the labrum, thereby increasing detection of subtle labral tears [20, 21]. An additional oblique axial fat-saturated T1 MR arthrogram sequence with the patient in FADIR positioning where the arm in the affected shoulder is flexed, adducted, and internally rotated has improved imaging of the posterior labrum because of tension/traction of the posterior capsulolabral structures [22]. This is helpful to evaluate for posterior glenohumeral instability which is much less common than anterior instability and thus the FADIR sequence is not routinely performed.

7.3 Normal Anatomy

7.3.1 Glenohumeral Joint

The glenohumeral joint is a ball-and-socket joint formed by the round articulating surface of the humeral head and the concave articular surface of the glenoid fossa (Fig. 7.1). This configuration allows the joint to have a wide range of motion including adduction, abduction, flexion, extension, internal rotation, external rotation, and 360° circumduction [23]. Although having such a tremendous range of motion can have the advantage of allowing for a wide variety of movements in the shoulder, it also comes at a disadvantage of being a very unstable joint and this is the major reason why shoulder instability and shoulder

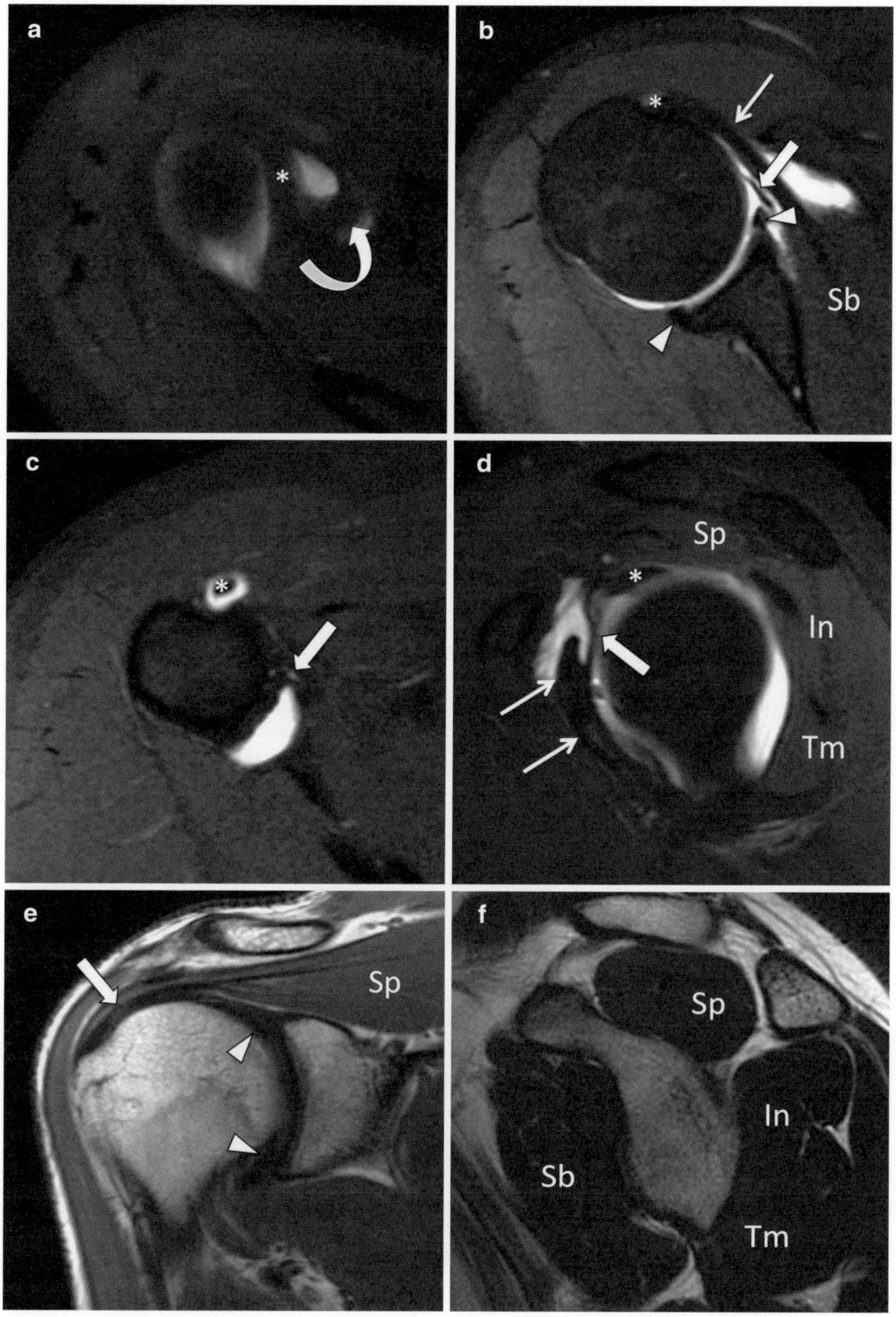

Fig. 7.1 Normal anatomy. Axial (**a–c**), sagittal (**d**), fat-saturated MR arthrographic, coronal nonfat-saturated T1-weighted (**e**), and sagittal nonfat-saturated T2-weighted MR images (**f**) demonstrating the normal MR appearance of the glenohumeral joint stabilizers. Long head of the biceps tendon = asterisk; superior glenohumeral ligament = curved arrow; middle glenohumeral ligament = thick arrows in (**b** and **d**); anterior band of the inferior glenohumeral ligament = thick arrow in (**c**); labrum = arrowheads; subscapularis tendon = thin arrows in (**b** and **d**); supraspinatus tendon = thick arrow in (**e**); Sb = subscapularis muscle; Sp = supraspinatus muscle; In = infraspinatus muscle; Tm = teres minor muscle

dislocation are very frequent in traumatic injuries such as falls and sports-related injuries [23]. The instability of the joint is partially alleviated by multiple reinforcing surrounding structures which include static stabilizers (glenohumeral joint capsule, glenohumeral ligaments, and labrum) and dynamic stabilizers (rotator cuff muscles and tendons, deltoid muscle, and long head of the biceps brachii muscle) working synchronously to maintain the articulation throughout the ranges of motion required by the shoulder.

The articular surface of the glenoid fossa is lined by a thin layer of hyaline cartilage. The glenoid normally has a slight retroversion angle of approximately 7° and has a distinct pear-shaped morphology which is best noted on sagittal CT or MR images, both of which are essential anatomic features that help maintain shoulder stability [24]. The humeral head articular surface is also covered by a thin layer of hyaline cartilage. The rounded morphology of the humeral head particularly along the posterosuperior aspect is also essential to maintain the stability of the glenohumeral joint.

7.4 Labrum and Glenohumeral Ligaments

The glenoid labrum is composed of fibrocartilage and is attached to the peripheral bony surface of the glenoid rim at the junction of the glenoid bone and hyaline cartilage articular surfaces, referred to as the chondrolabral junction. Normally, the labrum has uniformly low signal intensity on all MR pulse sequences attributable to a short T2 relaxation time because of its homogenous composition of fibrocartilage. However, there can be normal variations in signal intensity including globular and linear increased signal, particularly with intermediate-weighted proton density sequences and in elderly individuals, which is attributed to variations in the composition of fibrocartilage [25, 26]. The labrum usually has a triangular shape; however rounded, flat, cleaved, notched morphologies or even absence of the labrum has been described in normal asymptomatic individuals [27]. With the advancements made in MRI technology in the last decade, a routine MRI study without intra-articular contrast at a high magnetic field strength of 3 Tesla (3 T) will most likely be adequate to evaluate for a labral tear because of the high signal-to-noise ratio and anatomic detail obtained at 3 T. However, MR arthrography at any field strength (1.5 or 3 T) is still considered the imaging gold standard to evaluate the labrum [28] because it allows distension of the joint with contrast material increasing detection of labral tears.

The labrum increases the depth of the glenoid fossa by approximately 50% which contributes to the stability of the glenohumeral joint [27]. The labrum also provides points of attachment for the glenohumeral ligaments, joint capsule, and long head of the biceps tendon (LHBT). The superior glenohumeral ligament (SGHL) and the LHBT attach to the superior labrum. The attachment of the LHBT to the superior labrum is also referred to as the biceps labral complex. The middle glenohumeral ligament (MGHL) attaches to the anterior superior labrum. The inferior glenohumeral ligament (IGHL) complex includes an anterior band which attaches to the anterior inferior labrum, a posterior band which attaches to the posterior inferior labrum, and an intervening axillary pouch which forms the inferior part of the glenohumeral joint capsule. The labrum has a firm attachment along the posterior and inferior portions of the glenoid rim; however along the superior and anterior superior portions of the glenoid rim, the attachment is less firm and can have significant variation in the normal anatomy. If one is not familiar with such anatomic variants, this can be misinterpreted as a labral tear since these anatomic variants are often associated with physiologic joint fluid or contrast material extension around the labrum on MR images, mimicking a tear. The major anatomical variants of the labrum worth noting are [1] the sublabral recess or sublabral sulcus, [2] the sublabral foramen or sublabral hole, and [3] the Buford complex. These anatomic variants of the labrum involve the anterior half of the labrum which is also a common region of the labrum that is injured in anterior glenohumeral instability; therefore a detailed discussion of these variants is warranted.

The sublabral recess (Fig. 7.2), also referred to as a sublabral sulcus, is a normal anatomic potential space between the biceps-labral complex and the superior aspect of the glenoid rim, which is the result of a synovial reflection at the insertion of the long head biceps tendon on the supraglenoid tubercle, and it results in a physiologic loose attachment of the superior labrum to the superior glenoid cartilage [29]. Using the clock-face analogy to describe the portions of the labrum with 12:00 being located superiorly at the biceps-labral complex, 3:00 located anteriorly, 6:00 located inferiorly, and 9:00 located posteriorly, the sublabral recess is located between the 11 and 1 o'clock positions in the superior glenoid underlying the biceps labral complex. This is best appreciated on coronal MRI images, where the normal sublabral recess is located at the superior aspect glenoid rim and points toward the medial side of the glenoid. In contrast, a tear in this region of the labrum, which is referred to as superior labrum anteroposterior (SLAP) tear, the tear lesion, points toward the lateral aspect of the superior labrum [30].

The sublabral foramen (Fig. 7.2), also referred to as a sublabral hole, is a focal physiologic normal detachment of the anterosuperior labrum from the underlying glenoid rim, which is found in approximately 10% of asymptomatic subjects [31]. When present, it is located between the 1 and 3 o'clock positions of the glenoid, anterior to the biceps labral complex. This normal anatomic variant should not be confused with a tear of the anterosuperior labrum. Even though they can have a similar appearance, there are slight differences in morphology which are helpful to differentiate between the normal variant and a pathologic tear. A normal sublabral foramen is only located along the anterior superior labrum, should not be displaced by more than 1–2 mm, and should have smooth borders [27]. In contrast, a labral tear will usually be more prominent and have irregular borders and may or may not extend into other portions of the labrum.

The Buford complex (Fig. 7.2) is an anatomical variant characterized by a prominent or cord-like and thickened (sometimes even frayed appearing) MGHL in association with absence of the anterosuperior labrum. This normal variant is present in 1.5–2% of healthy subjects [32] and can mimic a tear of the anterosuperior labrum or MGHL if one is not familiar with this anatomical variant.

7.4.1 Rotator Cuff

The muscles of the rotator cuff include the supraspinatus, infraspinatus, subscapularis, and teres minor. The supraspinatus muscle has its origin along the supraspinatus fossa of the scapula. The infraspinatus muscle origin is at the infraspinatus fossa and the inferior surface of the spine of the scapula. The teres minor muscle originates at the lateral border of the scapula. The subscapularis muscle origin is at the subscapularis fossa. The rotator cuff muscles approximate each other along their tendinous insertion sites to the humeral head. The subscapularis tendon inserts at the lesser tuberosity of the humeral head and the supraspinatus, infraspinatus, and teres minor tendons insert at the greater tuberosity of the humeral head. The greater tuberosity is composed of superior, middle, and inferior facets for the rotator cuff tendons to insert at. The supraspinatus tendon predominantly inserts at the superior facet and the infraspinatus tendon predominantly inserts at the middle facet, keeping in mind that these two tendons have interdigitating fibers which fuse and have a partly continuous attachment at the margin of the superior and middle facets [30]. The teres minor tendon inserts along the inferior facet. The subscapularis tendon and supraspinatus tendon also have tendon fibers that interdigitate and fuse over the bicipital groove between the greater and lesser tuberosity, which helps to stabilize the LHBT in its anatomic location within the groove [33].

The rotator cuff muscles are the major dynamic stabilizers of the glenohumeral joint. The supraspinatus muscle abducts the humerus and functions synergistically with the deltoid muscle throughout the range of abduction. When

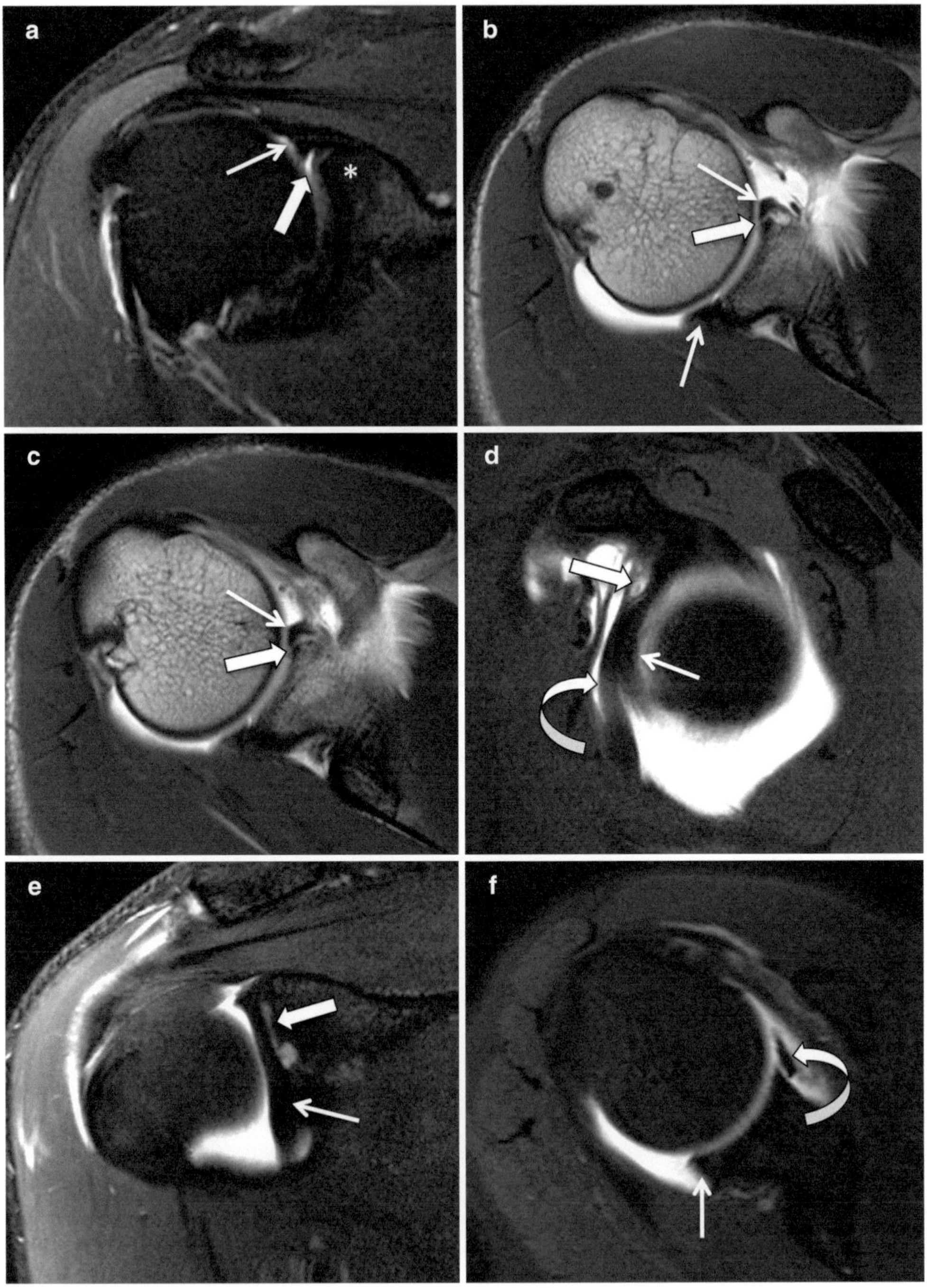

Fig. 7.2 Sublabral recess, sublabral foramen, and Buford complex. (**a**) Coronal fat-saturated T2-weighted MR image showing a fluid-filled sublabral recess (thick arrow) between the superior glenoid rim (asterisk) and the biceps-labral complex (thin arrow). Axial nonfat-saturated T1-weighted (**b** and **c**), sagittal fat-saturated T1-weighted (**d**), and coronal fat-saturated T2-weighted (**e**) arthrographic MR images demonstrating a sublabral foramen (thick arrows). The anterosuperior labrum is detached from the glenoid with a contrast-filled foramen (thick arrows). Superior and inferior to this foramen, the labrum (thin arrows) attaches normally to the glenoid. Axial fat-saturated T1-weighted arthrographic MR image (**f**) showing a Buford complex with a thickened middle glenohumeral ligament (curved arrows) and absence of the anterosuperior labrum

supraspinatus function is lost, such as through a tear, there is a substantial increase in the force required from the deltoid muscle to initiate arm abduction [34]. The infraspinatus and teres minor muscles function to externally rotate the humerus. The subscapularis muscle internally rotates and adducts the humerus.

The coupling of the forces of the rotator cuff and deltoid muscles in the coronal and transverse planes is important for stabilizing the glenohumeral joint. When the humerus is abducted and with overhead movement of the arm, the coupled forces of the deltoid muscle and the supraspinatus muscle are directed toward the glenoid, which physiologically "compresses" the humeral head onto the glenoid and thereby improves the stability of the joint by resisting superior humeral head displacement [35]. The additional coupling of forces between the subscapularis muscle anteriorly and infraspinatus muscle posteriorly also stabilizes the joint keeping it centered throughout the entire range of motion [35].

The tendons of the rotator cuff usually have low signal on all MR pulse sequences; however, there can be focally increased signal in the supraspinatus tendon at the distal tendon insertion where the tendon has an oblique course as it wraps over the greater tuberosity of the humeral head due to magic angle artifact. Magic angle artifact occurs in MR pulse sequences with a relative short-to-intermediate time to echo (TE) such as T1 and PD sequences; therefore, one should not see it on long TE sequences such as an FST2-weighted image. If one is not familiar with this common artifact, this can be confused with tendinopathy.

7.5 Imaging and Clinical Implications of Glenohumeral Instability

7.5.1 Mechanism of Injury

The wide range of motion of the glenohumeral joint predisposes it to inherent instability. Indeed, it is the most commonly subluxed and dislocated joint among all peripheral joints [36]. Dislocation of the glenohumeral joint is most commonly secondary to trauma but can also occur in a nontraumatic setting from underlying morphologic abnormalities or injuries of the static and dynamic stabilizing structures of the joint such as the glenoid labrum or rotator cuff tendons [37], chronic overuse, and congenital laxity [8]. The mechanism of injury in anterior glenohumeral dislocation involves an anterior-inferior movement of the humeral head relative to the glenoid usually caused by a direct blow to, or fall on, an outstretched arm and typically the patient's arm is in abduction and external rotation during the traumatic injury. Patients who suffer from such an initial traumatic dislocation event often have recurrent microtrauma in which minor repetitive injuries lead to recurring shoulder dislocations, which can also lead to injury to the soft-tissue stabilizers [36, 37]. Anterior shoulder dislocation is the most common form of traumatic shoulder instability, accounting for 90% of all dislocation events. Posterior dislocation is much less common, and is typically associated with seizure disorders [38].

7.5.2 Imaging of Glenohumeral Instability

When the clinical suspicion of glenohumeral joint dislocation arises, the initial imaging test that is performed is plain radiography to assess for dislocation of the glenohumeral joint and any possible associated fractures [36]. Cross-sectional imaging with CT and MRI is often also performed to further characterize the extent of injury and for surgical planning [39]. CT allows for the most accurate assessment of the osseous injuries associated with shoulder dislocation [40, 41], whereas MRI and MR arthrography is optimal to evaluate the associated soft-tissue injuries of the labrum, glenohumeral ligaments, and rotator cuff [42]. However, MRI can also provide useful information on the presence and size of osseous injury [43–45].

7.5.3 Capsulolabral Complex Injuries

With anterior dislocation, the inferior glenohumeral ligament (IGHL) pulls the anterior-inferior margin of the osseous glenoid rim, which results in an avulsion injury of the labrum and the anterior band of the inferior glenohumeral ligament, referred to as a soft-tissue Bankart injury [36]. The labrum can become detached off the glenoid at the chondrolabral junction, and often the labrum itself is torn and fragmented. When intra-articular contrast material is injected into the joint space during MR arthrography, this can help establish the diagnosis of a labral tear by demonstrating contrast extension between the labrum and the glenoid indicating detachment. Additional findings seen with tears of the labrum on conventional MRI or MR arthrography include abnormal morphology with fraying or fragmentation of the labrum, increased signal of the labrum, and displacement of torn labral tissue.

There are also numerous Bankart injury variants, which represent a spectrum of different types of injuries that can occur in the anteroinferior labrum and capsule with this mechanism of injury, including the Perthes lesion, anterior labral periosteal sleeve avulsion (ALPSA), and glenolabral articular disruption (GLAD).

A Perthes lesion (Fig. 7.3) refers to avulsion of the anterior labrum at the chondrolabral junction but the labrum remains attached to the glenoid because of an intact scapular periosteum [46, 47]. This injury is usually less conspicuous or can even be occult on standard axial MR images, typically becoming more apparent when the shoulder is in the ABER position [48].

ALPSA lesions (Fig. 7.4) are similar to Perthes lesions and can be acute or chronic. An acute ALPSA refers to detachment of the anterior labrum at the chondrolabral junction with stripping of the scapular periosteum but the labrum is non-displaced [49, 50]. A chronic ALPSA describes a chronic tear with scarring of the anterior labrum which is inferomedially displaced along the glenoid neck, but remains attached via a rim of scapular periosteum [8].

A GLAD lesion (Fig. 7.5) represents an anterior labral tear associated with an adjacent anterior glenoid articular cartilage defect [51]. Unlike the other mentioned Bankart variants, the GLAD lesion is not thought to typically predispose to recurrent shoulder dislocation [8].

A HAGL lesion (Fig. 7.6) is another type of avulsion injury that can occur with anterior shoulder dislocation and refers to a tear of the humeral attachment of the anterior glenohumeral joint capsule/glenohumeral ligaments [52, 53]. This is a relatively rare lesion that is usually found in the presence of other dislocation-related injuries. A study by Melvin et al. suggests that MRI may overestimate this type of injury, and thus definitive diagnosis should be reserved for arthroscopy [54]. If there is an osseous avulsion fragment of the humeral head attached to a HAGL lesion, this is referred to as a bony HAGL or BHAGL.

7.5.4 Osseous Injuries

If there is sufficient force applied to the anterior glenoid during an anterior dislocation event, this can also lead to fracture of the anteroinferior glenoid with associated bony defect in the glenoid rim referred to as a Bankart fracture. Alternatively, there can also be flattening of the anterior glenoid margin resulting from mechanical erosion or impaction from repeated dislocation events [8]. The glenoid bone loss that occurs from this injury gives the glenoid an inverted pear-shaped morphology on arthroscopy where the superior aspect of the glenoid is wider than the inferior portion [55]. This is in contrast to its normal appearance which resembles a pear with a wider inferior portion and narrower upper portion. With Bankart fractures, assessment of the morphology and size of the osseous defect of the glenoid bone loss are essential because substantial glenoid bone loss is associated with surgical failure [27]. Anterior glenohumeral dislocation injuries also often lead to an impaction fracture deformity of the posterior superior aspect of the humeral head referred to as a Hill-Sachs fracture. The mechanism of

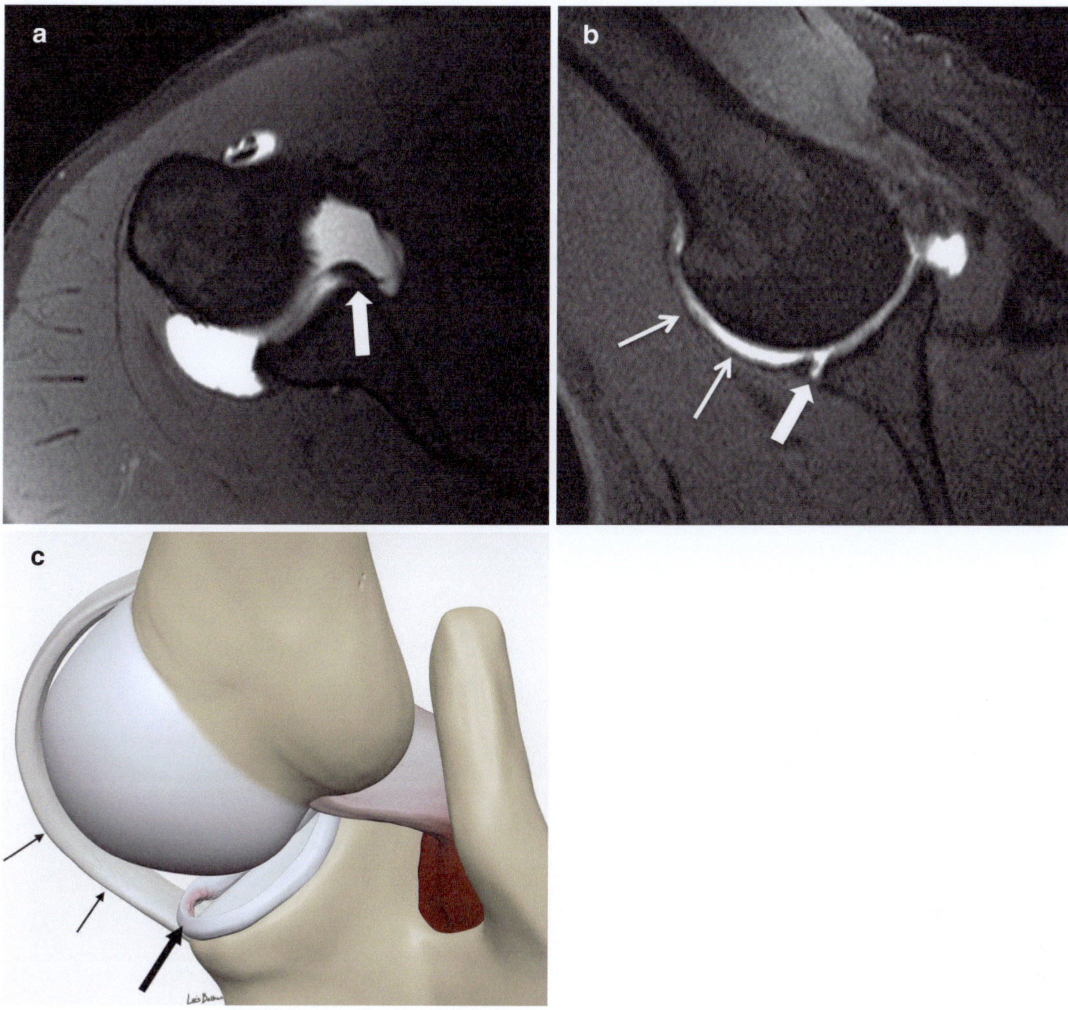

Fig. 7.3 Perthes lesion. Axial (**a**) and ABER (abduction and external rotation) fat-saturated T1-weighted (**b**) MR arthrographic images with illustration (**c**) showing a torn anteroinferior labrum (thick arrows). The labral tear is best demonstrated on abduction and external rotation as this position stretches the anterior band of the inferior glenohumeral ligament (thin arrows), revealing the lesion

injury is reciprocating impaction that occurs when the anteriorly translated humeral head contacts the anteroinferior glenoid rim. Assessment of the size and morphology of Hill-Sachs fractures is also important because they are associated with an increased risk of recurrent dislocation after surgical intervention [56, 57]. Furthermore, accurate preoperative characterization of combined glenoid and humeral bone loss (referred to as bipolar bone loss) followed by appropriate treatment has been shown to result in favorable postoperative outcomes with minimal risk of recurrent anterior shoulder instability [58–61]. In contrast, incorrect underestimation of glenoid and humeral bone loss and failure to intervene and correct such bone loss can lead to a higher risk of recurrent glenohumeral instability [8, 62, 63]. There are several studies supporting the use of 3D reconstructed CT and MR images to accurately quantify glenoid and humeral bone loss on [64–69] (Fig. 7.7).

Greater tuberosity fractures can also be seen in the setting of anterior shoulder dislocation with a prevalence of 15–35% of patients [70].

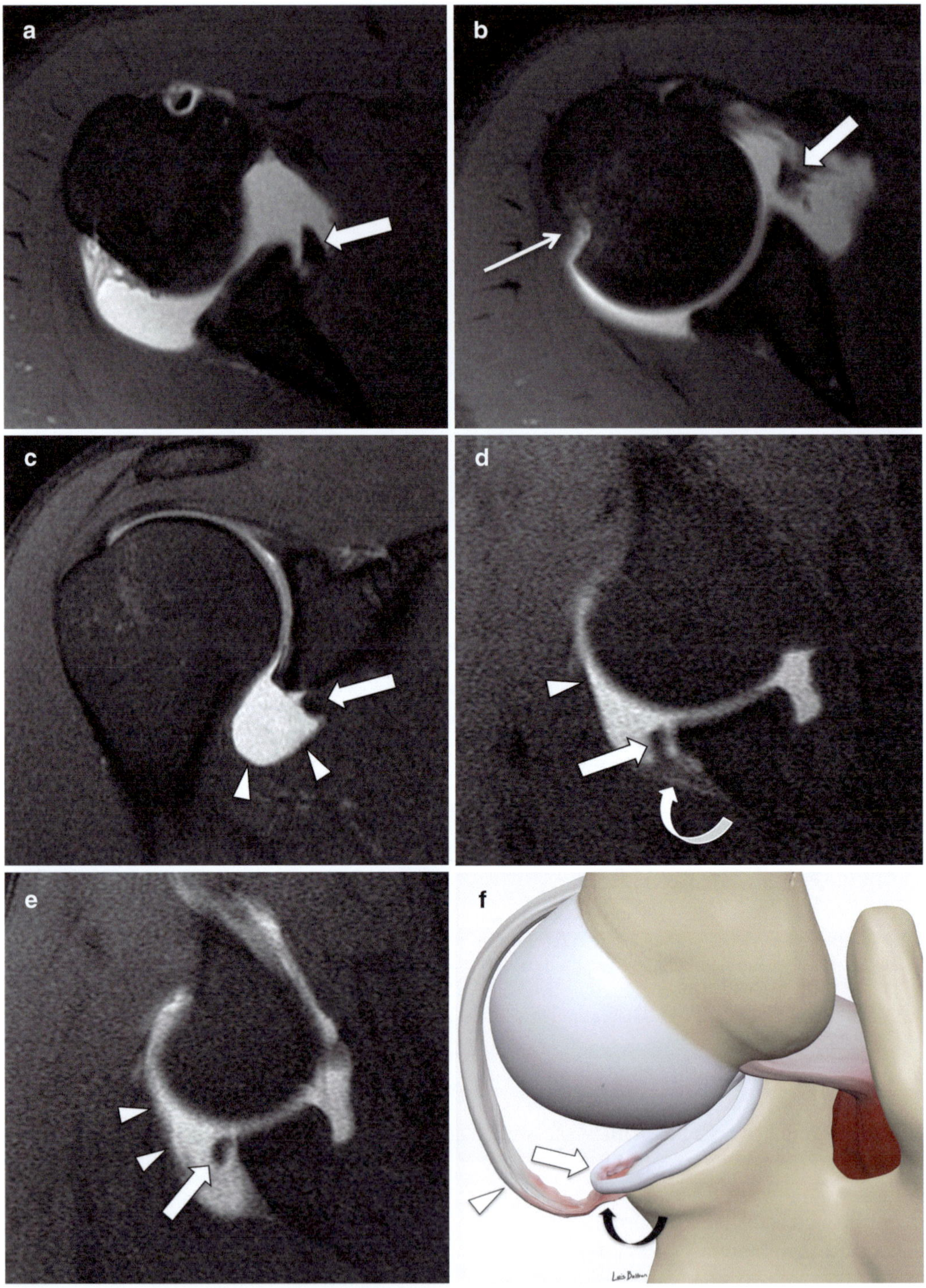

Fig. 7.4 Chronic anterior labral periosteal sleeve avulsion (ALPSA). Axial (**a** and **b**), coronal (**c**), and ABER fat-saturated T1-weighted (**d** and **e**) MR arthrographic images and illustration (**f**) demonstrating a detached anteroinferior labrum (thick arrows). There is inferomedial displacement of the torn labrum (thick arrows), which remains attached to the glenoid by the stripped scapular periosteum (curved arrow). Note the patulous anterior glenohumeral joint capsule (arrowheads) and associated humeral Hill-Sachs lesion (thin arrow). Inferior glenohumeral ligament = arrowheads

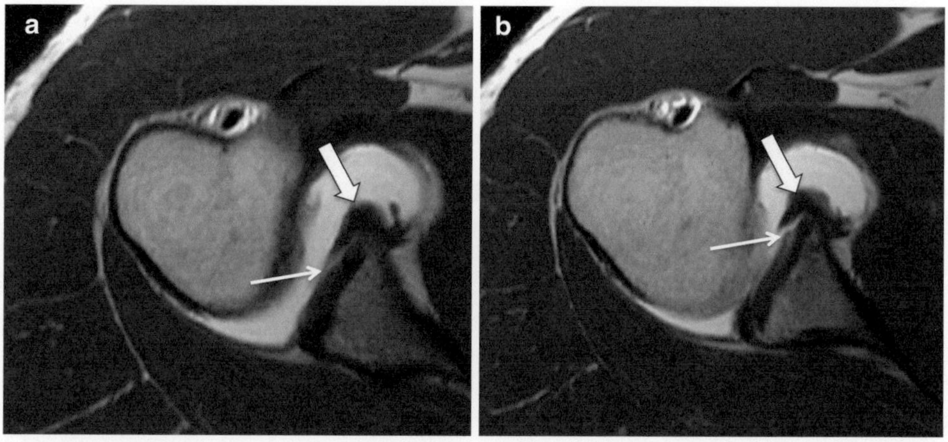

Fig. 7.5 Glenolabral articular disruption (GLAD). Axial (**a** and **b**) nonfat-saturated T1-weighted MR arthrographic MR images showing a tear or the anteroinferior labrum (thick arrows) with an adjacent defect in the articular cartilage (thin arrows)

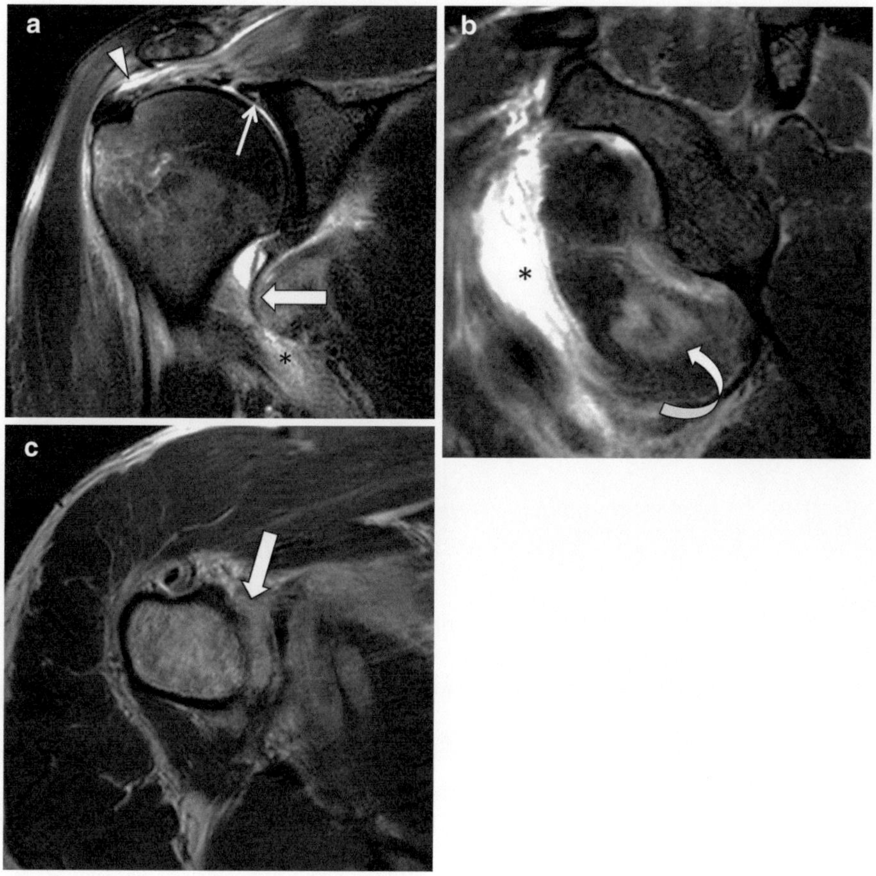

Fig. 7.6 Humeral avulsion of the inferior glenohumeral ligament (HAGL). Coronal (**a**), sagittal fat-saturated T2-weighted (**b**), and axial proton density (PD) MR images (**c**) demonstrating humeral avulsion of the inferior glenohumeral ligament (thick arrows) with leakage of joint fluid (asterisk) into the periarticular tissues. Note the associated intramuscular hematoma in the subscapularis (curved arrow), tear of the superior labrum or SLAP tear (thin arrow), and the high-grade tear of the supraspinatus tendon (arrowhead)

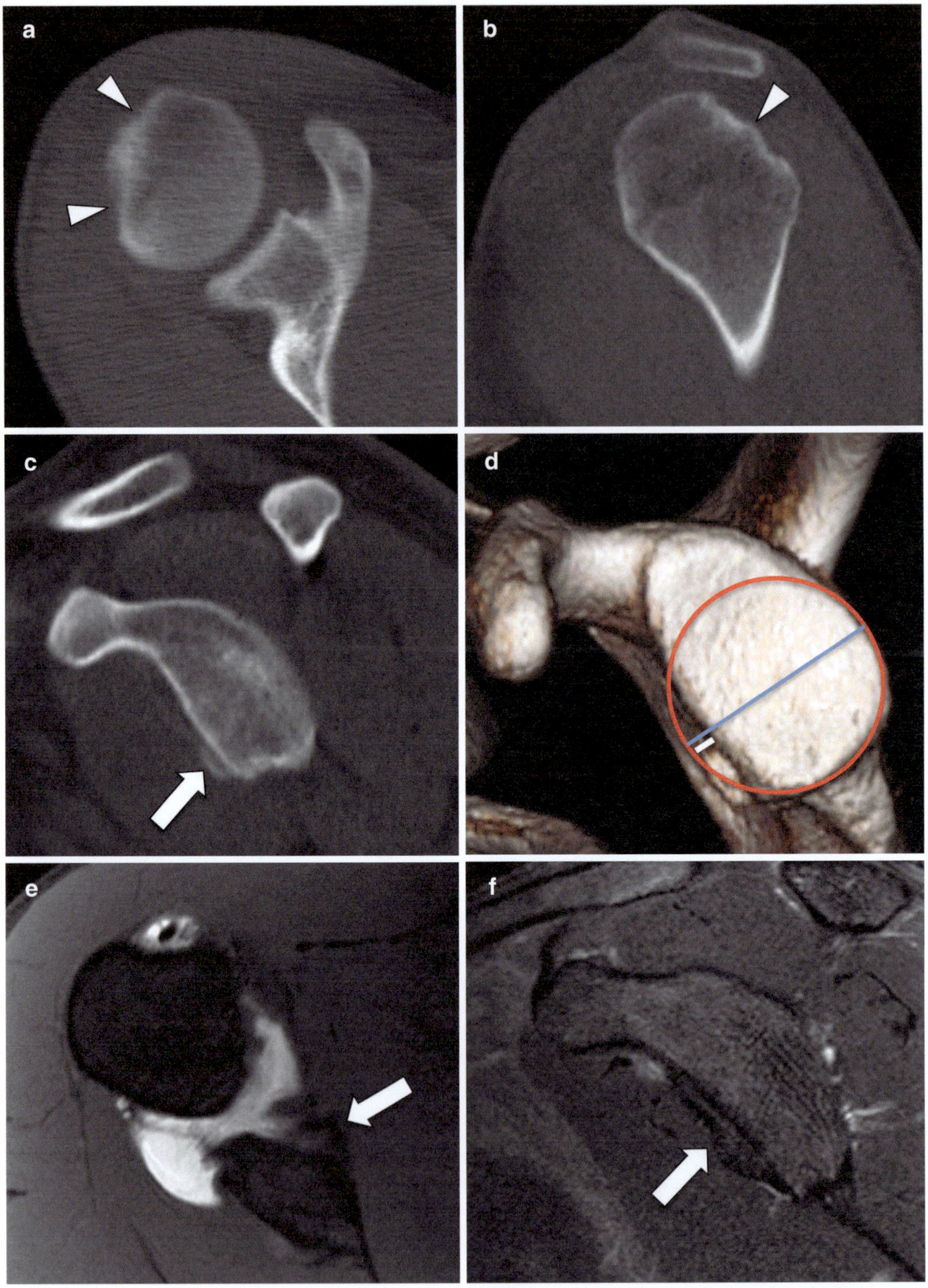

Fig. 7.7 Bankart and Hill-Sachs fractures. Axial (**a**), sagittal CT reformats (**b** and **c**), and 3D reconstruction of the glenoid (**d**) demonstrating Hill-Sachs (arrowheads) and Bankart fractures (thick arrows). Axial fat-saturated T1-weighted (**e**) and sagittal fat-saturated T2-weighted (**f**) arthrographic MR images showing a large osseous Bankart lesion (thick arrows). The best-fit circle method shown on the 3D reconstruction (**d**) is one of the methods used to quantify the amount of bone loss

Coracoid process fractures associated with glenohumeral dislocation are much less common [71, 72]. This type of fracture is more often found in the setting of acromioclavicular separation and clavicle fracture [73, 74].

7.5.5 Rotator Cuff Injuries

Injuries to the rotator cuff can be associated with glenohumeral dislocation although they are less common than the capsulolabral complex and osseous Bankart and Hill-Sachs injuries already discussed [75–82]. These injuries are more common in elderly patients; however it may be difficult to differentiate whether this association is due to preexisting rotator cuff degeneration from age-related factors or related to the dislocation episode itself [8]. The most commonly injured rotator cuff structure with glenohumeral instability is the subscapularis tendon, which is attributed to its location along the anterior aspect of the joint and its active and passive roles in glenohumeral joint stabilization (Fig. 7.8). Gyftopoulos et al. [83] demonstrated an association between tendon pathology (tendinosis and tearing) of the middle and inferior subscapularis tendon on MRI and prior anterior shoulder dislocation, and therefore noted that careful MR assessment of the subscapularis tendon is indicated in the setting of anterior shoulder dislocation as injury of this structure can be symptomatic and may be amenable to treatment. Tears of the supraspinatus and infraspinatus tendons in association with glenohumeral instability have also been described in elderly patients [8].

7.5.6 Nerve Injuries

The axillary nerve can be injured with anterior shoulder dislocation, occurring in a wide range of 5–54% of dislocation patients [84, 85]. Post-anterior shoulder dislocation axillary neuropathy is attributed to traction on the nerve as it is stretched when the humeral head dislocates anteriorly from the glenoid. Patients typically present with weakness on elevation and abduction of the arm and associated numbness and paresthesias along the lateral surface of the arm. The imaging findings can vary depending on the timing and extent of injury [86, 87]. In the acute setting, MR imaging may demonstrate no abnormality in the muscles innervated by the axillary nerve in the shoulder, which are the teres minor and posterior deltoid muscles. In the subacute stage of injury, MRI may show diffuse intramuscular edema within either muscle secondary to denervation injury, particularly if there is no space-occupying mass in the quadrilateral space to cause direct compression of the nerve [86, 87], and with chronic injury MRI can demonstrate atrophy with fat infiltration in the deltoid and teres minor muscles [86, 87]. Electrophysiologic studies are often performed to confirm nerve injury and to assess for recovery of nerve function [87].

7.5.7 Primary Versus Recurrent Dislocation

Differentiating between an acute first-time (primary) dislocation event and recurrent dislocation can be challenging. The patient's past medical history is helpful to differentiate the two; however this is often not possible as the patient may not be aware of or may fail to mention prior dislocations [8]. In general, various similar types of injuries can occur in both patient groups including anteroinferior labral pathology, Hill-Sachs and glenoid bone loss injuries, and rotator cuff tears [88].

Studies have demonstrated that anterior capsulolabral injuries (soft-tissue Bankart, Perthes, ALPSA, capsular tears, and capsular laxity) and osseous Bankart and Hill-Sachs lesions are found in both patients with primary dislocation and recurrent dislocation, but differ in prevalence [89, 90]. The presence of an inverted pear morphology of the glenoid appears to be the most reliable indicator of recurrent dislocation [8]. Indeed, this appearance of the glenoid has been found to represent a significant amount of glenoid bone loss of at least 25–27% of the inferior glenoid [91]. Hill-Sachs lesions also tend to be more common in recurrent dislocation [8]. Bankart lesions are

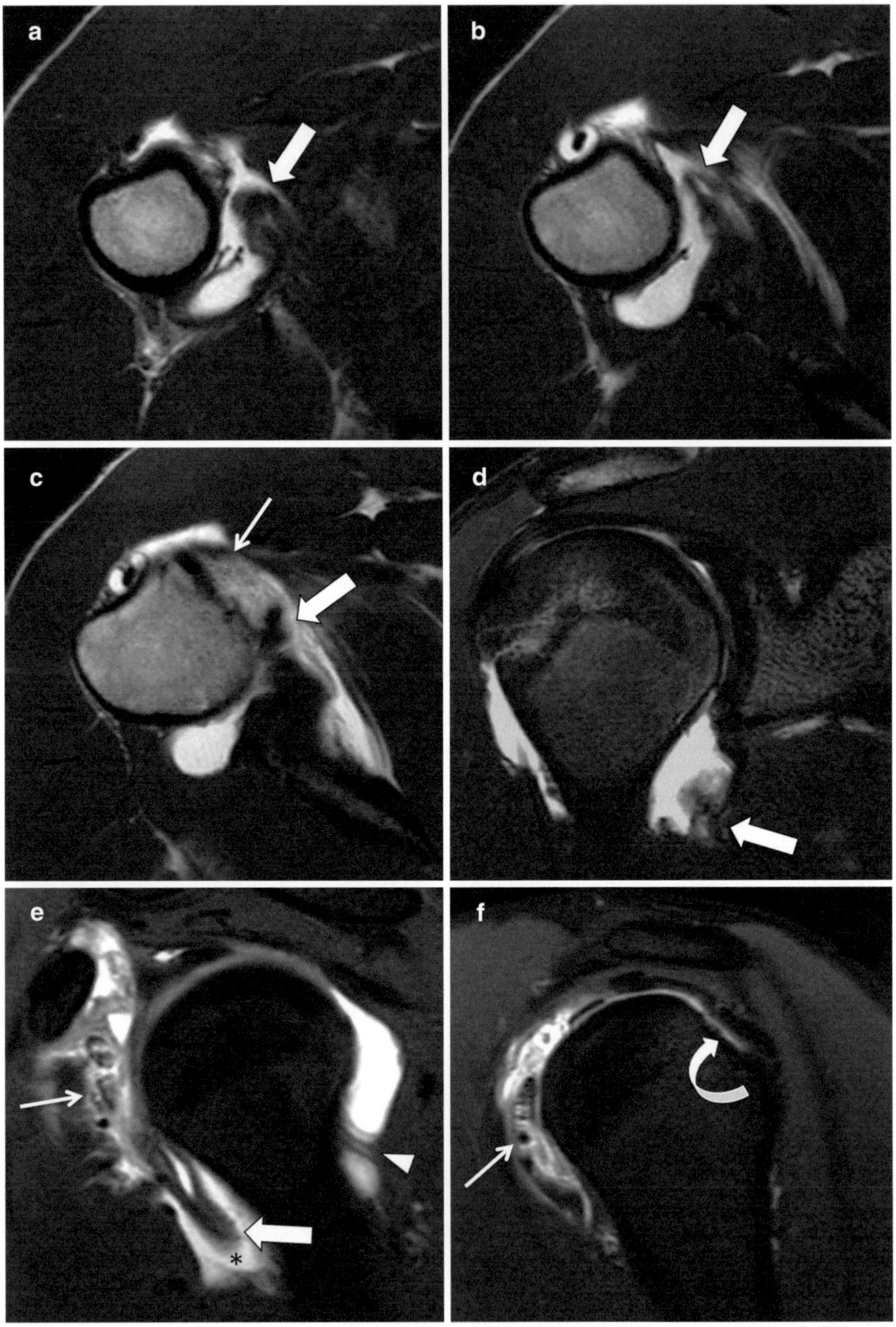

Fig. 7.8 Recurrent anterior glenohumeral dislocation associated with subscapularis tear. Axial nonfat-saturated T1-weighted (**a–c**), coronal fat-saturated T2-weighted (**d**), and sagittal fat-saturated T1-weighted (**e–f**) arthrographic MR images demonstrating humeral avulsion of the anterior band of the inferior glenohumeral ligament or HAGL lesion (thick arrows) with an intact posterior band (arrowhead). There is leakage of intra-articular contrast through the tear (asterisk). Note the associated Hill-Sachs lesion (curved arrow) and tear of the subscapularis tendon (thin arrows)

seen in high prevalence in both primary and recurrent dislocations [90]. Chronic ALPSA lesions are typically associated with recurrent dislocation, while acute ALPSA lesions are seen with primary dislocation. Gyftopoulos et al. [8] noted that the ALPSA lesion evolves from being a detached, non-displaced acute tear that over time retracts and scars down to the inferomedial aspect of the glenoid neck to become a chronic lesion and that this scarring and retraction can be, in part, related to and escalated by repeated anterior shoulder dislocation.

7.5.8 Posterior Instability

Posterior dislocation injuries of the glenohumeral joint are much less frequent than anterior dislocations and are typically associated with seizure disorders as the underlying cause of the posterior dislocation. Since the forces of injury in posterior dislocation are reversed relative to anterior dislocation injuries, the terms used to describe posterior shoulder dislocation injuries are prefixed with the phrase "reverse." Thus, in a posterior shoulder dislocation, a reverse Hill-Sachs injury refers to an impaction fracture of the anterior aspect of the humeral head, and a reverse Bankart fracture refers to a fracture of the posterior glenoid (Fig. 7.9). Bankart, Perthes, and ALPSA soft-tissue injuries can also be found in posterior dislocation and have the same imaging characteristics, but are found on the posteroinferior aspect of the joint and are usually referred to as a reverse Bankart, reverse Perthes, and/or reverse ALPSA lesions [92].

7.5.9 Postoperative Imaging

MR arthrography is the optimal modality to evaluate the integrity of the postoperative labrum [93–97]. In the postoperative setting following treatment of glenohumeral instability, it is important to evaluate the integrity of the repaired structures including the repaired labrum and repairs of glenoid and humeral osseous defects. In the normal postoperative labrum, there should be reattachment of the anteroinferior labrum and AIGHL to their normal anatomic position along the anteroinferior glenoid on MR arthrography [98]. There can normally be inhomogeneous signal and plump, rounded, enlarged, or irregular frayed morphology in the normal postoperative labrum and AIGHL; however these structures should be seen as continuous intact structures from the labrum to their osseous attachments [98]. Findings that indicate recurrent labral tear after Bankart labral repair on MR arthrography include detachment and fragmentation of the labrum with extension of contrast material into the labrum and/or contrast separating the labrum from the glenoid (Fig. 7.10) [99]. Recurrent tears of the labroligamentous complex can be partial or complete separation of the labrum and/or IGHL from the glenoid [98]. The use of the abduction external rotation (ABER) position on MR arthrography demonstrating pooling of contrast material between the anterior-inferior glenohumeral ligament (AIGHL) and glenoid at the site of surgical reattachment was shown to be a reliable sign of unstable detachment and recurrent labral tear which was confirmed on arthroscopy [95]. Additionally, patients who have recurrent dislocation after surgical intervention often also have associated signs of acute or worsening osseous Bankart and Hill-Sachs fractures which should also be inspected on postoperative MRI. Particularly, osseous signs of recurrent anterior shoulder instability in association with labral re-tear after failed Bankart labral repair include bone marrow edema along the anterior glenoid and posterior humeral head and/or increased size of glenoid and humeral bone loss compared to prior imaging if available [99]. It is also important to assess orthopedic fixation hardware for complications such as hardware fracture, loosening or displacement, and graft nonunion. Other postoperative complications to monitor for on postoperative imaging include osteonecrosis, infection, secondary osteoarthritis, and injury to the adjacent neurovascular structures.

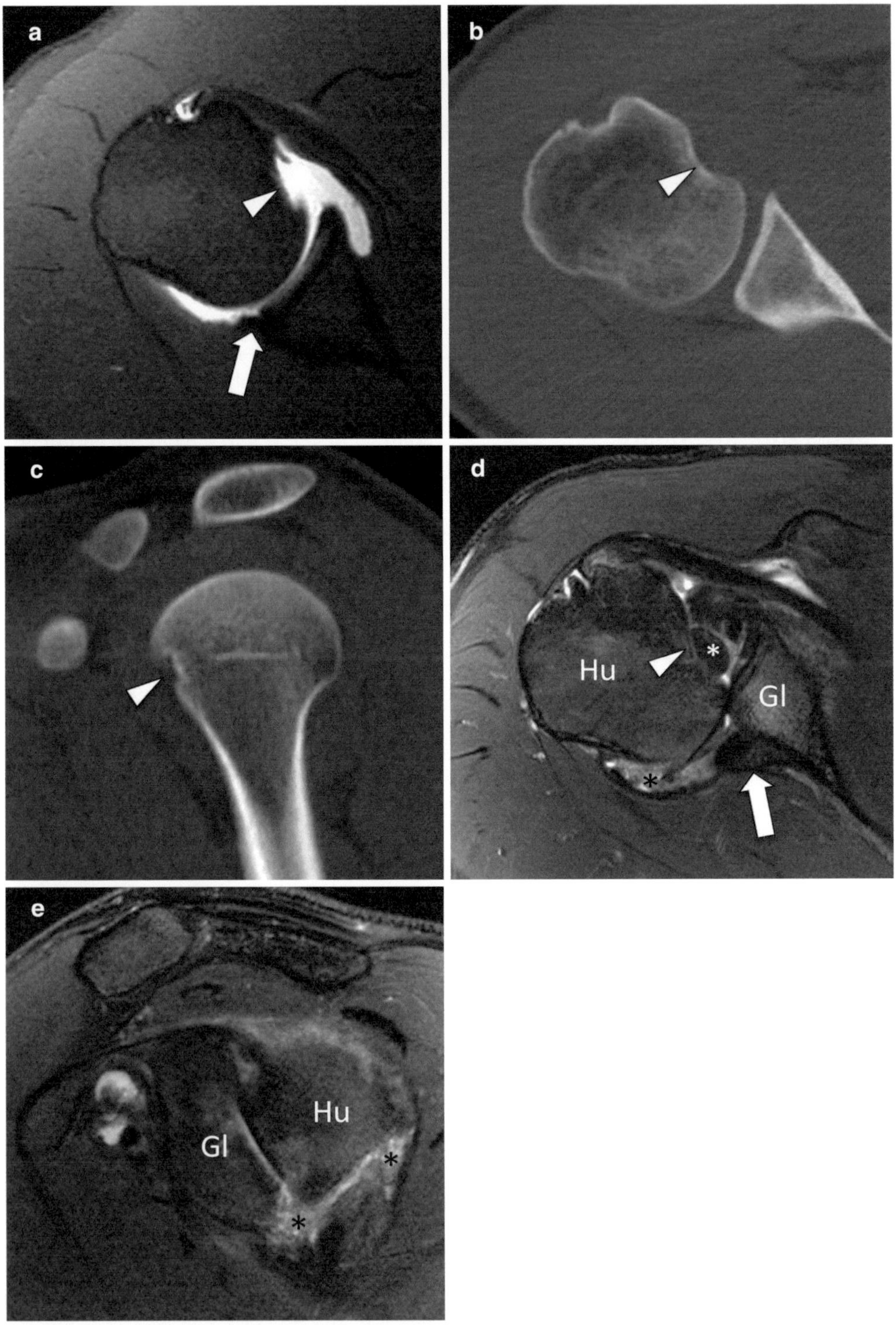

Fig. 7.9 Posterior glenohumeral dislocation. Axial fat-saturated T1-weighted MR arthrographic image (**a**), and axial (**b**) and sagittal (**c**) CT reformats showing a reverse soft-tissue Bankart lesion (thick arrow) and a reverse Hill-Sachs fracture (arrowheads). Axial (**d**) and sagittal (**e**) fat-saturated T2-weighted MR images demonstrating posterior subluxation of the glenohumeral joint with a large reverse osseous Bankart (thick arrow) and Hill-Sachs (arrowhead) fractures. Note the associated intra-articular body (white asterisk) and synovitis (black asterisks)

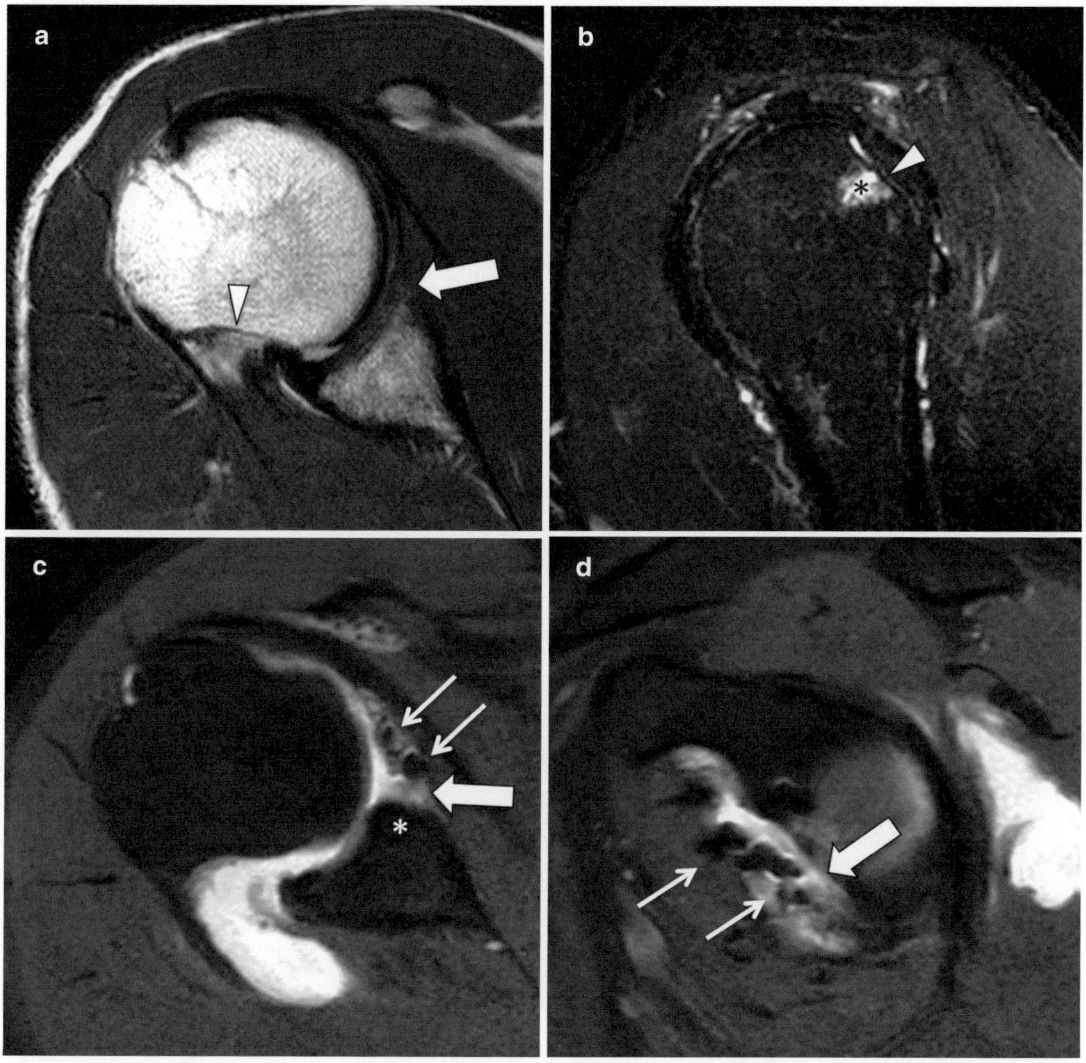

Fig. 7.10 Recurrent postoperative anterior glenohumeral instability. Preoperative axial nonfat-saturated PD (**a**) and sagittal fat-saturated T2-weighted MR images (**b**) demonstrating a Hill-Sachs lesion (arrowheads) with bone marrow edema (black asterisk) and a small soft-tissue Bankart lesion (thick arrow) for which the patient underwent Bankart repair. Axial (**c**) and sagittal (**d**) fat-saturated T1-weighted arthrographic MR images performed 3 years after surgery show an enlarging Bankart lesion (white asterisk) with contrast separating the repaired labrum (thin arrows) from the glenoid (thick arrow) suggestive of a recurrent tear

7.6 Summary

In summary, it is important to be familiar with the normal anatomical and pathologic imaging appearances of the structures in the shoulder to effectively diagnose and treat glenohumeral instability injuries. This chapter provides an up-to-date review of the normal shoulder anatomy and the various clinical and imaging features involved in glenohumeral instability with an emphasis on the MRI manifestations.

References

1. Kroner K, Lind T, Jensen J. The epidemiology of shoulder dislocations. Arch Orthop Trauma Surg. 1989;108(5):288–90.

2. Nordqvist A, Petersson CJ. Incidence and causes of shoulder girdle injuries in an urban population. J Shoulder Elbow Surg. 1995;4(2):107–12.
3. Simonet WT, Melton LJ III, Cofield RH, Ilstrup DM. Incidence of anterior shoulder dislocation in Olmsted County, Minnesota. Clin Orthop Relat Res. 1984;186:186–91.
4. Hovelius L. Shoulder dislocation in Swedish ice hockey players. Am J Sports Med. 1978;6(6):373–7.
5. Hovelius L. Incidence of shoulder dislocation in Sweden. Clin Orthop Relat Res. 1982;166:127–31.
6. Arciero RA, Wheeler JH, Ryan JB, McBride JT. Arthroscopic Bankart repair versus nonoperative treatment for acute, initial anterior shoulder dislocations. Am J Sports Med. 1994;22(5):589–94.
7. Wheeler JH, Ryan JB, Arciero RA, Molinari RN. Arthroscopic versus nonoperative treatment of acute shoulder dislocations in young athletes. Arthroscopy. 1989;5(3):213–7.
8. Gyftopoulos S, Bencardino J, Palmer WE. MR imaging of the shoulder: first dislocation versus chronic instability. Semin Musculoskelet Radiol. 2012;16(4):286–95.
9. Hovelius L, Lind B, Thorling J. Primary dislocation of the shoulder. Factors affecting the two-year prognosis. Clin Orthop Relat Res. 1983;176:181–5.
10. Simonet WT, Cofield RH. Prognosis in anterior shoulder dislocation. Am J Sports Med. 1984;12(1):19–24.
11. Hovelius L. Anterior dislocation of the shoulder in teen-agers and young adults. Five-year prognosis. J Bone Joint Surg Am. 1987;69(3):393–9.
12. Vermeiren J, Handelberg F, Casteleyn PP, Opdecam P. The rate of recurrence of traumatic anterior dislocation of the shoulder. A study of 154 cases and a review of the literature. Int Orthop. 1993;17(6):337–41.
13. Hovelius L, Augustini BG, Fredin H, Johansson O, Norlin R, Thorling J. Primary anterior dislocation of the shoulder in young patients. A ten-year prospective study. J Bone Joint Surg Am. 1996;78(11):1677–84.
14. Roberts SN, Taylor DE, Brown JN, Hayes MG, Saies A. Open and arthroscopic techniques for the treatment of traumatic anterior shoulder instability in Australian rules football players. J Shoulder Elbow Surg. 1999;8(5):403–9.
15. Kralinger FS, Golser K, Wischatta R, Wambacher M, Sperner G. Predicting recurrence after primary anterior shoulder dislocation. Am J Sports Med. 2002;30(1):116–20.
16. te Slaa RL, Brand R, Marti RK. A prospective arthroscopic study of acute first-time anterior shoulder dislocation in the young: a five-year follow-up study. J Shoulder Elbow Surg. 2003;12(6):529–34.
17. Rowe CR. Prognosis in dislocations of the shoulder. J Bone Joint Surg Am. 1956;38-A(5):957–77.
18. Milgrom C, Mann G, Finestone A. A prevalence study of recurrent shoulder dislocations in young adults. J Shoulder Elbow Surg. 1998;7(6):621–4.
19. Owens BD, Dawson L, Burks R, Cameron KL. Incidence of shoulder dislocation in the United States military: demographic considerations from a high-risk population. J Bone Joint Surg Am. 2009;91(4):791–6.
20. Beltran LS, Adler R, Stone T, Surace J, Beltran J, Bencardino JT. MRI and Ultrasound Imaging of the Shoulder Using Positional Maneuvers. AJR Am J Roentgenol. 2015;205(3):W244–54.
21. Cvitanic O, Tirman PF, Feller JF, Bost FW, Minter J, Carroll KW. Using abduction and external rotation of the shoulder to increase the sensitivity of MR arthrography in revealing tears of the anterior glenoid labrum. AJR Am J Roentgenol. 1997;169(3):837–44.
22. Chiavaras MM, Harish S, Burr J. MR arthrographic assessment of suspected posteroinferior labral lesions using flexion, adduction, and internal rotation positioning of the arm: preliminary experience. Skeletal Radiol. 2010;39(5):481–8.
23. Quillen DM, Wuchner M, Hatch RL. Acute shoulder injuries. Am Fam Physician. 2004;70(10):1947–54.
24. Di Giacomo G, Itoi E, Burkhart SS. Evolving concept of bipolar bone loss and the Hill-Sachs lesion: from "engaging/non-engaging" lesion to "on-track/off-track" lesion. Arthroscopy. 2014;30(1):90–8.
25. Arai R, Kobayashi M, Toda Y, Nakamura S, Miura T, Nakamura T. Fiber components of the shoulder superior labrum. Surgical and radiologic anatomy: SRA. 2012;34(1):49–56.
26. Gustas CN, Tuite MJ. Imaging update on the glenoid labrum: variants versus tears. Semin Musculoskelet Radiol. 2014;18(4):365–73.
27. Llopis E, Montesinos P, Guedez MT, Aguilella L, Cerezal L. Normal Shoulder MRI and MR Arthrography: Anatomy and Technique. Semin Musculoskelet Radiol. 2015;19(3):212–30.
28. Major NM, Browne J, Domzalski T, Cothran RL, Helms CA. Evaluation of the glenoid labrum with 3-T MRI: is intra-articular contrast necessary? AJR Am J Roentgenol. 2011;196(5):1139–44.
29. Kwak SM, Brown RR, Resnick D, Trudell D, Applegate GR, Haghighi P. Anatomy, anatomic variations, and pathology of the 11- to 3-o'clock position of the glenoid labrum: findings on MR arthrography and anatomic sections. AJR Am J Roentgenol. 1998;171(1):235–8.
30. Rudez J, Zanetti M. Normal anatomy, variants and pitfalls on shoulder MRI. Eur J Radiol. 2008;68(1):25–35.
31. Stoller DW. MR arthrography of the glenohumeral joint. Radiol Clin North Am. 1997;35(1):97–116.
32. Williams MM, Snyder SJ, Buford D Jr. The Buford complex--the "cord-like" middle glenohumeral ligament and absent anterosuperior labrum complex: a normal anatomic capsulolabral variant. Arthroscopy. 1994;10(3):241–7.
33. Boon JM, de Beer MA, Botha D, Maritz NG, Fouche AA. The anatomy of the subscapularis tendon insertion as applied to rotator cuff repair. J Shoulder Elbow Surg. 2004;13(2):165–9.
34. Opsha O, Malik A, Baltazar R, Primakov D, Beltran S, Miller TT, et al. MRI of the rotator cuff and internal derangement. Eur J Radiol. 2008;68(1):36–56.

35. Parsons IM, Apreleva M, Fu FH, Woo SL. The effect of rotator cuff tears on reaction forces at the glenohumeral joint. Journal of orthopaedic research: official publication of the Orthopaedic Research Society. 2002;20(3):439–46.
36. Demehri S, Hafezi-Nejad N, Fishman EK. Advanced imaging of glenohumeral instability: the role of MRI and MDCT in providing what clinicians need to know. Emerg Radiol. 2016;24(1):95–103.
37. Murray IR, Goudie EB, Petrigliano FA, Robinson CM. Functional anatomy and biomechanics of shoulder stability in the athlete. Clin Sports Med. 2013;32(4):607–24.
38. Shah AS, Karadsheh MS, Sekiya JK. Failure of operative treatment for glenohumeral instability: etiology and management. Arthroscopy. 2011;27(5):681–94.
39. Acid S, Le Corroller T, Aswad R, Pauly V, Champsaur P. Preoperative imaging of anterior shoulder instability: diagnostic effectiveness of MDCT arthrography and comparison with MR arthrography and arthroscopy. AJR Am J Roentgenol. 2012;198(3):661–7.
40. Fritz J, Fishman EK, Fayad LM. MDCT Arthrography of the Shoulder. Semin Musculoskelet Radiol. 2014;18(4):343–51.
41. Fritz J, Fishman EK, Small KM, Winalski CS, Horger MS, Corl F, et al. MDCT arthrography of the shoulder with datasets of isotropic resolution: indications, technique, and applications. AJR Am J Roentgenol. 2012;198(3):635–46.
42. Magee T. 3-T MRI of the shoulder: is MR arthrography necessary? AJR Am J Roentgenol. 2009;192(1):86–92.
43. Huijsmans PE, Haen PS, Kidd M, Dhert WJ, van der Hulst VP, Willems WJ. Quantification of a glenoid defect with three-dimensional computed tomography and magnetic resonance imaging: a cadaveric study. J Shoulder Elbow Surg. 2007;16(6):803–9.
44. Skendzel JG, Sekiya JK. Diagnosis and management of humeral head bone loss in shoulder instability. Am J Sports Med. 2012;40(11):2633–44.
45. Gyftopoulos S, Hasan S, Bencardino J, Mayo J, Nayyar S, Babb J, et al. Diagnostic accuracy of MRI in the measurement of glenoid bone loss. AJR Am J Roentgenol. 2012;199(4):873–8.
46. Perthes G. Zur therapie der habituellen schulterluxation. Med Zs. 1905;237:481.
47. Perthes G. Ueber operationen bei habitueller schulterluxation. Dtsch Z Chir. 1906;85:199.
48. Wischer TK, Bredella MA, Genant HK, Stoller DW, Bost FW, Tirman PF. Perthes lesion (a variant of the Bankart lesion): MR imaging and MR arthrographic findings with surgical correlation. AJR Am J Roentgenol. 2002;178(1):233–7.
49. Neviaser TJ. The anterior labroligamentous periosteal sleeve avulsion lesion: a cause of anterior instability of the shoulder. Arthroscopy. 1993;9(1):17–21.
50. Chung CB, Corrente L, Resnick D. MR arthrography of the shoulder. Magn Reson Imaging Clin N Am. 2004;12(1):25–38.. v-vi
51. Neviaser TJ. The GLAD lesion: another cause of anterior shoulder pain. Arthroscopy. 1993;9(1):22–3.
52. Wolf EM, Cheng JC, Dickson K. Humeral avulsion of glenohumeral ligaments as a cause of anterior shoulder instability. Arthroscopy. 1995;11(5):600–7.
53. Richards DP, Burkhart SS. Arthroscopic humeral avulsion of the glenohumeral ligaments (HAGL) repair. Arthroscopy. 2004;20(Suppl 2):134–41.
54. Melvin JS, Mackenzie JD, Nacke E, Sennett BJ, Wells L. MRI of HAGL lesions: four arthroscopically confirmed cases of false-positive diagnosis. AJR Am J Roentgenol. 2008;191(3):730–4.
55. Burkhart SS, De Beer JF. Traumatic glenohumeral bone defects and their relationship to failure of arthroscopic Bankart repairs: significance of the inverted-pear glenoid and the humeral engaging Hill-Sachs lesion. Arthroscopy. 2000;16(7):677–94.
56. Mascarenhas R, Rusen J, Saltzman BM, Leiter J, Chahal J, Romeo AA, et al. Management of humeral and glenoid bone loss in recurrent glenohumeral instability. Advances in orthopedics. 2014;2014:640952.
57. Ozaki R, Nakagawa S, Mizuno N, Mae T, Yoneda M. Hill-Sachs lesions in shoulders with traumatic anterior instability: evaluation using computed tomography with 3-dimensional reconstruction. Am J Sports Med. 2014;42(11):2597–605.
58. Provencher MT, Bhatia S, Ghodadra NS, Grumet RC, Bach BR Jr, Dewing CB, et al. Recurrent shoulder instability: current concepts for evaluation and management of glenoid bone loss. J Bone Joint Surg Am. 2010;92(Suppl 2):133–51.
59. Piasecki DP, Verma NN, Romeo AA, Levine WN, Bach BR Jr, Provencher MT. Glenoid bone deficiency in recurrent anterior shoulder instability: diagnosis and management. J Am Acad Orthop Surg. 2009;17(8):482–93.
60. Warner JJ, Gill TJ, O'Hollerhan JD, Pathare N, Millett PJ. Anatomical glenoid reconstruction for recurrent anterior glenohumeral instability with glenoid deficiency using an autogenous tricortical iliac crest bone graft. Am J Sports Med. 2006;34(2):205–12.
61. Provencher MT, Ghodadra N, LeClere L, Solomon DJ, Romeo AA. Anatomic osteochondral glenoid reconstruction for recurrent glenohumeral instability with glenoid deficiency using a distal tibia allograft. Arthroscopy. 2009;25(4):446–52.
62. Owens BD, DeBerardino TM, Nelson BJ, Thurman J, Cameron KL, Taylor DC, et al. Long-term follow-up of acute arthroscopic Bankart repair for initial anterior shoulder dislocations in young athletes. Am J Sports Med. 2009;37(4):669–73.
63. Crall TS, Bishop JA, Guttman D, Kocher M, Bozic K, Lubowitz JH. Cost-effectiveness analysis of primary arthroscopic stabilization versus nonoperative treatment for first-time anterior glenohumeral dislocations. Arthroscopy. 2012;28(12):1755–65.
64. Provencher MT, Frank RM, Leclere LE, Metzger PD, Ryu JJ, Bernhardson A, et al. The Hill-Sachs lesion: diagnosis, classification, and management. J Am Acad Orthop Surg. 2012;20(4):242–52.
65. Cho SH, Cho NS, Rhee YG. Preoperative analysis of the Hill-Sachs lesion in anterior shoulder instability:

how to predict engagement of the lesion. Am J Sports Med. 2011;39(11):2389–95.
66. Stillwater L, Koenig J, Maycher B, Davidson M. 3D-MR vs. 3D-CT of the shoulder in patients with glenohumeral instability. Skeletal Radiol. 2016;46(3):325–31.
67. Gyftopoulos S, Beltran LS, Bookman J, Rokito A. MRI Evaluation of Bipolar Bone Loss Using the On-Track Off-Track Method: A Feasibility Study. AJR Am J Roentgenol. 2015;205(4):848–52.
68. Gyftopoulos S, Beltran LS, Yemin A, Strauss E, Meislin R, Jazrawi L, et al. Use of 3D MR reconstructions in the evaluation of glenoid bone loss: a clinical study. Skeletal Radiol. 2014;43(2):213–8.
69. Gyftopoulos S, Yemin A, Beltran L, Babb J, Bencardino J. Engaging Hill-Sachs lesion: is there an association between this lesion and findings on MRI? AJR Am J Roentgenol. 2013;201(4):W633–8.
70. McLaughlin HL, MacLellan DI. Recurrent anterior dislocation of the shoulder. II. A comparative study. J Trauma. 1967;7(2):191–201.
71. Goss TP. Fractures of the coracoid process. J Bone Joint Surg Br. 1997;79(4):694.
72. McGinnis M, Denton JR. Fractures of the scapula: a retrospective study of 40 fractured scapulae. J Trauma. 1989;29(11):1488–93.
73. Cottalorda J, Allard D, Dutour N, Chavrier Y. Fracture of the coracoid process in an adolescent. Injury. 1996;27(6):436–7.
74. Ogawa K, Yoshida A, Takahashi M, Ui M. Fractures of the coracoid process. J Bone Joint Surg Br. 1997;79(1):17–9.
75. Symeonides PP. The significance of the subscapularis muscle in the pathogenesis of recurrent anterior dislocation of the shoulder. J Bone Joint Surg Br. 1972;54(3):476–83.
76. Hawkins RJ, Bell RH, Hawkins RH, Koppert GJ. Anterior dislocation of the shoulder in the older patient. Clin Orthop Relat Res. 1986;206:192–5.
77. Itoi E, Tabata S. Rotator cuff tears in anterior dislocation of the shoulder. Int Orthop. 1992;16(3):240–4.
78. DePalma AF, Cooke AJ, Prabhakar M. The role of the subscapularis in recurrent anterior dislocations of the shoulder. Clin Orthop Relat Res. 1967;54:35–49.
79. Neviaser RJ, Neviaser TJ, Neviaser JS. Concurrent rupture of the rotator cuff and anterior dislocation of the shoulder in the older patient. J Bone Joint Surg Am. 1988;70(9):1308–11.
80. Neviaser RJ, Neviaser TJ, Neviaser JS. Anterior dislocation of the shoulder and rotator cuff rupture. Clin Orthop Relat Res. 1993;291:103–6.
81. Berbig R, Weishaupt D, Prim J, Shahin O. Primary anterior shoulder dislocation and rotator cuff tears. J Shoulder Elbow Surg. 1999;8(3):220–5.
82. Edouard P, Degache F, Beguin L, Samozino P, Gresta G, Fayolle-Minon I, et al. Rotator cuff strength in recurrent anterior shoulder instability. J Bone Joint Surg Am. 2011;93(8):759–65.
83. Gyftopoulos S, Carpenter E, Kazam J, Babb J, Bencardino J. MR imaging of subscapularis tendon injury in the setting of anterior shoulder dislocation. Skeletal Radiol. 2012;41(11):1445–52.
84. Perlmutter GS. Axillary nerve injury. Clin Orthop Relat Res. 1999;368:28–36.
85. Robinson CM, Shur N, Sharpe T, Ray A, Murray IR. Injuries associated with traumatic anterior glenohumeral dislocations. J Bone Joint Surg Am. 2012;94(1):18–26.
86. May DA, Disler DG, Jones EA, Balkissoon AA, Manaster BJ. Abnormal signal intensity in skeletal muscle at MR imaging: patterns, pearls, and pitfalls. Radiographics. 2000;20:S295–315.
87. Linda DD, Harish S, Stewart BG, Finlay K, Parasu N, Rebello RP. Multimodality imaging of peripheral neuropathies of the upper limb and brachial plexus. Radiographics. 2010;30(5):1373–400.
88. Hintermann B, Gachter A. Arthroscopic findings after shoulder dislocation. Am J Sports Med. 1995;23(5):545–51.
89. Kim DS, Yoon YS, Yi CH. Prevalence comparison of accompanying lesions between primary and recurrent anterior dislocation in the shoulder. Am J Sports Med. 2010;38(10):2071–6.
90. Yiannakopoulos CK, Mataragas E, Antonogiannakis E. A comparison of the spectrum of intra-articular lesions in acute and chronic anterior shoulder instability. Arthroscopy. 2007;23(9):985–90.
91. Lo IK, Parten PM, Burkhart SS. The inverted pear glenoid: an indicator of significant glenoid bone loss. Arthroscopy. 2004;20(2):169–74.
92. Shah N, Tung GA. Imaging signs of posterior glenohumeral instability. AJR Am J Roentgenol. 2009;192(3):730–5.
93. Palmer WE, Caslowitz PL. Anterior shoulder instability: diagnostic criteria determined from prospective analysis of 121 MR arthrograms. Radiology. 1995;197(3):819–25.
94. Chandnani VP, Yeager TD, DeBerardino T, Christensen K, Gagliardi JA, Heitz DR, et al. Glenoid labral tears: prospective evaluation with MRI imaging, MR arthrography, and CT arthrography. AJR Am J Roentgenol. 1993;161(6):1229–35.
95. Sugimoto H, Suzuki K, Mihara K, Kubota H, Tsutsui H. MR arthrography of shoulders after suture-anchor Bankart repair. Radiology. 2002;224(1):105–11.
96. Jana M, Srivastava DN, Sharma R, Gamanagatti S, Nag HL, Mittal R, et al. Magnetic resonance arthrography for assessing severity of glenohumeral labroligamentous lesions. J Orthop Surg (Hong Kong). 2012;20(2):230–5.
97. Mutlu S, Mahirogullari M, Guler O, Ucar BY, Mutlu H, Sonmez G, et al. Anterior Glenohumeral Instability: Classification of Pathologies of Anteroinferior Labroligamentous Structures Using MR Arthrography. Advances in orthopedics. 2013;2013:473194.
98. Woertler K. Multimodality imaging of the postoperative shoulder. Eur Radiol. 2007;17(12):3038–55.
99. Beltran LS, Duarte A, Bencardino JT. Postoperative Imaging in Anterior Glenohumeral Instability. AJR Am J Roentgenol. 2018;211(3):528–37.

Imaging Diagnosis of SLAP Tears and Microinstability

8

Konstantin Krepkin, Michael J. Tuite, and Jenny T. Bencardino

8.1 Normal Labrum

8.1.1 Anatomy and Biomechanics

The glenohumeral joint is the most mobile joint in the body. Static and dynamic stabilizers play a vital role in maintaining the stability of the shoulder, negotiating the fine balance between physiologic mobility and pathologic laxity. The glenoid labrum is an important static stabilizer of the glenohumeral joint, consisting of a ring of fibrous and fibrocartilaginous tissue along the glenoid rim. The bulk of the labrum consists of dense fibrous tissue and collagen with a small amount of fibrocartilage at the chondrolabral junction [1, 2].

The labrum serves to increase the depth and surface area of the glenoid fossa, contributing 50% of the glenoid fossa depth and increasing the surface area of the glenoid by approximately one-third [3, 4]. In conjunction with intra-articular fluid, the labrum also creates a suction effect on the humeral head, helping to maintain the humeral head centered in the glenoid cavity [5]. It functions as a bumper-like mechanism to help protect the articular cartilage from compression and shear damage [1]. Perhaps even more importantly, the glenoid labrum allows other glenohumeral stabilizers to function by providing an attachment site for the glenohumeral ligaments and long head of the biceps tendon (LHBT).

The glenoid labrum can have a wide range of shapes. A study by Park and colleagues looking at labral morphology on MR arthrograms in asymptomatic volunteers found that triangular (64% anteriorly, 47% posteriorly) and round (17% anteriorly, 33% posteriorly) shapes were the most common [6]. Flat, cleaved, notched, or absent labral morphologies were also seen. Significant variability also exists in labral size, ranging from 2 to 14 mm in normal individuals [7]. Normally the labrum is larger at its superior and posterior aspects, compared to the inferior and anterior aspects [8]. The labrum typically has low signal intensity on all MRI sequences. However, increased linear or globular signal has been described in up to a third of arthroscopically normal labra [7].

The glenoid labrum is conventionally divided into four quadrants—anterosuperior, anteroinferior, posterosuperior, and posteroinferior—by a horizontal line bisecting the labrum into superior and inferior halves and a vertical line bisecting

K. Krepkin (✉)
Department of Radiology, New York University Langone Health, New York, NY, USA
e-mail: konstantin.krepkin@nyumc.org

M. J. Tuite
Department of Radiology, University of Wisconsin School of Medicine and Public Health, Madison, WI, USA
e-mail: mtuite@uwhealth.org

J. T. Bencardino
Department of Radiology, New York University Langone Health, New York, NY, USA

Penn Medicine, Department of Radiology, Perelman School of Medicine at the University of Pennsylvania, Philadelphia, PA, USA

J. T. Bencardino (ed.), *The Shoulder*, https://doi.org/10.1007/978-3-030-06240-8_8

the labrum into anterior and posterior halves. The labrum is also commonly divided into a clock face, with 12 o'clock designating superior and 3 o'clock anterior.

Significant variations exist between the labral quadrants, both in the incidence of labral pathology and normal variants. The posterior and inferior portions of the labrum are most firmly attached to the glenoid [9, 10]. This helps explain the preponderance of variants in labral attachment found in the superior and anterosuperior portions of the labrum. The superior labrum, and particularly the anterosuperior quadrant, is the site of attachment of the LHBT and most of the glenohumeral ligaments. The LHBT attaches at the level of the supraglenoid tubercle at approximately the 12 o'clock position. Both the superior (SGHL) and middle (MGHL) glenohumeral ligaments attach to the anterosuperior labrum. The anterior band of the inferior glenohumeral ligament (IGHL) has traditionally been thought to arise from the anteroinferior labrum. However, a recent cadaveric study by Ramirez Ruiz and colleagues found high origin of the anterior band of the IGHL at or above the 3 o'clock position in four of ten cadaveric shoulders [11]. The intimate relationship between the labrum and these vital capsular structures partly accounts for the disproportionate amount of pathology that occurs in the superior and anterosuperior labrum.

8.1.2 Superior Labral Variants

The superior and anterosuperior labrum are common sites for labral anatomic variants.

These same locations are also common sites for labral pathology, making the distinction between pathology and anatomic variant both difficult and clinically relevant. Knowledge of the array of anatomic variants that may occur here is crucial to avoid mistaking them for labral abnormalities.

8.1.2.1 Cartilage Undercutting

The glenoid hyaline cartilage may sometimes undercut the deep portion of the superior labrum, creating an extended chondrolabral interface (Fig. 8.1). This variant has been found in up to 32% of asymptomatic shoulders [6]. Superficially, this may resemble a superior labrum anterior-

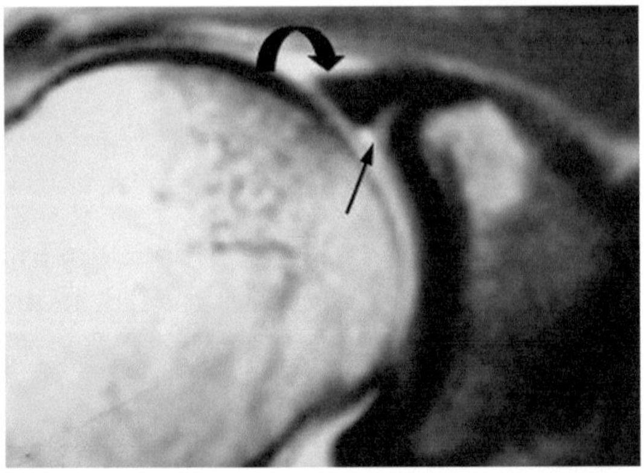

Fig. 8.1 Cartilage undercutting. Coronal proton density image demonstrates glenoid hyaline cartilage (arrow) undercutting the deep portion of the superior labrum (curved arrow). The cartilage parallels the contour of the glenoid rim and shows similar intermediate signal intensity to the rest of the glenoid articular cartilage

posterior (SLAP) tear. However, the cartilage has intermediate signal similar to the rest of the glenoid articular cartilage, compared to the high-signal-intensity fluid (on T2-weighted images) or gadolinium (on T1-weighted MR arthrogram images) insinuating into a labral tear. The cartilage also parallels the contour of the glenoid rim, unlike a SLAP tear, which typically curves laterally, away from the glenoid [12–14].

8.1.2.2 Sublabral Recess

The sublabral recess or sulcus is a small cleft found between the biceps labral complex and the glenoid cartilage (Fig. 8.2b, c). It is the most common anatomic variant of the superior labrum [15], present in up to 73% of shoulders and deeper than 2 mm in 39% [16, 17]. Like cartilage undercutting of the labrum, it can also be confused for a SLAP tear. However, a smooth contour cleft that parallels the curvature of the glenoid rim suggests a sublabral recess rather than a SLAP tear [14, 18, 19]. Although initially thought to never extend posterior to the LHBT insertion [9], studies have shown that a sublabral recess can extend posterior to the LHBT insertion in the absence of a SLAP tear [17, 20].

8.1.2.3 Biceps Labral Complex

Three distinct types of biceps labral complexes (BLC) have been described (Fig. 8.2) [10]. In

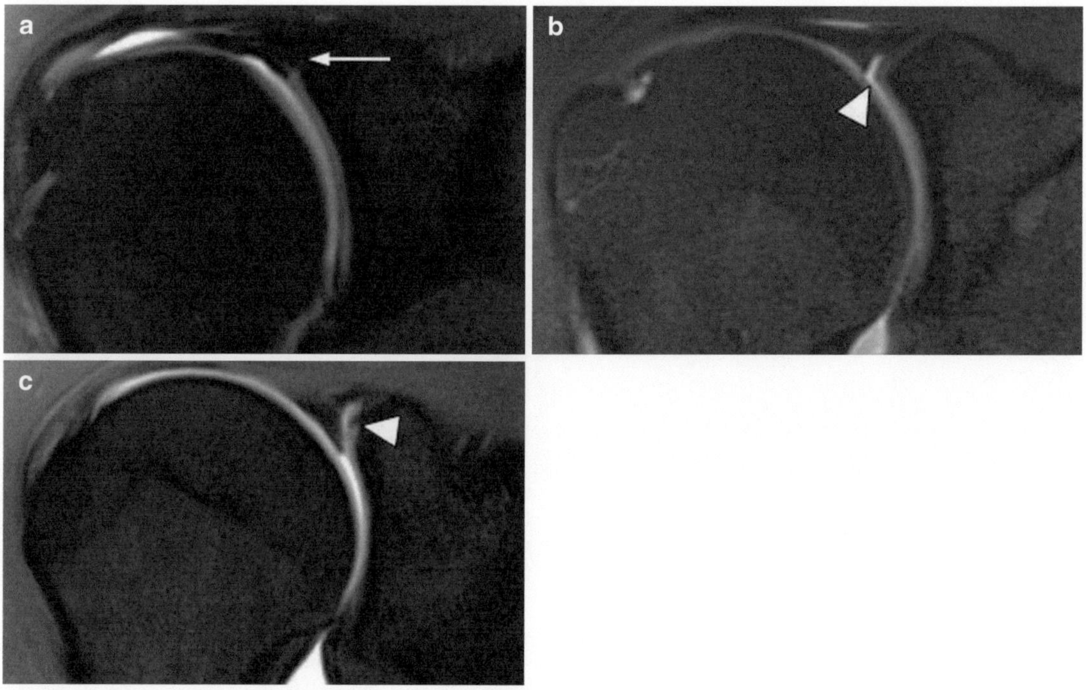

Fig. 8.2 Biceps labral complex (BLC). Coronal fat-suppressed T1-weighted MR arthrographic images demonstrate the three distinct types of biceps labral complexes. (**a**) Type I BLC with firm attachment of the labrum to the underlying glenoid cartilage without cartilage undercutting or sublabral recess (arrow). (**b**) Type II BLC with the labrum projecting slightly more medially over the glenoid articular cartilage and a small sublabral recess paralleling the contour of the glenoid (arrowhead). (**c**) Type III BLC with a meniscoid labrum projecting into the joint space and accompanied by a deep sublabral recess (arrowhead)

type I BLC, the labrum is firmly attached to the glenoid without cartilage undercutting or sublabral recess present. In type II BLC, the labrum projects more medially over the glenoid articular cartilage and there is a small sublabral recess paralleling the contour of the glenoid. In type III BLC, a prominent triangular meniscoid labrum projects into the joint space and is accompanied by a deep sublabral recess.

8.1.2.4 Bicipital Labral Sulcus

A shallow cleft can sometimes be found on the undersurface of the proximal intra-articular biceps tendon at the junction with the superior labrum (Fig. 8.3). This bicipital labral sulcus has been reported to have a prevalence of 30% on MR arthrography [6].

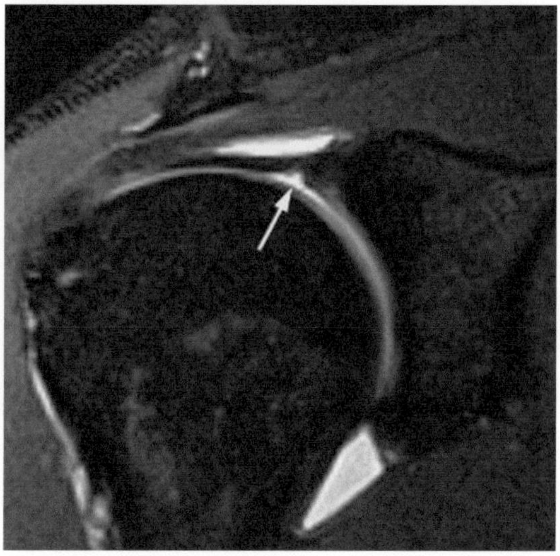

Fig. 8.3 Bicipital labral sulcus. Coronal fat-suppressed T1-weighted SPACE image from a direct MR arthrogram demonstrates a shallow cleft on the undersurface of the proximal intra-articular biceps tendon at the junction with the superior labrum (arrow)

8.1.2.5 Buford Complex

An absent or hypoplastic anterosuperior labrum accompanied by a thickened cordlike MGHL is

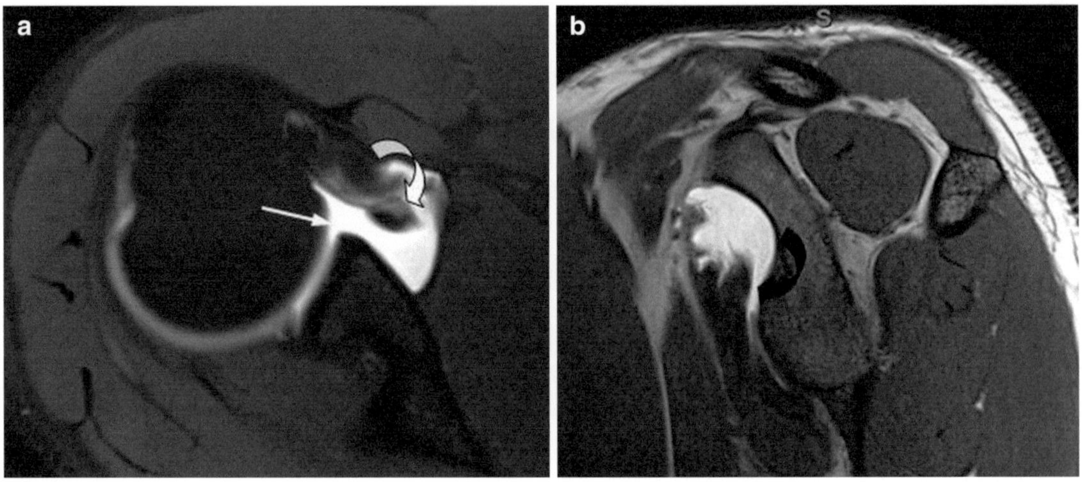

Fig. 8.4 Buford complex. (**a**) Axial fat-suppressed T1-weighted MR arthrographic images demonstrate an absent anterosuperior labrum (arrow) and a thickened cord-like MGHL (curved arrow). (**b**) Sagittal T1-weighted image from an MR arthrogram confirms a thickened MGHL (curved arrow) coursing deep to the subscapularis tendon

known as a Buford complex (Fig. 8.4). This relatively uncommon entity has been reported in 1.5–7.4% of patients [21, 22]. The Buford complex can sometimes be mistaken for a displaced labral tear. This pitfall can be avoided by following the thickened MGHL to its insertion on the humeral neck or as it blends with the anterior joint capsule beneath the subscapularis tendon. Correlating with the sagittal images is also important since the thickened MGHL can be well appreciated in the sagittal plane (Fig. 8.4b).

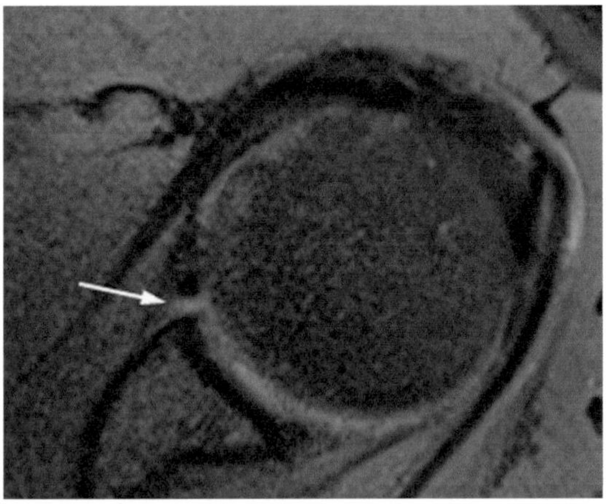

Fig. 8.5 Sublabral foramen. Axial fat-suppressed proton density image shows focal detachment of the anterosuperior labrum (arrow). There is a smooth labral contour and lack of significant labral displacement, differentiating the sublabral foramen from a labral tear

8.1.2.6 Sublabral Foramen

A sublabral foramen is a focal detachment of the anterosuperior labrum between the 1 o'clock and 3 o'clock positions (Fig. 8.5) [9]. It can be seen in up to 18.5% of shoulder arthroscopies and has been described in association with a thickened MGHL [23]. Although generally thought not to extend below the level of the midglenoid notch or glenoid equator, Tuite and colleagues have reported that a sublabral foramen may indeed extend to the anteroinferior labral quadrant [24]. The features distinguishing a sublabral foramen from a labral tear include focal detachment of the anterosuperior labrum without involvement of the biceps origin, labral displacement less than 1–2 mm, and a smooth labral contour [15]. Interestingly, although a sublabral foramen in and of itself is considered a normal labral variant, association between sublabral foramen and SLAP tears has been found [22, 23, 25]. This may be related to a sublabral foramen leading to alterations in biomechanics that produce greater forces on the superior labrum, thus predisposing to labral pathology.

8.2 Microinstability

8.2.1 Definition

Microinstability is a heterogeneous set of disorders with complex pathophysiology that presents a particular challenge both in its clinical and imaging evaluation. No universally accepted definition exists in the literature. Microinstability is generally understood to consist of poorly localized shoulder pain related to pathologic laxity without frank dislocation [26]. Historically, shoulder instability has been characterized as either TUBS (traumatic unidirectional Bankart lesion, responds to surgery) or AMBRII (atraumatic, multidirectional, bilateral, responds to rehabilitation, inferior capsular shift, and interval closure) [5, 27]. TUBS typically presents with the classic Bankart and Hill-Sachs lesions seen in anterior shoulder instability, whereas in AMBRII no obvious structural lesions are found. Microinstability encompasses the wide stretch of territory between the two extremes of TUBS and AMBRII. It is helpful to subdivide microinstability into two types, one associated with repetitive overhead motions—AIOS (acquired instability in overstressed shoulder)—and one without—AMSI (atraumatic minor shoulder instability) [27–30].

8.2.2 Classification and Pathophysiology

AIOS is a common type of microinstability typically seen in young overhead athletes, such as baseball pitchers, volleyball players, and tennis players. However, individuals whose professions require repetitive overhead motions, such as painters and builders, share a similar mechanism that predisposes them to the development of microinstability. Much of our knowledge of microinstability and AIOS is grounded in research performed to better understand the mechanics of the throwing athlete. It is this model that we will focus on to help understand the pathophysiology of AIOS.

The performance of an elite throwing athlete, the ability to throw both with high velocity and accuracy, relies on the complex interplay between static and dynamic stabilizers of the shoulder. Furthermore, the entire body is involved in the "kinetic chain" that transmits force from the ground up, coordinating the sequence of muscle contractions that culminate in tremendous force generation in the throwing shoulder. Imbalances in the components of the "kinetic chain" can contribute to the deleterious effects on the supporting structures of the shoulder seen in throwing athletes [29, 31–33]. Repetitive distracting forces on the throwing shoulder require internal adaptations that increase mobility to achieve peak performance. At the same time, shoulder stabilizers are tasked to prevent pathologic laxity and instability. The fine balance of these competing forces on the throwing shoulder is known as the "thrower's paradox" [34]. The disturbance of this balance can lead to injury.

8.2.2.1 Internal Impingement

There are two main theories that attempt to explain the mechanisms of injury and etiology of microinstability in the throwing athlete. In the anterior laxity internal impingement theory, repetitive abduction and external rotation experienced by the throwing shoulder during the late cocking and early acceleration phases of the throwing motion leads to adaptive changes in the anterior joint capsule. The anterior joint capsule stretches, causing anterior capsular laxity and leading to anterior instability [35–38]. The lax anterior capsule allows for increased external rotation of the shoulder, which leads to pathologic contact between the greater tuberosity, posterosuperior labrum, and rotator cuff in a process known as internal impingement. Internal impingement typically consists of the triad of posterosuperior labral tears, articular surface tearing of the posterior supraspinatus or anterior infraspinatus tendons, and cystic changes in the posterior aspect of the humeral head [39]. Posterior humeral head articular cartilage lesions can also be found in the setting of internal impingement [40].

8.2.2.2 Posterior Capsular Contracture/Glenohumeral Internal Rotation Deficit

The alternative theory that attempts to explain the spectrum of shoulder pathology seen in overhead athletes proposes that the initiating event occurs in the posterior capsule, rather than the anterior capsule as suggested by the anterior laxity internal impingement theory. The posterior capsule must withstand tensile forces of up to 750 N during the deceleration and follow-through phases of throwing [41]. This repetitive tensile loading on the posteroinferior capsule during the follow-through phase eventually causes posteroinferior capsular hypertrophy and contracture [41, 42]. Since the posterior band of the IGHL is located directly below the humeral head during maximum abduction and external rotation seen in the late cocking and early acceleration phases, a contracted posterior band causes posterosuperior shift of the humeral head relative to the glenoid [41, 43]. Such posterosuperior humeral shift allows for increased humeral external rotation due to increased clearance of the greater tuberosity over the glenoid, but also leads to more profound internal impingement between the humeral head, posterosuperior labrum, and rotator cuff. Thus, the ultimate result is the same as proposed by the internal impingement theory—pathology involving the posterosuperior labrum and adjacent rotator cuff. The posterior capsular contraction theory further suggests that the posterosuperior displacement of the humeral head causes functional redundancy and slackening of the anteroinferior capsule, producing a pseudolaxity that may simulate true laxity related to anterior capsular stretching.

Contraction of the posterior capsule also produces loss of internal rotation in the throwing shoulder compared to the non-throwing shoulder, a concept known as glenohumeral internal rotation deficit (GIRD). GIRD is defined as a loss of internal rotation >18° compared to the contralateral side, which can be easily assessed on physical examination [42]. Indeed, research has corroborated that GIRD has a significant association with pathology in the throwing shoulder. In a study by Verna of 38 overhead athletes with SLAP II tears, all were found to have significant GIRD, with an average of 33 degrees [44]. A study by Kibler assigned high-level tennis players to two groups, one that performed daily posteroinferior capsular stretching to minimize GIRD and one that did not [45]. During the 2-year follow-up period, the stretching group experienced both a significant increase in internal rotation and a 38% decrease in the incidence of shoulder injury compared to the control group.

8.2.2.3 Superior Labrum Anterior Cuff (SLAC) and MGHL Lesions

There are several types of microinstability not necessarily related to overhead activity. These are generally related to injuries to the supporting ligamentous structures of the shoulder, in particular the superior (SGHL) and middle (MGHL) glenohumeral ligaments, as well as the rotator interval. The rotator interval includes the SGHL, coracohumeral ligament, joint capsule, and biceps tendon [46]. The SGHL is particularly important in restraining anterior and superior translation of the humeral head in shoulder flexion and lesser degrees of abduction [47–49]. Injury to the SGHL can lead to pathologic anterosuperior translation of the humeral head with pathologic contact between the humeral head, anterosuperior labrum, and rotator cuff. The constellation of anterosuperior labral tears, articular surface tearing of the anterior supraspinatus tendon, and SGHL injury is known as the superior labrum anterior cuff (SLAC) lesion [50]. In the original work by Savoie and colleagues, 39 of 40 patients had avulsion of the SGHL, thought to be the inciting event precipitating a SLAC lesion [50].

The MGHL is the primary anterior stabilizer of the shoulder at 45 degrees of abduction and also serves to limit external rotation [27]. Dysfunction of the MGHL has long been recognized as a potential cause of microinstability [51]. In a study by Savoie and colleagues, 33 patients with isolated avulsions of the MGHL demonstrated evidence of anterior instability [52]. Subsequent arthroscopic repair led to improvement in pain and function in all patients.

8.2.2.4 Atraumatic Minor Shoulder Instability (AMSI)

A rare form of microinstability not related to overhead activity is atraumatic minor shoulder instability (AMSI). AMSI generally presents as shoulder pain after a period of inactivity, such as during pregnancy or immobilization [27]. These patients may have static anatomic variants of the MGHL, including absence, hypoplasia, or a large sublabral foramen or Buford complex [23, 25, 30].

8.2.3 Imaging Diagnosis of Microinstability

The findings of internal impingement are well depicted on MR imaging. The classic constellation of findings on MRI includes posterosuperior labral tears, articular surface tears of the posterior supraspinatus or anterior infraspinatus tendons, and cystic changes in the posterior aspect of the humeral head (Fig. 8.6) [39, 53]. However, not all findings may necessarily be present. MR arthrography with ABER (abduction external rotation) view is optimal for the evaluation of internal impingement since it has greater sensitivity for labral pathology and articular surface rotator cuff tears [53–55]. The ABER view may even depict impingement of the rotator cuff between the greater tuberosity and posterosuperior glenoid/labrum since ABER recreates the abduction and external rotation position in which internal impingement occurs. However, care must be taken not to misinterpret contact between the undersurface of the rotator cuff and the posterosuperior glenoid/labrum in the ABER position as internal impingement in the absence of other associated pathology, since such contact can be seen in normal individual placed in the ABER position [35, 56, 57].

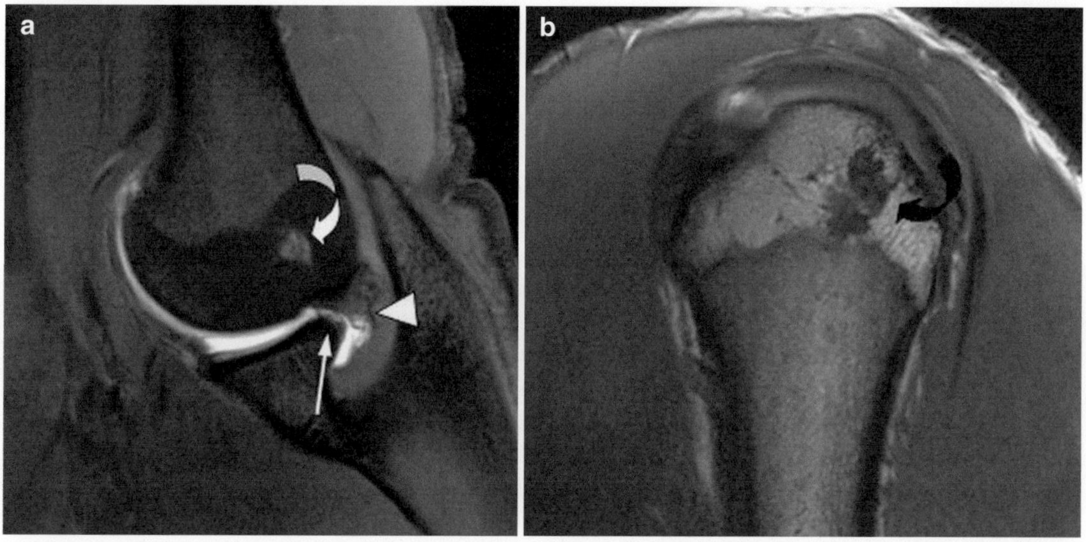

Fig. 8.6 18-Year-old baseball pitcher with shoulder pain. (**a**) Fat-suppressed T1-weighted abduction external rotation (ABER) view from an MR arthrogram of the shoulder demonstrates tearing of the posterosuperior labrum (arrow), articular surface tearing of the posterior supraspinatus tendon fibers (arrowhead), and cystic changes within the posterior aspect of the humeral head (curved arrow). Findings are consistent with posterosuperior internal impingement. (**b**) Sagittal T1-weighted image confirms that the cystic changes are present at the anterior aspect of the greater tuberosity middle facet (curved arrow)

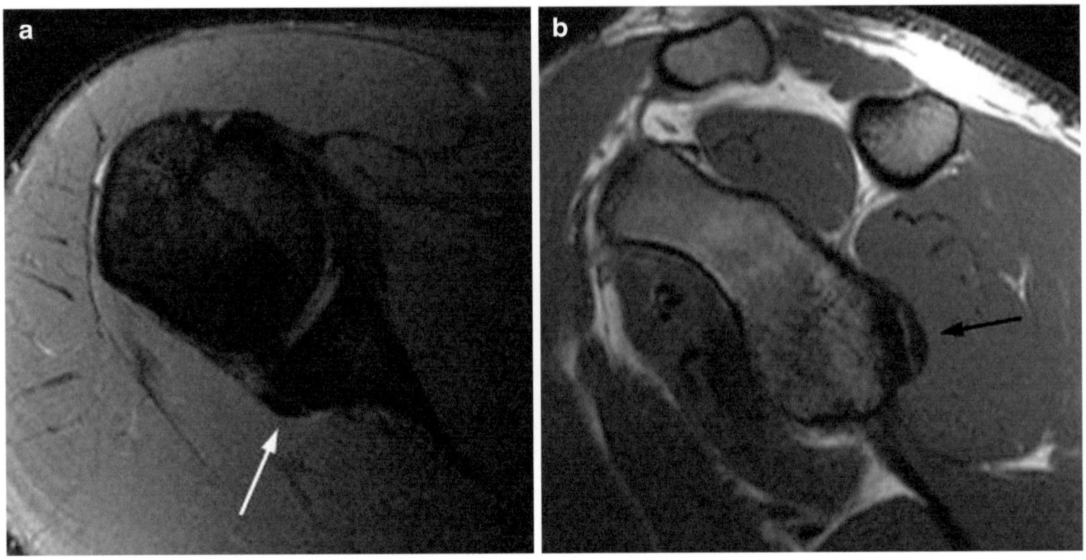

Fig. 8.7 21-Year-old baseball pitcher with shoulder pain. (**a**) Axial gradient-echo and (**b**) sagittal T1-weighted images demonstrate a crescent-shaped focus of low signal intensity adjacent to the posteroinferior aspect of the glenoid rim (arrow), consistent with mineralization in the setting of a Bennett lesion

Several theories exist that attempt to explain the occurrence of the posterior humeral head cysts. Traditionally, they have been thought to be the sequela of impaction injury as the humeral head abuts the posterosuperior glenoid during the late cocking and early acceleration phase of throwing. However, more recently, it has been proposed that inflammatory changes in the posterior humeral head secondary to internal impingement may lead to increased vascularity and result in cyst formation [39].

A number of imaging findings are associated with GIRD in the throwing athlete. A study by Tuite and colleagues found that patients with GIRD have a longer posteroinferior labrum, thicker posteroinferior capsule, and shallower posterior capsular recess [58]. In a study of professional baseball pitchers with GIRD, Tehranzadeh and colleagues also observed a thickened appearance of the posterior band of IGHL on MR imaging [59]. A variant of GIRD characterized by a thickened posteroinferior capsule is the Bennett lesion, a crescent-shaped focus of extra-articular mineralization at the posteroinferior aspect of the glenoid rim from calcification of the posterior band of IGHL and adjacent labrum (Fig. 8.7) [60, 61].

Imaging in the classic SLAC lesion reveals tears of the anterosuperior labrum, articular surface tearing of the anterior supraspinatus tendon, and injury of the SGHL. However, tears of the cranial fibers of the subscapularis tendon can also be seen in the setting of SLAC given their close proximity to the anterior supraspinatus tendon. SLAC lesions are also associated with lesions of the intra-articular biceps tendon and other components of the rotator interval, such as the coracohumeral ligament and rotator interval capsule (Fig. 8.8).

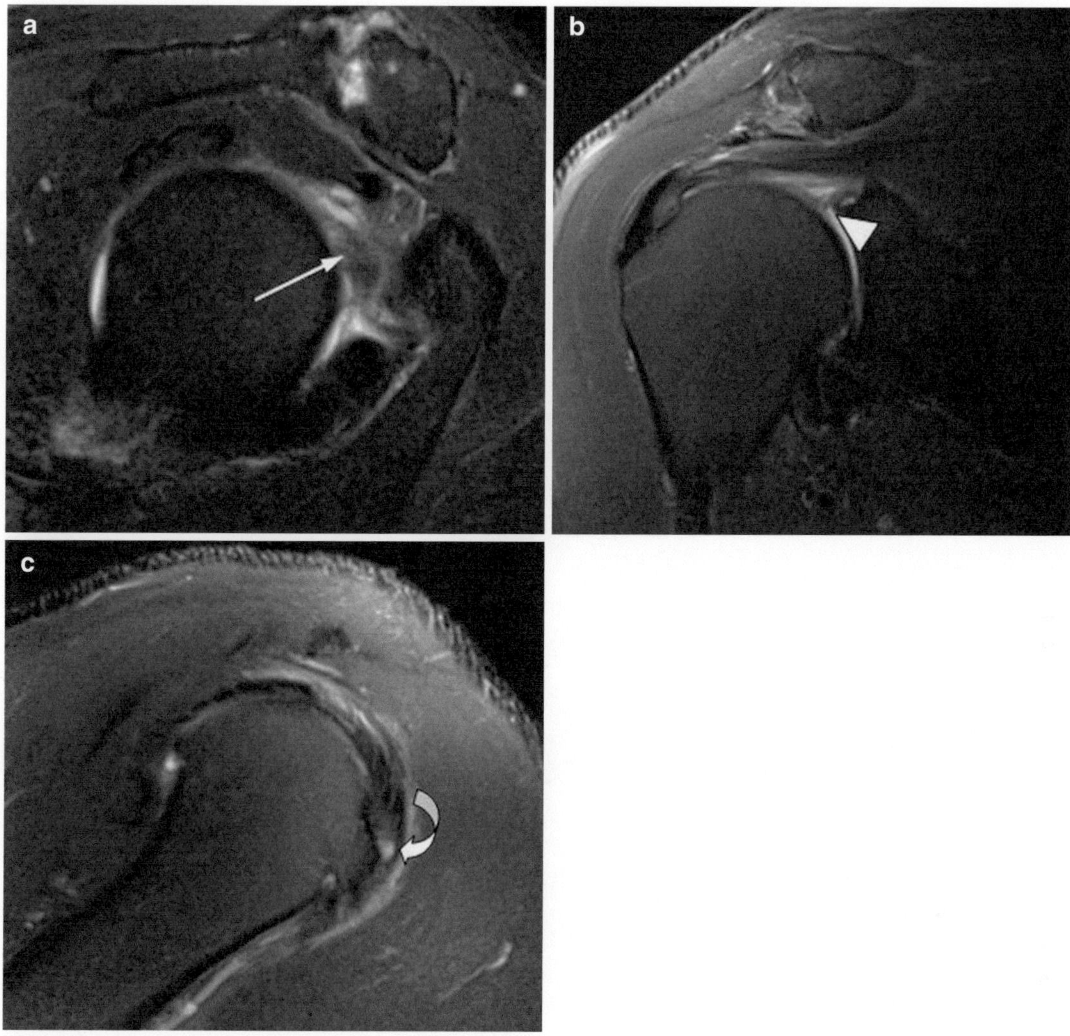

Fig. 8.8 60-Year-old male with shoulder pain. (**a**) Sagittal fat-suppressed T2-weighted image demonstrates absence of the biceps tendon, coracohumeral ligament, and superior glenohumeral ligament (SGHL) in the rotator interval (arrow), consistent with tears. Instead, debris and organizing hemorrhage fill the rotator interval. (**b**) Coronal fat-suppressed T2-weighted image demonstrates a superior labral tear (arrowhead). (**c**) Sagittal fat-suppressed T2-weighted image shows an articular surface tear of the far-anterior supraspinatus tendon (curved arrow). Constellation of findings can be seen in the setting of superior labrum anterior cuff (SLAC) lesion

8.3 SLAP Tears

8.3.1 Definition and Classification

Superior labral tears or SLAP (superior labrum anterior-posterior) lesions all involve the superior labrum at the level of the biceps origin, or approximately the portion of the labrum from 11 o'clock to 1 o'clock [62]. The significance of SLAP tears lies in their relationship to the biceps labral complex. As a result, many SLAP tears lead to instability of the biceps anchor and result in functional impairment and even microinstability of the glenohumeral joint.

Snyder and colleagues were the first to use the term SLAP lesion and described the original four types of SLAP lesions [63]. The classification system carries treatment implications, since the

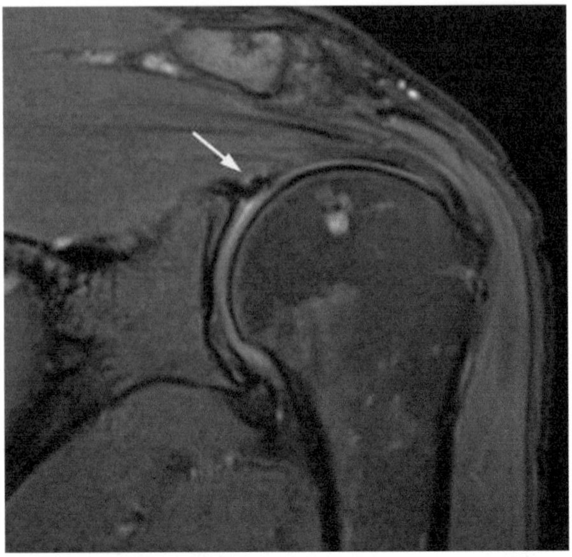

Fig. 8.9 SLAP I lesion. Coronal fat-suppressed T2-weighted image demonstrates degenerative fraying of the superior labrum (arrow), consistent with a SLAP I lesion

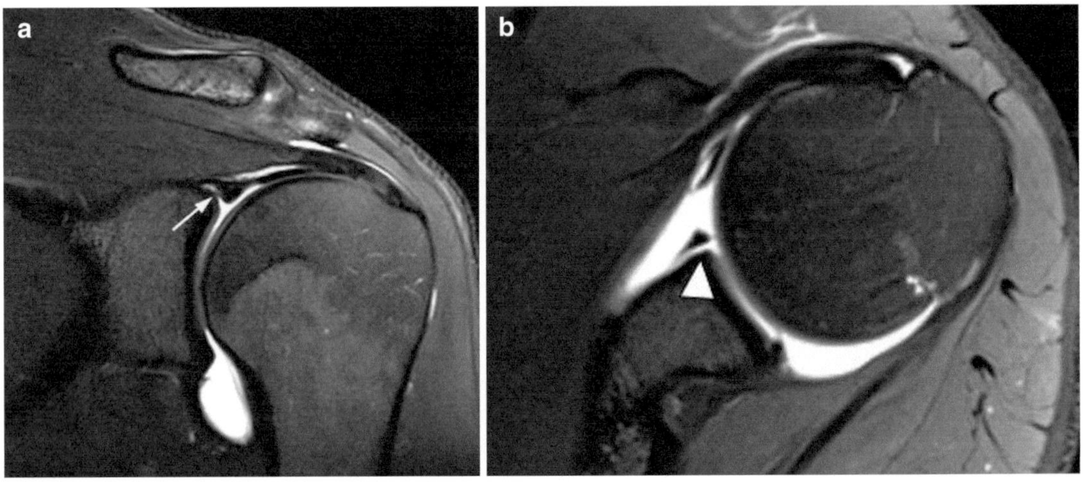

Fig. 8.10 SLAP II lesion. (**a**) Coronal fat-suppressed T2-weighted MR arthrographic image demonstrates detachment of the superior labrum and biceps anchor from the underlying glenoid with slightly irregular margins (arrow), consistent with a SLAP II lesion. (**b**) Axial fat-suppressed proton density MR arthrographic image at the level of the anterosuperior labrum demonstrates that the tear propagates to a sublabral foramen (arrowhead). Note that, in contrast to the SLAP tear, the sublabral foramen has smooth margins.

different types of SLAP lesions are treated via different surgical techniques. Furthermore, the different SLAP types have different implications for the stability of the biceps anchor. The four original types of SLAP tears include:

- Type I—Degenerative fraying of the superior labrum with an intact biceps anchor (Fig. 8.9).
- Type II—The superior labrum and biceps anchor are detached from the underlying glenoid (Fig. 8.10). This results in an unstable biceps anchor.
- Type III—Bucket-handle tear of the superior labrum without extension to the biceps tendon (Fig. 8.11). The central portion of the tear may or may not be displaced inferiorly into the joint. The biceps anchor remains attached to the glenoid.
- Type IV—Bucket-handle tear of the superior labrum with extension of the tear to the biceps

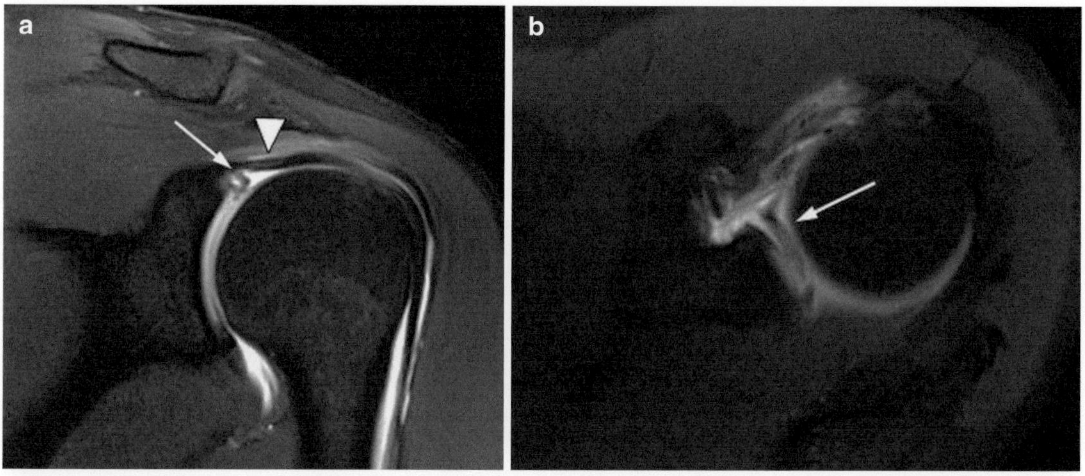

Fig. 8.11 SLAP III lesion. Coronal (**a**) and axial (**b**) fat-suppressed T1-weighted MR arthrographic images demonstrate a bucket-handle tear of the superior labrum, with the detached labrum surrounded by intra-articular contrast (arrow). Note a normal biceps tendon (arrowhead)

tendon. The biceps tendon and the attached labral flap may displace into the joint. This type of tear renders the biceps anchor unstable.

The passage of synovial fluid through the cleft created by a labral tear may result in the formation of a paralabral cyst (Fig. 8.12).

There is discrepancy in the frequency of the different SLAP lesions reported in the literature. In part, this is related to differences in patient demographics across studies, particularly since there is increasing prevalence of degenerative labral fraying with age [64]. However, considerable variability also exists in the threshold used by arthroscopists in classifying the different SLAP lesions. The original study by Snyder and colleagues reported the type II SLAP lesion as the most common (41%), followed by type III (33%), with only 11% of patients having a type I SLAP lesion [63]. However, this study looked at a relatively young patient population, with an average age of 37.5 years, and had stringent criteria for classifying type I SLAP lesions. In a relatively older patient population, with an average age of 44.2 years, Kim and colleagues found that the type I SLAP lesion was most common, accounting for 74% of SLAP lesions, followed by type II (21%) [64].

In the years following the classification of the original four SLAP lesions, six additional SLAP categories have been described [65–67]. Also known as extended SLAP, this group of SLAP lesions encompasses superior labral tears that also propagate to other labral quadrants or capsuloligamentous structures (Table 8.1), including a superior labral tear propagating to a Bankart lesion of the anteroinferior labrum (SLAP V) (Fig. 8.13), SLAP tear extending to the posterior labrum (SLAP VIII), circumferential tear of the labrum (SLAP IX), and a SLAP lesion that extends into the rotator interval, including the SGHL, coracohumeral ligament, or rotator interval capsule (SLAP X).

8.3.2 Pathophysiology

The pathophysiology of SLAP lesions can be divided into those that are caused by repetitive overhead activity and those that are not related to overhead activity, although there is overlap between the two. One of the more common mechanisms for the development of a SLAP lesion in the non-overhead athlete is a fall on an outstretched hand. This mechanism causes compression of the biceps-labral complex between the humeral head and glenoid [63]. A biomechanical study by Clavert and colleagues demonstrated that in the setting of a fall on an

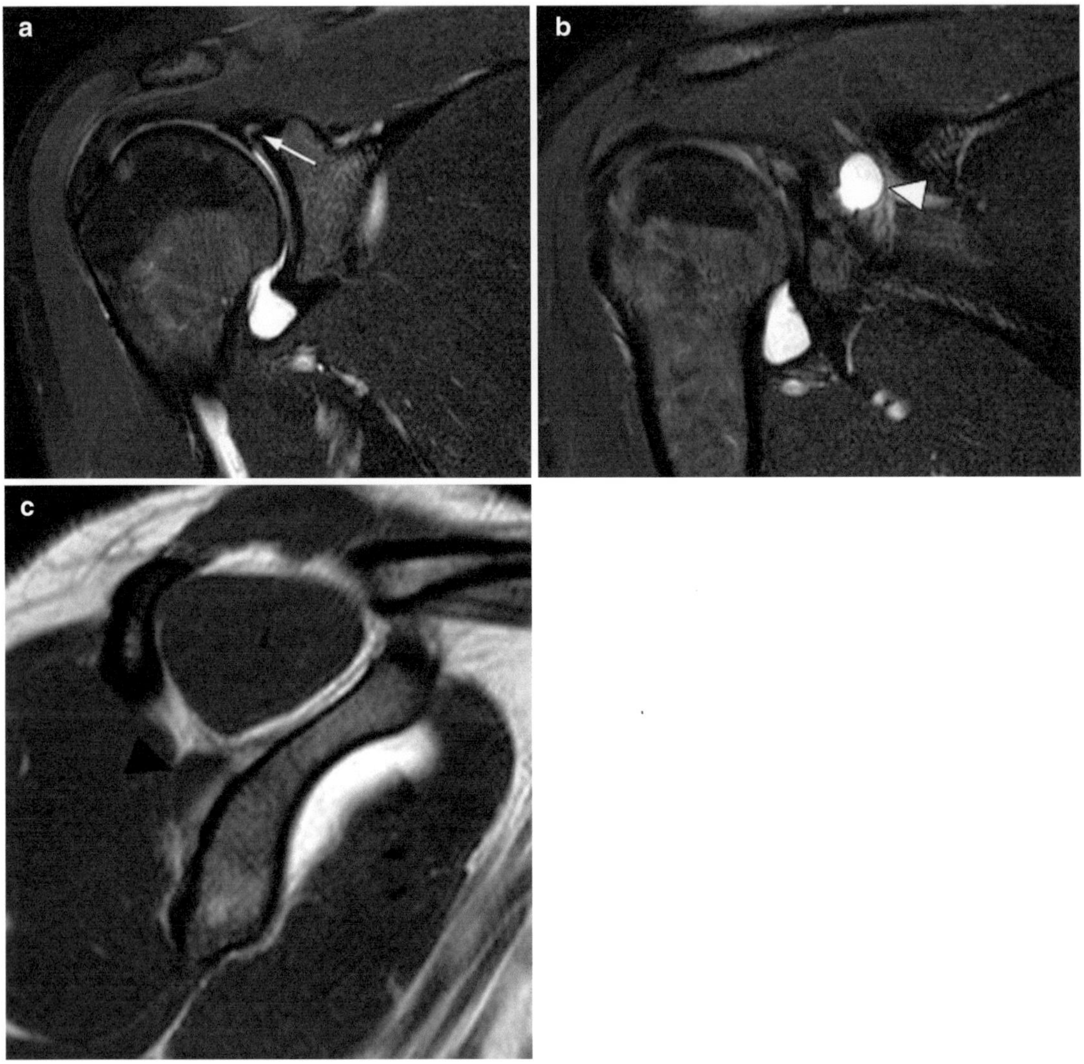

Fig. 8.12 SLAP II lesion with paralabral cyst. (**a**) Coronal fat-suppressed T2-weighted MR arthrographic image demonstrates detachment of the superior labrum and biceps anchor from the underlying glenoid (arrow), consistent with a SLAP II lesion. (**b**) Coronal fat-suppressed T2-weighted and (**c**) sagittal T1-weighted MR arthrographic images demonstrate an associated paralabral cyst in the spinoglenoid notch (arrowhead). Note that the cyst is hypointense on the T1-weighted sequence since it does not fill with intra-articular contrast

outstretched hand, SLAP tears are more likely with a forward fall (shoulder flexed) compared to a backward fall (shoulder extended) [68].

Another important mechanism responsible for the pathogenesis of some SLAP lesions is traction on the biceps-labral complex by forceful contraction of the biceps tendon, such as when lifting a heavy object. A biomechanical study by Bey and colleagues found that the generation of SLAP lesions by traction from the biceps tendon is facilitated by inferior subluxation of the humeral head [69]. In some circumstances, a combination of mechanisms may be responsible for the development of SLAP lesions in the setting of a single traumatic event. For example, a forceful contraction of the biceps tendon during a fall on an outstretched hand can combine both compressive and tensile forces on the superior labrum and biceps anchor.

In the overhead-throwing athlete, several factors contribute to the development of SLAP lesions. As previously discussed, internal impingement in the shoulder is caused by excessive external rotation, which leads to abnormal contact between the greater tuberosity, posterosuperior labrum, and rotator cuff. This mechanism produces posterosuperior SLAP lesions. Posterior capsular contracture/GIRD also contributes to posterosuperior labral lesions since the associated posterosuperior shift of the humeral head relative to the glenoid places increased stress on the posterosuperior labrum. Finally, another important component of the cascade of biomechanical factors resulting in SLAP lesions in the throwing athlete is known as the peel-back mechanism [41, 70]. In the position of maximal shoulder abduction and external rotation experienced during the late cocking and early acceleration phases of throwing, the biceps tendon exerts significant tensile and torsional forces on the biceps-labral anchor. These forces result in stripping and tearing of the biceps-labral anchor which may propagate posteriorly, or both posteriorly and anteriorly. The combination of the above mechanisms results in SLAP lesions in throwing athletes that almost always extend to the posterosuperior

Table 8.1 Classification of SLAP lesions

SLAP lesion	Description
Type I	Degenerative fraying of the superior labrum
Type II	Detachment of the superior labrum and biceps anchor from the glenoid
Type III	Bucket-handle tear of the superior labrum without extension to the biceps tendon
Type IV	Bucket-handle tear of the superior labrum with extension to the biceps tendon
Type V	Superior labral tear continuous with a Bankart lesion of the anteroinferior labrum
Type VI	Unstable flap tear of the superior labrum
Type VII	Superior labral tear that extends anteriorly to involve the middle glenohumeral ligament
Type VIII	Superior labral tear extending to the posterior labrum (to at least 9 o'clock)
Type IX	Circumferential tear of the labrum
Type X	Superior labral tear extending into the rotator interval

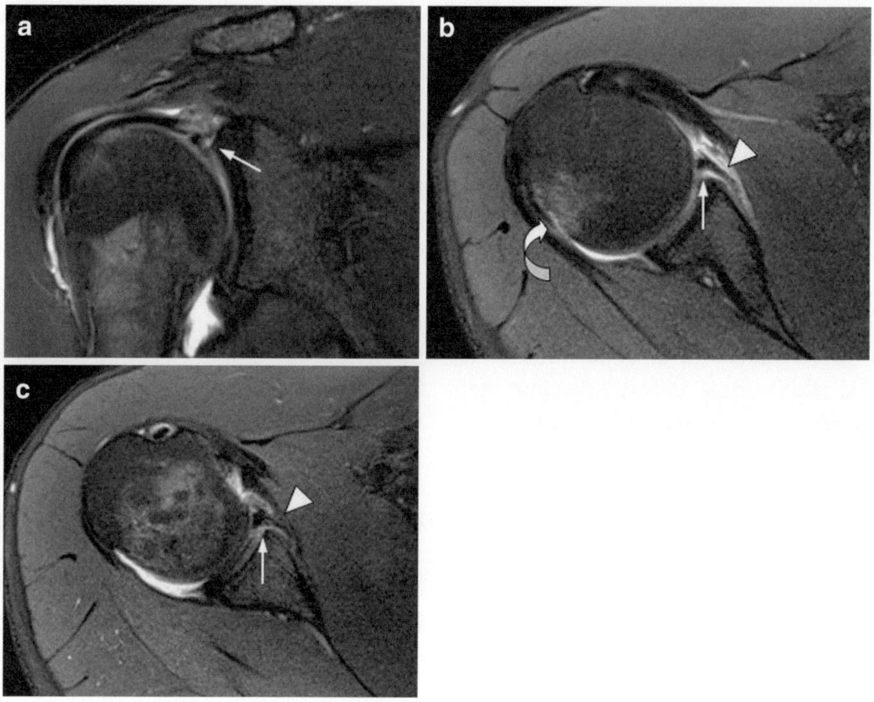

Fig. 8.13 SLAP V lesion. (**a**) Coronal fat-suppressed T2-weighted image demonstrates superior labral tear (arrow). Axial fat-suppressed proton density images at the level of the equator (**b**) and anteroinferior labrum (**c**) demonstrate propagation of the tear to the anterior and anteroinferior labrum (arrow) with stripping of the periosteal sleeve (arrowhead), consistent with anterior labral periosteal sleeve avulsion (ALPSA), a labral Bankart variant. There is also a Hill-Sachs impaction fracture of the posterolateral humeral head (curved arrow)

quadrant. Indeed, SLAP lesions of the anterosuperior labrum without posterior extension are rare in throwing athletes [41].

SLAP lesions also contribute to microinstability of the shoulder, particularly the lesions that cause instability of the biceps anchor. A study by Pagnani and colleagues found that SLAP lesions that destabilized the biceps anchor resulted in increased anteroposterior and superoinferior glenohumeral translation compared to SLAP lesions that did not [71]. Hantes and colleagues found a higher rate of preoperative shoulder dislocations in patients with combined Bankart and SLAP lesions compared to those with Bankart lesions alone [72]. Indeed, SLAP lesions can be found in both acute and recurrent glenohumeral dislocations [73–75]. In this setting, SLAP lesions are believed to be contributors to instability rather than the primary lesions responsible for instability.

8.3.3 Technical Considerations: Conventional MRI Versus MR Arthrography

MR arthrography is a technique whereby contrast material is introduced into a joint to help visualize both normal anatomy and pathology. There are two methods to perform MR arthrography—direct and indirect. In direct MR arthrography, dilute contrast material is injected directly into a joint via an 18–22 gauge needle [76]. For the shoulder, approximately 10–15 mL of a gadolinium solution is diluted to a concentration of 1–2 mmol/L with normal saline, lidocaine, and iodinated contrast if fluoroscopic guidance is used [76, 77]. Although injection can be done without direct visualization, sonographic or fluoroscopic guidance is preferred to help insure instillation of the contrast mixture into the joint. Multiple approaches for needle placement can be used, including anterior, posterior, and rotator interval approaches [78–80]. The approach is generally chosen to avoid crossing structures that are suspected of having pathology. MR imaging should be performed within 1 h of intra-articular injection to maintain adequate contrast-to-noise ratio, as the intra-articular gadolinium diffuses out of the joint with time [81].

Indirect MR arthrography involves the intravenous injection of gadolinium-based contrast media in a concentration of 0.1 mmol/kg [77]. The intravenous contrast diffuses into the joint space over time. The rate of diffusion depends on the permeability of the joint which is increased in infectious and inflammatory conditions, the pressure differential between the intravascular and joint spaces, and the viscosity of joint fluid [82, 83]. Exercising the joint prior to imaging increases both vascular permeability and vascular pressure, thereby increasing the amount of contrast diffusing into the joint. For the shoulder, imaging is generally performed with a delay of 15 min after contrast injection [83].

For both direct and indirect MR arthrography, the imaging protocol consists of fat-suppressed T1-weighted sequences in multiple planes to visualize the contrast material and intra-articular structures. At least one fluid-sensitive sequence, such as a STIR, fat-suppressed T2, or fat-suppressed proton density, is also acquired to evaluate for extra-articular fluid collections, T2 hyperintense periarticular mass lesions, or bone marrow edema.

One of the main advantages of direct MR arthrography compared to indirect arthrography or conventional MRI consists of superb joint distention. This helps separate intra-articular structures, which delineates anatomy and allows contrast to outline defects and tears. The disadvantages of direct MR arthrography include its relatively invasive nature, which may make some patients hesitant to undergo the procedure, and the additional amount of time necessary to perform the intra-articular injection. Although indirect MR arthrography is not invasive and also allows contrast to outline intra-articular structures, it lacks the capability to create the joint distention that may be necessary in some cases to fully evaluate the joint. Furthermore, since the contrast is not introduced selectively into the joint of interest with indirect arthrography, other extra-articular structures can enhance as well, including blood vessels and synovial lined spaces, such as bursae and tendon sheaths.

A number of studies have looked at the diagnostic performance of MR arthrography compared to conventional MRI and arthroscopic/surgical findings in diagnosing SLAP lesions. In a study evaluating direct MR arthrography with surgical findings as the reference standard, Bencardino and colleagues found a high sensitivity (89%), specificity (91%), and accuracy (90%) for MR arthrography in diagnosing SLAP lesions [84]. MR arthrography correctly classified 76% of SLAP lesions that it identified. A study by Waldt and colleagues found that MR arthrography had sensitivity of 82%, specificity of 98%, and accuracy of 94% in diagnosing SLAP lesions [85]. A study by Chandnani and colleagues comparing MR arthrography to conventional MR imaging in the evaluation of labral tears found similar sensitivities, 96% and 93%, respectively [86]. However, direct MR arthrography performed better at detecting detached labral fragments—96% compared to 46% for conventional MRI. Amin and Youssef found that in 34 patients who had normal conventional MRIs, MR arthrography was able to detect 18 SLAP lesions that were confirmed by arthroscopy [87]. In a study of 20 athletes by Magee and colleagues, MR arthrography detected 9 labral tears that were not seen on conventional MRI, 6 of which were SLAP lesions [88].

Comparing indirect MR arthrography to conventional MRI in detecting SLAP lesions, Herold and colleagues found a higher sensitivity (91% vs. 73%), the same specificity (85% vs. 85%), and higher accuracy (89% vs. 77%) for indirect MR arthrography [89]. Dinaeur and colleagues found that indirect arthrography had higher sensitivity (84–91% vs. 66–85%), a slightly higher accuracy (78–86% vs. 70–83%), but lower specificity (58–71% vs. 75–83%) compared to conventional MRI in detecting SLAP lesions [90]. In a head-to-head comparison of indirect and direct MR arthrography, Jung and colleagues found no statistically significant difference in the sensitivity and specificity of both methods in diagnosing labral tears [91].

8.3.4 The Role of Field Strength: 1.5 T Versus 3 T

With the continued evolution of MR magnets and coils, 3 T MR imaging is becoming widely available. High-field-strength 3 T MR imaging offers unique benefits and challenges compared to lower field strength systems. The main advantage of 3 T imaging lies in the higher signal-to-noise ratio (SNR) afforded by higher field strength systems. SNR increases linearly with field strength for frequencies less than 250 MHz [92, 93]. This means that, with all other parameters held constant, the SNR at 3 T is twice that compared to 1.5 T. The extra SNR allows imaging at smaller voxel sizes (larger matrix), thus improving spatial resolution, and has the potential to decrease imaging time, since the same amount of signal can be acquired in a shorter imaging period. As a result, 3 T imaging has the potential to afford improved evaluation of small, signal-poor structures, such as the shoulder labrum, that require both high spatial resolution and SNR to accurately diagnose tears.

3 T imaging also allows the implementation of a wide array of novel imaging techniques and pulse sequences. Parallel imaging, a technique that uses spatial information from individual radiofrequency coil elements to decrease imaging time, can only be performed on high-field-strength systems, since there is inherent loss of signal associated with this technique [94]. High-field-strength imaging is also necessary to perform functional imaging, such as T2 mapping, a technique that has been studied extensively in the evaluation of articular cartilage and is gaining new applications [95, 96].

The multiple advantages of 3 T imaging do not come without a cost. The hardware and radiofrequency coils from a 1.5 T system cannot be simply transposed to a 3 T system; 3 T systems require their own dedicated hardware and coils. 3 T imaging accentuates MRI artifacts, alters image contrast, and presents unique safety challenges compared to lower field strength systems. Susceptibility artifact, which causes signal loss and geometric distortion around paramagnetic materials, such as metal, air, and blood products, is much more pronounced at 3 T. This artifact is particularly problematic when imaging orthopedic hardware. Chemical shift artifact is also greater at 3 T due to the doubling of the frequency separation between fat and water [97]. This produces spatial misregistration at fat-water interfaces that is proportional to the frequency shift between fat and water.

Apart from the exaggeration of artifacts, another important effect of high-field-strength imaging is the alteration of T1 contrast due to the increase in the T1 relaxation time of tissues [97]. This leads to loss of signal unless there is compensatory increase in the repetition time (TR). Finally, increased field strength also causes increased energy deposition in the patient, which can cause tissue heating [94]. This issue can be a particular challenge at 3 T that has required substantial technical advances to overcome and must be addressed with each exam by the careful selection of sequence parameters. Ultimately, the adjustment of sequence parameters necessary to overcome significant artifacts, alteration of image contrast, and problem of increased energy deposition may partially offset the increased SNR afforded by 3 T imaging.

As far as the evaluation of the diagnostic performance of 3 T MRI in the detection of SLAP lesions, Magee and Williams found a sensitivity of 90% and specificity of 100% for conventional 3 T MRI compared to arthroscopy [98]. This is as good or better than the sensitivity (41–98%) and specificity (75–100%) reported for 1.5 T imaging [89, 90, 99–102]. To address whether the advantages of 3 T imaging may obviate the need for MR arthrography, Magee looked at the diagnostic performance of conventional MRI compared to MR arthrography at 3 T [103]. MR arthrography had a statistically significantly higher sensitivity (98%) than conventional MRI (83%), with the same specificity (99%), for the detection of SLAP lesions. On the other hand, Major and colleagues showed the same sensitivity (75%) and specificity (100%) for MR arthrography and conventional MRI at 3 T in the diagnosis of SLAP lesions, although MR arthrography performed better than conventional MRI in the other labral quadrants [104].

8.3.5 Imaging Diagnosis of SLAP Tears, and Differentiating Variants from Tears

The distinction between normal labral variants and tears is particularly challenging in the case of SLAP lesions, since the majority of labral variants occur in the superior and anterosuperior labral quadrants. The distinction is important clinically since operating on a normal labral variant will not address the source of a patient's pain and may lead to adverse consequences. A number of distinguishing features between variants and tears have been proposed, although they are not always absolute, and correlation with the clinical scenario is essential, especially in cases that are ambiguous on imaging.

Increased signal can often be seen in the posterosuperior labrum in the absence of labral pathology (Fig. 8.14). This is attributed to magic angle phenomenon, with the orientation of the labral collagen fibers in this position relative to the main magnetic field generating spurious increased signal on short TE (echo time) sequences, such as T1 and proton density [105, 106]. Adjusting the TE and positioning can help overcome this artifact (Fig. 8.14) [106]. Knowledge of this artifact is especially important in the context of the overhead-throwing athlete, given the posterosuperior location of labral tears in posterosuperior internal impingement.

The two most common normal variants of the superior labrum include cartilage undercutting and sublabral recess. Cartilage undercutting can be distinguished from a SLAP tear by its intermediate linear signal, similar to the rest of the hyaline articular cartilage, that is medially oriented, paralleling the contour of the glenoid rim (Fig. 8.1). A SLAP tear, on the other hand, often curves laterally away from the glenoid and demonstrates irregular margins. Cartilage undercutting also demonstrates smooth margins, width less than 2 mm, and normal adjacent labral signal [107]. Similarly, a smooth contour fluid signal cleft that parallels the curvature of the glenoid and is less than 2 mm in width is highly suggestive of a sublabral recess rather than a SLAP tear (Fig. 8.2b, c) [108]. The sublabral recess was initially thought to never extend posterior to the LHBT insertion [9]. However, given the variability in the superior labral attachment of the LHBT, studies have shown that a sublabral recess can indeed extend posterior to the LHBT insertion in the absence of a SLAP tear [17, 20, 108].

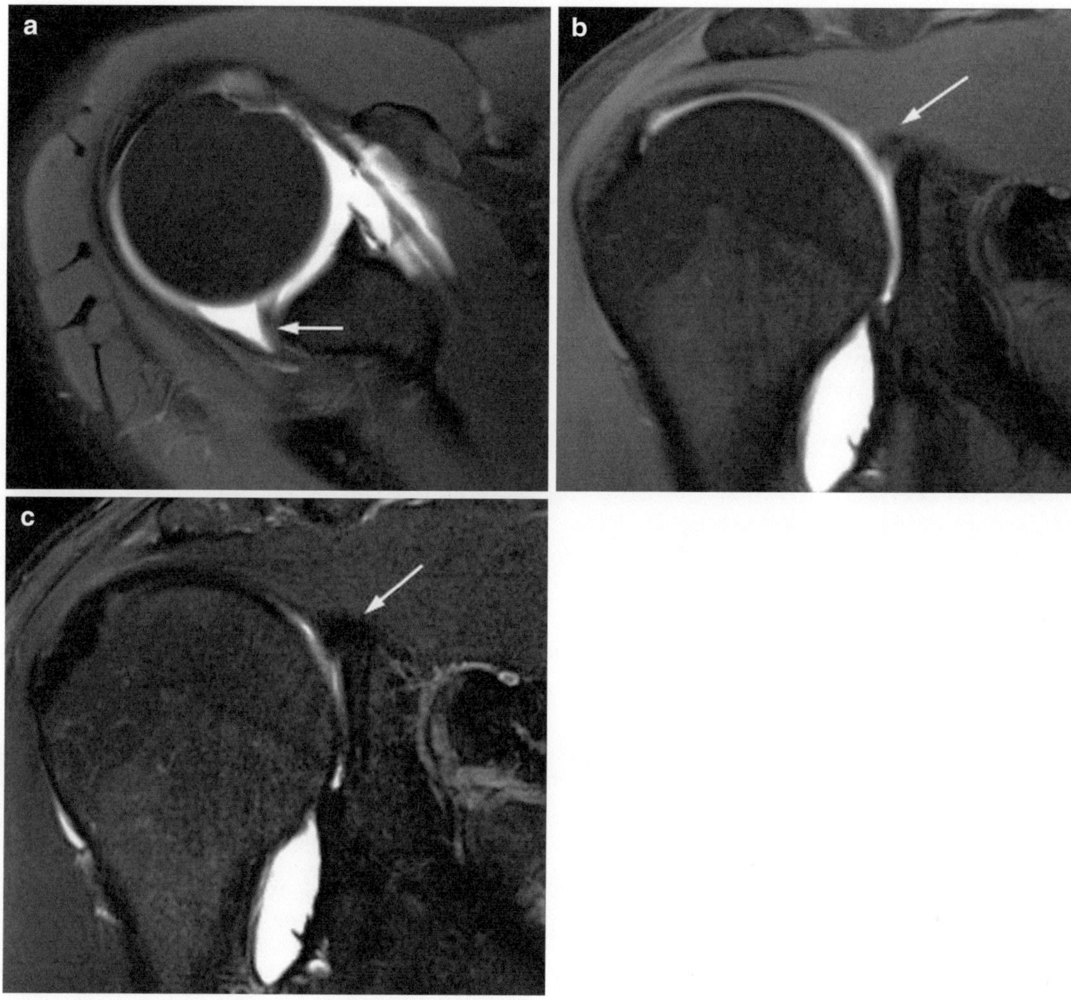

Fig. 8.14 Magic angle phenomenon in the posterosuperior labrum. (**a**) Axial and (**b**) coronal fat-suppressed T1-weighted MR arthrographic images demonstrate intermediate signal in the posterosuperior labrum (arrow). (**c**) Coronal T2-weighted image, which has a longer TE (echo time), shows a hypointense posterosuperior labrum (arrow), confirming that the increased signal on the T1-weighted sequences is an artifact. No posterosuperior labral injury was found on arthroscopy

The variants in the anterosuperior labral quadrant that can be confused for a SLAP tear include the sublabral foramen and Buford complex. The features distinguishing a sublabral foramen from a SLAP tear include focal detachment of the anterosuperior labrum without involvement of the biceps origin, labral displacement less than 1–2 mm, and a smooth labral contour (Fig. 8.5) [15]. The sublabral foramen is often associated with a sublabral recess [109–111]. The Buford complex represents an absent or a hypoplastic anterosuperior labrum accompanied by a thickened cordlike MGHL (Fig. 8.4). The Buford complex can sometimes be mistaken for a displaced labral tear. This pitfall can be avoided by following the thickened MGHL to its insertion on the humeral neck or as it blends with the anterior joint capsule. Correlating with the sagittal images is also important since the thickened MGHL can be well appreciated in the sagittal plane (Fig. 8.4b). Although it was previously thought that the anterosuperior labral variants cannot extend below the 3 o'clock position, studies have shown that both the sublabral foramen and

Buford complex can extend into the anteroinferior labrum to the level of the anterior band of the IGHL [24, 112].

References

1. Nishida K, Hashizume H, Toda K, Inoue H. Histologic and scanning electron microscopic study of the glenoid labrum. J Shoulder Elb Surg. 1996;5(2 Pt 1):132–8.
2. Huber WP, Putz RV. Periarticular fiber system of the shoulder joint. Arthrosc J Arthrosc Relat Surg. 1997;13(6):680–91.
3. Howell SM, Galinat BJ. The glenoid-labral socket. A constrained articular surface. Clin Orthop Relat Res. 1989;243:122–5.
4. Hertz H, Weinstabl R, Grundschober F, Orthner E. Macroscopic and microscopic anatomy of the shoulder joint and the limbus glenoidalis. Acta Anat (Basel). 1986;125(2):96–100.
5. Rockwood CA, Matsen FA, editors. The shoulder. 4th ed. Philadelphia, PA: Saunders/Elsevier; 2009.
6. Park YH, Lee JY, Moon SH, Mo JH, Yang BK, Hahn SH, et al. MR arthrography of the labral capsular ligamentous complex in the shoulder: imaging variations and pitfalls. AJR Am J Roentgenol. 2000;175(3):667–72.
7. Zanetti M, Carstensen T, Weishaupt D, Jost B, Hodler J. MR arthrographic variability of the arthroscopically normal glenoid labrum: qualitative and quantitative assessment. Eur Radiol. 2001;11(4):559–66.
8. De Maeseneer M, Van Roy P, Shahabpour M. Normal MR imaging anatomy of the rotator cuff tendons, glenoid fossa, labrum, and ligaments of the shoulder. Radiol Clin N Am. 2006;44(4):479–87.. vii
9. Cooper DE, Arnoczky SP, O'Brien SJ, Warren RF, DiCarlo E, Allen AA. Anatomy, histology, and vascularity of the glenoid labrum. An anatomical study. J Bone Joint Surg Am. 1992;74(1):46–52.
10. Stoller DW. Magnetic resonance imaging in Orthopaedics and sports medicine. 3rd ed. Philadelphia, PA: Lippincott Williams & Wilkins; 2006.
11. Ramirez Ruiz FA, Baranski Kaniak BC, Haghighi P, Trudell D, Resnick DL. High origin of the anterior band of the inferior glenohumeral ligament: MR arthrography with anatomic and histologic correlation in cadavers. Skelet Radiol. 2012;41(5):525–30.
12. Chloros GD, Haar PJ, Loughran TP, Hayes CW. Imaging of glenoid labrum lesions. Clin Sports Med. 2013;32(3):361–90.
13. Chaipat L, Palmer WE. Shoulder magnetic resonance imaging. Clin Sports Med. 2006;25(3):371–86.. v
14. Lin E. Magnetic resonance arthrography of superior labrum anterior-posterior lesions: a practical approach to interpretation. Curr Probl Diagn Radiol. 2009;38(2):91–7.
15. Dunham KS, Bencardino JT, Rokito AS. Anatomic variants and pitfalls of the labrum, glenoid cartilage, and Glenohumeral ligaments. Magn Reson Imaging Clin N Am. 2012;20(2):213–28.
16. Smith DK, Chopp TM, Aufdemorte TB, Witkowski EG, Jones RC. Sublabral recess of the superior glenoid labrum: study of cadavers with conventional nonenhanced MR imaging, MR arthrography, anatomic dissection, and limited histologic examination. Radiology. 1996;201(1):251–6.
17. Waldt S, Metz S, Burkart A, Mueller D, Bruegel M, Rummeny EJ, et al. Variants of the superior labrum and labro-bicipital complex: a comparative study of shoulder specimens using MR arthrography, multislice CT arthrography and anatomical dissection. Eur Radiol. 2006;16(2):451–8.
18. Tuite MJ, Orwin JF. Anterosuperior labral variants of the shoulder: appearance on gradient-recalled-echo and fast spin-echo MR images. Radiology. 1996;199(2):537–40.
19. Modarresi S, Motamedi D, Jude CM. Superior labral anteroposterior lesions of the shoulder: part 2, mechanisms and classification. AJR Am J Roentgenol. 2011;197(3):604–11.
20. Jin W, Ryu KN, Kwon SH, Rhee YG, Yang DM. MR arthrography in the differential diagnosis of type II superior labral anteroposterior lesion and sublabral recess. AJR Am J Roentgenol. 2006;187(4):887–93.
21. Williams MM, Snyder SJ, Buford D. The Buford complex--the "cord-like" middle glenohumeral ligament and absent anterosuperior labrum complex: a normal anatomic capsulolabral variant. Arthrosc J Arthrosc Relat Surg. 1994;10(3):241–7.
22. Ilahi OA, Cosculluela PE, Ho DM. Classification of anterosuperior glenoid labrum variants and their association with shoulder pathology. Orthopedics. 2008;31(3):226.
23. Ilahi OA, Labbe MR, Cosculluela P. Variants of the anterosuperior glenoid labrum and associated pathology. Arthrosc J Arthrosc Relat Surg. 2002;18(8):882–6.
24. Tuite MJ, Blankenbaker DG, Seifert M, Ziegert AJ, Orwin JF. Sublabral foramen and Buford complex: inferior extent of the unattached or absent labrum in 50 patients. Radiology. 2002;223(1):137–42.
25. Rao AG, Kim TK, Chronopoulos E, McFarland EG. Anatomical variants in the anterosuperior aspect of the glenoid labrum: a statistical analysis of seventy-three cases. J Bone Joint Surg Am. 2003;85-A(4):653–9.
26. Wilk KE, Reinold MM, Andrews JR. The Athlete's shoulder. 2nd ed. Philadelphia, PA: Churchill Livingstone/Elsevier; 2009.
27. Castagna A, Nordenson U, Garofalo R, Karlsson J. Minor shoulder instability. Arthrosc J Arthrosc Relat Surg. 2007;23(2):211–5.
28. Silliman JF, Hawkins RJ. Classification and physical diagnosis of instability of the shoulder. Clin Orthop. 1993;291:7–19.

29. Burkhart SS, Morgan CD, Kibler WB. Shoulder injuries in overhead athletes. The "dead arm" revisited. Clin Sports Med. 2000;19(1):125–58.
30. Steinbeck J, Liljenqvist U, Jerosch J. The anatomy of the glenohumeral ligamentous complex and its contribution to anterior shoulder stability. J Shoulder Elb Surg. 1998;7(2):122–6.
31. McQuade KJ, Dawson J, Smidt GL. Scapulothoracic muscle fatigue associated with alterations in scapulohumeral rhythm kinematics during maximum resistive shoulder elevation. J Orthop Sports Phys Ther. 1998;28(2):74–80.
32. Paletta GA, Warner JJ, Warren RF, Deutsch A, Altchek DW. Shoulder kinematics with two-plane x-ray evaluation in patients with anterior instability or rotator cuff tearing. J Shoulder Elb Surg. 1997;6(6):516–27.
33. Warner JJ, Micheli LJ, Arslanian LE, Kennedy J, Kennedy R. Scapulothoracic motion in normal shoulders and shoulders with glenohumeral instability and impingement syndrome. A study using Moiré topographic analysis. Clin Orthop Relat Res. 1992;285:191–9.
34. Wilk KE, Arrigo C. Current concepts in the rehabilitation of the athletic shoulder. J Orthop Sports Phys Ther. 1993;18(1):365–78.
35. Walch G, Boileau P, Noel E, Donell ST. Impingement of the deep surface of the supraspinatus tendon on the posterosuperior glenoid rim: an arthroscopic study. J Shoulder Elb Surg. 1992;1(5):238–45.
36. Jobe FW, Kvitne RS, Giangarra CE. Shoulder pain in the overhand or throwing athlete. The relationship of anterior instability and rotator cuff impingement. Orthop Rev. 1989;18(9):963–75.
37. Jobe CM. Posterior superior glenoid impingement: expanded spectrum. Arthrosc J Arthrosc Relat Surg. 1995;11(5):530–6.
38. Chung CB, Steinbach LS. MRI of the upper extremity: shoulder, elbow, wrist and hand. Philadelphia, PA: Lippincott Williams & Wilkins; 2009.
39. Giaroli EL, Major NM, Higgins LD. MRI of internal impingement of the shoulder. AJR Am J Roentgenol. 2005;185(4):925–9.
40. Kaplan LD, McMahon PJ, Towers J, Irrgang JJ, Rodosky MW. Internal impingement: findings on magnetic resonance imaging and arthroscopic evaluation. Arthrosc J Arthrosc Relat Surg. 2004;20(7):701–4.
41. Burkhart SS, Morgan CD, Kibler WB. The disabled throwing shoulder: spectrum of pathology part I: pathoanatomy and biomechanics. Arthrosc J Arthrosc Relat Surg. 2003;19(4):404–20.
42. Kibler WB, Kuhn JE, Wilk K, Sciascia A, Moore S, Laudner K, et al. The disabled throwing shoulder: spectrum of pathology-10-year update. Arthrosc J Arthrosc Relat Surg. 2013;29(1):141–61.
43. Grossman MG, Tibone JE, McGarry MH, Schneider DJ, Veneziani S, Lee TQ. A cadaveric model of the throwing shoulder: a possible etiology of superior labrum anterior-to-posterior lesions. J Bone Joint Surg Am. 2005;87(4):824–31.
44. Verna C. Shoulder flexibility to reduce impingement. Im: Presented at the 3rd Annual PBATS (Professional Baseball Athletic Trainer Society) Meeting. Mesa, AZ; 1991.
45. Kibler WB. The relationship of glenohumeral internal rotation deficit to shoulder and elbow injuries in tennis players: a prospective evaluation of posterior capsular stretching. In: Presented at the Annual closed meeting of the American Shoulder and Elbow Surgeons. New York, NY; 1998.
46. Petchprapa CN, Beltran LS, Jazrawi LM, Kwon YW, Babb JS, Recht MP. The rotator interval: a review of anatomy, function, and normal and abnormal MRI appearance. AJR Am J Roentgenol. 2010;195(3):567–76.
47. Chang EY, Fliszar E, Chung CB. Superior labrum anterior and posterior lesions and microinstability. Magn Reson Imaging Clin N Am. 2012;20(2):277–94.
48. Bowen MK, Warren RF. Ligamentous control of shoulder stability based on selective cutting and static translation experiments. Clin Sports Med. 1991;10(4):757–82.
49. Speer KP. Anatomy and pathomechanics of shoulder instability. Clin Sports Med. 1995;14(4):751–60.
50. Savoie FH, Field LD, Atchinson S. Anterior superior instability with rotator cuff tearing: SLAC lesion. Orthop Clin North Am. 2001;32(3):457–61.. ix
51. Townley CO. The capsular mechanism in recurrent dislocation of the shoulder. J Bone Joint Surg Am. 1950;32A(2):370–80.
52. Savoie FH, Papendik L, Field LD, Jobe C. Straight anterior instability: lesions of the middle glenohumeral ligament. Arthrosc J Arthrosc Relat Surg. 2001;17(3):229–35.
53. Tirman PF, Bost FW, Garvin GJ, Peterfy CG, Mall JC, Steinbach LS, et al. Posterosuperior glenoid impingement of the shoulder: findings at MR imaging and MR arthrography with arthroscopic correlation. Radiology. 1994;193(2):431–6.
54. Flannigan B, Kursunoglu-Brahme S, Snyder S, Karzel R, Del Pizzo W, Resnick D. MR arthrography of the shoulder: comparison with conventional MR imaging. AJR Am J Roentgenol. 1990;155(4):829–32.
55. Palmer WE, Brown JH, Rosenthal DI. Rotator cuff: evaluation with fat-suppressed MR arthrography. Radiology. 1993;188(3):683–7.
56. Barber FA, Morgan CD, Burkhart SS, Jobe CM. Current controversies. Point counterpoint. Labrum/biceps/cuff dysfunction in the throwing athlete. Arthrosc J Arthrosc Relat Surg. 1999;15(8):852–7.
57. Gold GE, Pappas GP, Blemker SS, Whalen ST, Campbell G, McAdams TA, et al. Abduction and external rotation in shoulder impingement: an open MR study on healthy volunteers initial experience. Radiology. 2007;244(3):815–22.
58. Tuite MJ, Petersen BD, Wise SM, Fine JP, Kaplan LD, Orwin JF. Shoulder MR arthrography of the posterior labrocapsular complex in overhead throwers

with pathologic internal impingement and internal rotation deficit. Skelet Radiol. 2007;36(6):495–502.
59. Tehranzadeh AD, Fronek J, Resnick D. Posterior capsular fibrosis in professional baseball pitchers: case series of MR arthrographic findings in six patients with glenohumeral internal rotational deficit. Clin Imaging. 2007;31(5):343–8.
60. Bennett GE. Elbow and shoulder lesions of baseball players. Am J Surg. 1959;98:484–92.
61. De Maeseneer M, Jaovisidha S, Jacobson JA, Tam W, Schils JP, Sartoris DJ, et al. The Bennett lesion of the shoulder. J Comput Assist Tomogr. 1998;22(1):31–4.
62. Andrews JR, Carson WG, McLeod WD. Glenoid labrum tears related to the long head of the biceps. Am J Sports Med. 1985;13(5):337–41.
63. Snyder SJ, Karzel RP, Del Pizzo W, Ferkel RD, Friedman MJ. SLAP lesions of the shoulder. Arthrosc J Arthrosc Relat Surg. 1990;6(4):274–9.
64. Kim TK, Queale WS, Cosgarea AJ, McFarland EG. Clinical features of the different types of SLAP lesions: an analysis of one hundred and thirty-nine cases. J Bone Joint Surg Am. 2003;85-A(1):66–71.
65. Maffet MW, Gartsman GM, Moseley B. Superior labrum-biceps tendon complex lesions of the shoulder. Am J Sports Med. 1995;23(1):93–8.
66. Powell SE, Nord KD, Ryu RKN. The diagnosis, classification, and treatment of SLAP lesions. Oper Tech Sports Med. 2004;12(2):99–110.
67. Mohana-Borges AVR, Chung CB, Resnick D. Superior labral anteroposterior tear: classification and diagnosis on MRI and MR arthrography. Am J Roentgenol. 2003;181(6):1449–62.
68. Clavert P, Bonnomet F, Kempf JF, Boutemy P, Braun M, Kahn JL. Contribution to the study of the pathogenesis of type II superior labrum anterior-posterior lesions: a cadaveric model of a fall on the outstretched hand. J Shoulder Elb Surg. 2004;13(1):45–50.
69. Bey MJ, Elders GJ, Huston LJ, Kuhn JE, Blasier RB, Soslowsky LJ. The mechanism of creation of superior labrum, anterior, and posterior lesions in a dynamic biomechanical model of the shoulder: the role of inferior subluxation. J Shoulder Elb Surg. 1998;7(4):397–401.
70. Burkhart SS, Morgan CD. The peel-back mechanism: its role in producing and extending posterior type II SLAP lesions and its effect on SLAP repair rehabilitation. Arthrosc J Arthrosc Relat Surg. 1998;14(6):637–40.
71. Pagnani MJ, Deng XH, Warren RF, Torzilli PA, Altchek DW. Effect of lesions of the superior portion of the glenoid labrum on glenohumeral translation. J Bone Joint Surg Am. 1995;77(7):1003–10.
72. Hantes ME, Venouziou AI, Liantsis AK, Dailiana ZH, Malizos KN. Arthroscopic repair for chronic anterior shoulder instability: a comparative study between patients with Bankart lesions and patients with combined Bankart and superior labral anterior posterior lesions. Am J Sports Med. 2009;37(6):1093–8.
73. Taylor DC, Arciero RA. Pathologic changes associated with shoulder dislocations. Arthroscopic and physical examination findings in first-time, traumatic anterior dislocations. Am J Sports Med. 1997;25(3):306–11.
74. Yiannakopoulos CK, Mataragas E, Antonogiannakis E. A comparison of the spectrum of intra-articular lesions in acute and chronic anterior shoulder instability. Arthrosc J Arthrosc Relat Surg. 2007;23(9):985–90.
75. Antonio GE, Griffith JF, Yu AB, Yung PSH, Chan KM, Ahuja AT. First-time shoulder dislocation: high prevalence of labral injury and age-related differences revealed by MR arthrography. J Magn Reson Imaging. 2007;26(4):983–91.
76. Sebro R, Oliveira A, Palmer WE. MR arthrography of the shoulder: technical update and clinical applications. Semin Musculoskelet Radiol. 2014;18(4):352–64.
77. La Rocca VR, Rybak LD, Recht M. Technical update on magnetic resonance imaging of the shoulder. Magn Reson Imaging Clin N Am. 2012;20(2):149–61.
78. Chung CB, Dwek JR, Feng S, Resnick D. MR arthrography of the glenohumeral joint: a tailored approach. AJR Am J Roentgenol. 2001;177(1):217–9.
79. Farmer KD, Hughes PM. MR arthrography of the shoulder: fluoroscopically guided technique using a posterior approach. AJR Am J Roentgenol. 2002;178(2):433–4.
80. Dépelteau H, Bureau NJ, Cardinal E, Aubin B, Brassard P. Arthrography of the shoulder: a simple fluoroscopically guided approach for targeting the rotator cuff interval. AJR Am J Roentgenol. 2004;182(2):329–32.
81. Wagner SC, Schweitzer ME, Weishaupt D. Temporal behavior of intra-articular gadolinium. J Comput Assist Tomogr. 2001;25(5):661–70.
82. Vahlensieck M, Sommer T, Textor J, Pauleit D, Lang P, Genant HK, et al. Indirect MR arthrography: techniques and applications. Eur Radiol. 1998;8(2):232–5.
83. Bergin D, Schweitzer ME. Indirect magnetic resonance arthrography. Skelet Radiol. 2003;32(10):551–8.
84. Bencardino JT, Beltran J, Rosenberg ZS, Rokito A, Schmahmann S, Mota J, et al. Superior labrum anterior-posterior lesions: diagnosis with MR arthrography of the shoulder. Radiology. 2000;214(1):267–71.
85. Waldt S, Burkart A, Lange P, Imhoff AB, Rummeny EJ, Woertler K. Diagnostic performance of MR arthrography in the assessment of superior labral anteroposterior lesions of the shoulder. Am J Roentgenol. 2004;182(5):1271–8.
86. Chandnani VP, Yeager TD, DeBerardino T, Christensen K, Gagliardi JA, Heitz DR, et al. Glenoid labral tears: prospective evaluation with MRI imaging, MR arthrography, and CT arthrography. Am J Roentgenol. 1993;161(6):1229–35.

87. Amin MF, Youssef AO. The diagnostic value of magnetic resonance arthrography of the shoulder in detection and grading of SLAP lesions: comparison with arthroscopic findings. Eur J Radiol. 2012;81(9):2343–7.
88. Magee T, Williams D, Mani N. Shoulder MR arthrography: which patient group benefits most? AJR Am J Roentgenol. 2004;183(4):969–74.
89. Herold T, Hente R, Zorger N, Finkenzeller T, Feuerbach S, Lenhart M, et al. Indirect MR-arthrography of the shoulder-value in the detection of SLAP-lesions. RöFo Fortschritte Auf Dem Geb Röntgenstrahlen Nukl. 2003;175(11):1508–14.
90. Dinauer PA, Flemming DJ, Murphy KP, Doukas WC. Diagnosis of superior labral lesions: comparison of noncontrast MRI with indirect MR arthrography in unexercised shoulders. Skelet Radiol. 2007;36(3):195–202.
91. Jung JY, Yoon YC, Yi S-K, Yoo J, Choe B-K. Comparison study of indirect MR arthrography and direct MR arthrography of the shoulder. Skelet Radiol. 2009;38(7):659–67.
92. Collins CM, Smith MB. Signal-to-noise ratio and absorbed power as functions of main magnetic field strength, and definition of "90 degrees " RF pulse for the head in the birdcage coil. Magn Reson Med. 2001;45(4):684–91.
93. Edelstein WA, Glover GH, Hardy CJ, Redington RW. The intrinsic signal-to-noise ratio in NMR imaging. Magn Reson Med. 1986;3(4):604–18.
94. Ramnath RR. 3T MR imaging of the musculoskeletal system (part I): considerations, coils, and challenges. Magn Reson Imaging Clin N Am. 2006;14(1):27–40.
95. Matzat SJ, van Tiel J, Gold GE, Oei EHG. Quantitative MRI techniques of cartilage composition. Quant Imaging Med Surg. 2013;3(3):162–74.
96. Anz AW, Lucas EP, Fitzcharles EK, Surowiec RK, Millett PJ, Ho CP. MRI T2 mapping of the asymptomatic supraspinatus tendon by age and imaging plane using clinically relevant subregions. Eur J Radiol. 2014;83(5):801–5.
97. Mosher TJ. Musculoskeletal imaging at 3T: current techniques and future applications. Magn Reson Imaging Clin N Am. 2006;14(1):63–76.
98. Magee TH, Williams D. Sensitivity and specificity in detection of labral tears with 3.0-T MRI of the shoulder. Am J Roentgenol. 2006;187(6):1448–52.
99. Legan JM, Burkhard TK, Goff WB, Balsara ZN, Martinez AJ, Burks DD, et al. Tears of the glenoid labrum: MR imaging of 88 arthroscopically confirmed cases. Radiology. 1991;179(1):241–6.
100. Murray PJ, Shaffer BS. Clinical update: MR imaging of the shoulder. Sports Med Arthrosc Rev. 2009;17(1):40–8.
101. Gusmer PB, Potter HG, Schatz JA, Wickiewicz TL, Altchek DW, O'Brien SJ, et al. Labral injuries: accuracy of detection with unenhanced MR imaging of the shoulder. Radiology. 1996;200(2):519–24.
102. Connell DA, Potter HG, Wickiewicz TL, Altchek DW, Warren RF. Noncontrast magnetic resonance imaging of superior labral lesions. 102 cases confirmed at arthroscopic surgery. Am J Sports Med. 1999;27(2):208–13.
103. Magee T. 3-T MRI of the shoulder: is MR arthrography necessary? Am J Roentgenol. 2009;192(1):86–92.
104. Major NM, Browne J, Domzalski T, Cothran RL, Helms CA. Evaluation of the glenoid labrum with 3-T MRI: is intra-articular contrast necessary? Am J Roentgenol. 2011;196(5):1139–44.
105. Gustas CN, Tuite MJ. Imaging update on the glenoid labrum: variants versus tears. Semin Musculoskelet Radiol. 2014;18(4):365–73.
106. Sasaki T, Yodono H, Prado GLM, Saito Y, Miura H, Itabashi Y, et al. Increased signal intensity in the normal glenoid labrum in MR imaging: diagnostic pitfalls caused by the magic-angle effect. Magn Reson Med Sci. 2002;1(3):149–56.
107. Chang D, Mohana-Borges A, Borso M, Chung CB. SLAP lesions: anatomy, clinical presentation, MR imaging diagnosis and characterization. Eur J Radiol. 2008;68(1):72–87.
108. Tuite MJ, Rutkowski A, Enright T, Kaplan L, Fine JP, Orwin J. Width of high signal and extension posterior to biceps tendon as signs of superior labrum anterior to posterior tears on MRI and MR arthrography. AJR Am J Roentgenol. 2005;185(6):1422–8.
109. De Maeseneer M, Van Roy F, Lenchik L, Shahabpour M, Jacobson J, Ryu KN, et al. CT and MR arthrography of the normal and pathologic anterosuperior labrum and labral-bicipital complex. Radiographics. 2000;20:S67–81.
110. Kwak SM, Brown RR, Trudell D, Resnick D. Glenohumeral joint: comparison of shoulder positions at MR arthrography. Radiology. 1998;208(2):375–80.
111. Yeh L, Kwak S, Kim YS, Pedowitz R, Trudell D, Muhle C, et al. Anterior labroligamentous structures of the glenohumeral joint: correlation of MR arthrography and anatomic dissection in cadavers. Am J Roentgenol. 1998;171(5):1229–36.
112. Palmer WE, Brown JH, Rosenthal DI. Labral-ligamentous complex of the shoulder: evaluation with MR arthrography. Radiology. 1994;190(3):645–51.

Part IV

Trauma and Arthropathies

Imaging Diagnosis of Shoulder Girdle Fractures

9

Joseph S. Yu

9.1 Introduction

The shoulder is vulnerable to both direct and indirect trauma, and fractures and dislocations are relatively common [1]. The shoulder girdle refers to a complex region of the skeleton that consists of numerous muscular and osseous structures, several joints containing fibrocartilage and hyaline cartilage, and ligaments and tendons that attach and suspend the arm to the thorax allowing for maximum mobility of the upper extremity. Muscles act synergistically to optimize motion.

Evaluation of the shoulder typically begins with a radiographic inspection of the osseous structures and joints. There are limitations associated with the radiographic evaluation. Certain fractures are difficult to visualize unless specific projections are performed. Complex fractures or fracture-dislocation complexes often are difficult to characterize owing to displacement of osseous fragments. Multi-detector CT has enabled rapid and accurate assessment of osseous and articular injuries. Depiction in an infinite number of imaging planes and three-dimensional (3D) images has rendered CT an indispensable modality for assessment of acute shoulder trauma.

Ultrasound is not routinely utilized in patients presenting with shoulder fractures but it is a useful follow-up modality for assessing the rotator cuff, vascular structures, and fluid collections that may have developed as a result of acute trauma. MRI is preferred for shoulder instability, but in the setting of acute trauma its role is limited to depicting marrow edema that is associated with acute contusions and occult fractures as well as for patients presenting with significant soft-tissue injuries.

J. S. Yu (✉)
Department of Radiology, The Ohio State University
Wexner Medical Center, Columbus, OH, USA
e-mail: joseph.yu@osumc.edu

9.2 Clavicle

9.2.1 Pertinent Imaging Findings

The clavicle is an S-shaped bone that is unique, functioning as an osseous connection between the arm and the trunk. It is therefore vulnerable to trauma especially in children and adolescents. It is one of the first bones to ossify, though the medial epiphysis does not fuse until the second decade of life. Radiographic examination typically includes an AP view and a 35- to 40-degree cephalad-angled projection called the *serendipity* view. Owing to the curved contour of the bone, the serendipity view offers better visualization of the clavicle in its entirety and the sternoclavicular joints. Medially, it is tubular with a broad head that articulates with the manubrium and the first rib. Laterally, the clavicle becomes flatter with a discoid end that forms a gliding synovial joint with the acromion process. The AP view allows ideal inspection of the middle-third of the bone while the Zanca view (10-degree cephalad view) optimizes the acromioclavicular joint region.

J. T. Bencardino (ed.), *The Shoulder*, https://doi.org/10.1007/978-3-030-06240-8_9

When evaluating complex or comminuted fractures, CT is optimal for assessment of displacement, angulation, and injury to the adjacent neurovascular structures. In general, thin-section protocols are recommended. MRI is occasionally employed to evaluate trauma to the muscles that insert on the clavicle including the pectoralis major, deltoid, trapezius, and sternocleidomastoid muscles.

9.2.2 Clavicular Fractures

9.2.2.1 Definition

Typically, young people are at risk for clavicle fractures. Children and adolescents engage in activities that subject them to accidents and falls. In one study, falls during play or an athletic activity were the etiology of a fracture in greater than 90% of cases [2]. The point of the shoulder was usually the site of impact. Additional mechanisms of injury include direct impaction on the clavicle from assault or motor vehicle accidents and rarely a fall on an outstretched hand. Birth trauma may place excessive pressure of the shoulder against the maternal symphysis pubis producing a characteristic fracture at the junction of the middle and lateral thirds of the bone [3].

9.2.2.2 Radiographic and CT Findings

The Allman classification divides the clavicle into thirds [4]. About 80% of clavicle fractures involve the middle third of the bone (Fig. 9.1). The majority of fractures are simple and transversely oriented; however, comminuted fractures associated with butterfly fragments are not uncommon. In children, fractures may be either a greenstick or bowing-type injury. Angulation and displacement occur from the pull of the sternocleidomastoid muscle on the medial fragment and depression of the lateral fragment from the weight of the arm [5]. The degree of displacement is usually more conspicuous on the serendipity or Zanca view than on the AP view (Fig. 9.1). When a fracture is severely comminuted, CT may be indicated to assess for a concomitant injury to the subclavian artery, particularly in the setting of a rapidly growing hematoma, or to the subclavian vein and brachial plexus (Fig. 9.2).

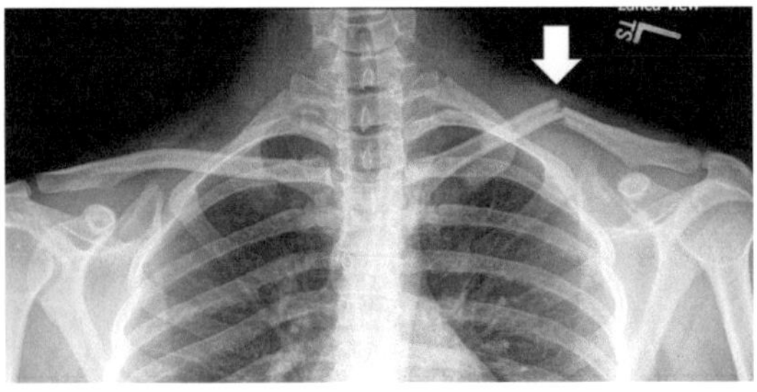

Fig. 9.1 Clavicle fracture, nondisplaced. The majority of clavicle fractures involve the middle one-third of the clavicle (arrow). Imaging both clavicles with 10° of cephalad angulation optimizes assessment of the angular deformity

Lateral third fractures account for 15% of clavicle fractures (Fig. 9.3) [6]. The Neer classification is dependent on the location of the fracture with respect to the coracoclavicular (CC) ligament which consists of a conoid (medial) and trapezoid (lateral) component. A type 1 fracture is located lateral to the CC ligament and has minimal displacement. A type 2a fracture occurs medial to the conoid component where a type 2b occurs between the fibers of the CC ligament, disrupting the conoid component. Type 2 injuries can lead to significant separation between the coracoid process and the clavicle. Because it has the highest risk for nonunion, it generally requires surgical fixation. A type 3 fracture is intra-articular, thus predisposing to arthritis. A type 4 fracture occurs in pediatric patients with the displacement at the junction of the metaphysis and the growth plate. A type 5 fracture is comminuted but contains a small inferior fragment that remains attached to the CC ligament and is similar to a type 2 variant.

Less than 5% of clavicle fractures involve the medial third (Fig. 9.4). These are difficult to visualize if not displaced owing to the overlap of the ribs and spine. Since these fractures are caused by direct trauma, CT is useful to further characterize the fracture to assess the surrounding structures and to evaluate the sternoclavicular joint. There are two types: transverse fractures and intra-articular fractures.

9.2.2.3 Ultrasound Findings

Currently, sonography is not routinely used in adults with clavicle fractures except to diagnose vascular complications such as a pseudoaneurysm or the formation of a hematoma. Sonography, however, is commonly utilized in neonates to visualize clavicular birth fractures [7].

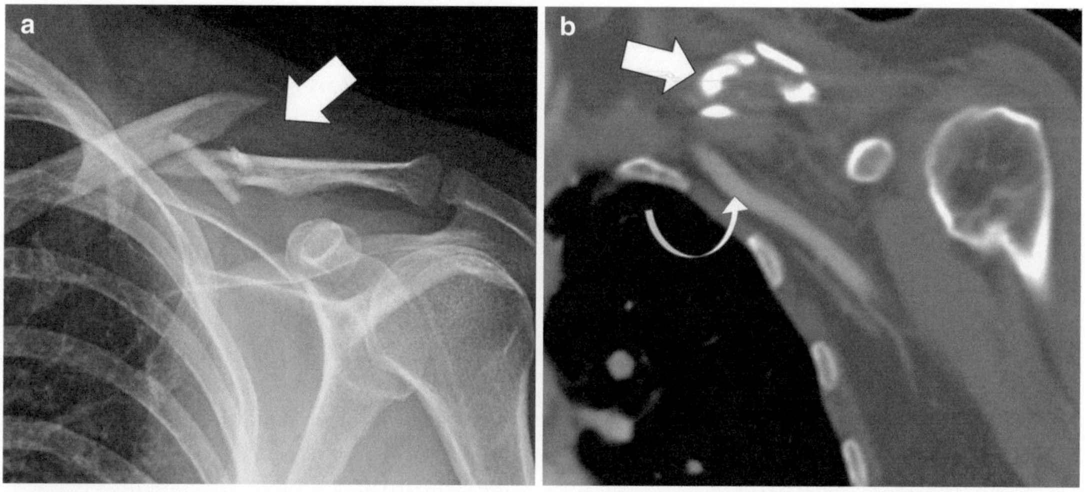

Fig. 9.2 Clavicle fracture, comminuted. (**a**) A comminuted mid-clavicular fracture (arrow) is frequently displaced from the pull of the sternocleidomastoid muscle on the medial fragment while the weight of the arm depresses the lateral fragment. (**b**) CT is recommended when there is significant displacement of the clavicle fragments (arrow) to evaluate the vascular structures (curved arrow) and the brachial plexus

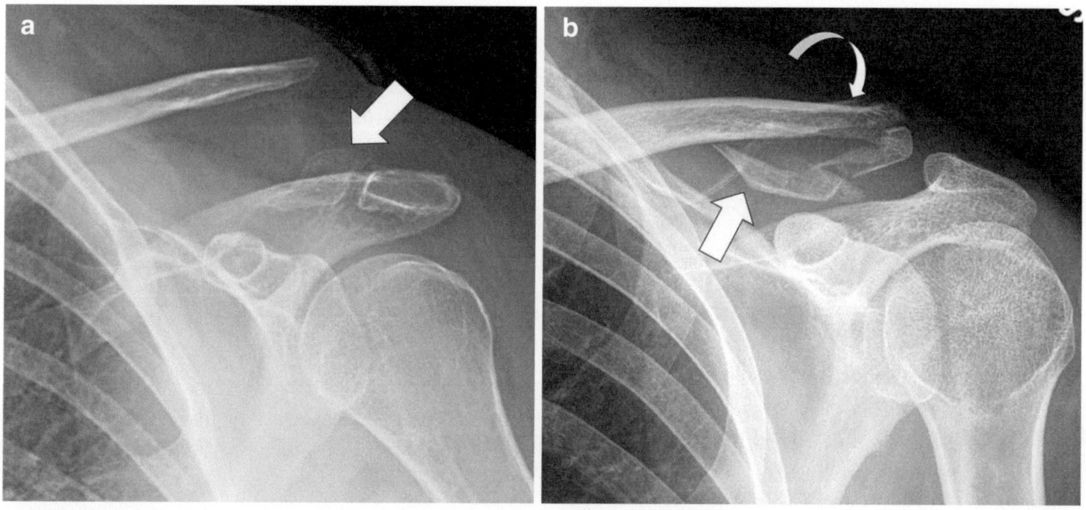

Fig. 9.3 Distal clavicular fractures. (**a**) This patient had a Neer type 2 fracture occurring medial to the coracoclavicular (CC) ligament, resulting in a fragment in anatomic alignment with the acromioclavicular (AC) joint (arrow) and marked superior migration of the rest of the clavicle from the coracoid process. (**b**) A different patient with a type 5 fracture with an inferior fragment still attached to the CC ligament, another fragment attached to the AC joint, and the rest of the clavicle (curved arrow) displacing superiorly

9.2.2.4 MR Findings

On occasion, MRI may be used to evaluate a clavicle fracture when there is a simultaneous muscle injury or accumulation of a pathologic fluid collection. When the soft tissues protrude above the clavicle or into the axilla, for example, it may be an indication that there is an enlarging hematoma from an occult vascular injury.

9.2.3 Postoperative Imaging

Most clavicular fractures heal without sequela although a nonunion occurs in 1–4% of patients [8]. When fixation is required, radiographic follow-up is sufficient with standard clavicle projections. There are two common fixation techniques employed. For midshaft fractures, uni-cortical

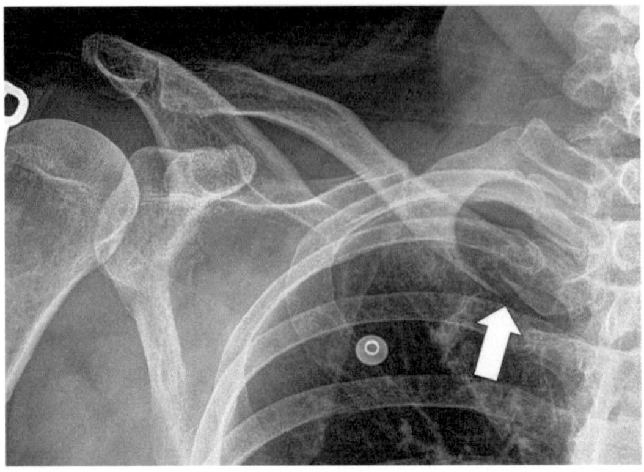

Fig. 9.4 Medial clavicle fracture. Fractures involving the medial clavicle (arrow) are uncommon but are frequently overlooked owing to the overlap of the spine and ribs

plate fixation is common with the plate on the superior cortical margin with screws directed inferiorly in order to avoid the neurovascular structures [9]. For distal type 2 clavicle fractures, it is not uncommon to see a variation of a clavicle hook plate that has an S-shaped contour so that the lateral end can be placed underneath the inferior margin of the acromion process [10].

9.3 Sternoclavicular Joint

9.3.1 Pertinent Imaging Findings

The sternoclavicular (SC) joint is a di-arthrodial joint at the medial end of the clavicle. The disc within the SC joint divides the gliding synovial joint into medial and lateral compartments. Supporting the joint are the interclavicular, costoclavicular, anterior sternoclavicular, and posterior sternoclavicular ligaments. Radiographic evaluation consists of a PA view of both SC joints with the beam centered over the manubrium, and bilateral PA oblique projections. It is important to confirm symmetric position of the clavicular head and when in doubt CT is confirmatory. The rhomboid fossa is a variant that occurs in the inferomedial aspect of the clavicle corresponding to the insertion of the costoclavicular ligament. It is depicted by an irregular concavity located lateral to the head of the clavicle and is seen commonly in males.

9.3.2 Sternoclavicular Joint Injuries

9.3.2.1 Definition

Dislocation of the SC joint is uncommon accounting for 2–3% of all shoulder girdle dislocations [11]. Anterior dislocations are overwhelmingly more common than posterior dislocations but the latter type can be more severe because of associated injuries to adjacent structures. The mechanism of injury for anterior dislocations is most often indirect trauma with impaction to the anterior shoulder with the clavicle acting as a fulcrum. Posterior dislocation usually occurs as a result of a direct blow against the medial clavicle. Complete disruption of the SC joint may result in scapulothoracic dissociation.

9.3.2.2 Radiographic and CT Findings

Diagnosis of a SC joint dislocation is challenging on AP radiographs and this abnormality is frequently missed on initial inspection. Detection requires asymmetry of the joint space which may not be evident with minor subluxation unless there is also superior subluxation (Fig. 9.5). The Allman classification defines three types [3]. In a type 1 dislocation, there is partial disruption of the SC ligaments. In type 2, there is complete rupture of the SC ligaments. In type 3, the SC ligaments and the costoclavicular ligament are torn.

The modality of choice for confirmation is CT. Rapidly acquired images display the direction of the dislocation, degree of osseous displacement, presence of any associated fracture, as well as any potential complication to the adjacent structures such as the great vessels. Approximately 25% of posterior dislocations are associated with a laceration of the superior vena cava, thoracic outlet syndrome from venous compression, compression of the recurrent laryngeal nerve, pneumothorax or pneumomediastinum from esophageal or tracheal rupture, or injury to the subclavian or carotid artery [12].

9.3.2.3 Ultrasound Findings

Ultrasound has been described as a potential screening tool to assess possible sternoclavicular dislocation [13].

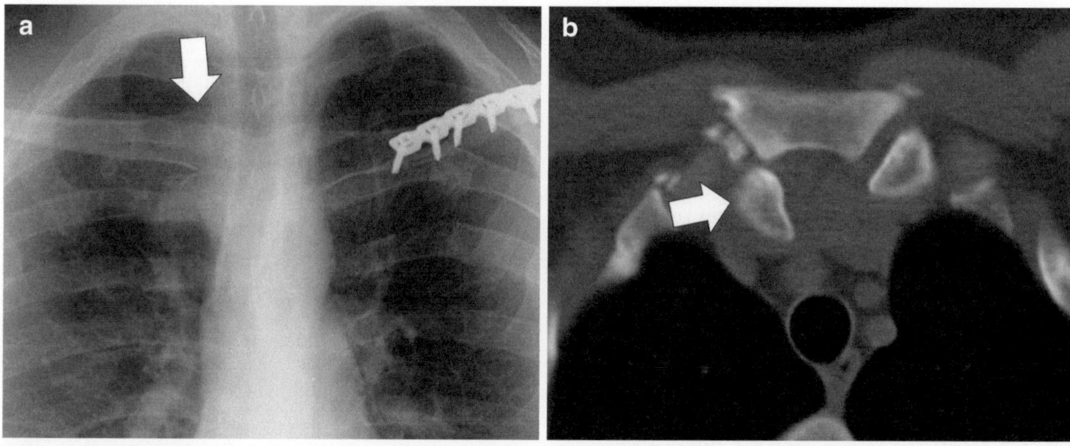

Fig. 9.5 Sternoclavicular joint (SC) separation. (**a**) Frontal radiograph of the chest shows asymmetric elevation of the right clavicular head (arrow) compared to the left. (**b**) Axial CT image shows that the asymmetry is caused by posterior dislocation of the right clavicular head (arrow). When this occurs, it is important to thoroughly evaluate the vascular structures

9.3.2.4 MR Findings

The multiplanar capabilities of MRI along with its superior soft tissue resolution have made this modality particularly effective for characterizing ligamentous tears and cartilaginous injuries [14]. MR angiography is very helpful in elucidating occult vascular injury as well.

9.3.3 Postoperative Imaging

The treatment of choice for SC dislocations is closed reduction and immobilization of the arm with a sling [15]. Delay in diagnosis may lead to instability; stabilization procedures of the SC joint with a trans-osseous tension band or ligamentous reconstruction are potential long-term solutions. However, in some patients, resection arthroplasty of the medial end of the clavicle is the only option for treating persistently painful SC joints.

9.4 Acromioclavicular Joint

9.4.1 Pertinent Imaging Findings

The acromioclavicular (AC) joint is a diarthrodial gliding joint at the lateral end of the clavicle containing a variably developed intra-articular disc. This synovial joint is supported by the capsule, the AC ligaments, and the CC ligament. Radiographic evaluation consists of an AP view of the upper thorax including AC joints and a 15-degree cephalad-angled view and symmetry with the contralateral joint is a key observation. If findings are equivocal or surgery is contemplated, bilateral weight-bearing stress views may be performed to confirm the severity of pathology. The normal width of the AC joint is 2–6 mm and it decreases with age [16]. Any discrepancy of the CC distance greater than 3–4 mm, or asymmetry of the AC joint space greater than 2 mm, may indicate a rupture of the CC ligament. An axillary view is useful especially when there is concern of a posterior subluxation. Though not routinely used, MRI is an excellent modality that enables comprehensive evaluation of the osseous structures and soft-tissue stabilizers of this joint.

9.4.2 Acromioclavicular Joint Injuries

9.4.2.1 Definition

The AC joint is the second most commonly dislocated joint in the shoulder accounting for about

12% of all shoulder dislocations [17]. Two injury mechanisms are responsible, either a direct fall on the shoulder or a fall on an outstretched hand. The force applied determines the spectrum of pathology. The initial injury is a strain of the AC ligaments. As the force increases, the trapezoid component of the CC ligament ruptures then followed by the conoid component as the force is increased. With complete rupture of the CC ligament, the clavicle is allowed to detach resulting in injuries to the insertion of the deltoid and trapezius muscles.

9.4.2.2 Radiographic and CT Findings

A six-point grading system is used to classify and treat AC joint injuries [18]. A grade 1 separation indicates stretching of the AC ligaments without capsular disruption. Radiographs appear normal or may show mild soft-tissue swelling over the joint. A grade 2 separation results in disruption of the AC ligaments and an incomplete tear of the CC ligament (Fig. 9.6). The clavicle elevates superiorly but usually less than 50% of the width of the clavicle and the AC joint widens compared to the contralateral joint, particularly with weight-bearing views. A grade 3 separation is a true dislocation with complete rupture of the AC and CC ligaments (Fig. 9.7). A variation can occur in people younger than 25 years of age depicted by an avulsion fracture at the base of the coracoid process but with an intact CC ligament.

The three latter grades are uncommon. In grade 4 injuries, the clavicle displaces posteriorly into or through the trapezius muscle. In grade 5 injuries, elevation of the clavicle is more severe than in a grade 3 separation. In grade 6 injuries, the clavicle dislocates inferiorly below the coracoid or acromion process often occurring with associated rib fractures.

9.4.2.3 Ultrasound Findings

Ultrasound may be used to screen for AC joint separation but it is suggested only if CT or MRI is not available.

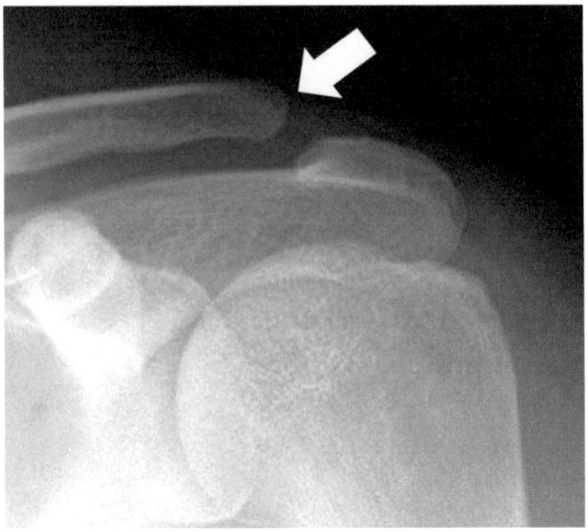

Fig. 9.6 Acromioclavicular (AC) joint separation, type 2. The distal clavicle (arrow) elevates superiorly by about half of the shaft width relative to the acromion process owing to a rupture of the AC ligament and partial tears of the coracoclavicular ligaments

9.4.2.4 MR Findings

MRI is a useful tool for assessment of AC joint pain and it has recently been advocated for evaluation of acute AC joint separations [19]. The main limitation of radiography is accuracy in the categorization of the injury and this may have an effect on the treatment. MR enables distinction between grade 2 and 3 injuries and also has been shown to reclassify radiographic grading to a lesser type in as many as 36% of patients and to a more severe type in greater than 11% of patients [20].

9.4.3 Postoperative Imaging

There are several surgical options in the management of AC joint dislocations [21, 22]. Current evidence suggests that operative management of type 3 fractures has better results. Early surgery has been reported to have better cosmetic and radiologic outcomes and a lower risk for infection, and reduce the overall incidence of failed surgery.

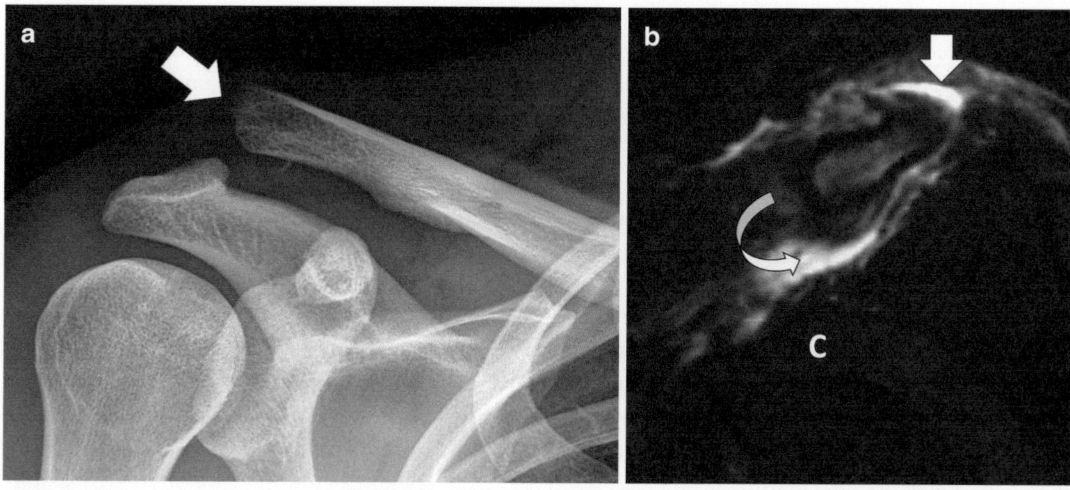

Fig. 9.7 Acromioclavicular (AC) joint separation, type 3. (**a**) Frontal radiograph shows complete disarticulation of the clavicle (arrow) from the acromion process and an abnormally wide distance between the clavicle and the coracoid process. (**b**) Sagittal T2-weighted MR image shows complete disruption of the coracoclavicular ligaments (curved arrow) and a hematoma (arrow) where the superior AC ligament is typically visualized. [C—coracoid]

9.5 Scapula

9.5.1 Pertinent Imaging Findings

The scapula is a large, triangular flat bone located in the dorsolateral aspect of the thorax that is almost entirely surrounded by muscles. Because the body of the scapula is anteverted 30–40° with respect to the coronal plane of the body, a true AP view of the scapula is actually an AP oblique radiograph of the shoulder. This projection allows visualization of the superior and inferior angles in the medial aspect of the blade, the superior and lateral borders, the tip of the coracoid process, the majority of the spine, the portion of the acromion that articulates with the clavicle, and the glenoid neck and fossa. A lateral projection, or Y-view, allows assessment of the body, acromion, and base of the spine. An axillary view depicts the acromion and coracoid processes as well as the glenoid fossa and neck. CT, on the other hand, is preferred when there is a complex fracture of the scapula particularly when performed with 3D reconstruction.

Ossification centers have a typical radiographic appearance and should not be mistaken for a fracture. An os acromiale represents failure of fusion of an apophysis (which generally occurs by 25 years of age) appearing as a transverse lucency. It is common and occurs in 7–10% of people [23]. True fractures of the acromion process usually occur at the junction of the spine and the acromion. One pitfall is a chronic fracture with nonunion which may be impossible to differentiate from a basi-acromial type of os acromiale unless there are comparison radiographs.

9.5.2 Scapular Fractures

9.5.2.1 Definition

Scapular fractures account for 3–5% of fractures in the shoulder girdle [24]. Fractures of the scapula require major trauma with either axial loading on an outstretched arm or direct forces aimed at the scapula such as those that occur from a fall from a height, motor vehicular trauma, or crushing injury. Fractures of the glenoid rim and coracoid process may also occur with glenohumeral joint dislocations. There are numerous classification systems for describing scapular fractures but none predominate; thus, fractures often are described according to the anatomic area involved including the acromion process, coracoid process, scapular neck, and glenoid fossa/rim with the latter subdivided into extra- and intra-articular types. The majority of fractures involve the body and inferior glenoid neck and over 20% enters the spinoglenoid notch [25].

9.5.2.2 Radiographic and CT Findings

Fractures of the body constitute the most common fracture of the scapula. The Grashey and lateral projections are useful since these fractures, though often comminuted, have conspicuous vertical and/or horizontal components. Fractures through the scapular neck are frequently displaced and are unstable if the clavicle and CC ligament are also disrupted.

Coracoid fractures are categorized according to where the fracture is located with respect to the CC ligament attachment (Fig. 9.8). A type 1 fracture occurs proximal to the CC ligament and may be associated with AC joint separation, fractures of the clavicle, and/or other scapular fractures involving the superior scapula and glenoid [26]. A type 2 fracture occurs distal to the CC ligament. Acromion process fractures are usually transversely oriented at its base. Three types have been described by Kuhn et al. A type 1 fracture is not displaced and has two subtypes: avulsive type 1a and impactive type 1b. A type 2 fracture is displaced but does not encroach on the subacromial space. A type 3 fracture is either inferiorly displaced or associated with a superiorly displaced glenoid fracture. Coracoid and acromion fractures may be radiographically occult or difficult to visualize. Axillary views and trans-scapular Y views are considered essential projections for depicting fractures of either bony tubercle.

Glenoid fractures are categorized as either extra-articular or intra-articular [27]. In extra-articular fractures, the integrity of the clavicle and AC joint is important (Fig. 9.9). Intra-articular fractures comprise about 10% of scapular fractures and is most commonly classified according to the classification described by Ideberg (Fig. 9.10) [28]. Type 1a is most common and represents an anterior chip fracture of the glenoid rim. Type 1b is through the posterior glenoid rim. Type 2 is a transverse or an oblique fracture through the inferior glenoid fossa with inferior displacement. Type 3 is a transverse fracture through the superior glenoid fossa and extending to the superior border. Type 4 is a transverse fracture through the body extending to

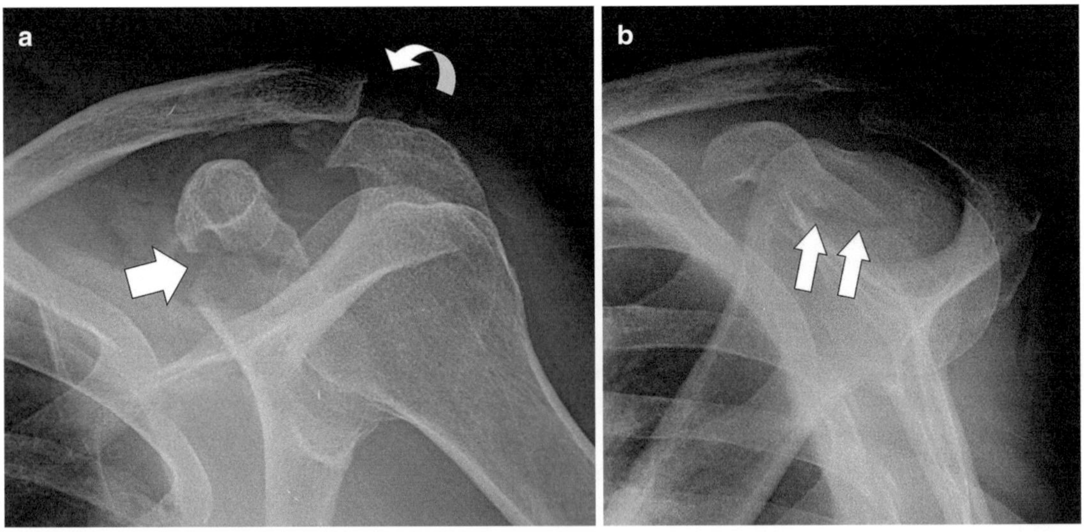

Fig. 9.8 Coracoid fracture, type 1. (**a**) Frontal radiograph shows cortical disruption near the base of the coracoid process (arrow). There is also a type 3 AC separation (curved arrow). (**b**) The scapular Y-view offers a second opportunity to observe this fracture (arrows) since it is often obscured in the frontal projection owing to bony overlap

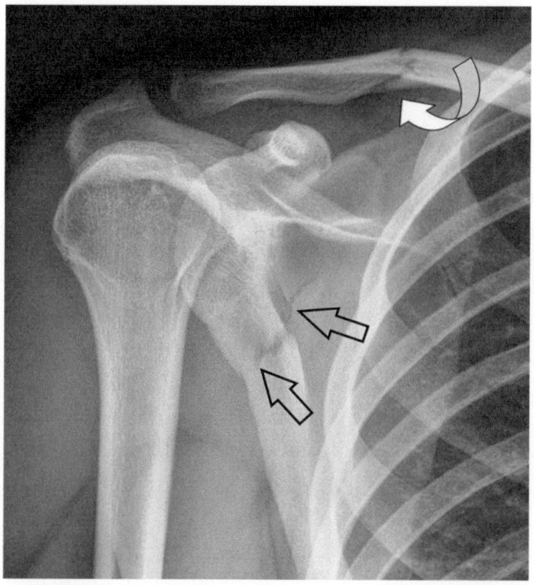

Fig. 9.9 Scapular fracture, extra-articular type. Extra-articular fractures (arrows) are frequently associated with concomitant injuries of the clavicle (curved arrow) and acromioclavicular joint

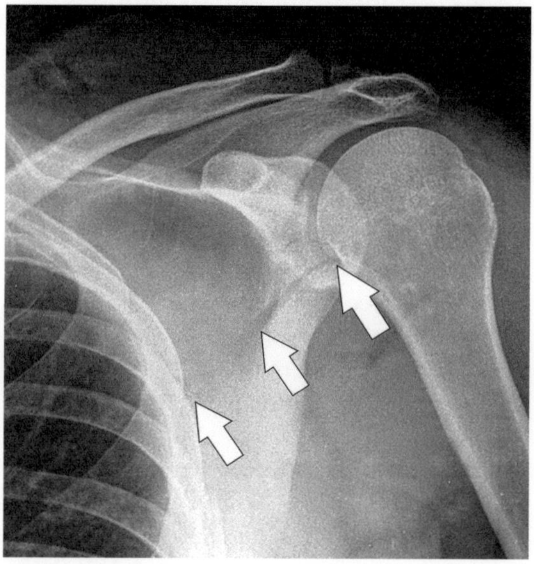

Fig. 9.10 Scapular fracture, intra-articular type. Fractures that involve the glenoid fossa and rim are considered intra-articular. The location of the fracture in the fossa is useful for its characterization. This patient has an Ideberg type 4 fracture extending from the fossa to the medial border

the medial border. Type 5 is a type 4 with separation of the glenoid. Type 6 is a comminuted fracture.

Approximately 25–43% of scapular fractures are not detected initially [29]. Scapular fractures are frequently associated with other injuries to the rib, clavicle, spine, extremities, lung, vascular structures, and brachial plexus or central nervous system. These injuries have been reported in 81–98% of scapular fractures [24, 30]. 3DCT is optimal for evaluating these fractures since it reliably identifies extension to the superior, medial, and lateral borders which are clinically relevant [31].

9.5.2.3 Ultrasound Findings

Ultrasound has been useful for diagnosing occult coracoid fractures but otherwise is not generally employed for assessment of this bone [32].

9.5.2.4 MR Findings

MRI allows simultaneous inspection of the bone and the ligaments of the shoulder girdle but is best reserved as a follow-up study after the osseous injuries have been ascertained acutely. It is useful for the evaluation of compartment syndrome of the scapula.

9.5.3 Postoperative Imaging

The majority of scapular fractures are treated conservatively but because closed reduction is not possible malalignment is a common outcome. Intra-articular fractures that are complex do well with surgery [33, 34]. The goal is to restore stability to the glenoid when fractures are displaced more than 1 cm or more than 25% of the articular surface is involved. Scapular neck fractures may be repaired if medially displaced more than 1 cm or angulated more than 40°.

9.6 Glenohumeral Joint

9.6.1 Pertinent Imaging Findings

The glenohumeral joint is a spheroidal joint that has the distinction of being the most mobile articulation in the body. The range of motion afforded by this joint is related to the disproportionate sizes of the articulating surfaces and the relative lack of osseous constriction. What this joint has in mobility, however, it lacks in stability. It is the most commonly dislocated joint in the skeleton with 50% of dislocations affecting this articulation [35]. Reportedly, shoulder dislocations occur at a rate of 1–2% in the general population and have an incidence of as high as 7% in selected groups of athletes [36]. Anterior dislocations are most common. Posterior dislocations are often difficult to diagnose. Inferior dislocations, referred to as luxatio erecta, are caused by either hyperabduction of the arm or a direct blow against the length of the arm with the shoulder maximally abducted. Superior dislocations are rare and caused by forces directed cephalad along an adducted arm.

Evaluation of trauma usually begins with a three- or four-view radiographic series that include an AP, oblique AP (Grashey), lateral Y, and axillary projections. It is generally recommended that the AP view be performed with the arm in neutral position or internally rotated, and the Grashey view be performed with the humerus externally rotated to allow a more complete depiction of the humeral head. Internal rotation depicts the anterior and posterior articular surfaces and brings the lesser tuberosity cortex into profile. External rotation, on the other hand, brings the greater tuberosity into full profile and enables much of the medial articular surface to be visualized. An advantage of the Grashey view over the AP shoulder projection is that it eliminates the overlap of the glenoid rim and the humeral joint. The nearly spherical head articulates with the glenoid fossa much like a golf ball sitting on a tee. The axial view is optimal in showing subtle decentering of the humerus that may not be detectable on other radiographic projections and to depict hypertrophic osseous changes in the glenoid rim that may herald an underlying labral abnormality.

When there is an injury of the glenohumeral joint, CT is an excellent imaging tool for further characterizing the humeral head and glenoid. However, it does not show the connective and cartilaginous tissues as well as MRI, even in the setting of arthrography. When MRI is necessary, it can depict injuries involving the joint capsule, labrum, articular cartilage, tendons and supporting ligaments, as well as marrow edema that are associated with bone contusions and occult fractures.

9.6.2 Anterior Glenohumeral Joint Dislocation

9.6.2.1 Definition

Anterior dislocation accounts for about 95% of all glenohumeral joint dislocations. Four types of anterior dislocations have been described depending on the location of the humeral head after it has become dislocated: subcoracoid, subclavicular, subacromial, and intrathoracic. The majority of anterior dislocations are caused by abduction with forced external rotation of the arm, although a direct blow to the back of the shoulder may be an occasional cause [37].

9.6.2.2 Radiographic and CT Findings

Radiographic diagnosis of an anterior dislocation is not difficult. The most common type of anterior dislocation is a subcoracoid dislocation characterized by anterior, inferior, and medial displacement of the humeral head beneath the coracoid process (Fig. 9.11). A subglenoid dislocation is characterized by anterior, inferior, and more medial displacement of the humeral head so that it comes to rest beneath the inferior rim of the glenoid. A subclavicular dislocation results in anterior, inferior, and even more medial displacement so that the humeral head terminates beneath the clavicle. Lastly, an intrathoracic anterior dislocation occurs when the humeral head penetrates an intercostal space.

The shoulder girdle must be scrutinized for certain injuries after a dislocation. A Hill-Sachs lesion, an impaction fracture of the posterolateral aspect of the humeral head, occurs when the humeral head becomes perched against the inferior aspect of the anterior glenoid rim [38]. It is detectable as a wedge-shaped or concave defect in the posterolateral aspect of the head when it is internally rotated. It is best depicted on an AP shoulder view but a Stryker notch view is also

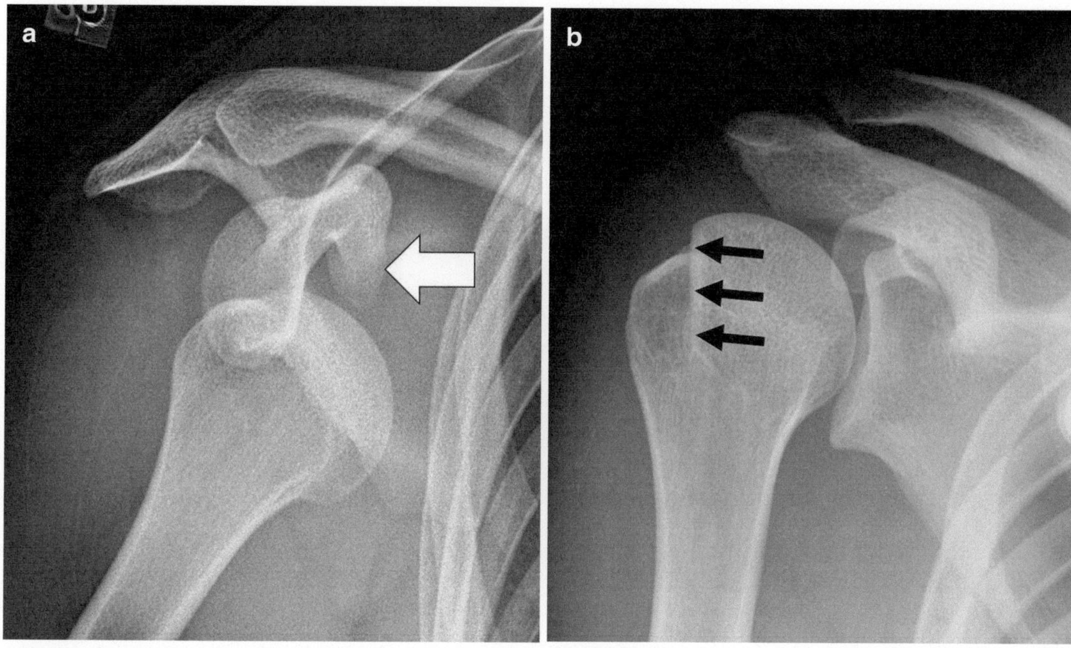

Fig. 9.11 Anterior glenohumeral joint dislocation. (**a**) The humeral head has dislocated anteriorly from the glenoid fossa and is located beneath the coracoid process (arrow). The subcoracoid type of anterior dislocation is the most common type. (**b**) After reduction, a sclerotic linear abnormality (arrows) seen on an internally rotated view of the humerus defines the posteromedial border of the Hill-Sachs lesion

useful. If the defect is sufficiently large, a linear sclerotic band may be seen vertically oriented on the head which defines the posterior edge of the impaction fracture. CT is reliable for diagnosis and characterization. A Hill-Sachs lesion is differentiated from the normal trough by its more superior location [39].

In about 8% of patients, a concomitant fracture of the anteroinferior glenoid rim (osseous Bankart lesion) occurs but the reported incidence has been as high as 31% (Fig. 9.12) [40]. Close scrutiny on AP and lateral radiographs is required since the fragment of bone may be quite small but a well-positioned lateral view is most optimal. An uncommon avulsion fracture may occur at the humeral attachment of the inferior glenohumeral ligament referred to as a BHAGL (bony humeral avulsion of the glenohumeral ligament) lesion (Fig. 9.13). An osteochondral defect of the glenoid has also been associated with anterior dislocations and is usually occult unless large [41].

About 15–25% of anterior dislocations are associated with a fracture of the greater tuberosity which can be displaced or comminuted (Fig. 9.14) [40]. Another 2% of dislocations are associated with a fracture of the surgical neck of the humerus, scapular body, acromion process, and clavicle.

9.6.2.3 Ultrasound Findings

Sonography is a useful modality for evaluating the rotator cuff in patients with shoulder instability and for identifying Hill-Sachs lesions but is overall inferior to MRI for characterization of osseous lesions, capsular and ligamentous injuries, and labral tears [42, 43].

9.6.2.4 MR Findings

MRI has become indispensable for the evaluation of shoulder instability [44]. Acute dislocations are characterized by bone marrow edema surrounding a Hill-Sachs lesion and in the anterior glenoid rim as well. Pathologic entities that are occult or not easily seen on radiographs or CT include avulsions and tears of the subscapularis tendon, stripping of the capsule, and soft-tissue Bankart

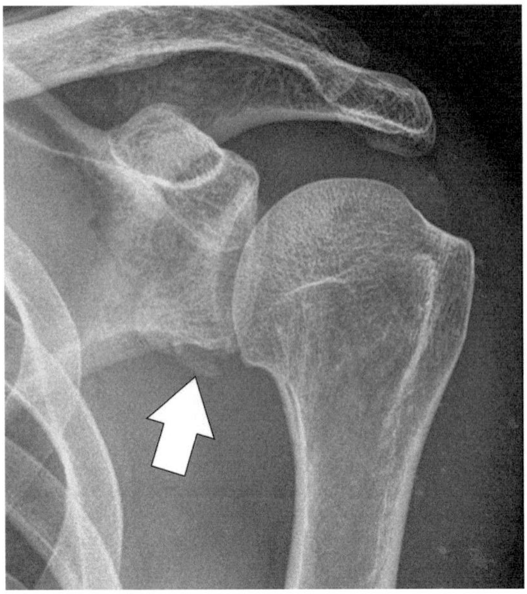

Fig. 9.12 Osseous Bankart lesion. There is a displaced fragment of bone arising from the anteromedial aspect of the glenoid rim (arrow). The size of the fragment correlates with the degree of instability and if more than 25% of the articular surface is involved surgical repair with the Latarjet-Bristow (coracoid transfer) procedure

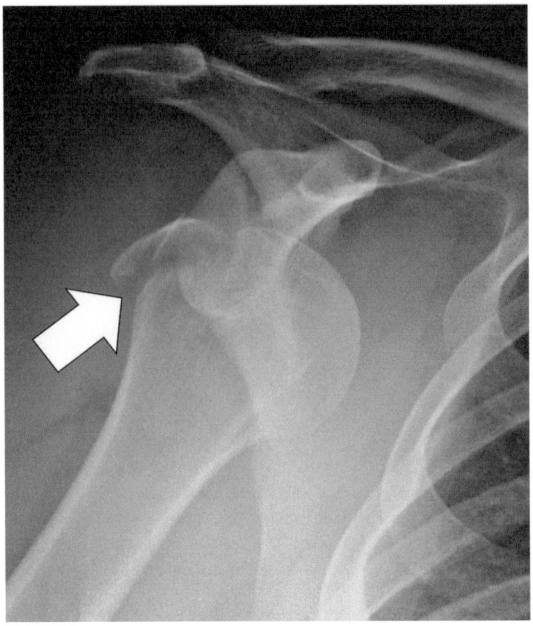

Fig. 9.14 Anterior shoulder dislocation with greater tuberosity fracture. As the humeral head dislocates anteriorly, the force of impaction against the anterior glenoid rim can produce a fracture through the greater tuberosity (arrow) which often is displaced or comminuted

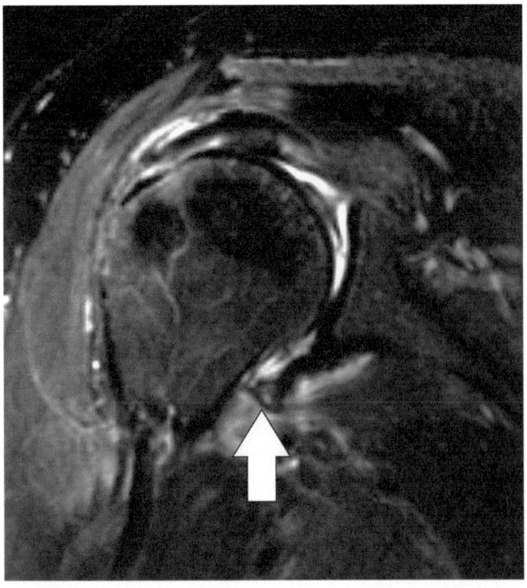

Fig. 9.13 Bony humeral avulsion of the glenohumeral ligament (BHAGL) lesion. Coronal T2-weighted MR image shows an avulsed fragment of bone (arrow) arising from the humeral attachment of the anterior band of the inferior glenohumeral ligament. This lesion may mimic an osseous Bankart lesion on radiographs

lesions, defined as an avulsion of the anterior labrum by the anterior band of the inferior glenohumeral ligament associated with disruption of the anterior periosteum. Bankart variants with the acronyms HAGL, ALPSA (anterior labroligamentous periosteal sleeve avulsion), and GLAD (glenoid labral articular disruption) lesions are best characterized with MR arthrography [45].

9.6.3 Posterior Glenohumeral Joint Dislocation

9.6.3.1 Definition

Posterior dislocations are much less common than anterior dislocations accounting for less than 5% of glenohumeral dislocations [46]. The mechanism of injury is either a fall on an outstretched hand or a direct trauma to a flexed, adducted, and internally rotated shoulder which forces the humeral head posteriorly. There are three types of posterior shoulder dislocations. Nearly all, about 98%, are the subacromial type.

The posterior subglenoid and subspinous types are uncommon. Bilateral dislocations are typically associated with seizures.

9.6.3.2 Radiographic and CT Findings

The radiographic features of posterior dislocations often are subtle so that over one-half of dislocations are still missed on initial inspection [47]. When the humeral head dislocates posteriorly, the stretched anterior musculature pulls it back forcing it to impact against the posterior glenoid rim. This creates a wedge-shaped impaction, referred to as a trough lesion, in the anteromedial aspect of the humeral head that is similar to a Hill-Sachs lesion (Fig. 9.15) [48]. It appears as a vertically oriented dense linear band that parallels the medial cortex of the humeral head on internally rotated frontal radiographs of the shoulder. An axillary view is useful in characterizing the size of the lesion. The incidence of a trough lesion has been estimated to occur in 29–75% of all dislocations [48, 49]. Reverse osseous Bankart lesions are generally difficult to detect radiographically and usually require CT for confirmation (Fig. 9.16).

There are several important radiographic signs that are associated with posterior shoulder dislocations [50]. These radiographic observations underscore the difficulty in making this diagnosis (Fig. 9.17). The *lightbulb* sign is a persistently internally rotated arm on all views of a shoulder series when the head is perched on the glenoid. The *rim* sign indicates a widened glenohumeral joint exceeding 6 mm in width. The *crescent* (absent half-moon) sign is absence of the normal overlap between the glenoid and humeral head. A disrupted scapulohumeral arch indicates humeral head subluxation.

A lesser tuberosity fracture (25% incidence) (Fig. 9.18) and humeral head fracture (10% incidence) are two additional observations that should elicit a search for other indicators of a posterior dislocation [48].

9.6.3.3 Ultrasound Findings

Sonography has a limited role in patients with acute posterior shoulder instability.

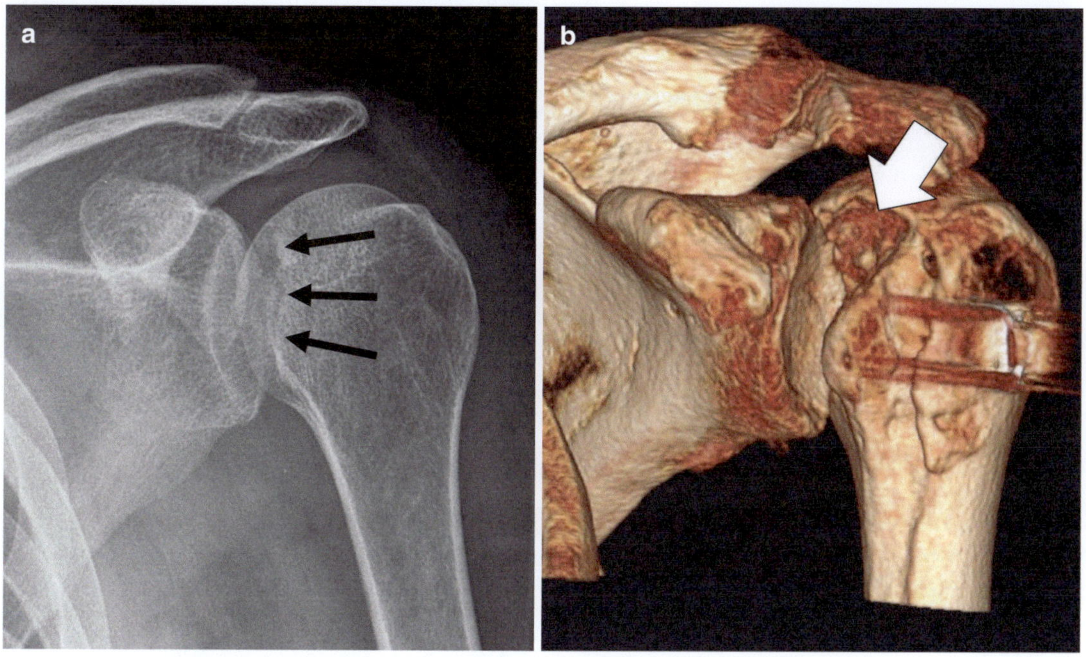

Fig. 9.15 Trough lesions in posterior glenohumeral joint dislocations. (**a**) This patient shows a posteriorly dislocated humerus with an impaction fracture in the anterior surface of the humeral head manifested as a linear vertically oriented area of sclerosis (arrows). (**b**) A 3D CT image in another patient shows the effect of a chronic dislocation with the formation of a pseudoarthrosis with widening of the trough lesion (arrow) as it toggles on the posterior glenoid rim

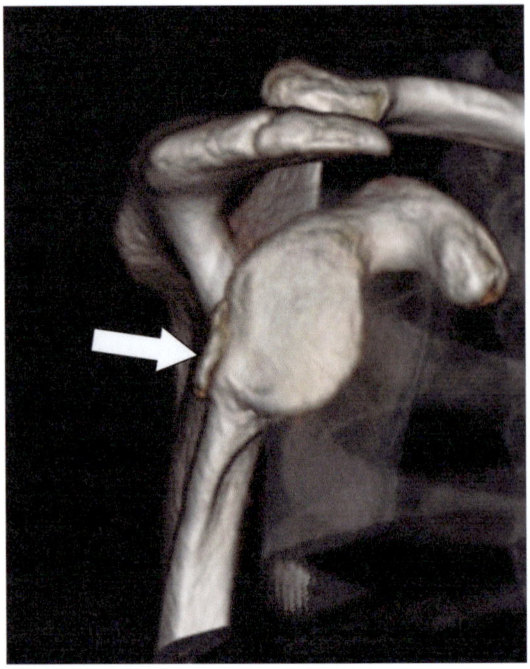

Fig. 9.16 Reverse osseous Bankart lesion. A disarticulated 3D CT image of the scapula shows a fracture of the posterior glenoid rim with a displaced fragment (arrow) in a patient who had sustained a posterior glenohumeral joint dislocation

9.6.3.4 MR Findings

The presence of bone marrow edema in the anterior humeral head is consistent with an acute impaction injury [51]. A reverse soft-tissue Bankart lesion represents damage to the posterior labrum that occurs either when the humeral head displaces posteriorly or when it impacts the posterior glenoid rim. The labrum may appear detached or fragmented, and the capsule may be stripped or torn.

9.6.4 Postoperative Imaging

The focus of this section is treatment of fractures that have been sustained during a glenohumeral joint dislocation. 3DCT and MRI are both useful for assessing the size of glenoid and humeral defects [52, 53].

Glenoid defects that exceed 25% of the fossa usually require surgical management for best results. The Latarjet-Bristow procedure is performed in patients with large osseous Bankart fractures and has been popularized owing to excellent outcomes and a low risk for recurrence [54]. In this open surgical proce-

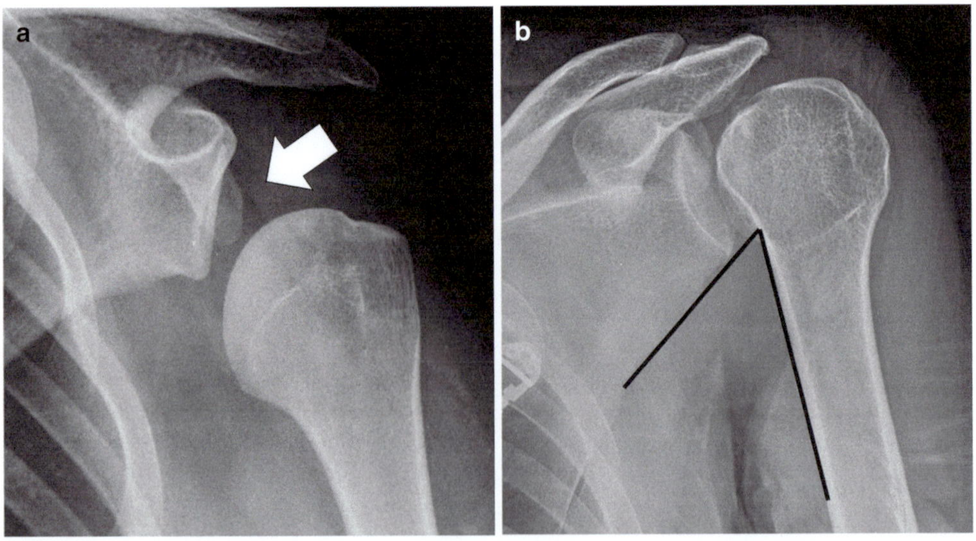

Fig. 9.17 Radiographic signs associated with a posterior shoulder dislocation. (**a**) A rim sign is present when the glenohumeral joint measures greater than 6 mm in width (arrow). The humeral head does not have to sublux inferiorly or superiorly for this sign to be present. (**b**) This scapulohumeral arch is formed by the smooth transition of the cortical margins formed by the lateral scapula, inferior glenoid neck, surgical neck of the humerus, and medial margin of the humeral shaft. In this patient, there is a break in the arch producing an angular deformity (black lines). Note that there is a rim sign as well

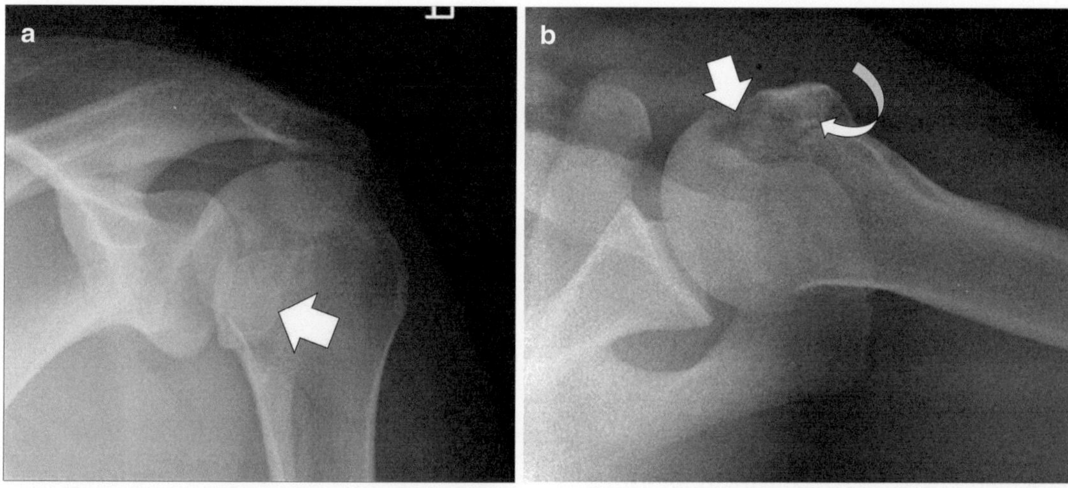

Fig. 9.18 Lesser tuberosity fracture in a posterior shoulder dislocation. (**a**) Frontal radiograph shows that the humeral head is perched against the posterior glenoid rim and there is double density seen in the region of the lesser tuberosity (arrow). (**b**) The axillary view shows a prominent trough defect (arrow) just medial to the lesser tuberosity fracture (curved arrow)

dure, a portion of the coracoid process is harvested as a bone graft and then transferred to the anterior glenoid along with the attached muscles, thus simultaneously replacing the absent bone and providing an additional muscular strut which stabilizes the anterior capsule and reinforces the subscapularis tendon. Patients with large posterior glenoid defects can be effectively treated using the McLaughlin procedure which transfers the lesser tuberosity with the attached subscapularis tendon into the defect [55].

Patients with large impaction defects of the humeral head show a dramatically lower incidence of recurrence with surgery. Several procedures have been effective including transferring the infraspinatus tendon (remplissage procedure), allograft humeral head reconstruction, and partial resurfacing arthroplasty [56]. Allograft reconstruction utilizing cryopreserved femoral head allografts or bone blocks has been performed with either anterior or posterior defects when the defect involves greater than 40% of the articular surface. In severe cases, total arthroplasty may be the option to prevent future dislocations.

9.7 Proximal Humerus

9.7.1 Pertinent Imaging Findings

In order to evaluate the humeral head and proximal shaft, shoulder radiographs performed with both internal and external rotation are necessary. The proximal humerus is divided into four anatomic regions: the head, anatomic neck, surgical neck, and greater and lesser tuberosities. When a fracture occurs in the surgical neck, the axillary view is most useful for demonstrating both angulation and displacement. Complex fractures often require additional imaging with CT to further assess fracture orientation, displacement and rotation of bone fragments, angulation, and impaction/overriding for treatment and preoperative planning. When the rotator cuff attachment is involved, MRI or ultrasound may be useful for follow-up.

9.7.2 Pathologic Conditions

9.7.2.1 Definition

People who are in their sixth and seventh decades of life are susceptible to fractures of the proximal humerus [57]. In this age group, the most common mechanism of injury is a fall on the outstretched hand. In younger people, more severe trauma like those that occur from a motor vehicle accident is responsible for humeral fractures. The muscular insertions are noteworthy since the actions of the rotator cuff, pectoralis, latissimus dorsi, and teres major muscles can influence the degree and direction of displacement of osseous fragments.

9.7.2.2 Radiographic and CT Findings

Radiography is usually sufficient for diagnosis but CT is superior for fracture characterization particularly with 3D reconstruction. Isolated fractures of the greater (Fig. 9.19) and lesser tuberosities are uncommon and may be associated with rotator cuff insufficiency. The surgical neck is the most common location for fractures in the proximal humerus (Fig. 9.20). Frequently, these fractures are impacted and extend to the greater tuberosity. Anterior and medial displacement of the shaft may occur in about 15–20% of patients owing to the action of the pectoralis major muscle while the rest usually are not significantly displaced [58]. Fractures of the anatomic neck are less common but can be complicated by avascular necrosis from disruption of the blood supply to the humeral head.

The Neer classification is a widely used classification because it provides predictive value to treatment plans [59]. The classification takes into account the number of fragments and the degree of angulation and/or displacement, roughly following the anatomic lines of epiphyseal union. Displacement from its anatomic position by more than 1 cm or angulation by more than 45° is significant. About 80% of fractures under this classification are one-part fractures without significant displacement or angulation. Another 10% are two-part fractures with displacement of shaft anteromedially with respect to the neck. Three-part fractures constitute about 3% of fractures with displacement of the surgical neck and one of the tuberosities but as long as one of the tubercles remains attached to the humeral head, the blood supply to the head is likely to remain intact. Rotator cuff tears are common with this pattern of injury as well. About 4% of fractures are four-part fractures and osteonecrosis is a common complication.

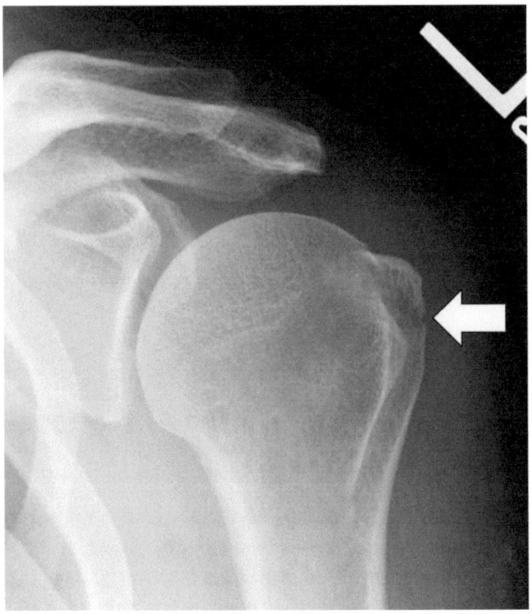

Fig. 9.19 Avulsion fracture of the greater tuberosity. An avulsion fracture of the greater tuberosity may be subtle if not displaced. An externally rotated view that depicts the footplate is optimal. When displaced, it is important to measure the separation since displacement can contribute to rotator cuff insufficiency

9.7.2.3 Ultrasound Findings

Sonography has a role in the diagnosis of humeral fractures in the neonatal period but in adults it has limited application in osteoporotic patients and for evaluation of occult fractures of the tuberosity [60].

9.7.2.4 MR Findings

MRI is useful for further assessment of symptomatic patients with an occult proximal humeral fracture [61]. These include two important groups of patients: adolescents with Salter-Harris injuries and severely osteoporotic patients. MRI depicts areas of marrow edema and areas of disrupted trabeculation.

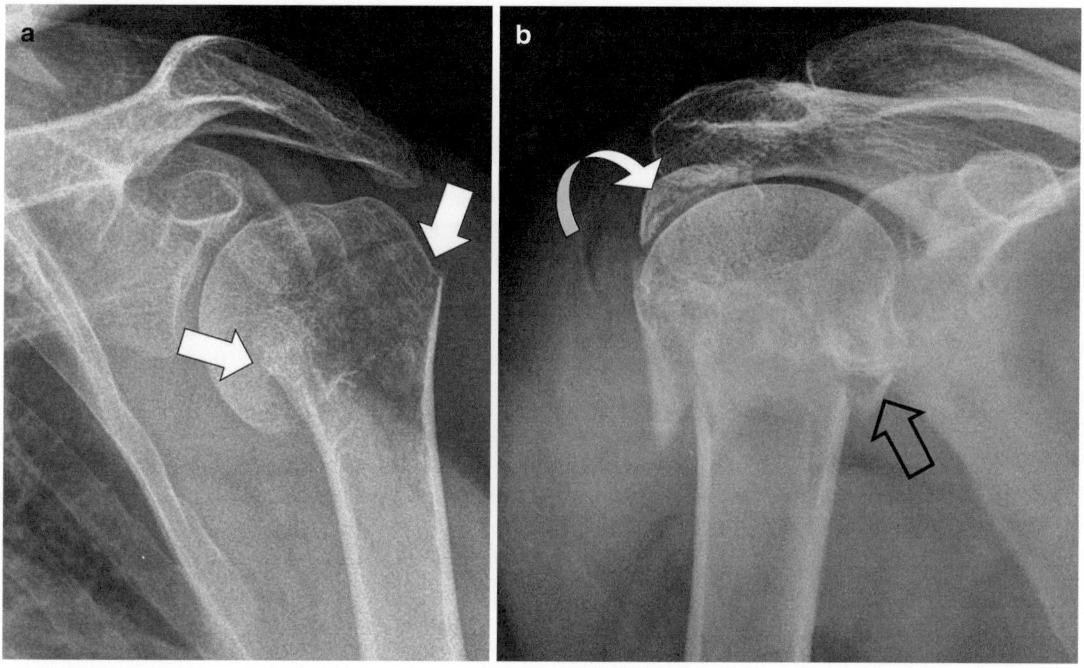

Fig. 9.20 Humerus fracture, surgical neck. (**a**) Fractures located at the surgical neck of the humerus are frequently impacted and can extend to the greater tuberosity or lesser tuberosity. (**b**) When multiple fragments are affected, the Neer classification is useful. This patient had a lesser tuberosity fracture (arrow) and a displaced greater tuberosity fragment (curved arrow), in addition to a surgical neck fracture

9.7.3 Postoperative Imaging

Radiographic findings of a greater tuberosity fractures repair is much like a rotator cuff repair. There are a variety of open reduction and internal fixation techniques using intramedullary devices for surgical neck two-part fractures. Three- and four-part fractures in elderly patients usually involve either a hemiarthroplasty, reverse shoulder arthroplasty, or complete conventional arthroplasty [62, 63].

References

1. Sheehan SE, Gaviola G, Sacks A, Gordon R, Shi LL, Smith SE. Traumatic shoulder injuries: a force mechanism analysis of complex injuries to the shoulder girdle and proximal humerus. AJR Am J Roentgenol. 2013;201:W409–24.
2. Sankarankutty M, Turner BW. Fractures of the clavicle. Injury. 1975;7:101–6.
3. Madsen ET. Fractures of the extremities in the newborn. Acta Obstet Gynecol Scand. 1955;34:41–7.
4. Allman FL. Fractures and ligamentous injuries of the clavicle and its articulations. J Bone Joint Surg Am. 1967;49:774–84.
5. Ridpath CA, Wilson AJ. Shoulder and humerus trauma. Semin Musculoskelet Radiol. 2000;4:151–70.
6. Neer CS II. Fractures of the distal third of the clavicle. Clin Orthop. 1968;58:43–50.
7. Mavrogenis AF, Mitsiokapa EA, Kanellopoulos AD, Ruggieri P, Papagelopoulos PJ. Birth fracture of the clavicle. Adv Neonatal Care. 2011;11:328–31.
8. Barger WL, Marcus RE, Ittleman FP. Late thoracic outlet syndrome secondary to pseudoarthrosis of the clavicle. J Trauma. 1984;24:847–59.
9. Donnelly TD, Macfarlane RJ, Nagy MT, Ralte P, Waseem M. Fractures of the clavicle: an overview. Open Orthop J. 2013;7:329–33.
10. Renger RJ, Roukema GR, Reurings JC, Raams PM, Font J, Verleisdonk EJ. The clavicle hook plate for Neer type II lateral clavicle fractures. J Orthop Trauma. 2009;23:570–4.
11. Sewell MD, Al-Hadithy N, Le Leu A, Lambert SM. Instability of the sternoclavicular joint: current concepts in classification, treatment and outcomes. Bone Joint J. 2013;95-B:721–31.
12. Gove N, Ebraheim NA, Glass E. Posterior sternoclavicular dislocations: a review of management and complications. Am J Orthop. 2006;35:132–6.

13. Ferri M, Finlay K, Popowich T, Jurriaans E, Friedman L. Sonographic examination of the acromioclavicular and sternoclavicular joints. J Clin Ultrasound. 2005;33:345–55.
14. Emberg LA, Potter HG. Radiographic evaluation of the acromioclavicular and sternoclavicular joints. Clin Sport Med. 2003;22:255–75.
15. Balcik BJ, Monseau AJ, Krantz W. Evaluation and treatment of sternoclavicular, clavicular, and acromioclavicular injuries. Prim Care. 2013;40:911–23.
16. Petersson CJ, Redlnd-Johnell I. Radiographic joint space in normal acromioclavicular joint. Acta Orthop Scand. 1983;54:431–3.
17. Neviaser RJ. Injuries to the clavicle and acromioclavicular joint. Orthop Clin North Am. 1987;18:433–8.
18. Melenevsky Y, Yablon CM, Ramappa A, Hochman MG. Clavicle and acromioclavicular joint injuries: a review of imaging, treatment, and complications. Skelet Radiol. 2011;40:831–42.
19. Alyas F, Curtis M, Speed C, Saifuddin A, Connell D. MR imaging appearances of acromioclavicular joint dislocation. Radiographics. 2008;28:463–79.
20. Nemec U, Oberleitner G, Nemec SF, Gruber M, Weber M, Czerny C, et al. MRI versus radiography of acromioclavicular joint dislocation. AJR Am J Roentgenol. 2011;197:968–73.
21. Modi CS, Beazley J, Zywiel MG, Lawrence TM, Veillette CJ. Controversies relating to the management of acromioclavicular joint dislocations. Bone Joint J. 2013;95-B:1595–602.
22. Babhulkar A, Pawaskar A. Acromioclavicular joint dislocations. Curr Rev Musculoskeletal Med. 2014;7:33–9.
23. Yammine K. The prevalence of os acromiale: a systematic review and meta-analysis. Clin Anat. 2014;27:610–21.
24. Imatani RJ. Fractures of the scapula: a review of 53 fractures. J Trauma. 1975;15:473–8.
25. Armitage BM, Wijdicks CA, Tarkin IS, Schroder LK, Marek DJ, Zlowodzki M, et al. Mapping of scapular fractures with three-dimensional computed tomography. J Bone Joint Surg Am. 2009;91:2222–8.
26. Ogawa K, Yoshida A, Takahashi M, Ui M. Fractures of the coracoid process. J Bone Joint Surg Br. 1997;79:17–9.
27. van Oostveen DP, Temmerman OP, Burger BJ, van Noort A, Robinson M. Glenoid fractures: a review of pathology, classification, treatment and results. Acta Orthop Belg. 2014;80:88–98.
28. Ideberg R, Grevsten S, Larsson S. Epidemiology of scapular fractures. Incidence and classification of 338 fractures. Acta Orthop Scand. 1995;66:395–7.
29. Harris RD, Harris JH. The prevalence and significance of missed scapular fractures in blunt chest trauma. AJR Am J Roentgenol. 1988;151:747–50.
30. Thompson DA, Flynn TC, Miller PW, Fischer RP. The significance of scapular fractures. J Trauma. 1985;25:974–7.
31. Audigé L, Kellam JF, Lambert S, Madsen JE, Babst R, Andermahr J, et al. The AO Foundation and Orthopaedic Trauma Association (AO/OTA) scapula fracture classification system: focus on body involvement. J Shoulder Elb Surg. 2014;23:189–96.
32. Botchu R, Lee KJ, Bianchi S. Radiographically undetected coracoid fractures diagnosed by sonography. Report of seven cases. Skelet Radiol. 2012;41:693–8.
33. Anavian J, Gauger EM, Schroder LK, Wijdicks CA, Cole PA. Surgical and functional outcomes after operative management of complex and displaced intra-articular glenoid fractures. J Bone Joint Surg Am. 2012;94:645–53.
34. Cole PA, Gauger EM, Herrera DA, Anavian J, Tarkin IS. Radiographic follow-up of 84 operatively treated scapula neck and body fractures. Injury. 2012;43:327–33.
35. Gyftopoulos S, Bencardino J, Palmer WE. MR imaging of the shoulder: first dislocation versus chronic instability. Semin Musculoskelet Radiol. 2012;16:286–95.
36. Hovelius L. Incidence of shoulder dislocation in Sweden. Clin Orthop. 1982;166:127–31.
37. Bencardino JT, Gyftopoulos S, Palmer WE. Imaging in anterior glenohumeral instability. Radiology. 2013;269:323–37.
38. Provencher MT, Frank RM, Leclere LE, Metzger PD, Ryu JJ, Bernhardson A, et al. The Hill-Sachs lesion: diagnosis, classification, and management. J Am Acad Orthop Surg. 2012;20:242–52.
39. Richards RD, Sartoris DJ, Pathria MN, Resnick D. Hill-Sachs lesion and normal humeral groove: MR imaging features allowing their differentiation. Radiology. 1994;190:665–8.
40. Kummel BM. Fractures of the glenoid causing chronic dislocation of the shoulder. Clin Orthop. 1970;69:189–91.
41. Yu JS, Greenway G, Resnick D. Osteochondral defect of the glenoid fossa: cross-sectional imaging features. Radiology. 1998;206:35–40.
42. Pavic R, Margetic P, Bensic M, Brnadic RL. Diagnostic value of US, MR and MR arthrography in shoulder instability. Injury. 2013;44(Suppl 3):S26–32.
43. Cicak N, Bilic R, Delimar D. Hill-Sachs lesion in recurrent shoulder dislocation: sonographic detection. J Ultrasound Med. 1998;17:557–60.
44. Zlatkin MB, Sanders TG. Magnetic resonance imaging of the glenoid labrum. Radiol Clin N Am. 2013;51:279–97.
45. Omoumi P, Teixeira P, Lecouvet F, Chung CB. Glenohumeral joint instability. J Magn Reson Imaging. 2011;33:2–16.
46. Shah N, Tung GA. Imaging signs of posterior glenohumeral instability. AJR Am J Roentgenol. 2009;192:730–5.
47. Arndt JH, Sears AD. Posterior dislocation of the shoulder. AJR Am J Roentgenol. 1965;94:639–45.
48. Cisternino SJ, Rogers LF, Stufflebam BC, Kruglik GD. The trough line: a radiographic sign of posterior shoulder dislocation. AJR Am J Roentgenol. 1978;130:951–4.

49. Mok DW, Fogg AJ, Hokan R, Bayley JI. The diagnostic value of arthroscopy in glenohumeral instability. J Bone Joint Surg Br. 1990;72:698–700.
50. Kowalsky MS, Levine WN. Traumatic posterior glenohumeral dislocation: classification, pathoanatomy, diagnosis, and treatment. Orthop Clin North Am. 2008;39:519–33.
51. Saupe N, White LM, Bleakney R, Schweitzer ME, Recht MP, Jost B, et al. Acute traumatic posterior shoulder dislocation: MR findings. Radiology. 2008;248:185–93.
52. Lee RK, Griffith JF, Tong MM, Sharma N, Yung P. Glenoid bone loss: assessment with MR imaging. Radiology. 2013;267:496–502.
53. Griffith JF, Yung PS, Antonio GE, Tsang PH, Ahuja AT, Chan KM. CT compared with arthroscopy in quantifying glenoid bone loss. AJR Am J Roentgenol. 2007;189:1490–3.
54. Bhatia S, Frank RM, Ghodadra NS, Hsu AR, Romeo AA, Bach BR Jr, et al. The outcomes and surgical techniques of the latarjet procedure. Arthroscopy. 2014;30:227–35.
55. Kokkalis ZT, Mavrogenis AF, Ballas EG, Papanastasiou J, Papagelopoulos PJ. Modified McLaughlin technique for neglected locked posterior dislocation of the shoulder. Orthopedics. 2013;36:e912–6.
56. Giles JW, Elkinson I, Ferreira LM, Faber KJ, Boons H, Litchfield R, et al. Moderate to large engaging Hill-Sachs defects: an in vitro biomechanical comparison of the remplissage procedure, allograft humeral head reconstruction, and partial resurfacing arthroplasty. J Shoulder Elb Surg. 2012;21:1142–51.
57. Roux A, Decroocq L, El Batti S, Bonnevialle N, Moineau G, Trojani C, et al. Epidemiology of proximal humerus fractures managed in a trauma center. Orthop Traumatol Surg Res. 2012;98:715–9.
58. Neer CS II. Displaced proximal humeral fractures. I. Classification and evaluation. J Bone Joint Surg Am. 1970;52:1077–89.
59. Neer CS II. Displaced proximal humeral fractures. II. Treatment of three-part and four-part displacement. J Bone Joint Surg Am. 1970;52:1090–103.
60. Rutten MJ, Jager GJ, de Waal Malefijt MC, Blickman JG. Double line sign: a helpful sonographic sign to detect occult fractures of the proximal humerus. Eur Radiol. 2007;17:762–7.
61. Berger PE, Ofstein RA, Jackson DW, Morrison DS, Silvino N, Amador R. MRI demonstration of radiographically occult fractures: what have we been missing? Radiographics. 1989;9:407–36.
62. Thanasas C, Kontakis G, Angoules A, Limb D, Giannoudis P. Treatment of proximal humerus fractures with locking plates: a systematic review. J Shoulder Elb Surg. 2009;18:837–44.
63. Bufquin T, Hersan A, Hubert L, Massin P. Reverse shoulder arthroplasty for the treatment of three- and four-part fractures of the proximal humerus in the elderly: a prospective review of 43 cases with a short-term follow-up. J Bone Joint Surg Br. 2007;89:516–20.

Imaging Diagnosis of Shoulder Arthropathy

10

Mingqian Huang and Mark Schweitzer

10.1 Introduction

The shoulder is a quite interesting joint. It is highly mobile and maintains an exquisite balance in order to maintain its range of motion. In fact, two of the most common disorders of the shoulder (adhesive capsulitis and instability) are demonstrative of alterations in the balance. Articular disorder also may be the end result of this loss of stability regulation. Additionally, articular disorders may be the presentation of loss of motion.

Also interesting is that articular disorders of the shoulder are proportionally less common in the shoulder than the other major joints. Although various theories have been proposed for this incongruence, none of them are terribly satisfying.

Nonetheless, these disorders are far from infrequent, and are debilitating, and as mentioned above can mimic clinically more acute shoulder disorders.

In the following pages we discuss arthropathies of the shoulder. We discuss how osteoarthritis presents on imaging, differently than other large joints such as knee or hip. Differently, since secondary osteoarthritis is much common in the shoulder, this secondary osteoarthritis can be related to cuff tear or instability.

Next, we discuss infections of the shoulder. As with any monoarthropathy, we clinicians should keep this diagnosis in mind. We also should remember that disordered joints of any disease, especially those effected by rheumatoid, are predisposed to infections.

Following this we discuss the interrelationship of rheumatoid of the glenohumeral, acromioclavicular joints with each other and with the rotator cuff.

Perhaps the most interesting of the articular disorders of the shoulder are those related to crystals. Some of these are overwhelmingly more common in the shoulder (HADD), and others present with complex and unique imaging appearances, such as the Milwaukee shoulder.

10.2 Osteoarthritis

10.2.1 Definition

Osteoarthritis (OA) is the most common form of arthritis, and it is a leading cause of chronic disability in the elderly population [1]. More than half of people over 60 will have symptoms of osteoarthritis.

Altman et al. [2] defined OA as "a heterogeneous group of conditions that lead to joint symptoms and signs which are associated with defective integrity of articular cartilage, in

M. Huang (✉) · M. Schweitzer
Department of Radiology, Stony Brook University Hospital, Stony Brook School of Medicine, Stony Brook, NY, USA
e-mail: Mingqian.Huang@stonybrookmedicine.edu; Mark.Schweitzer@stonybrookmedicine.edu

J. T. Bencardino (ed.), *The Shoulder*, https://doi.org/10.1007/978-3-030-06240-8_10

addition to related changes in the underlying bone and at the joint margins." It is important to recognize the difference between idiopathic (primary) OA and OA that is related to an underlying condition (secondary). It is also important to recognize that it is becoming increasingly accepted that OA likely represents multiple different diseases with similar imaging appearances.

In terms of OA of the shoulder, primary OA was historically believed to be rare. However, Philip and Kattapuram [3] noted that primary OA on radiographic examination is seen in about 1 in 1000 individuals of advanced age and noted that the condition "may not be as rare as many observers have stated." OA could also occur secondarily, such as sequelae of chronic rotator cuff tears, fractures, dislocations, rheumatoid, CPPD arthropathy, avascular necrosis, or congenital skeletal variants and deformities [3].

In recent years, shoulder degenerative disease is becoming more recognized and at the same time therapeutic options for treatment are increasing, both medically and surgically. Hence, there is a need to develop systematic, reliable, and noninvasive means to accurately diagnose shoulder degenerative disease, especially at the early stages.

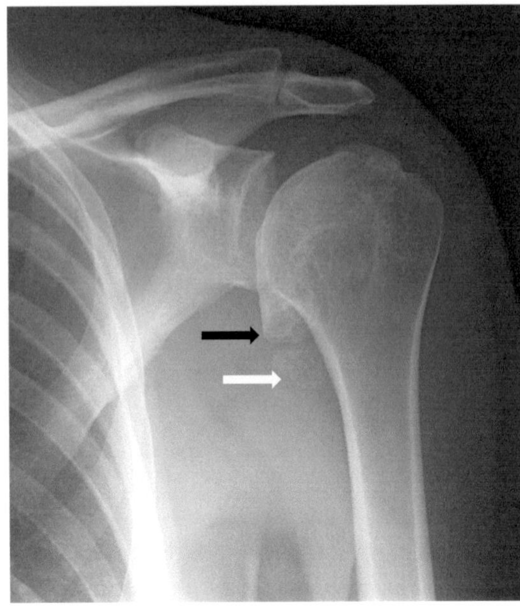

Fig. 10.1 Osteoarthritis. Frontal view of the left shoulder demonstrates a typical medial osteophyte of the anatomic neck of proximal left humerus, "beard-like" (black arrow) with an inferior intra-articular body (white arrow)

10.2.2 Radiographic and CT Findings

On radiographs, the findings of primary OA of the shoulder are similar to OA findings in large joints, elsewhere in the body. Noted are osteophytes, cartilage loss with space narrowing, occasional subchondral sclerosis, and infrequent cystic changes. Specifically, the marginal osteophytes tend to develop along the anatomic neck of the proximal humerus and are nearly always more prominent medially, often with a "beard-like" appearance (Fig. 10.1). In more advanced cases, the humeral head becomes pseudo-flattened (due to lateral humeral head osteophytes) and positioned posteriorly, due to the asymmetric joint space loss. There is occasional posterior glenoid subchondral cystic changes and even less frequent subchondral sclerosis.

In a study by Roger Kerr [4] and colleagues, they compared cadaveric specimens and patient radiographs to establish the pattern and distribution of degenerative alterations of the glenohumeral joint. They found that the most frequent degenerative abnormality was the formation of osteophytes along the articular margin of the humeral head at the line of attachment of the labrum to the glenoid. This is probably due to functional stress provided by capsular traction [5, 6]. However, routine radiographs tend to underestimate the degree of osteophyte formation involving both the humeral head and the glenoid [4]. This underestimation is true for all joints, however. The second degenerative-like finding in their study is focal or global eburnation of the articular surface of the humeral head. This is most evident in the middle and superior parts of the humeral head, consistent with that described by Neer [7]. They also found that the degree of enthesopathic change generally parallels that of osteophyte formation. Such changes consist predominantly of bony proliferation with occasional areas of pitting or cystic change, involving the

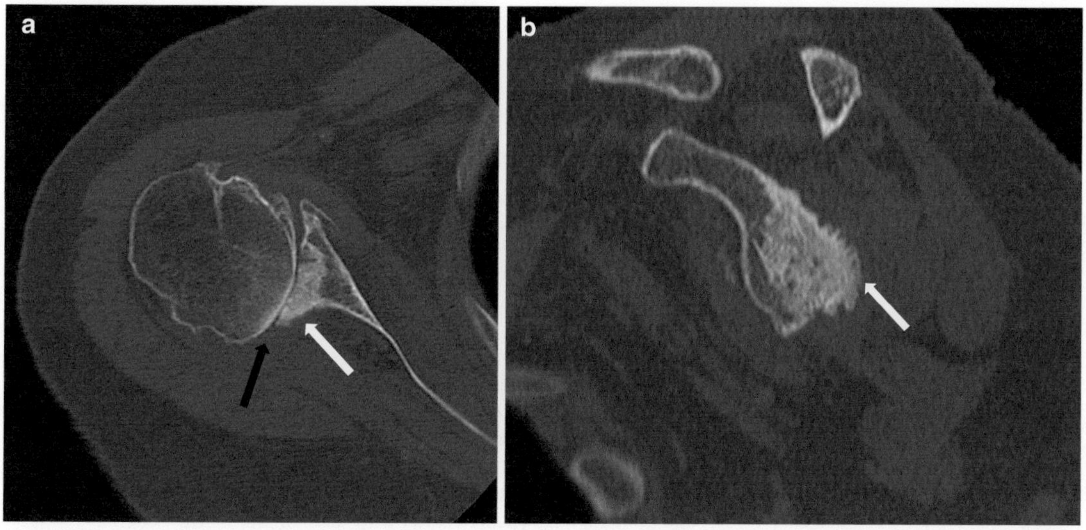

Fig. 10.2 Advanced osteoarthritis. Axial (**a**) and sagittal (**b**) reformatted images demonstrate posterior displacement of the humeral head over the glenoid (black arrow), joint-space loss, related subchondral sclerosis, and cystic changes at the posterior glenoid (white arrow)

anatomic neck and extending over the tuberosities and bicipital groove [4]. A strong association was found between the changes of OA and those related to deterioration of the rotator cuff [4]. This is likely related to epidemiologic overlap in the populations involved.

With multiplanar capability, CT scan can depict posterior glenoid wear and posterior humeral subluxation (Fig. 10.2) in primary degenerative joint disease (Fig. 10.2). CT is also useful in preoperative planning to assess glenoid bone stock and degree of posterior bone loss (Fig. 10.2) [8, 9].

10.2.3 MR Findings

Radiographic findings of glenohumeral joint degenerative changes are well recognized, though they tend to occur late in the course of the disease when therapeutic options are more limited and less effective. MR can provide information on early pre-structural changes, especially cartilage loss. MR imaging is also superior to plain radiograph in helping identify other causes that may cause patient chronic shoulder pain.

MR imaging with multiplanar capability and soft-tissue resolution depicts the chondral erosions, osteophyte formation, subchondral cysts, and sclerosis and synovitis in more detail. Central and posterior glenoid wear with sclerosis and cartilage loss is typically seen in shoulder OA. This is better seen on axial proton density (PD) and FS (fat-suppressed) PD fast spin-echo (FSE) images (Fig. 10.3). Humeral head sclerosis and cartilage loss are usually central or superior in glenohumeral osteoarthritis. Peripheral osteophytes projecting from the humeral head are directed inferiorly on coronal images. Glenoid peripheral osteophytes tend to involve the lower two-thirds of the glenohumeral joint. Subchondral cysts can be seen in both glenoid and humeral head. The inferior capsule may be enlarged and the anterior capsule contracted. Intra-articular bodies can frequently be seen in the subscapularis recess or within the biceps tendon sheath. A secondary chondromatosis is associated with full-thickness chondral loss of the humerus or glenoid. An intraosseous ganglion is a less common finding in degenerative OA.

Imaging of articular cartilage in the shoulder is challenging for MR imaging due to the deep shoulder joint, relatively thin glenoid cartilage, and difficulty placing the joint isocenter in the imaging system. But improvements have been made in contrast and resolution. Progress has

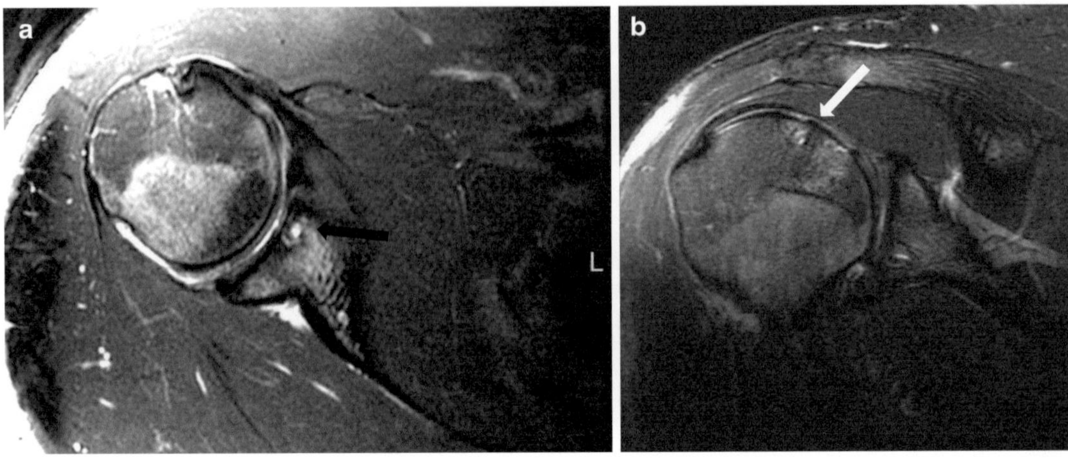

Fig. 10.3 Cartilage loss. Axial (**a**) and coronal oblique (**b**) fat-suppressed fluid-sensitive MR images demonstrate cartilage loss along the glenoid (black arrow) and humeral head (white arrow) with subchondral marrow edema

been made in understanding cartilage physiology and ability to detect proteoglycan and collagen loss.

MR is effective at assessing the degree of damage to cartilage and adjacent bone, and effectiveness of treatment. Arthroscopy is invasive, but the gold standard for monitoring cartilage damage in shoulder with optical resolution and ability to probe the cartilage surface. With the advancement of technology, more MR sequences have been developed to enable better evaluation of the glenoid cartilage. Cartilage volumes in the shoulder can be measured using 3D spoiled gradient-echo 3D-SPGR [10]. However, there are two main disadvantages of limited contrast between cartilages and fluid that outlines the surface defects and long scanning time. Steady-state free precession (SSFP) MR imaging has shown to be a promising method for cartilage imaging in the knee [11, 12].

Advanced MR imaging of articular cartilage composition takes advantage of the fact that articular cartilage is approximately 70% water and rest are type II collagen fibers and proteoglycans. Gadolinium-enhanced imaging has the potential to allow monitoring of glycosaminoglycan content within the cartilage [13, 14] and thus monitoring physiologic state of the cartilage repair. T2 mapping of T2 relaxation time of articular cartilage is a function of the water content of the tissue. Measurement of the spatial distribution of the T2 relaxation time may reveal areas of increased or decreased water content, correlating with cartilage damage. Sodium MR imaging has shown some promising results recently of imaging articular cartilage. This is based on the ability of sodium imaging to depict regions of proteoglycan depletion [15]. Another innovative physiologic imaging alternative is spin-lattice relaxation in the rotating (T1 rho). This technique exploits the low-frequency interactions between macromolecules and bulk water and has been applied to articular cartilage [16]. Ultrashort TE imaging has also demonstrated good delineation of cartilage lesions [17].

10.2.4 Ultrasound Findings

In shoulder osteoarthritis, the progressive disintegration of the articular surfaces leads to the formation and release of intra-articular loose bodies which, once freed into the joint cavity, can progressively worsen the damage to the joint surfaces. Osteochondral bodies usually remain trapped in the most dependent portions of the glenohumeral joint, such as the axillary pouch and the long head of the biceps tendon sheath.

Most of the intra-articular bodies appear as hyperechoic areas with posterior acoustic shadowing. In some cases, however, a thin layer of hypoechoic cartilage may be seen overlying the echogenic interface of the subchondral bone [18]. The size and position of a fragment can be reliably evaluated with US, but the exact number of fragments cannot always be established.

10.3 Rotator Cuff Arthropathy

10.3.1 Definition

Cuff deficient arthritis of the glenohumeral joint encompasses a number of pathologies including osteoarthritis without a competent rotator cuff, rheumatoid arthritis, degenerative joint disease secondary to failed rotator cuff repair, and cuff tear arthropathy (CTA).

Robert Adams first described the clinical findings of CTA in 1857. Charles Neer [19] coined the term "cuff tear arthropathy" in 1977 and went on to provide the first detailed description in 1983. It is characterized by a rotator cuff tear, proximal migration of the humerus with femoralization of the humeral head and acetabularization of the acromion, glenoid erosion, loss of glenohumeral articular cartilage, osteoporosis of the humeral head, and eventually humeral head collapse. Neer et al. [19] estimated that only 4% of patients with a complete tear of the rotator cuff go on to develop CTA based on their experience over the 8-year period from 1975 to 1983.

There were debates over the years about the pathophysiology of CTA. Especially since "Milwaukee shoulder," this was considered by Neer as the same condition as CTA initially. And the etiology of this condition is considered to be under the hydroxyapatite crystal-mediated theory. In 1997, Collins and Harryman [20] synthesized Neer's theory on CTA pathogenesis with the crystal-mediated theory. Superior humeral migration that results from the loss of rotator cuff dynamic stability leads to abnormal trauma of the glenohumeral articular cartilage and the coracoacromial arch. This trauma releases particulate debris into the joint, setting off the crystal-mediated inflammatory cascade.

CTA tends to afflict the elderly, with women more likely to be affected than men [21–25]. Patients often present with complaints of chronic, progressive shoulder pain that is worse at night and with use of shoulder.

10.3.2 Radiographic and CT Findings

Glenohumeral joint degenerative changes, osteopenia of the humeral head, and superior migration of the humeral head are the common findings. Humeral migration leads to changes in the acromion, acromioclavicular joint, coracoid, and glenoid. Abnormal contact between the humerus and the acromion can lead to rounding off of the greater tuberosity (femoralization) and concave erosion of the undersurface of the acromion (acetabularization) [26, 27]. Superior glenoid erosion is another common sequela of superior humeral head migration.

Migration results in a decreased acromiohumeral interval (AHI) on anteroposterior (AP) radiographs, which is the distance from the undersurface of the acromion to the superior aspect of the humeral head. Hamada et al. [28] used the AHI on AP radiographs as the basis for radiographic classification system of massive rotator cuff tears. In grade 1, the AHI is greater than 6 mm; in grade 2, the AHI is 5 mm or less. In grade 3, there is acetabularization of the acromion in addition to the findings of grade 2. In grade 4, there is glenohumeral joint space narrowing in addition to the findings of grade 3. In grade 5, there is humeral head collapse.

The massive loss of the rotator cuff and the associated superior humeral migration lead to destabilization of the glenohumeral center of rotation. The amount of decentralization depends on the extent of the rotator cuff tear, the integrity of the coracoacromial (C-A) arch, and the degree and direction of the glenoid bone erosion. Analysis of cuff tear arthropathy and failed treatments has led to a biomechanical classification of cuff tear arthropathy by Seebauer [26]. Four distinct groups have been formed on the basis of the biomechanics and clinical outcomes of arthroplasty. The four types are distinguished by the degree of superior migration from the center of rotation and the amount of instability of the center of rotation. This classification was proposed for benefits in surgical decision-making for optimal implant type, goals of reconstruction, and outcomes.

- Type 1A: centered stable, minimal superior migration, C-A arch acetabularization
- Type 1B: centered medialized, minimal superior migration, medial glenoid erosion, C-A arch acetabularization
- Type 2A: decentered limited stable, superior translation, superior-medial erosion, significant C-A arch acetabularization.
- Type 2B: decentered unstable, anterior superior escape, C-A arch and anterior structures deficient.

Based upon the preoperative radiological appearance, four types of glenoid erosion were defined by Sirveaux [29]. In type E0, the head of the humerus migrated upwards without erosion of the glenoid. Type E1 was defined by a concentric erosion of the glenoid. In type E2 there was an erosion of the superior part of the glenoid and in type E3 the erosion extended to the inferior part of the glenoid.

The geyser phenomenon that soft-tissue mass is superior to the acromioclavicular joint is a well-recognized finding related to underlying rotator cuff tear.

CT can provide a more detailed view of the bony architecture that can be used for determining the extent of the bone erosion when planning treatment.

10.3.3 MRI Findings

MRI provides detailed information of the soft-tissue structures of the shoulder (Fig. 10.4), such as the extent of the rotator cuff tear, the location of the tear, and the quality of the rotator cuff muscles and tendons.

Saupe et al. [30] showed that the size of rotator cuff tendon tears and the extent of fatty infiltration of the rotator cuff muscles have a significant negative correlation with the AHI ($p < 0.05$).

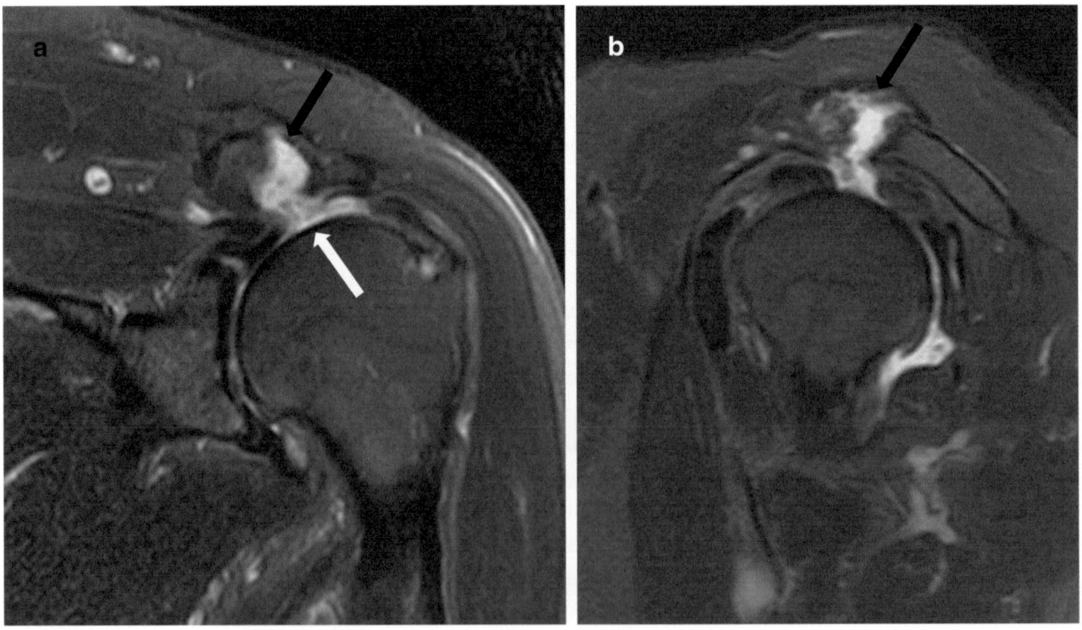

Fig. 10.4 Rotator cuff arthropathy with early geyser phenomenon. Coronal oblique (**a**) and sagittal oblique (**b**) fat-suppressed fluid-sensitive sequences of the shoulder. Note is made of the full-thickness supraspinatus tear (white arrow) with superior migration of the humeral head and narrowing of the acromiohumeral space. Fluid is noted extending superior through the acromioclavicular joint superior, delineating an early geyser formation (black arrows)

10.3.4 Ultrasound Findings

Superior humeral migration can be seen at coronal ultrasound as a reduced acromiohumeral distance. The humeral head shows loss of the hypoechoic layer of articular cartilage and bone irregularities; the greater tuberosity has a smooth appearance and blends with the humeral epiphysis. In these circumstances, it might be hard to identify the bicipital groove. Reduced thickness of the acromion may be seen.

Superior humeral migration can lead to secondary damage of the inferior acromioclavicular joint capsule and passage of joint fluid through the acromioclavicular joint, producing a cyst in the soft tissue at the superior aspect of the shoulder ("geyser sign"), and a finding that may be considered pathognomonic for long-standing massive rotator cuff tears. During passive movements of the arm or exertion of pressure on the cyst with the probe, debris may be seen moving to and fro across the acromioclavicular joint.

10.4 Septic Arthritis

10.4.1 Definition

Septic arthritis of the shoulder is rare. Recent reviews from both Europe and the United States have reported a similar low incidence, with 21, 17, and 23 cases over 8-, 11-, 15-year periods, respectively [31–33]. Most cases of septic arthritis tend to occur in patients with underlying articular disease. Septic arthritis of the shoulder rarely develops in young adults or in healthy individuals of any age [34]. In the series of Leslie et al. [34] and Pfeiffenberger et al. [35], the average age of patients suffering from septic arthritis of the shoulder was 65 years and 61 years, respectively. Although the overall incidence is low, there is an apparent increase of septic shoulder arthritis. This is possibly due to increased aging of the general population and hence more frequent underlying, predisposing shoulder articular disease.

Septic arthritis is rare between late infancy and young adulthood. This is thought to be related to the evolution of vascularity within developing bones. Diaphyseal vessels in the newborn traverse the physis, allowing hematogenous agents ready access to the epiphysis and joint. Beginning at approximately 8–18 months of age, the diaphyseal vessels instead terminate in sinusoidal lakes situated in the metaphysis, effectively obliterating any hematogenous pathway to the epiphysis. This accounts for the metaphyseal predilection of infections such as Brodie abscesses in adolescence. After the closure of the growth plate in adulthood, infection can more easily extend to the epiphysis and joint [36]. Even in the neonatal age group, incidentally, the knee and hip are much more common sites of infection than is the shoulder.

The potential sources for shoulder joint infection include (1) hematogenous spread either secondary to hematogenous seeding of the synovial membrane from a distant focus or spread from an adjacent epiphyseal area of osteomyelitis by means of vascular continuity between the epiphysis and the synovial membrane; (2) spread from a contiguous source of infection (e.g., such as in the diabetic foot); (3) direct implantation; and (4) postprocedural implantation often following local corticosteroid injection [37]. Following joint injections, the incidence of septic arthritis is approximately 1/1000. The complexity and increasing performance of orthopedic procedures, including arthroscopy and joint replacement, have resulted in an increase in postoperative shoulder infections. It has been suggested that the infection rate following total shoulder joint arthroplasty is around 2% for constrained systems, and of less than 1% for unconstrained systems or for humeral prosthetic placement alone [38, 39]. Infection may occur in the early postoperative period, or after months and years following the initial surgery.

Staphylococcus aureus and *Neisseria gonorrhoeae* are examples of bacteria that have a high degree of selectivity for the synovium, probably related to their adherence characteristics and toxin production [34, 35, 39]. Thus, the most common causative organism in all age groups combined for shoulder septic arthritis is *Staphylococcus aureus* [40–42]. Group D streptococcus is an important cause of septic arthritis in neonates and infants, whereas *Haemophilus influenzae* and *Staphylococcus aureus* are important causes, respectively, in young children and adults, the former only in those without immunization [37].

In recent years, an increasing number of *Staphylococcus aureus* infections have been attributable to methicillin-resistant *S. aureus* (MRSA) strains. In Cleeman and colleagues' series of 23 cases of glenohumeral infections, for instance, 70% of cases were due to *S. aureus* and of these 17% were MRSA [33].

Multifocal septic arthritis in young adults is suggestive of gonococcal arthritis. Certain patient populations are more susceptible to specific bacteria. Patients with sickle cell anemia are more prone to Salmonella infection, although this remains less frequent in these patients than staph infections. Septic arthritis caused by *Mycobacterium tuberculosis* is rare [34]; however, with the increasing number of immunocompromised patients (AIDS, immunosuppressive therapy), tuberculous involvement of the shoulder is becoming more frequent. Despite the above tendency, staphylococcus is still the most common causative organism in nearly all patient populations.

Degenerative joint disease, rheumatoid arthritis, and corticosteroid therapy are the most common predisposing conditions for shoulder septic arthritis. In particular, patients with severe rheumatoid arthritis with significant functional impairments are at greater risk of septic arthritis as a complication of the disease [43]. Patients with diabetes mellitus, leukemia, liver cirrhosis, cancer, hypogammaglobulinemia, and intravenous drug abuse have also an increased incidence of septic arthritis [34]. AIDS patients and stem cell recipients are illustrative examples of hosts with impaired immune responses and susceptible to infections caused by uncommon microorganisms.

There is no specific presentation or physical examination sign for septic arthritis. There is considerable clinical and imaging overlap with any inflammatory arthropathy. An acute onset with fever and chills is common. Pain, tenderness, redness, heat, and soft-tissue swelling about the involved joint are the usual complaints and findings. However, there is considerable variation in the presentation depending on the causative bacterial agent, the patient's immune status, and the presence of preexisting joint abnormality. In general, there are no reliable clinical signs for septic arthritis at clinical examinations, and the lack of a visible inflammatory response should not exclude the diagnosis of a septic shoulder. In a series of Leslie et al. [34], in one-third of the patients with shoulder septic arthritis the diagnosis had been delayed more than 6 months.

Leukocytosis and positive blood and joint cultures are important laboratory parameters of pyogenic arthritis [44, 45]. However, leukocytosis is an unreliable indicator, as it may be absent in immunocompromised patients. Increased C-reactive protein levels and erythrocyte sedimentation rates may be present. However, they are not very specific, since elevated levels can also be seen in other inflammatory conditions such as rheumatoid arthritis.

Because of the devastating sequelae of septic arthritis, any monoarticular arthritis should be regarded as infection until proven otherwise. Increasing number of septic arthritis is occurring due to the increasing immunocompromised population and microorganisms that are resistant to common drugs [46]. It is imperative for clinicians and radiologists to provide a prompt and accurate diagnosis. Septic arthritis is ultimately a clinical diagnosis that hinges on appropriate synovial fluid analysis. Direct sampling of joint fluid remains as the most important diagnostic step.

10.4.2 Radiographic and CT Findings

Radiographs usually are the first-line imaging modality used in patients with suspected shoulder septic arthritis. Unfortunately, initially, radiographs can be normal, which does not exclude infection. Initial radiographs can also be used to determine associated conditions, such as osteoarthritis and inflammatory arthropathy, or may be used as a baseline image in monitoring the response of treatment.

The first detectable abnormalities are soft-tissue swelling with hyperemia and joint distention secondary to effusion. However, both of these imaging findings tend to be occult on shoulder radiography. The hyperemia can result in osteopenia on radiographs and followed by uniform joint space narrowing and erosions usually at the joint margins. Advanced cases of infection are associated with subluxation or dislocation and massive bone destruction. During recovery, bones recalcify and although marginal erosions do not disappear such erosions become well demarcated and sclerotic. In severe cases, fibrous or bony ankylosis may occur.

Arthrography in the evaluation of joint infection should be used only in conjunction with joint aspiration to obtain fluid for bacteriologic examination. Injection of contrast material into the joint should be performed only after fluid aspiration due to the bacteriostatic properties of contrast agents. Radiographs obtained after injection of contrast material may reveal destruction of the articular cartilage and hypertrophic alterations in the synovium. In chronic septic arthritis, arthrography may display an irregular or contracted joint capsule [47].

Complications of septic arthritis are subluxation and dislocation, osteonecrosis, fibrous or bony ankylosis, chronic degenerative arthritis, and bone growth disturbance (lengthening, shortening, and angulation) [37].

Radiographs lack specificity in demonstrating nonpyogenic infection of the shoulder, especially tuberculosis (TB). The cardinal features of mycobacterial infection are osteoporosis, marginal subchondral erosions (usually occurring later), and gradual and delayed cartilage destruction: the triad of Phemister [48]. An appearance similar to chronic pyogenic osteomyelitis can be seen, including sclerosis, periostitis, and synovial membrane thickening [49].

On CT images, joint effusion, synovial thickening, and soft-tissue swellings are early manifestations of septic arthritis. Later on, destruction of the articular cartilage, irregularity and narrowing of joint, articular erosion, and subchondral bone destruction can be seen.

10.4.3 MR Findings

Synovial inflammation and joint effusion are the earliest signs in septic arthritis and can be easily identified on MR imaging. With chronicity the synovium thickens, the fluid becomes more complex, and joint recess becomes increasingly distended.

Thick and/or frond-like rim-enhancing synovium on postcontrast fat-suppressed T1-weighted images are typical findings of synovial inflammation in septic arthritis. Because the synovium normally enhances with gadolinium, careful examination of intensity of the enhancement, as well as the character of the synovium, should be performed. Comparison with other visible synovial structures should be performed. On postcontrast images, the acromioclavicular joint can be used as a standard of reference for normal enhancement in the absence of complete communicating rotator cuff tears.

In the normal glenohumeral joint, almost no fluid is present. In a review of 20 shoulder MR imaging studies of 12 asymptomatic patients, Recht and colleagues [50] found joint fluid in 14 shoulders, but not exceeding 2 mL in any cases. MR imaging can provide an assessment of the fluid volume in the joint. The following criteria have been proposed: grade 0 reflects scant fluid not distending any joint recesses; grade 1 demonstrates a small amount of fluid in the subscapularis recess, axillary recess (marked by a U-shaped inferior capsule), or biceps tendon sheath on at least two coronal-oblique images; grade 2 demonstrates distention of at least two of these recesses; and grade 3 demonstrates fluid in all three recesses [51]. The effusion tends to be homogenous, although loculation and inhomogeneity may be seen in more chronic septic process [37]. The effusions of glenohumeral septic arthritis frequently dissect into the subscapularis recess. From there, they frequently lead to synovial outpouching into the muscles of the rotator cuff. Rotator cuff tears often occur with subacute infections, and in this case the infection often spreads to the acromioclavicular joint.

Bone marrow edema is common. Reactive bone marrow edema, in the absence of osteomyelitis, may be present in up to 50% of patients [37]. This reactive edema tends to involve both sides of the articulation, and be subtle on T1-weighted images. The edema pattern is patchy and ill defined. When the marrow edema is quite obvious on T1-weighting images consider concomitant osteomyelitis. Bone erosions and cartilage destruction in more advanced cases are well demonstrated with MR imaging. Using animal experiments, Bremell et al. [52] have shown that cartilage loss and subchondral bone erosions may develop within days. With protracted subchondral loss, the infection may progress to subacute phase, when subchondral marrow edema and subchondral cyst formation occur.

In the chronic stages of glenohumeral septic arthritis, joint destruction will ultimately lead to ankylosis. Osteomyelitis may occur and the differentiation by MR of reactive marrow edema changes from osteomyelitis is often challenging, because both can show edematous-enhancing marrow changes. There tends to be more overt and confluent marrow changes on T1-weighted images in patients with osteomyelitis.

Overall, synovial enhancement, peri-synovial edema, and joint effusion (Fig. 10.5) are the MR

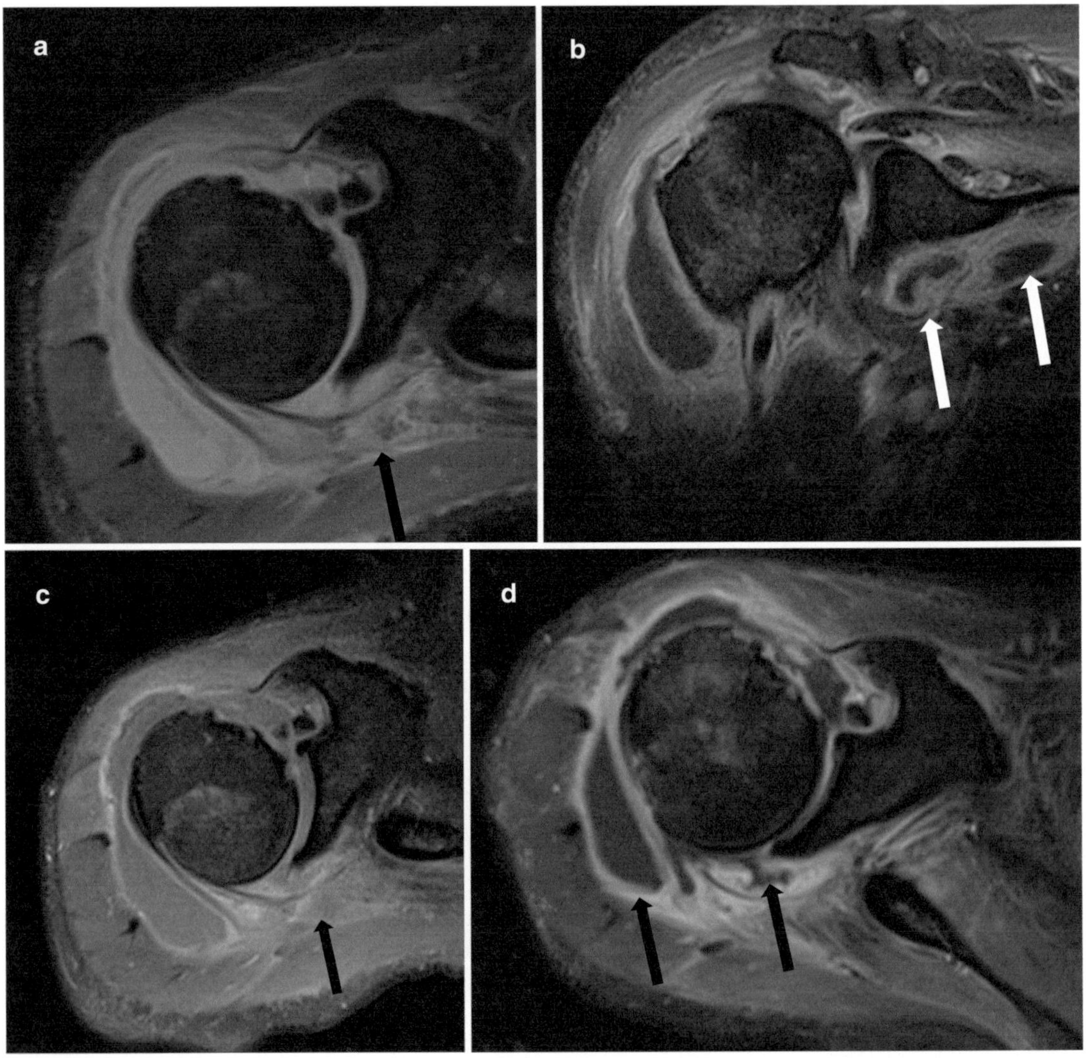

Fig. 10.5 56-Year-old patient with septic glenohumeral arthritis and history of recent discitis and osteomyelitis of the lumbar spine. Axial fat-suppressed proton density (**a**), coronal oblique postcontrast (**b**), axial fat-suppressed T1 precontrast (**c**), and axial postcontrast MR images demonstrate thick synovial enhancement (black arrows) of the glenohumeral joint effusion and subacromial subdeltoid bursa and periarticular soft-tissue enhancement. Fat-suppressed proton density axial image (**a**) and precontrast (**c**) demonstrates surrounding deep soft-tissue edema (black arrows). Coronal oblique postcontrast image (**d**) demonstrates additional peripheral enhancing small collections in the subscapularis muscle (white arrows)

findings that correlate most with septic arthritis. Karchevsky and colleagues [53] reported the presence of these findings in 98, 84, and 70%, respectively, of 50 consecutive subjects with joint infection (the study was not restricted to glenohumeral infection).

In everyday practice, differentiation of septic arthritis of the shoulder versus nonseptic inflamed joint is very difficult. Graif et al. [54] have shown that no single MR sign, including joint effusion, fluid outpouching, fluid heterogeneity, synovial thickening, peri-synovial edema, synovial enhancement, cartilage loss, bone erosions, bone erosion enhancement, bone marrow edema with and without enhancement, soft-tissue edema with and without enhancement, and periosteal edema, reliably distinguishes between the two entities. The combination of bone erosions with marrow edema is highly suggestive of septic arthritis; however joint aspiration is required for confirmation.

With high spatial resolution and soft-tissue contrast, MRI is our current best clinical imaging tool at monitoring treatment and disease progression in patients with septic arthritis. Bierry G and colleagues [55] reported their findings after comparing patients MRI before and after surgical debridement and antibiotic treatment and correlation with microbiological and clinical data. They found that the sizes of joint effusions and abscesses both decreased following successful treatment. However, synovial thickening and enhancement, periarticular myositis/cellulitis, and bone marrow edema can persist even after resolution of the infection.

Macrophage MR imaging with sequences enhanced with ultrasmall superparamagnetic iron oxide (USPIO) particles has been widely investigated and has demonstrated its ability to help demonstrate joint inflammation or infection [56, 57]. USPIO particles undergo macrophage phagocytosis with persistent T2 or T2* effects on delayed postcontrast MR images in tissues with macrophage infiltration [58]. Macrophages are recruited in infected joints in the early phases of infection and decrease with infection resolution [59]. It has recently been shown that the number of dark pixels observed on T2-weighted gradient-echo images after iron nanoparticle infection is correlated with the number of USPIO-loaded cells [60, 61]. Lefevre S and colleagues [62] using USPIO-enhanced macrophage MR technique imaged rabbits with knee septic arthritis in acute phase of infection and after antibiotic treatment and compared with histological specimen and gadoterate dimeglumine-enhanced fat-suppressed T1-weighted MR images. They concluded that USPIO-enhanced macrophage MR can demonstrate resolution of experimental bacterial joint infection.

It is important to be mindful of nonpyogenic infections when evaluating for shoulder septic arthritis, especially those caused by *Mycobacterium tuberculosis* and other mycobacteria, for they can present with quite different clinical and imaging pictures. Skeletal TB is encountered in 1–3% of extrapulmonary cases of TB, and of these skeletal cases 1–10% involve the shoulder [49]. Nonpyogenic infection can smolder in the joint for years. Richter and colleagues [63] found an average 15-month delay from time of symptom onset to correct diagnosis of TB of the shoulder. Periostitis and synovial membrane thickening are features that can be demonstrated on MR imaging. Large effusion and osteolysis are other associated features. T2-intermediate intraosseous tubercles are sometimes encountered.

Tuberculous bursitis has been well described, most commonly in the bursae of the shoulder, hands, ischium, and gluteal muscles [48]. TB often has a predisposition to the subacromial/subdeltoid bursa. Intrabursal rice bodies can be seen in TB, or any kind of chronic bursitis, appearing to be no more than several millimeters in size and isointense to muscle on both T1-weighted and T2-weighted images [64]. These bodies can often calcify and show signal voids as well as bloom on gradient-echo images. In advanced stages of nonpyogenic infection, there are significant bone and joint destructions similar to pyogenic septic arthritis.

In patients with a history of shoulder arthroplasty or with metallic implants, artifacts from the metallic prostheses and radiopaque cement pose big challenges for detection of underlying septic arthritis. Field distortion can be minimized by using lower field strength scanners, wider bandwidths, smaller voxels, and/or higher gradients. Frequency-selective fat suppression and gradient-echo sequences should be avoided. STIR and water excitation can be used instead for less distortion. Recent advancement in MR imaging technology has also enabled better results in this area. Fast spin-echo (FSE) metal artifact reduction sequences (MARS), and newer multi-acquisition variable-resonance image combination (MAVRIC) and slice-encoding metal artifact reduction (SEMAC) sequences, are among the new developments. Initial studies on patients undergoing shoulder, hip, and knee arthroplasty have demonstrated improved visualization of synovitis, periprosthetic bone, supraspinatus tendon fibers, and supraspinatus tendon tears with MAVRIC sequences [65–67].

10.4.4 US Findings

Ultrasonography has a growing role in the evaluation of septic arthritis of the shoulder. The main ultrasound findings are superior bulging of the joint capsule, widening of the joint space with erosion of the bony edges, and debris moving freely within the joint space (new [68]).

Both joint effusion and synovial hypertrophy can be well depicted on US. Synovial hypertrophy usually appears as hypoechoic intra-articular material that lacks compressibility and mobility and often demonstrates flow on Doppler images [69]. Septic effusions may be completely anechoic or associated with septations and debris. However, neither the size nor the relative echogenicity of the fluid can be used to distinguish an infected inflammatory effusion from an uninfected inflammatory effusion [70]. Although US is unable to confirm the diagnosis of septic arthritis, it may be effective in guiding needle aspiration of the joint.

There are two different locations where effusions can be easily seen of the shoulder: the bicipital groove and the posterior joint recess. The bicipital groove is best seen by the anterior view, looking for the long biceps tendon. The effusion is gravity dependent so the probe must be walked up to the musculotendinous junction. When there is joint effusion, usually the biceps tendon can be seen completely surrounded by fluid. Posteriorly, the effusion will displace the capsule and the infraspinatus tendon. In one review of 30 glenohumeral joint effusions, fluid was consistently identified by US in the posterior joint recess in 100% of the patients and in the biceps tendon sheath in 97% [71].

10.5 Rheumatoid Arthritis

10.5.1 Definition

Rheumatoid arthritis (RA) is a chronic systemic disorder that can lead to significant disability, morbidity, and even decreased life expectancy [72]. RA affects 1–3% of the adult population in Europe and the United States [73]. RA is the most common type of inflammatory arthritis treated by rheumatologists and comprises up to 25% of all referrals to rheumatology clinics and 75% of follow-up work [74]. The peak onset is between fourth and sixth decades of life. Women are two to three times more likely to be affected by RA than men [75].

RA is a chronic inflammatory process that characteristically targets the synovial lining of diarthrodial joints. As the disease progresses, destruction of the structural components of the joints follows. As a systemic disorder RA is also frequently associated with a variety of extra-articular manifestations.

The pathogenesis of RA is multifactorial including genetic, immunoregulatory, and environmental factors [76]. One of the few voluntary risk factors is heavy cigarette smoking. Among the newer advances in this area is an association between major histocompatibility complex, class II, DR beta 1 (HLA-DRB1), and disease severity [77]. The HLA-DRB1 gene provides instructions for making a protein that plays a critical role in the immune system and is part of a family of genes called the human leukocyte antigen (HLA) complex. The HLA complex helps the immune system distinguish the body's own proteins from proteins made by foreign invaders such as viruses and bacteria. Several studies have implicated the oral cavity bacterium *Porphyromonas gingivalis* in the pathogenesis of the disease, noting that RA patients have high antibodies to the organism [78]. It is thought that the bacterium's ability to citrullinate enolase molecules at a site slightly different from that which is citrullinated physiologically may produce the autoantigen central to the inception of RA. Anticitrullinated protein antibodies (ACPAs) have been found in the serum of RA patients and are thus considered a fundamental part of the disease pathway [79]. Autoantibodies (rheumatoid factor and ACPA) result in synovial inflammation, pannus formation, and bone and cartilage destruction with systemic manifestations.

Autoimmune factors are well-recognized components in the pathogenesis of RA. Native B cells accumulate in synovium where select clones are continuously activated [78]. Synovial tissue T cells that express transcription factors are also important for maintaining the inflammatory response. The synovium, congested with immune cells, becomes progressively inflamed under the influence of monocyte and macrophage-secreted cytokines such as interleukins (IL)-1, IL-6, and IL-17, and tumor necrosis factor alpha (TNFα) [78, 80, 81]. These cytokines can cause synovial neovascularization and cartilage damage.

Recent studies have emphasized the importance of fibroblast-like synoviocytes (FLSs) that predominate in the synovium of RA patients, in the spread of RA from one joint to the other [82].

RA can involve any synovial joints in either the peripheral or the axial skeleton. However, there is a preference for the metacarpophalangeal (MCP), metatarsophalangeal (MTP), and proximal interphalangeal (PIP) joints of the hands and feet, the distal radioulnar joint, and radiocarpal joints.

Swelling of the PIP joints is one of the most common early clinical signs. The severity of the shoulder joint involvement is related to the general severity of the disease. Sparing of the distal interphalangeal joint is a useful sign to distinguish it from osteoarthritis or psoriatic arthritis. The shoulder joint is one of the most commonly involved large joints in RA, and RA is the most common inflammatory arthropathy to involve the shoulder. Shoulder involvement can be seen in 70% of patients with RA. However, the shoulder joint becomes involved later than other upper limb joints in RA patients. During the first 2 years of the disease, nearly 50% of patients suffer from shoulder symptoms, and during the first 14 years 83% of patients have similar shoulder complaints [83].

RA of the shoulder frequently involves both glenohumeral and acromioclavicular (AC) joints. In a study of 148 shoulders at 15 years of follow-up, Lehtinen and colleagues [84] found erosive change in the acromioclavicular joint alone in 17% of the shoulders, in the glenohumeral joint alone in 6%, and in both joints in 42%. The bursae surrounding the shoulder, particularly the subacromial subdeltoid bursa, are also commonly involved. This could present clinically as mass-like lesion and may be mistaken for a soft-tissue neoplasm.

In patients with inflammatory arthritis, the pain may limit the use of the affected shoulder. If no appropriate physical therapy is conducted, the joint capsule and ligaments may shorten and result in adhesive capsulitis/"frozen shoulder." The joint contracture leads to greater pain and even less motion, and eventually substantial atrophy of the rotator cuff musculature [85]. With the progression of this atrophy, the humeral head becomes superiorly migrated which causes impingement of the rotator cuff between the humerus and acromion, predisposing to tear. Additional cytokines in both the inflamed bursa and joint lead to collagen breakdown in the rotator cuff. Up to 80% of RA patients have significant thinning of the rotator cuff, and up to 20% have full-thickness tears [85, 86]. This thinning of the cuff may easily be confused with a cuff tear, and special care should be paid in the interpretation of these images. Although cuff repair is an option, benefits are limited. One review over a 15-year period demonstrated significant improvements in pain and patient satisfaction after repair, but functional gains (defined as an increased rage of abduction) were only obtained in the partial-thickness tear group [87].

10.5.2 Radiographic and CT Findings

Radiography has for a long time been the standard for assessing joint damages in RA. The earliest finding on radiographs is periarticular osteoporosis, followed by erosions and subchondral cysts at the articular margins of the humeral head, followed later by central or peripheral glenoid erosions [88]. Glenohumeral joint space narrowing is a late finding in RA, and this slower progression of cartilage destruction by synovial pannus may be related to either the absence of weight bearing or the relatively high cartilage-to-synovial ratio [84]. Erosion in shoulder is most prominent along the superolateral portion of the humerus, adjacent to the greater tuberosity (Fig. 10.6). This is the bare area between the articular cartilage of the humeral head and the reflection of the joint capsule. Deep, bony erosion may also develop at an opposite side, at the medial aspect of the surgical neck of the humerus, related to pressure exerted by the glenoid margin. Rarely, these large erosions can result in a pathologic fracture of the humeral neck. Continued destruction can lead to extension of bony erosions, resulting in destruction of the entire anatomic neck, the greater tuberosity, and the glenoid cavity. At the end, the destruction pattern may mimic a neuropathic joint or severe crystal deposition disease, such as Milwaukee shoulder.

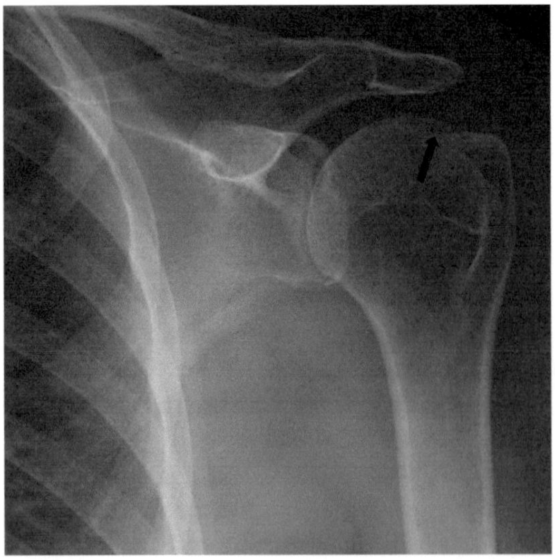

Fig. 10.6 47-Year-old patient with RA. Frontal radiograph demonstrates the erosion at the humeral head at the typical location of bare area (black arrow)

Upward migration index (UMI) evaluates proximal humeral migration which is secondary to rotator cuff tear and fatty atrophy of the rotator cuff muscles. This is measured by a ratio of the distance from center of humeral head to acromion (CA) to radius of humeral head, as UMI = CA/R. An UMI >1 0.35 indicates normal rotator cuff and UMI <1.25 indicates severe proximal migration of humeral head and rotator cuff tear. Van der Zwaal et al. [89] studied 44 shoulders over an 8-year period of time. They demonstrated that a plain anteroposterior radiograph of the shoulder is sufficient to assess any progression of rheumatoid disease and to predict functional outcome in the long term by using the UMI as an indicator of rotator cuff degeneration.

Widening of the acromioclavicular joint space with inferior clavicular erosions and secondary osteoarthritic changes are the common manifestations of AC joint involvement. In a series of 49 patients with RA, Petersson [90] assessed clinical and radiographic findings and noted radiographic changes to the acromioclavicular joint in 85% of cases.

Radiography can assess the joint damage at the onset of RA and document the progression and response to treatment during the course of the disease. The benefits of radiography are low costs, high availability, and possibility of standardization and blinded centralized reading, reasonable reproducibility, and existence of validated assessment methods [91]. Thus, radiography findings are part of the American College of Rheumatology (ACR) classification criteria for RA [92], and is recommended as obligatory in clinical trials with a duration of 1 year [93].

There are have been several proposed radiological classification systems for shoulder involvement in RA and each emphasized on different aspects of the disease.

The Larsen classification was proposed in 1977 [94] to introduce standard reference films for RA evaluation in the joints and numerical scores for each individually involved joint.

- Grade 0: Normal conditions, abnormalities not related to arthritis may be present.
- Grade 1: Slight abnormality, periarticular soft-tissue swelling, osteoporosis, or joint-space narrowing.
- Grade 2: Definite early abnormality, erosion, and joint-space narrowing present, erosion obligatory except in weight-bearing joint.
- Grade 3: Medium destructive abnormality, erosion, and joint-space narrowing present, erosion obligatory in all joints.
- Grade 4: Severe destructive abnormality, erosion, and joint-space narrowing present, bone deformation in weight-bearing joints.
- Grade 5: Mutilating abnormality, gross bony destruction, dislocation, and ankylosis.

The Laine [95] classification from 1954 has three stages based on clinical and radiographic findings:

- Stage I is slight limitation of shoulder motion, with mild-to-moderate pain and tenderness to palpation. Crepitation may be appreciated on range of motion. Radiographs show only generalized osteopenia.
- Stage II is characterized by moderate limitation of shoulder motion, moderate-to-severe pain, and crepitus. Radiographic findings include osteoporosis, erosive bony changes, and joint-space narrowing.
- Stage III is where severe functional deficits are present; range of motion is painful and limits activities of daily living. Radiographs show advanced erosive changes of the humeral head and glenoid.

Neer [96] later classified RA of the shoulder into three categories based on clinical and radiographic findings; his dry, wet, and resorptive stages are approximately equivalent to those of Laine et al.

Levigne and Franceschi [97] proposed three radiographic patterns of RA. These three patterns were distinguished by sphericity of the humeral head and upward migration of the head in relation to the glenoid. There is similarity of these three patterns with the three categories described by Neer. They found that the three patterns do not have the same functional prognosis after insertion of prosthesis.

1. Ascending pattern: Most frequent, upward migration of humeral head with retained sphericity, head initially ascends and then medializes, inferior glenoid notches the humeral neck at late stage.
2. Center pattern: No upward migration, uniform glenoid wear, humeral head pushes into glenoid, and progressive head medialization with eventual reduction of the acromio-humeral distance.
3. Destructive pattern: Destruction of the humeral head with loss of sphericity and notching of the humeral neck and simultaneous glenoid destruction.

Levigne and Franceschi further classified humeral head and glenoid wear in RA in the same paper. For humeral head wear, stage 1: subchondral bone intact; stage 2: anatomical neck deformed by notch >10 mm; and stage 3: loss of spherical form of the head. For glenoid wear, stage 1: subchondral bone intact or minimally deformed; stage 2: erosion reaching the base of coracoid; and stage 3: erosion going beyond the base of coracoid.

Computed tomography (CT) may be indicated when preoperative analysis of humeral head defects and glenoid articular erosions is necessary [88]. Albertson et al. reported agreement between preoperative CT results and intraoperative findings, concluding that CT could characterize osseous defects and bone loss more accurately than standard radiography. This is particularly important in evaluating glenoid erosion to determine whether implantation of a glenoid component is possible.

As the current therapeutic goal is to minimize joint destruction so as to obviate salvage procedures, radiographs and CT are of limited use in early disease detection as they are opaque to synovial inflammation.

10.5.3 MRI Findings

MR features of shoulder RA involvement include synovial thickening, joint effusion, joint-space narrowing, erosions of glenoid, greater tuberosity and posterolateral humeral head, supraspinatus and cuff tendon tears, subacromial subdeltoid bursitis, biceps tenosynovitis, and acromioclavicular joint involvement.

A standard RA scoring system has been developed, most notably the rheumatoid arthritis MRI scoring (RAMRIS) system, developed as part of the Outcome Measures in Rheumatoid Arthritis Clinical Trials (OMERACT) international initiative [98]. Generally, they propose standard field strength (1.5 T) contrast-enhanced MR imaging of the wrist and metacarpophalangeal joints to assign numeric scores for the severity of each of the three findings: synovitis, marrow edema, and erosion. Studies have demonstrated good intra-reader variability but less reliable interreader performance with this staging method [36].

MR imaging is considered to be the gold standard for synovial imaging [99]. Currently, two findings are used as indicators for synovial inflammation: volume of enhancing synovial tissue and enhancement of the synovium after injection of contrast. Thickened synovium demonstrates low-to-intermediate signal intensity on T1-weighted images and high signal intensity on T2-weighted images (Figs. 10.7 and 10.8). Easily identifiable synovium is usually thickened synovium. Synovitis and joint effusion are the earliest findings in RA on MR images (Figs. 10.7 and 10.8). Synovitis is usually appreciated as avid or thick enhancement with frond-like morphology, similar to septic arthritis. The signal characteristics of the synovial fluid tend to be heterogeneous. In more advanced stages, portions of the synovium may even fail to enhance or demonstrate relative hypoenhancement and T2 intermediate-to-low signal intensity, reflecting fibrous synovitis, although small amounts of fibrotic pannus can even be seen earlier in the disease course [100]. Later on, the synovium can turn fatty.

Active synovitis is best visualized on fat-suppressed T1-weighted images with contrast

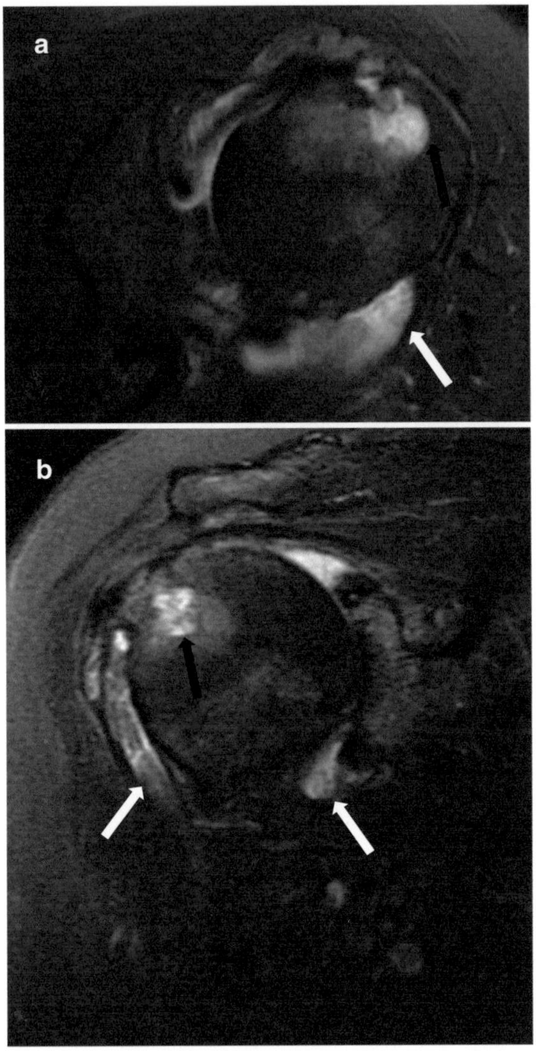

Fig. 10.7 47-Year-old patient with RA, same patient as in Fig. 10.1. Axial (**a**) and coronal oblique (**b**) fat-suppressed fluid-sensitive sequence images of the shoulder. Typical erosion of the humeral head (black arrows) with adjacent synovitis and pannus. Glenohumeral joint effusion and synovitis (white arrow), which extend distally within the biceps tendon sheath (white arrow)

[101]. Based on the OMERACT guidelines, synovitis is defined as enhancement greater than the width of the joint capsule. New efforts have made using dynamic contrast-enhanced (DCE) MR imaging. A gadolinium dose of 0.05–0.3 mmol/kg is used and typically short repetition time and short echo time T1-weighted gradient-echo images were acquired every few seconds over a period of minutes [36]. A curve can be

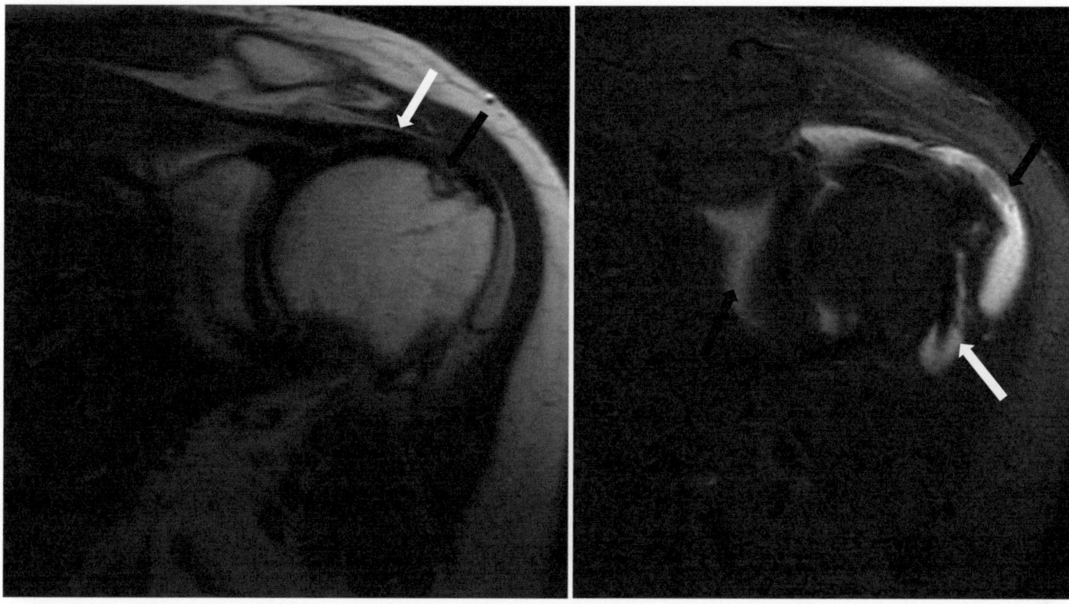

Fig. 10.8 53-Year-old female patient with RA. Coronal oblique proton density-weighted image (**a**) demonstrates attenuated caliber of the supraspinatus tendon (white arrow) and small erosions at the humeral head (black arrow). Fat-suppressed T2-weighted image (**b**) demonstrates glenohumeral joint effusion (black arrow), synovitis (black arrow), and extending to the biceps tendon sheath (white arrow)

obtained by plotting signal intensity over time. DCE MR imaging of the knees and wrist joints has yielded promising results. Cimmino and colleagues [102] demonstrated that the enhancement rate of wrist synovium can be used to distinguish between active and inactive disease. DCE MR imaging findings have also correlated well with histopathologic findings. Active research is focusing on the potential role for DCE MR imaging in monitoring and helping to appropriately time RA treatment with new disease-modifying anti-rheumatoid drugs (DMARDs) such as anti-TNFα. Response to more established agents such as corticosteroids and methotrexate is also under investigation [98, 103]. Since the shoulder tends to be involved later in the disease process, the more recent MRI scoring methods and dynamic enhancement protocols have not yet, to our knowledge, been applied to the glenohumeral and acromioclavicular joints.

Bone marrow edema is an increased signal intensity on fat-suppressed fluid-sensitive sequences (Fig. 10.6), representing increased amount of water in the marrow, and may represent the internal bony response to external attack by the inflamed synovium [99]. Bone marrow edema seems to be the strongest predictor of future erosion [104]. One study showed that if bone edema was present at a specific site at baseline, it was associated with a sixfold increase in the chance of erosion occurrence at the same site after 1 year [105].

Erosion is defined on MR images as focal loss of normal signal intensity from cortical or subchondral bone on T1-weighted images or focal regions of high signal on T2-weighted sequences [106]. Erosion enhances on a T1-weighted image with gadolinium contrast, implying the presence of inflamed synovium within the defect. Erosions can be distinguished from intraosseous cyst or cyst-like lesion, because the latter does not enhance. Marginal erosions in shoulder RA are usually seen at the posterolateral aspect of the humeral head (Fig. 10.7). In Lehtinen and colleagues' [107] series of 148 glenohumeral joints, MR imaging revealed erosive changes in 71 (48%) of the joints; and erosions were seen on the superolateral articular surface of the humeral head in 61 of the 71 joints. Glenoid involvement was only seen in 28 joints. Alasaarela and colleagues [108] demonstrated the superiority of MR imaging to ultrasound, CT, and radiograph at identifying humeral head erosions in their prospective multimodality study.

Rotator cuff pathology is very common in patients with RA. This may be related to the destructive effects of the synovitis around the supraspinatus and infraspinatus tendon at their footprints. MR imaging can depict the tendinosis, partial tear, full-thickness tear, and related fatty muscle atrophy (Fig. 10.8). Rotator cuff tears with muscle atrophy indicated chronicity of the disease and correlate with functional impairment. Both morphologic and functional information are important to guide treatment, especially in helping identify which patients would benefit from arthroplasty. With recent more wide use of reversed shoulder arthroplasty, MR imaging evaluation for rotator cuff and integrity of the deltoid muscle are increasingly common.

Acromioclavicular involvement is common in RA. On MR imaging, distention of the acromioclavicular joint capsule with extension of pannus into the joint may be seen at any stage of the disease. With early distal clavicular osteolysis, there is subchondral marrow edema disproportionate to the acromion. Erosions can enlarge over time to cause osteolysis of the distal clavicle or even the acromion. The erosive changes tend to be more pronounced at the caudal aspect of the distal clavicle. Widening of the joint is common but dislocation and subluxation are uncommon [109]. Although it is traditionally taught that acromioclavicular joint is involved early and more severely than glenohumeral joint in RA, this has not been our experience. However, when presented with differentiating RA and septic arthritis which can be quite similar, involvement of the acromioclavicular joint, regardless of severity, makes the diagnosis of RA more likely.

Synovial cyst formation and subacromial subdeltoid bursitis are other common findings in RA. The synovial cysts develop in the surrounding soft tissue of the shoulder joint and frequently dissect along tendon sheaths. Extension along the biceps tendon sheath is characteristic. The cysts may also develop under the subscapularis or around the axillary recess. However, these two locations are more commonly seen in patients with septic arthritis. Rarely, a cyst may grow large enough to be masslike [110]. Subacromial subdeltoid bursa fluid can accumulate from direct inflammation or rotator cuff tear. Chronic proliferative synovium can over time infarct and shed into the bursae or joint, forming fibrinous joint bodies known as rice bodies with varying signal intensity (although generally isotense to muscle).

10.5.4 Ultrasound Findings

Within the past decade, musculoskeletal ultrasound (US) has become an established imaging technique for the diagnosis and follows-up of patients with rheumatic disease [111, 112]. Its role in diagnostic imaging is continuing to expand with the development of further clinical applications and with the advancement of ultrasound technology. Owing to the better axial and lateral resolution of US, even minute bone surface abnormalities may be depicted. Thus destructive and/or reparative hypertrophic changes on the bone surface may be seen before they are apparent on plain radiography and comparable to magnetic resonance imaging [113]. The "real-time" capability of US allows dynamic assessment of joint and tendon movements. Advantages of US include its noninvasiveness, portability, relatively low cost, lack of ionizing radiation, and its ability to be repeated as often as necessary, making it particularly useful for the monitoring of treatment [114].

The sonographic features of RA in shoulder include joint effusions, active synovitis best seen on color Doppler images, biceps tenosynovitis, synovial cysts, subacromial subdeltoid bursitis and rotator cuff tears, bone erosions, and muscle atrophy. To detect inflammatory lesions the anterior, lateral and posterior, and longitudinal and transverse scans with rotation of the shoulder are most helpful. A sensitive technique for finding even very small shoulder effusion is the axillary longitudinal scan, but elevation of the arm may not be possible for patients with advanced disease [114].

Biceps tenosynovitis demonstrated as thickening of the tendon with anechoic or hypoechoic fluid accumulation in the tendon sheath. Alasaarela and Alasaarela found biceps tendinitis (57%) and changes in the supraspinatus tendon (33%) to be the most frequent tendinopathy changes in patients with painful rheumatoid shoulder [115]. Long head of the biceps tendon and supraspinatus tendon lesions were also the most common findings of the rheumatic shoulder in the work of Keysser and Osthus [116].

Erosions are visualized as steplike or contour deformities at the humeral head. The humeral articular cartilage can be seen between the supraspinatus and infraspinatus tendons and the humeral head. For the visualization of the joint effusion, distance between joint capsule and inferior margin of infraspinatus tendon above 2 mm was considered as a positive sign [117]. Combination of glenohumeral joint effusion, bone cartilage reduction, and humeral erosions was a significant predictor of inflammatory nature of the painful shoulder syndrome [117].

Synovial inflammation in active arthritis leads to synovial thickening and hyperemia, which can be identified on both grayscale and color Doppler images. Synovial thickening usually is hypoechoic, noncompressible, or poorly compressible which allows for differentiation from fluid. Color Doppler images can demonstrate vascularity indicating active inflammation. Thus, color Doppler images should be included at all US exams to help target therapy early in the diagnosis and to aid in the assessment of treatment responses.

Real-time imaging capability of US is a particularly advantageous feature, permitting dynamic evaluation of a system on movement. Nevien El-Liethy et al. proposed that dynamic US for the diagnosis of shoulder impingement in RA should be done in addition to the standard protocol to improve management [118]. The stress position they used is arm semiflexed, semi-abducted, and hand pronated. The acromiohumeral distance (AHD) is measured as the minimum distance from the inferior aspect of the acromion to the point of entry of the tendon into the acoustic shadow of the humeral head on neutral position. The stress position brings the greater tuberosity of the humeral head underneath the acromion. If there is a considerable reduction in its dimensions, then the repeated shearing force will cause damage to the rotator cuff. They found that in cases of subacromial impingement, the AHD measures less than 6 mm in neutral position and shows further reduction (about 25%) in stress position.

The involvement of acromioclavicular joint is also a common feature although a small study found it to be more common in spondyloarthritis compared to RA [119]. Patients with RA have higher incidence of joint effusions, bursitis, and erosions compared to spondyloarthritis.

10.6 CPPD and HAD

10.6.1 Definition

Calcium pyrophosphate dihydrate (CPPD) disease comprises a spectrum of clinical and imaging disorders. The nomenclature of CPPD and related conditions can seem confusing. The four terms that are often confused, since some mistakenly believe that they are synonymous, are 1. CPPD disease, 2. chondrocalcinosis, 3. CPPD arthropathy, and 4. pseudogout.

1. CPPD disease is an overarching term that refers to the pathologic articular alterations and destruction that is believed to be the response to CPPD crystals within a joint.
2. Chondrocalcinosis refers to cartilage calcification seen on radiography, pathologically or on fluid examination. On radiography calcification must be seen in at least two locations to differentiate systemic disease from dystrophic calcification.
3. Pyrophosphate or CPPD arthropathy refers to structural changes of cartilage and bone in the setting of CPPD deposition [120] that are macroscopically visible or seen radiographically. The patterns of joint disease can closely mimic osteoarthritis or less commonly have more specific patterns. Notably, cartilage calcification may be absent on

radiographs in patients with pyrophosphate arthropathy [121].

4. Pseudogout is not a radiologic diagnosis, but a clinical syndrome produced by CPPD crystal deposition disease with intermittent acute attacks similar to gouty arthritis. Other clinical patterns described included pseudo-OA and pseudo-RA, for patients whose clinical presentation mimics osteoarthritis or rheumatoid.

Ryan and McCarty proposed several diagnostic criteria for the diagnosis of CPPD crystal deposition disease [122], including the identification of CPPD crystal in tissues or synovial fluid by definite means (for example, chemical analysis) or by compensated polarized light microscopy as well as radiographic findings [123, 124]. Hence they described the "disorder" as a combination of pathologically visible crystals with corresponding structures/radiographic changes.

At the cellular level, CPPD disease is defined by the accumulation of CPPD crystals in soft tissues, most commonly within the extracellular matrix of midzonal articular cartilage [125]. It is thought that the initial insult may be a derangement in chondrocyte function that impairs maintenance of the extracellular matrix. This will lead to buildup of excess adenosine triphosphate (ATP), subsequently, of the inorganic extracellular pyrophosphate (ePPi) that results from its cleavage [126]. The ePPi in turn binds calcium, producing crystals. The symptomatic forms of CPPD disease (and other crystal deposition disease) reflect a complex inflammatory cascade that occurs subsequently. These cascades manifest at synovial and chondral levels and are mediated by matrix metalloproteinases, prostaglandins, toll-like receptors, and ILs, among other factors [126].

CPPD disease is classified based on its etiology into hereditary, idiopathic, and secondary types associated with metabolic disease and trauma [122].

10.6.2 Radiographic and CT Findings

Chondrocalcinosis is commonly seen in older patients. There is no strong gender predilection. Most of these cases, even when multifocal, are dystrophic. Richette and colleagues noted that chondrocalcinosis has been reported in 7–10% of individuals around age 60 years [120] and other studies have found it in up to 60% of individuals over the age of 85 years [127, 128]. Hence it becomes increasingly difficult in the aging patients to use radiographic findings of chondrocalcinosis as differential diagnostic criteria.

In addition to CPPD disease and dystrophic causes, such metabolic disorders as hemochromatosis and ochronosis and other heritable genetic mutations should be considered in patients less than 55 years of age and in patients with significant polyarticular involvement. In patients more than 55 years of age, hyperparathyroidism warrants some consideration when chondrocalcinosis is seen [120].

The most commonly affected sites are menisci of the knee, triangular fibrocartilage of the wrist, labra of the acetabulum and symphysis pubis, and annulus fibrosus of the intervertebral disk. Also noted may be hyaline cartilage, various ligaments (most commonly the scapholunate and lunatotriquetral), and joint capsule. For some peculiar reasons the latter two are still termed chondrocalcinosis even though the structures calcified are not cartilage.

Chondrocalcinosis is usually apparent on radiographs. Hence a chondrocalcinosis survey may be requested. This survey consists of three exposures: a frontal view of the pelvis, a frontal view encompassing both knees, and one exposure with both wrists. Occasionally CPPD arthropathy can precede radiographically detectable cartilage calcification, although crystals should be seen on fluid aspiration [124, 129]. In one study of 3228 patients, who underwent knee arthroscopy, of patients who had pathologically proved CPPD crystal deposition, only 39.2% of them had radiographic diagnosis of chondrocalcinosis [130].

CT scan is of higher soft-tissue contrast and cross-sectional capability and thus can detect more subtle chondrocalcinosis as compared to radiographs. However, due to comparatively high radiation dose, CT is rarely used for the identification of chondrocalcinosis alone.

The majority of chondrocalcinosis is caused by CPPD crystal deposition. However, in 5% of the cases, it can be related to dicalcium phosphate dihydrate and calcium hydroxyapatite [121]. In terms of shoulder, occasionally, deposition can be seen along the glenoid labra as linear density paralleling the glenoid contour or within the humeral head articular cartilage. The acromioclavicular (AC) joint contains fibrocartilage intra-articular disc. CPPD crystal deposition preferentially involves fibrocartilage. Thus, chondrocalcinosis can occur at the AC joint.

Tendon calcifications are frequently seen in patients with CPPD crystal deposition disease [124, 131, 132]. An incidence of 13.5% was reported in one study [132]. The most commonly involved tendon in the shoulder is supraspinatus. It appears as linear or punctate calcifications near the tendon attachment while the calcium hydroxyapatite crystal deposition tends to be more homogeneous, discrete, and nodular and also extends distant from the tendon attachment [123]. There is a high correlation between presence of tendon calcifications and extent and intensity of calcific deposits in other joints [131]. Direct translocation of CPPD crystals from the articular or bursal surfaces may be responsible for some of the tendinous calcification [133]. Additionally calcification of joint capsules can be seen as well. Even though it is an oxymoron, calcifications of capsules, ligaments, and even sometimes tendons are commonly called "chondrocalcinosis."

Pyrophosphate arthropathy is more common in elderly women. The radiocarpal, first and second metacarpophalangeal joints, and knee are the most common sites of involvement. In all joints, the most common appearance is similar to typical osteoarthritis, but more specific changes may be seen such as second and third metacarpal phalangeal involvement in the hand and lateral and patellofemoral involvement in the knee. Shoulder involvement is not uncommon.

The clinical presentation of CPPD crystal deposition disease is highly variable, and thus it has been called a "great mimicker" of other arthritides [134]. Ryan and McCarty [135] described six patterns of joint involvement in their classic textbook in 1985. Several of these clinical patterns can present at different times during the course of the arthritis. Significant number of patients with CPPD crystal deposition disease is asymptomatic. The absence of symptoms occurs in at least 10–20% of documented cases of CPPD crystal deposition disease. Recently in 2001, Canhao and colleagues [136] proposed five clinical presentations based on a study of 50 patients with confirmed CPPD disease: pseudogout, pseudo-osteoarthritis, pseudo-osteoarthritis with synovitis, monoarthropathy, and pseudo-rheumatoid.

Pseudogout presentation accounts for about 25% of CPPD clinical presentations. Usually, the diagnosis is made based on symptoms of acute onset of pain, similar to acute gouty flares, in patients with known CPPD disease. It is believed that shedding of CPPD crystals into joint fluid incited an inflammatory response. This can develop spontaneously or triggered by direct trauma concomitant medical condition such as myocardial infarction, stroke, joint lavage, granulocyte colony-stimulating factor therapy, bisphosphonates, and intra-articular hyaluronic acid injections [120].

The pseudo-osteoarthritic patterns account for roughly 50% of pyrophosphate arthropathy. The imaging findings in these patients greatly resemble degenerative osteoarthritis, however affecting non-weight-bearing joints such as radiocarpal, metacarpophalangeal joints, glenohumeral joints, and elbow specifically. It is usually bilateral and symmetric. The spectrum of radiographic findings of osteoarthritis such as narrowing of the joint space, subchondral sclerosis and subchondral cystic changes, and osteophyte formation can be present. However, subchondral cysts are one of the hallmarks of this condition. They tend to be bigger, numerous, and more widespread when compared to those in osteoarthritis. This can go on leading to fragmentation and collapse of the articular surface. Intra-articular osteochondral bodies thus are quite common in patients who suffer from CPPD arthropathy [137]. Osteophytosis occurs less frequently in pyrophosphate arthropathy than in usual osteoarthrosis [138].

In terms of the glenohumeral joint, primary shoulder osteoarthrosis is commonly worse posteriorly with posterior translation of the humeral head over the glenoid. In patients with pyrophosphate arthropathy, when there is associated secondary cuff arthropathy, the joint space loss may be worse anteriorly.

Pseudo-rheumatic arthropathy accounts for 5–8% of pyrophosphate arthropathies. Similar to rheumatoid arthritis, the patient may present with fatigue, flexion contractures, and bilateral shoulder stiffness, often worse in the mornings [136, 139]. Laboratory testing often demonstrates elevated ESR. Resnick and colleagues observed that the key radiographic distinction between pseudo-rheumatic arthropathy and true rheumatoid arthritis in the setting of coexisting CPPD disease is that the former lacks erosions [140].

Occasionally, tumoral deposits of CPPD can be seen, especially at the smaller joints (such as acromioclavicular and temporomandibular joints). These deposits may actually be within the small articular discs noted in these locations. In the shoulder, the deposits can cause pressure erosion or frank destruction of subjacent bone [141]. The deposits tend to be less than 10 cm in size. Lobulated margins and location near a joint without intra-articular extension are characteristic features.

Neuropathic type arthropathy can occur in as many as 2% of patients [123, 142, 143] with osseous fragmentation, sclerosis, and disorganization. Thus, pyrophosphate arthropathy should be considered in the differential diagnosis of rapidly progressive destruction of large joints.

10.6.3 MR Findings

MR imaging is often used for the evaluation of a painful joint. Thus, it is quite common to encounter CPPD crystal deposition disease in older patients who are studied with routine MR imaging. Due to its inherent low signal on both T1- and T2-weighted images, calcification is difficult to detect on MR imaging. In this instance, correlation with radiograph if available would be very helpful. Usually, the calcification would be seen as linear or punctate hypointense areas. This is present on spin-echo, fast spin-echo (FSE), and STIR images [144]. Sometimes, a small halo of hyperintense signal intensity would be seen surrounding the hypointense area, which could be related to magnetic susceptibility artifacts. The cartilage calcification is best seen on gradient-echo images (with an echo time greater than 5 ms) which produce "blooming" effect to highlight the cartilage calcification. This is from the local magnetic field inhomogeneity produced by magnetic susceptibility of hyaline cartilage and CPPD crystals. Low signal intensity in the hyaline cartilage of chondrocalcinosis should be included in the search pattern, especially in older patients.

Crystal disease should always be a consideration in cases of full-thickness and massive rotator cuff tears in younger patients (as well as secondary impingement in unstable shoulders). CPPD crystal that accumulates in bursal linings may trigger or exacerbate a bursitis. In the synovium, they may mimic other deposition or synovial based processes. The differential diagnosis for this pattern includes hemosiderin, pigmented villonodular synovitis (PVNS), hemophilia, gas related to vacuum phenomenon, and various causes of magnetic susceptibility artifacts [138].

A combination of significant joint-space narrowing and chondrocalcinosis suggests pyrophosphate arthropathy. In pyrophosphate arthropathy, the hallmark of afore-mentioned cyst formation can precede joint-space narrowing and be easily identified on MR imaging. Thus, on MR imaging with relatively less dramatic cartilage loss but prominent osseous and synovial cysts will raise concern for pyrophosphate arthropathy.

10.6.4 Ultrasound Findings

High-frequency ultrasound (US) is rapidly growing in popularity as a diagnostic means for evaluation of crystal-related arthropathies. By virtue of both high resolution and degree of sonic reflectivity, even minimal deposits of calcium pyrophosphate crystals can be detected by US when the radiograph is otherwise normal [145].

High-frequency US can be used to detect articular and juxta-articular alterations and calcific deposits in crystal-related disease with proven accuracy [145, 146].

The normal sonographic appearance of articular cartilage is characterized by two sharply defined hyperechoic margins delineating an anechoic and homogeneous layer. The superficial margin is typically thinner than the deeper one and is optimally visualized when the direction of the US beam is perpendicular to the cartilage surface. CPPD crystals tend to lie within the substance of the hyaline cartilage. The sparkling reflectivity of CPPD crystals allows the clear depiction of even minimal aggregates within cartilage. The crystal deposition can be focal or diffuse, leading to "double-contour" sign, which is created by the permeability of crystal permitting US waves to penetrate and depict the bone profile beneath. Calcification of tendons in CPPD is typically linear and extensive and may generate an acoustic shadow. A study by Filippucci and colleague on patients with established diagnosis of gout or CPPD demonstrated high specificity of US findings and indicating supraspinatus tendon and fibrocartilage of the AC joint are the most frequence affected structures in the shoulder [147].

The ability of US to detect CPPD crystals in joints with aspirated synovial fluid containing CPPD crystals has been investigated with excellent results [148]. Furthermore, US guidance permits aspiration of even minimal amounts of fluid within joint, peri-tendinous, or bursal. The obtained fluid analysis is of utmost importance in establishing the diagnosis of crystal deposition.

10.7 Calcium Hydroxyapatite Deposition Disease (HAD)

10.7.1 Definition

HAD is characterized by periarticular calcifications, usually in tendons near their osseous attachments. Bursae, ligaments, and peri-tendinous soft tissues are other common sites involved. Although the most recognized manifestation of HAD is calcific tendinitis, calcific periarthritis is the more preferred phrase due to the inclusive nature of the phrase.

The deposition of hydroxyapatite and related calcium phosphate crystals is divided into primary and secondary processes [149]. For example, collagen vascular diseases, end-stage renal disease, and vitamin D intoxication can all result in secondary deposition of hydroxyapatite. The exact etiology of the primary or idiopathic form is not yet known. There has been extensive studies on the pathophysiology of periarticular HAD, with most of the research focused on rotator cuff tendons, one of the most commonly involved sites.

One earlier theory favored that calcifications preferentially deposit in degenerated tendons over the health tendon. This proposal was originally championed by Codman [150] that calcification arises within necrotic and dystrophic tendon fibers that occur naturally with aging. Recently, the reactive hypothesis proposed by Uhthoff and colleagues argues that hydroxyapatite deposits in healthy tissue via cell-mediated processes and that the calcifications of HAD pass three distinct stages [151]. The first or pre-calcific stage is marked by fibrocartilaginous metaplasia of tenocytes into chondrocytes. This metaplasia may be stimulated by decreased local oxygen tension, which in turn may be secondary to repetitive compression of tendon fibers. The second, calcific stage is further divided into formative, resting, and resorptive phases. Chalky deposits develop during the formative phase, and then are bordered by fibrocollagenous tissues during the resting phase when calcium hydroxyapatite accumulation ceases. In the resorptive phase, vascular channels form around the deposit and provide access to macrophages and multinucleated giant cells. Then phagocytosis removes the calcium. Uhthoff and Loehr [151] noted that, during the resorptive phase, the calcification has a toothpaste-like, creamy quality and is often under pressure. The third, post-calcific stage is marked by fibroblast proliferation and partial or complete tendon reconstitution.

This disorder is usually monoarticular and most commonly presents between the ages of 40 and 70 years and peaks in the fifth decade of life with a slight male predilection. Gondos made the interesting observation that the frequency of involvement of a joint roughly paralleled its physiologic range of motion. In his series, calcifications about the shoulder occurred in 69% of all cases, followed by the hip, elbow, wrist, and knee [152]. This is in contrast to its much less common involvement of shoulder by CPPD deposition disease. However, clinical findings in both HAD and CPPD can be quite similar.

Bosworth reviewed more than 6000 shoulders and found HAD deposits in 2.7%; but of these only 30% were symptomatic. Half of the affected cases showed bilateral calcifications [153].

When symptomatic, patients present with pain, erythema, swelling, and limitation of motion of the neighboring joint [154]. The most symptomatic of the HAD stages is the calcific stage, specifically during its resorptive phase. These effects are thought to result from rupture of a calcific deposit into an adjacent soft-tissue space or bursa, causing an acute self-limited inflammatory reaction. Phagocytosis of hydroxyapatite crystals by neutrophils and macrophages results in the release of lysosomal enzymes and other inflammatory mediators [155, 156]. This condition is known as acute calcific periarthritis. The pain often mimics subacromial impingement, being elicited or exacerbated by recurrent or prolonged abduction. Clinically, HAD can be accompanied by fever and can mimic an infection, especially in the resorptive stage. Normal erythrocyte sedimentation rate and leukocyte count are distinguishing characteristics that differentiate HAD from infection [154]. More chronic and dull pain is seen in patients during other stages of HAD.

The definitive diagnosis of HAD is made by identifying hydroxyapatite and related calcium phosphate crystals (such as octacalcium phosphate, carbonate apatite, and calcium triphosphate) in the affected joint. Since this requires electron microscopy, electron diffraction studies, or a specialized alizarin red S stain which are all impractical diagnostic tools in the routine clinical setting, radiographic findings play a major role in the diagnosis of HAD [149].

Treatment is often directed at symptom relief, with most symptoms subsiding in less than 2–3 weeks. NSAIDs are the main treatments [157]. Local corticosteroid injections and oral or parenteral steroids can be used for patients who cannot tolerate NSAIDs.

Symptomatic deposits can be removed under ultrasound with needle puncture, aspiration, and lavage and steroid injection if symptoms do not resolve quickly. Extracorporeal shockwave therapy has been advocated by some; a recent meta-analysis by Lee and colleagues [158] concluded level B support for this technique in recalcitrant cases [159]. Surgical debridement remains the definitive treatment for refractory calcific tendinitis, with postoperative physical therapy identified as a critical component expediting return to baseline activity levels. Concomitant subacromial decompression has fallen out of favor because of longer recovery times and no demonstrable added benefit on 5-year outcome analysis [160].

10.7.2 Radiographic and CT Findings

Initially, HAD presents as a thin, cloudlike, poorly defined clump of calcification in periarticular soft tissues such as tendons, ligaments, bursae, or synovium. Later the calcifications become denser and more homogenous with well-defined margins. Deposits can remain static over the years. They also can enlarge, change shape, or disappear. Rarely, the crystals can deposit in the joint [161]. Recognition of the dynamic nature of the process is very important in avoiding some diagnostic pitfalls. The region of hydroxyapatite deposition may show variable consistency and may spontaneously decrease or increase in size and may cause local intense inflammatory reaction in the soft tissues and occasionally erosion in adjacent bone (Fig. 10.9).

Several authors have proposed various classification systems based on the size of the deposits on the radiograph, stage of the disease process, and its morphological appearances.

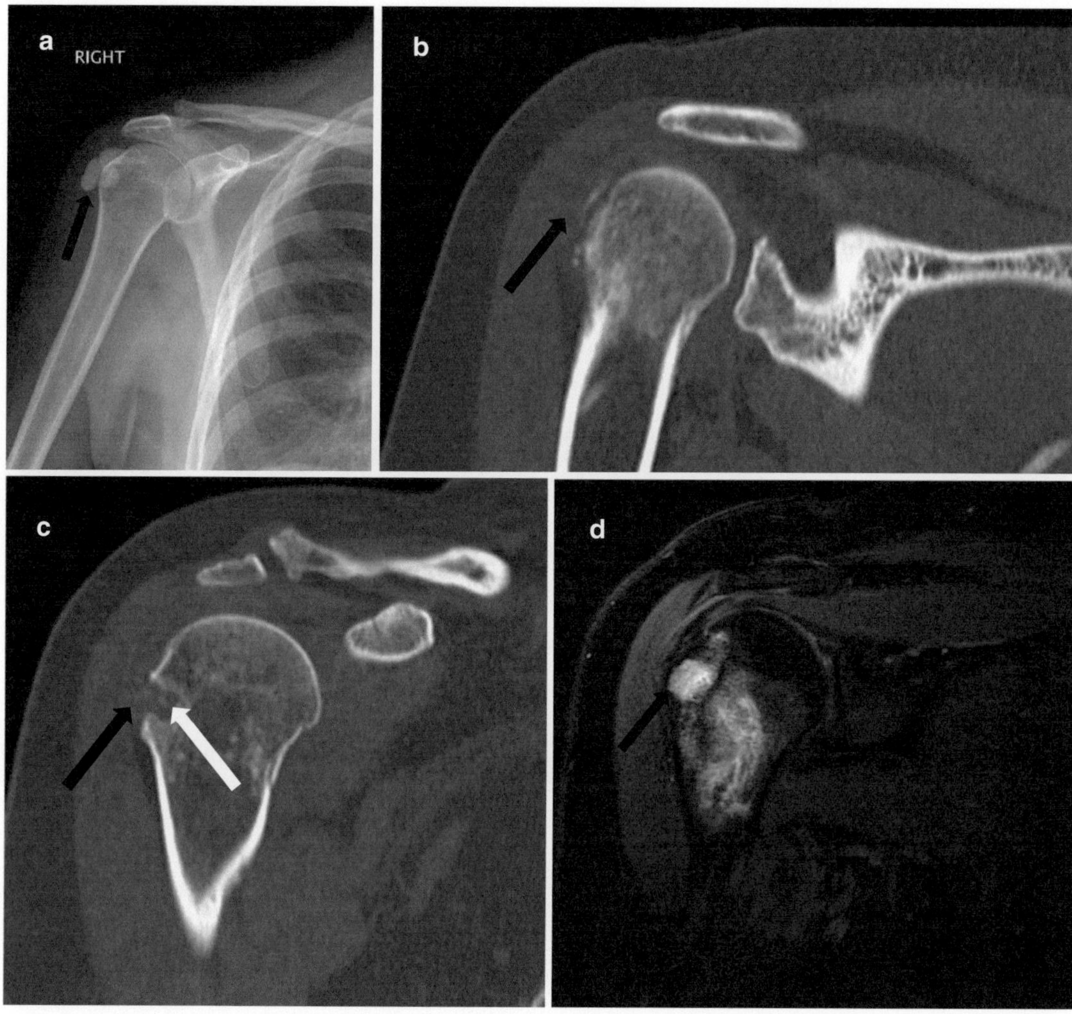

Fig. 10.9 Calcific tendinitis with possible secondary osseous involvement. Frontal view radiograph of the right shoulder (**a**), sagittal reformatted CT images of the right shoulder (**b**, **c**), and coronal oblique fat-suppressed fluid-sensitive MR image (**d**) of the same patient. The CT and MRI images were obtained about 4 months later after the radiograph. Frontal radiograph A demonstrates globular HAD (black arrow) around the humeral head. CT of the right shoulder (**b**, **c**) approximately 4 months later demonstrates interval change to linear calcification along the humeral head (black arrow) and underlying cystic erosions (black arrow) with some vague calcification within (white arrow), indicating migration of the calcification into the osseous structure. Coronal oblique MR image (**d**) demonstrates the erosion at the humeral head (black arrow). Incidentally noted is a chondroid lesion in the proximal humerus

Bosworth proposed the classification based on the size of the deposits [162]. Large deposits are the ones measuring 1.5 cm or more in their greatest profile dimension, medium-size deposits are the ones measuring less than 1.5 cm, and tiny deposits are the ones that can be seen only on fluoroscopy.

De Palma and Kruper had classified these appearances into two main types: Type 1 has a fluffy, fleecy appearance that corresponds to the resorptive phase. Occasionally, there is crescentic shaped streaky density above the fluffy deposits; this suggests extrusion into the overlying bursa (Fig. 10.10). Type 2 deposits correspond to the

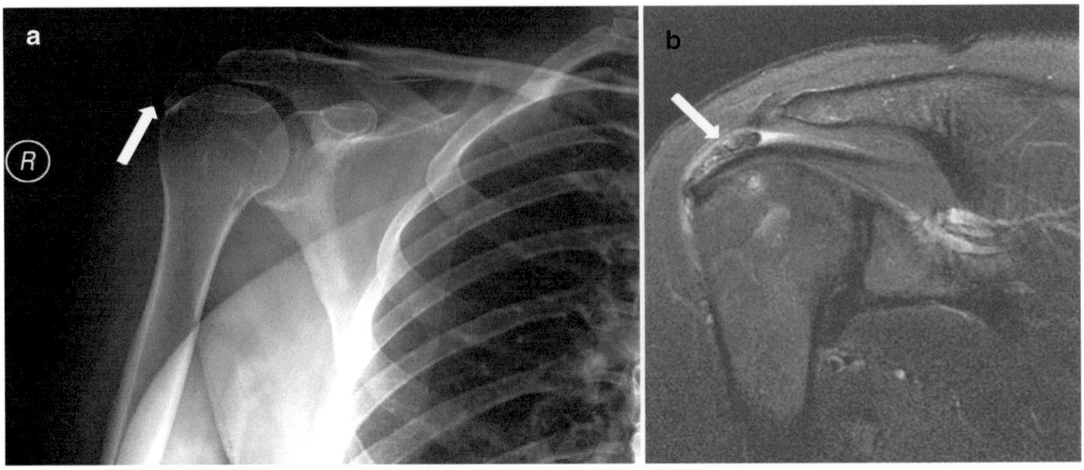

Fig. 10.10 Calcific tendinitis/bursitis. Frontal view of the right shoulder (**a**) and coronal oblique fat-suppressed fluid-sensitive weighted (**b**) images of the same patient. Subacromial subdeltoid bursa calcification usually appears as teardrop or crescent-shaped radiodense area (white arrows) below acromion and deltoid (**a**) and confirmed on MRI image (**b**)

late formative stage, and are marked by homogeneous, more defined calcific densities. It is usually ovoid in shape, and occasionally triangular and linear shape can be seen [163].

Mole developed the classification system based on the morphology [164]:

- Type A: Calcification dense, homogenous with clear contours
- Type B: Calcification dense split/separated with clear contours
- Type C: Calcification nonhomogeneous serrated contours
- Type D: Calcification as dystrophic calcification of the insertion in continuity with the tuberosity

The shoulder is the most common site of HAD, accounting for 60% of cases of acute calcific periarthritis [165]. Periarticular calcifications in one or both shoulders occur in as many as 7.5% of adults [165].

Calcifications can be seen in any of the rotator cuff tendons, with the supraspinatus tendon being the most common site. In order of decreasing frequency, the infraspinatus, teres minor, and subscapularis may be affected [166]. These calcific deposits around supraspinatus tend to be around the greater tuberosity on anteroposterior external rotation views of the shoulder and move medially on the internal rotation view. Calcifications of the infraspinatus and teres minor tendons are best seen in profile on internal rotation anteroposterior views, lateral to the humeral head. The former moves laterally on external rotation views. Subscapularis tendon calcifications are better seen on the axillary view, close to the lesser tuberosity of the humeral head. In contrast, subacromial subdeltoid bursa calcification appears as oval or teardrop-shaped radio-dense area superior to the humeral head but below the acromion (Fig. 10.10).

In the study by Loew and colleagues, they found that the site with the highest incidence of HAD deposits was broadened to include not only the supraspinatus tendon but also the adjoining, cranial portion of the subscapularis [167]. The study further reported that most supraspinatus deposits lie in the midportion of the tendon or just subjacent to its acromial surface. Uhthoff and Loehr [151] observed that it is uncommon for intratendinous HAD deposits to contract the bone surface because they are generally 1.5 or 2 cm away from it. In the case of the supraspinatus, this corresponds to the critical zone thought to be the region most susceptible to tears because of its relatively diminished vascularity and/or lower oxygen tension. However, rotator cuff tears are not common in the setting of calcific periarthritis. In their study population, only one patient had a coexistent partial-thickness tear, and only one patient had intraosseous extension of the calcification. Multiple other studies have corroborated this lack of correlation between HAD and rotator cuff tears. When tears do occur, they tend to occur more often in the setting of small rather than large deposits [168]. The characteristic location of calcifications within the critical zone can be used to distinguish HAD from degenerative calcifications.

HAD can also be seen in the origin of the long head of the biceps above the glenoid fossa, and below the coracoid at the origin of the short head of the biceps and coracobrachialis tendons. Calcifications adjacent to the inferior margin of the glenoid indicate HAD at the origin of the triceps tendon.

The pectoralis major tendon calcifications are seen along the anterior margin of the proximal humeral shaft, specifically along the lateral lip of the distal aspect of the bicipital groove. Erosions within the humerus are rare when HAD involves rotator cuff, although sometimes they can be seen in cases of pectoralis calcific tendinitis. Cortical erosion at the tendinous insertion may occur, and the juxtaposition of the erosive change and the insertional HAD deposit can radiographically mimic a destructive juxtacortical, partially mineralized mass. The few reported cases in the literature have noted that the HAD deposit spontaneously resolved over 6–10 weeks [169–171]. In worrisome cases, biopsy may be performed, and psammomatous bodies can confirm HAD and exclude neoplasm.

10.7.3 MR Findings

The calcification of HAD is hard to identify on MR due to its inherent low signal (Fig. 10.11). Zubler and colleagues concluded from a study of 62 MR shoulder arthrograms that MR imaging alone is unreliable for diagnosis of HAD [172]. However, sometimes there is edema in the adjacent marrow and soft tissue (Fig. 10.11), which increases its conspicuity, and raises the concern for differential diagnosis of infection, injury, or neoplasm [173]. Image interpreters need to be vigilant for detection of ovoid-shaped low signal foci around the rotator cuff tendon in our search

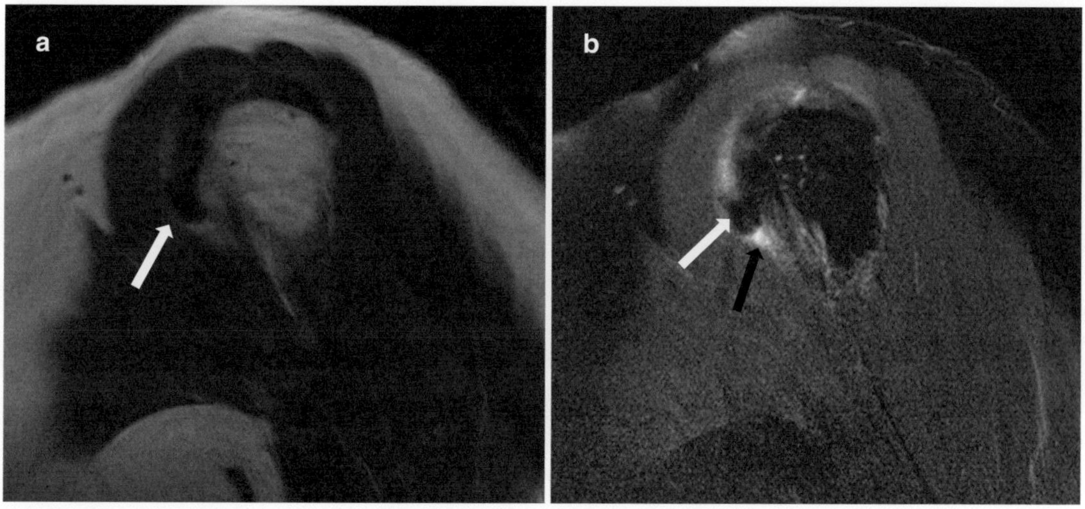

Fig. 10.11 Calcific tendinitis. Sagittal oblique proton density (**a**) and sagittal oblique fat-suppressed, fluid-sensitive weighted (**b**) MR images. **a** demonstrates focal low signal circumscribed HAD deposits (white arrow) along the subscapularis tendon anteriorly. **b** demonstrates thin rim of signal hyperintensity (black arrow) around the HAD deposit (white arrow) compatible with peri-tendon edema and highlights the focal calcification which was less obvious on the proton density images of (**a**)

pattern. In the resorptive and inflammatory stages adjacent high T2 signal and bursitis are frequent.

Loew and colleagues [167] set out attempting to determine whether MR imaging appearances of calcific tendinitis in 76 patients correlated with the feature of osseous subacromial impingement. They concluded that there was no significant correlation, but did observe three distinct MR imaging morphologies of rotator cuff HAD in 71 of their patients. Type A (54%) appearance is a compact, homogenous, single deposit with a defined outline. Type B (38%) appearances were subdivided rather than solitary but remained homogenous and well defined. Type C (7%) appearance is diffuse low signal intensity without a defined outline. In 45 patients in their study, a band of T2 signal hyperintensity surrounded the calcification and was thought to represent perifocal edema.

Osseous involvement as cortical erosion and bone marrow edema is gaining more recognition recently. Hayes and colleagues [174] first described this phenomenon in 1987, presenting a case series of five patients with calcific tendinosis in pectoralis major, gluteus maximus, and adductor magnus tendons with associated cortical erosion at the tendon insertion sites. This author hypothesized that bone resorption may be secondary to increased vascularity and inflammation at the tendon site or alternatively may be due to adjacent mass effect. Recently, Flemming and colleagues [175] retrospectively reviewed 50 cases of osseous involvement in calcific tendinosis and found 11 patients with cortical erosions in the shoulder. Even less commonly described is the associated bone marrow edema, which may occur with or without cortical erosion (Fig. 10.9) [176]. This may lead to difficulties in differentiating this entity from other diagnostic considerations such as neoplasm and infection [176].

10.7.4 Ultrasound Findings

Ultrasound can accurately depict the location, morphology, and size of the calcific deposits on the rotator cuff. Additionally, with sonography, the calcification can be localized by depth so that bursal or tendon calcification can be distinguished. In this assessment, the sensitivity of ultrasound diagnosis was reported at 94% with specificity at 99% and accuracy at 99% [177].

Calcification along the rotator cuff can be seen as hyperechoic focus with acoustic shadow, no shadow, or faint shadow [177]. The more discrete and well-defined calcification of the resting phase on radiograph tends to create more acoustic shadowing on ultrasound. During the resorptive phase, the calcification on radiograph is ill defined and usually shows no or very little acoustic shadowing on ultrasound.

Ultrasound has been shown to detect most of the big and small scattered calcifications around the rotator cuff. However, the shadow of acromion makes the subacromial calcification hard to detect on ultrasound. However, this kind of calcification around the myotendinous junction is rare. Calcifications can interference diagnosis of rotator cuff tear on ultrasound because the calcification can obscure the structure behind.

Larger calcifications located at the location of the confluence of the supraspinatus and infraspinatus tendon are found to be most symptomatic [178]. The symptomatic calcific tendinitis may cause adjacent focal thickening of the tendon on ultrasound images. The advantage of ultrasound diagnosis is that when probed percutaneously, there may be elicited pain. A concomitant subacromial subdeltoid bursa formation can be easily identified on the ultrasound. Some authors have showed that the presence of a power Doppler signal near the tendon calcification is more common in patients with symptomatic calcifications than in individuals with asymptomatic calcifications [179].

10.8 Milwaukee Shoulder

10.8.1 Definition

Milwaukee shoulder is a destructive arthropathy that results from the less common intra-articular accumulation of hydroxyapatite crystals. Symptoms are usually comparatively mild, despite rapid and marked progression seen radiographically.

The term Milwaukee shoulder syndrome was first used in 1981 by McCarty and colleagues [180] to describe four elderly women from Milwaukee, Wisconsin, who presented with recurrent bilateral shoulder joint effusions, radiographic findings of severe destructive changes of the glenohumeral joints, and massive tears of the rotator cuff.

The knees are affected in 50% of the cases with pyrophosphate-like arthropathy [181]. There is some contention about whether the entity purely involves HAD crystals or also involves coexistent intra-articular CPPD deposition [138]. The classic features described by McCarty [182, 183] include pain, loss of joint function, and effusion. In their original series of 30 patients and through their analysis of 42 additional patients who had been reported in other studies, they noted that Milwaukee shoulder favored female patients by a 4:1 ratio. The mean age is 72 years of age. Bilaterality of involvement was observed in 82% of the cases. The dominant arm was always involved and the nondominant arm, when involved, often demonstrated less dramatic changes. However, this pattern is common in most arthropathies. In their series, the patient's pain tended to be mild or intermittent, but restricted range of motion was more universal. Potential predisposing factors were previous trauma (nine patients), CPPD disease (eight patients), neuroarthropathy (three patients), dialysis-associated arthropathy (one patient), and idiopathic (ten patients).

The precise cause of Milwaukee shoulder is unknown. However, intra-articular HA crystals are thought to incite a chronic synovitis that eventually triggers the release of proteases and collagenases. These substances degrade both cartilage and bone. Secondary destabilization of the joint resulting from these processes may promote subclinical destruction [184]. Periarticular calcifications frequently accumulate as well over the course of the disease, and in time the periarticular tissues can also undergo significant destruction.

The treatment of Milwaukee shoulder is usually supportive; resting the affected joint and use of nonsteroidal anti-inflammatory agents have shown to be effective. Colchicine has been shown to be effective in the management [185]. Physiotherapy also has a major role, which provides the required exercise to help the patient to maintain the range of motion and strengthen the surrounding muscles. For large effusions, arthrocentesis is beneficial. Surgical intervention, such as partial or total arthroplasty, is considered in severe or advanced cases, provided that there are no contraindications. More recent studies have suggested some benefits from tidal irrigation [186].

10.8.2 Radiographic and CT Findings

Imaging features of Milwaukee shoulder overlap with those of other arthropathies and not infrequently resemble neuropathic joint. The main imaging differential diagnoses include rapidly destructive or progressing arthropathy, septic arthritis, neuropathic arthropathy, osteonecrosis, inflammatory arthropathy, crystal-associated arthropathy, and arthropathy of late syphilis.

Joint-space narrowing and destruction of subchondral bone are the hallmarks of the Milwaukee shoulder. Joint effusion is a cardinal feature and these tend to be large. Superior migration of the humeral head can be seen as a secondary sign of underlying, related, rotator cuff tear. There are associated scalloping of the undersurface of the acromion, forming pseudoarticulation. This feature can be seen in all causes of rotator cuff arthropathy, and is termed acetabularization of the acromion; the changes in the humeral head are called femurization.

Soft-tissue swelling, capsular calcification, and intra-articular bodies can be seen. Severe and focal osteoporosis of the humeral head is typical. Glenohumeral osteophytes tend to be small or absent. Subchondral cystic changes are not as prominent as in pure pyrophosphate arthropathy.

10.8.3 Ultrasound Findings

Ultrasonography of the shoulder usually shows fluid collection and synovial proliferation.

10.8.4 MRI Findings

Full-thickness rotator cuff tear is common. McCarty even noted that original descriptions of HAD dating to the mid-nineteenth century identified loss of the intra-articular segment of the long head of the biceps tendon as another typical feature [182].

Large joint effusion, thinning of the glenoid cartilage, and subchondral destructions are other finds that can be well documented on MRI.

References

1. Lawrence RC, Felson DT, Helmick CG, et al. Estimates of the prevalence of arthritis and other rheumatic conditions in the United States. II. Arthritis Rheum. 2008;58(1):26–35.
2. Altman R, Asch E, Block D, Bole G, Borenestein D, Brankt K, et al. Development of criteria for the classification and reporting of osteoarthritis. Classification of osteoarthritis of the knee. Diagnostic and therapeutic criteria committee of the American Rheumatism Association. Arthritis Rheum. 1986;29(8):1039–49.
3. Philips WC Jr, Kattapuram SV. Osteoarthritis: with emphasis on primary osteoarthritis of the shoulder. Del Med J. 1991;63(10):609–13.
4. Kerr R, Resnick D, Pineda C, Haghighi P. Osteoarthritis of the glenohumeral joint: a radiologic-pathologic study. AJR. 1985;144:967–72.
5. dePalma AF. Surgery of the shoulder. 3rd ed. Philadelphia: Lippincott; 1983. p. 211–41.
6. Kernwein GA. Roentgenographic diagnosis of shoulder dysfunction. JAMA. 1965;194:179–83.
7. Neer CS. Replacement arthroplasty for glenohumeral osteoarthritis. J Bone Joint Surg Am. 1974;56:1–13.
8. Green A, Norris TR. Imaging techniques for glenohumeral arthritis and glenohumeral arthroplasty. Clin Orthop Rel Res. 1994;307:7–17.
9. Walch G, Boulahia A, Boileau P, Kempf JF. Primary glenohumeral osteoarthritis: clinical and radiographic classification. The Aequalis Group. Acta Orthop Belg. 1998;64(Suppl 2):46–52.
10. Graichen J, Jakob J, von Eisenhart-Rothe R, et al. Validation of cartilage volume and thickness measurements in the human shoulder with quantitative magnetic resonance imaging. Osteoarthr Cartil. 2003;11:475–82.
11. Vasnawala SS, Pauly JM, Nishimura DG, Gold GE. MR imaging of knee cartilage with FEMR. Skelet Radiol. 2002;31:574–80.
12. Hargreaves BA, Gold GE, Beaulieu CF, et al. Comparison of new sequences for high-resolution cartilage imaging. Magn Reson Med. 2003;49:700–9.
13. Bashir A, Gray ML, Boutin RD, Burstein D. Glycosaminoglycan in articular cartilage: in vivo assessment with delayed Gd (DTPA) (2-)-enhanced MR imaging. Radiology. 1997;205:551–8.
14. Bashir A, Gray ML, Harke J, Burstein D. Nondestructive imaging of human cartilage glycosaminoglycan concentration by MRI. Magn Reson Med. 1999;41:857–65.
15. Reddy R, Insko EK, Noyszewski EA, et al. Sodium MRI of human articular cartilage in vivo. Magn Reson Med. 1998;39:697–701.
16. Regatte RR, Akella SV, Borthakur A, Kneeland JB, Reddy R. In vivo proton MR three-dimensional T1ρ mapping of human articular cartilage: initial experience. Radiology. 2003;229(1):269–74.
17. Brossmann J, Frank LR, Pauly JM, et al. Short echo time projection reconstruction MR imaging of cartilage: comparison with fat-suppressed spoiled GRASS and magnetization transfer contrast MR imaging. Radiology. 1997;203:501–7.
18. Bianchi S, Martinoli C. Detection of loose bodies in joint. Radiol Clin N Am. 1999;37:679–90.
19. Neer CS 2nd, Craig EV, Fukuda H. Cuff-tear arthropathy. J Bone Joint Surg Am. 1983;65(9):1232–44.
20. Collins DN, Harryman DT 2nd. Arthroplasty for arthritis and rotator cuff deficiency. Orthop Clin North Am. 1997;28(2):225–39.
21. Macaulay AA, Greiwe RM, Bigliani LU. Rotator cuff deficient arthritis of the glenohumeral joint. Clin Orthop Surg. 2010;2(4):196–202.
22. Ecklund JK, Lee TQ, Tibone J, Gupta R. Rotator cuff tear arthropathy. J Am Acad Orthop Surg. 2007;15(6):340–9.
23. Feeley BT, Gallo RA, Craig EV. Cuff tear arthropathy: current trends in diagnosis and surgical management. J Shoulder Elb Surg. 2009;18(3):484–94.
24. Jensen KL, Williams GR Jr, Russell IJ, Rockwood CA Jr. Rotator cuff tear arthropathy. J Bone Joint Surg Am. 1999;81(9):1312–24.
25. Zeman CA, Arcand MA, Cantrell JS, Skedros JG, Burkhead WZ Jr. The rotator cuff-deficient arthritic shoulder: diagnosis and surgical management. J Am Acad Orthop Surg. 1998;6(6):337–48.
26. Visotsky JL, Basamania C, Seebauer L, Rockwood CA, Jensen KL. Cuff tear arthropathy: pathogenesis, classification, and algorithm for treatment. J Bone Joint Surg Am. 2004;86(Suppl 2):35–40.
27. Nam D, Maak TG, Raphael BS, Kepler CK, Cross MB, Warren RF. Rotator cuff tear arthropathy: evaluation, diagnosis, and treatment: AAOS exhibit selection. J Bone Joint Surg Am. 2012;94(6):e24.
28. Hamada K, Fukuda H, Mikasa M, Kobayashi Y. Roentgenographic findings in massive rotator cuff tears: a long-term observation. Clin Orthop Relat Res. 1990;254:92–6.
29. Sirveaux F, Favard L, Oudet D, Huquet D, Walch G, Molé D. Grammont inverted total shoulder arthroplasty in the treatment of glenohumeral osteoarthritis with massive rupture of the cuff. Results

of a multicentre study of 80 shoulders. JBJS. 2004;86(3):388–95.
30. Saupe N, Pfirrmann CW, Schmid MR, Jost B, Werner CM, Zanetti M. Association between rotator cuff abnormalities and reduced acromiohumeral distance. AJR. 2006;187(2):376–82.
31. Klinger HM, Baums MH, Freche S, et al. Septic arthritis of the shoulder joint: an analysis of management and outcome. Acta Orthop Belg. 2010;76(5):598–603.
32. Mehta P, Schnall SB, Zalavras CG. Septic arthritis of the shoulder, elbow, and wrist. Clin Orthop Relat Res. 2006;451:42–5.
33. Cleeman E, Auerbach JD, Klingenstein GG, et al. Septic arthritis of the glenohumeral joint: a review of 23 cases. J Surg Orthop Adv. 2005;14(2):102–7.
34. Leslie BM, Harris JM III, Driscoll D. Septic arthritis of the shoulder in adults. J Bone Joint Surg Am. 1989;71(10):1516–22.
35. Peiffenberger J, Meiss L. Septic conditions of the shoulder- an up-dating of treatment strategies. Arch Orthop Trauma Surg. 1996;115(6):325–31.
36. Sussmann AR, Cohen J, Nomikos GC, Schweitzer ME. Magnetic resonance imaging of shoulder arthropathies. Magn Reson Imaging Clin N Am. 2012;29(2):349–71.
37. Resnick D, Niwayama G. Osteomyelitis, septic arthritis, and soft tissue infection. In: Resnick D, Niwayama G, editors. Diagnosis of bone and joint disorders, vol. 3. 4th ed. Philadelphia: WB Saunders; 2002. p. 2419–35.
38. Cofield RH. The shoulder: results of complications. In: Morey BF, Cooney WPI, editors. Joint replacement arthroplasty. New York: Churchill Livingstone; 1991. p. 437–53.
39. Silliman JF, Hawkins RJ. Complications following shoulder arthroplasty. In: Friedman RJ, editor. Arthroplasty of the shoulder. New York: Thieme; 1994. p. 242–53.
40. Mohana-Borges AV, Chung CB, Resnick D. Monoarticular arthritis. Radiol Clin N Am. 2004;42(1):135–49.
41. Shirtliff ME, Mader JT. Acute septic arthritis. Clin Microbiol Rev. 2002;15(4):527–44.
42. Dubost JJ, Soubrier M, De Champs C, et al. No changes in the distribution of organisms responsible for septic arthritis over a 20 year period. Ann Rheum Dis. 2002;61(3):267–9.
43. Ho G Jr. Bacterial arthritis. Curr Opin Rheumatol. 2001;13(4):310–4.
44. Stimmler MM. Infectious arthritis: tailoring initial treatment to clinical findings. Postgrad Med. 1996;99(4):127–31.. (discussion 135-9)
45. Swan A, Amer H, Dieppe P. The value of synovial fluid assays in the diagnosis of joint disease: a literature survey. Ann Rheum Dis. 2002;61: 493–8.
46. Yoshikawa TT. Antimicrobial resistance and aging: beginning of the end of the antibiotic era? J Am Geriatr Soc. 2002;50(7 suppl):S226–9.
47. Greenspan A, Tehranzadeh J. Imaging of infectious arthritis. Radiol Clin N Am. 2001;39(2):267–76.
48. Rutten MJ, van den Berg JC, van den Hoogen FH, et al. Nontuberculous mycobacterial bursitis and arthritis of the shoulder. Skelet Radiol. 1998;27(1):33–5.
49. Kapukaya A, Subasi M, Burke Y, et al. Tuberculosis of the shoulder joint. Joint Bone Spine. 2006;73(2):177–81.
50. Recht MP, Kramer J, Petersilge CA, et al. Distribution of normal and abnormal fluid collections in the glenohumeral joint: implications for MR arthrography. J Magn Reson Imaging. 1994;4(2):173–7.
51. Schweitzer ME, Magbalon MJ, Fenlin JM, et al. Effusion criteria and clinical importance of glenohumeral joint fluid: MR imaging evaluation. Radiology. 1995;194(3):821–4.
52. Bremell T, abdelnour A, Tarkowski A. Histopathological and serological progression of experimental *Staphylococcus aureus* arthritis. Infect Immun. 1992;60(7):2976–85.
53. Karchevsky M, Schweitzer ME, Morrison WB, et al. MRI findings of septic arthritis and associated osteomyelitis in adults. AJR Am J Roentgenol. 2004;182(1):119–22.
54. Graif M, Schweitzer ME, Deely D, Matteucci T. The septic versus nonseptic inflamed joint: MRI characteristics. Skelet Radiol. 1999;28(11):616–20.
55. Bierry G, Huang AJ, Chang CY, Torriani M, Bredella MA. MRI findings of treated bacterial septic arthritis. Skelet Radiol. 2012;41(12):1509–16.
56. Lutz AM, Seemayer C, Corot C, et al. Detection of synovial macrophages in an experimental rabbit model of antigen-induced arthritis: ultrasmall superparamagnetic iron oxide-enhanced MR imaging. Radiology. 2004;233(1):149–57.
57. Bierry G, Jehl F, Neuville A, et al. MRI of macrophages in infectious knee synovitis. AJR Am J Roentgenol. 2010;194(6):W521–6.
58. Lutz AM, Weishaupt D, Persohn E, et al. Imaging of macrophages in soft-tissue infection in rats: relationship between ultrasmall superparamagnetic iron oxide dose and MR signal characteristics. Radiology. 2005;234(3):765–75.
59. Heale JP, Speert DP. Macrophages in bacterial infection. In: Burke B, Lewis CE, editors. The macrophage. 2nd ed. Oxford: Oxford University Press; 2002. p. 210–52.
60. Sigovan M, Boussel L, Sulaiman A, et al. Rapid-clearance iron nanoparticles for inflammation imaging of atherosclerotic plaque: initial experience in animal model. Radiology. 2009;252(2):401–9.
61. Hyafil F, Laissy JP, Mazighi M, et al. Ferumoxtran-10-enhanced MRI of the hypercholesterolemic rabbit aorta: relationship between signal loss and macrophage infiltration. Arterioscler Thromb Vasc Biol. 2006;26(1):176–81.
62. Lefevre S, Ruimy D, Neuville A, et al. Septic arthritis: monitoring with USPIO-enhanced macrophage MR imaging. Radiology. 2011;258(3):722–8.

63. Richter R, Hahn H, Nubling W, et al. Shoulder girdle and shoulder joint tuberculosis. Z Rheumatol. 1985;44(2):87–92.. (in German)
64. Griffith JF, Peh WC, Evans NS, et al. Multiple rice body formation in chronic subacromial/subdeltoid bursitis: MR appearances. Clin Radiol. 1996;51(7):511–4.
65. Hayter CL, Koff MF, Shah P, et al. MRI after arthroplasty: comparison of MAVRIC and conventional fast spin-echo techniques. AJR Am J Roentgenol. 2011;197(3):W405–11.
66. Chen CA, Chen W, Goodman SB, et al. New MR imaging methods for metallic implants in the knee: artifact correction and clinical impact. J Magn Reson Imaging. 2011;33(5):1121–7.
67. Koch KM, Brau AC, Chen W, et al. Imaging near metal with a MAVRIC-SEMAC hybrid. Magn Reson Med. 2011;65(1):71–82.
68. Widman DS, Craig JG, van Holsbeeck MT. Sonographic detection, evaluation and aspiration of infected acromioclavicular joints. Skelet Radiol. 2001;30:388–92.
69. Garcia-De La Torre I. Advances in the management of septic arthritis. Infect Dis Clin N Am. 2006;20(4):773–88.
70. Gordon JE, Huang M, Dobbs M, et al. Causes of false-negative ultrasound scans in the diagnosis of septic arthritis of the hip in children. J Pediatr Orthop. 2002;22:312–6.
71. Zubler V, Mamisch-Saupe N, Pfirrmann CW, et al. Detection and quantification of glenohumeral joint effusion: reliability of ultrasound. Eur Radiol. 2011;21(9):1858–64.
72. Michel BA, Bloch DA, Wolfe F, Fries JF. Fractures in rheumatoid arthritis: an evaluation of associated risk factors. J Rheumatol. 1993;20:1666–9.
73. Kirwan JR, Silman AJ. Epidemiological, sociological and environmental aspects of rheumatoid arthritis and osteoarthrosis. Baillieres Clin Rheumatol. 1987;1(3):467–89.
74. Kirwan JR. Rheumatology out-patient workload increases inexorably. Br J Rheumatol. 1997;36(4):481–6.
75. Arnett FC. Goldman: Cecil text-book of medicine. In: Rheumatoid arthritis. 21st ed. Philadelphia: W. B. Saunders Co; 2000.
76. McInnes IB, Schett G. The pathogenesis of rheumatoid arthritis. N Engl J Med. 2011;365(23): 2205–19.
77. Felson DT, Klareskog L. The genetics of rheumatoid arthritis: new insights and implications. JAMA. 2015;313(16):1623–4.
78. Cooles FA, Isaacs JD. Pathophysiology of rheumatoid arthritis. Curr Opin Rheumatol. 2011;23(3): 233–40.
79. Hitchon CA, Chandad F, Ferucci ED, et al. Antibodies to porphyromonas gingivalis are associated with anticitrullinated protein antibodies in patients with rheumatoid arthritis and their relatives. J Rheumatol. 2010;37(6):1105–12.
80. van den Berg WB. Lessons from animal models of osteoarthritis. Curr Opin Rheumatol. 2001;13(5):452–6.
81. Tak PP, Bresnihan B. The pathogenesis and prevention of joint damage in rheumatoid arthritis: advances from synovial biopsy and tissue analysis. Arthritis Rheum. 2000;43(12):2619–33.
82. Philippe L, Alsaleh G, Suffert G, Meyer A, Georgel P, Sibilia J, Wachsmann D, Pfeffer S. TLR2 expression is regulated by microRNA miR-10 in rheumatoid fibroblast-like synoviocytes. J Immunol. 2012;188(1):454–61.
83. Hämälainen N. Epidemiology of upper limb joint affections in rheumatoid arthritis. In: Baumgartner H, Dvorak J, Grob D, Munzinger U, Simmen B, editors. Rheumatoid arthritis: current trends in diagnostics, conservative treatment, and surgical reconstruction. Stuttgart: Georg Thieme Verlag; 1995. p. 158–61.
84. Lehtinen JT, Lehto MU, Kaarela K, Kautiainen HJ, Belt EA, Kauppi MJ. Radiographic joint space in rheumatoid glenohumeral joints. A 15-year prospective follow-up study in 74 patients. Rheumatology (Oxford). 2000;39:288–92.
85. Cruess RL. Corticosteroid-induced osteonecrosis of the humeral head. Orthop Clin North Am. 1985;16(4):789–96.
86. Ennevaara K. Painful shoulder joint in rheumatoid arthritis. A clinical and radiological study of 200 cases, with special reference to arthrography of the glenohumeral joint. Acta Rheumatol Scand. 1967;Suppl 11:11–116.
87. Smith AM, Sperling JW, Cofield RH. Arthroscopic rotator cuff debridement in patients with rheumatoid arthritis. J Shoulder Elb Surg. 2007;16(1):31–6.
88. Chen AL, Joseph TN, Zuckerman JD. Rheumatoid arthritis of the shoulder. J Am Acad Orthop Surg. 2003;11:12–24.
89. van der Zwaal P, Pijls BG, Thomassen BJ, Lindenburg R, Nelissen RG, van de Sande MA. The natural history of the rheumatoid shoulder: a prospective long-term follow-up study. Bone Joint J. 2014;96-B(11):1520–4.
90. Petersson CJ. The acromioclavicular joint in rheumatoid arthritis. Clin Orthop Relat Res. 1987;223:86–93.
91. van der Heijde DM. Plain X-rays in rheumatoid arthritis: overview of scoring methods, their reliability and applicability. Baillieres Clin Rheumatol. 1996;10(3):435–53.
92. Arnett FC, Edworthy SM, Bloch DA, McShane DJ, Fries JF, Cooper NS, et al. The American rheumatism association 1987 revised criteria for the classification of rheumatoid arthritis. Arthritis Rheum. 1988;31(3):315–24.
93. Tugwell P, Boers M. OMERACT conference on outcome measures in rheumatoid arthritis clinical trials: introduction. J Rheumatol. 1993;20(3):528–30.
94. Larsen A, Dale K, Eek M. Radiographic evaluation of rheumatoid arthritis and related conditions

by standard reference films. Acta Radiol Diagn. 1977;18:481–91.

95. Laine VAI, Vainio KJ, Pekanmäki K. Shoulder affections in rheumatoid arthritis. Ann Rheum Dis. 1954;13:157–60.
96. Neer CS. The rheumatoid shoulder. In: Crubbs RL, Mitchell NS, editors. The surgical management of rheumatoid arthritis. Philadelphia: JB Lippincott; 1971. p. 117–27.
97. Levigne, Ranceschi F. Shoulder arthroplasty. In: Walch, Boileau, editors. Rheumatoid arthritis of the shoulder: radiological presentation and results of arthroplasty. Berlin, Heidelberg: Springer; 1999. p. 221–30.
98. Conaghan PG, McQueen FM, Bird P, et al. Update on research and future directions of the OMERACT MRI inflammatory arthritis group. J Rheumatol. 2011;38(9):2031–3.
99. McQueen FM. Magnetic resonance imaging in early inflammatory arthritis: what is its role? Rheumatology (Oxford). 2000;39(7):700–6.
100. Narvaez JA, Narvaez J, De Lama E, et al. MR imaging of early rheumatoid arthritis. Radiographics. 2010;30(1):143–63.. (discussion:163-5)
101. Sugimoto H, Takeda A, Hyodoh K. MR imaging for evaluation of early rheumatoid arthritis. Semin Musculoskelet Radiol. 2001;5(2):159–65.
102. Cimmino MA, Innocenti S, Livrone F, et al. Dynamic gadolinium-enhanced magnetic resonance imaging of the wrists in patients with rheumatoid arthritis can discriminate active from inactive disease. Arthritis Rheum. 2003;48(5):1207–13.
103. Hodgson RJ, O'Connor P, Moots R. MRI of rheumatoid arthritis image quantitation for the assessment of disease activity, progression and response to therapy. Rheumatology (Oxford). 2008;47(1):13–21.
104. McQueen FM, Stewart N, Crabbe J, Robinson E, Yeoman S, Tan PL, et al. Magnetic resonance imaging of the wrist in early rheumatoid arthritis reveals a high prevalence of erosions at four months after symptom onset. Ann Rheum Dis. 1998;57(6):350–9.
105. McQueen FM, Stewart N, Crabbe J, Robinson E, Yeoman S, Tan PL, et al. Magnetic resonance imaging of the wrist in early rheumatoid arthritis reveals progression of erosions despite clinical improvement. Ann Rheum Dis. 1999;58(3):156–63.
106. Foley-nolan D, Stack JP, Ryan M, Redmond U, Barry C, Ennis J, et al. Magnetic resonance imaging in the assessment of rheumatoid arthritis: a comparison with plain film radiographs. Br J Rheumatol. 1991;31:101–6.
107. Lehtinen JT, Kaarela K, Belt EA, et al. Incidence of glenohumeral joint involvement in seropositive rheumatoid arthritis. A 15 year endpoint study. J Rheumatol. 2000;27(2):347–50.
108. Alasaarela E, Suramo I, Tervonen O, et al. Evaluation of humeral head erosions in rheumatoid arthritis: a comparison of ultrasonography, magnetic resonance imaging, computed tomography and plain radiography. Br J Rheumatol. 1998;37(11):1152–6.
109. Lehtinen JT, Lehto MU, Kaarela K, et al. Acromioclavicular joint subluxation is rare in rheumatoid arthritis. A radiographic 15-year study. Rev Rhum Engl Ed. 1999;66(10):462–6.
110. Cuende E, Vesga JC, Barrenengoa E, et al. Synovial cyst as differential diagnosis of supraclavicular mass in rheumatoid arthritis. J Rheumatol. 1996;23(8):1432–4.
111. Gibbon WW, Wakefield RJ. Ultrasound in inflammatory disease. Radiol Clin N Am. 1999;37:633–51.
112. Wakefield RJ, Gibbon WW, Emery P. The current status of ultrasonography in rheumatology. Rheumatology (Oxford). 1999;38:195–8.
113. Backhaus M, Kamradt T, Sandrock D, Loreck D, Fritz J, Wolf KJ, et al. Arthritis of the finger joints: a comprehensive approach comparing conventional radiography, scintigraphy, ultrasound, and contrast-enhanced magnetic resonance imaging. Arthritis Rheum. 1999;42:1232–45.
114. Backhaus M, Burmester G-R, Gerber T, et al. Guidelines for musculoskeletal ultrasound in rheumatology. Ann Rheum Dis. 2001;60(7):641–9.
115. Alasaarela EM, Alasaarela EL. Ultrasound evaluation of painful rheumatoid shoulders. J Rheumatol. 1994;21:1642–8.
116. Keysser P, Osthus H, Jacobi E. Ultrasound of the shoulder in patients with rheumatoid arthritis. Ann Rheum Dis. 2003;62:519.
117. Sanja MR, Mirjana ZS. Ultrasonographic study of the painful shoulder in patients with rheumatoid arthritis and patients with degenerative shoulder disease. Acta Rheumatol Port. 2010;35(1):50–8.
118. Nevien EL, Heba K, et al. Value of dynamic sonography in the management of shoulder pain in patients with rheumatoid arthritis. Egypt J Radiol Nucl Med. 2014;45(4):1171–82.
119. Ottaviani S, Gill G, Palazzo E, Meyer O, Dieudé P. Ultrasonography of shoulders in spondyloarthritis and rheumatoid arthritis: a case-control study. Joint Bone Spine. 2014;81(3):247–9.
120. Richette P, Bardin T, Doherty M. An update on the epidemiology of calcium pyrophosphate dihydrate crystal deposition disease. Rheumatology (Oxford). 2009;48(7):711–5.
121. McCarty DJ, Hogan JM, Gatter RA, et al. Studies on pathological calcifications in human cartilage. I. Prevalence and types of crystal deposits in the menisci of two hundred fifteen cadavers. J Bone Joint Surg. 1966;48A:309–25.
122. Ryan LM, McCarty DJ. Calcium pyrophosphate crystal deposition disease, pseudogout and articular chondrocalcinosis. In: McCarty DJ, Koopman WJ, editors. Arthritis and allied conditions. 13th ed. Philadelphia: Lea and Febiger; 1997. p. 2103–25.
123. Resnick D, Niwayama G, Georgen TG, et al. Clinical, radiographic and pathologic abnormalities in calcium pyrophosphate dihydrate deposition disease (CPPD): pseudogout. Radiology. 1977;122:1–15.
124. Martel W, McCarter DK, Solsky MA, et al. Further observation of the arthropathy of calcium

pyrophosphate dihydrate crystal deposition disease. Radiology. 1981;141:1–15.
125. Rosenthal AK. Crystals, inflammation, and osteoarthritis. Curr Opin Rheumatol. 2011;23(2):170–3.
126. Ea HK, Liote F. Advances in understanding calcium-containing crystal disease. Curr Opin Rheumatol. 2009;21(2):150–7.
127. McCarty DJ. Calcium pyrophosphate dihydrate crystal deposition disease --1975. Arthritis Rheum. 1976;19(Suppl 3):275–85.
128. Doherty M, Dieppe P. Clinical aspects of calcium pyrophosphate dihydrate crystal deposition. Rheum Dis Clin N Am. 1998;14(2):395–414.
129. Resnick D, Utsinger PD. The wrist arthropathy of "pseudogout" occurring with and without chondrocalcinosis. Radiology. 1974;113:633–41.
130. Fisseler-Eckhoff A, Muller KM. Arthroscopy and chondrocalcinosis. Arthroscopy. 1992;8:98–104.
131. Kanterewicz E, Sanmarti R, Panella D, Brugures J. Tendon calcifications of the hip adductors in chondrocalcinosis: a radiological study of 75 patients. Br J Rheumatol. 1993;32:790–3.
132. Gerster JC, Baud CA, Lagier R, Boussina I, Fallet GH. Tendon calcifications in chondrocalcinosis: a clinical, radiologic, histologic and crystallographic study. Arthritis Rheum. 1977;20:717–22.
133. Foldes K, Lenchik L, Jaovisidha S, Clopton P, Sartoris DJ, Resnick D. Association of gastrocnemius tendon calcification with chondrocalcinosis of the knee. Skelet Radiol. 1996;25:621–4.
134. Martel W, Champion CK, Thompson GR, Carter TL. A roentgenologically distinctive arthropathy in some patients with the pseudogout syndrome. AJR Am J Roentgenol. 1970;109:587–605.
135. Ryan LM, McCarty DJ. Calcium pyrophosphate crystal deposition disease: pseudogout; articular chondrocalcinosis. In: McCarty DJ, editor. Arthritis and allied conditions. Philadelphia: Lea & Febiger; 1985. p. 1515–46.
136. Canhao H, Fonseca JE, Leandro MJ, et al. Cross-sectional study of 50 patients with calcium pyrophosphate dihydrate crystal arthropathy. Clin Rheumatol. 2001;20(2):119–22.
137. Ellman MH, Krieger MI, Brown N. Pseudogout mimicking synovial chondromatosis. J Bone Joint Surg. 1975;57:863–5.
138. Steinbach LS. Calcium pyrophosphate dihydrate and calcium hydroxyapatite crystal deposition diseases: imaging perspectives. Radiol Clin N Am. 2004;42(1):185–205.. vii
139. Schumacher HR Jr, Klippel JH, Koopman WJ. Calcium pyrophosphate dihydrate crystal deposition disease. In: Schumacher HR Jr, Klippel JH, Koopman WJ, Primer on the rheumatic disease. Atlanta Arthritis Foundation; 1993 219–222.
140. Resnick D, Williams G, Weisman MH, et al. Rheumatoid arthritis and pseudo-rheumatoid arthritis in calcium pyrophosphate dihydrate crystal deposition disease. Radiology. 1981;140(3): 615–21.
141. Mizutani H, Ohba S, Mizutani M, et al. Tumoral calcium pyrophosphate dihydrate deposition disease with bone destruction in the shoulder. CT and MR findings in two cases. Acta Radiol. 1998;39(3):269–72.
142. Richards AJ, Hamilton EBD. Destructive arthropathy in chondrocalcinosis articularis. Ann Rheum Dis. 1973;33:196.
143. Jacobelli S, McCarty DJ, Silcox DC, et al. Calcium pyrophosphate dihydrate crystal deposition in neuropathic joints: four cases of polyarticular involvement. Ann Intern Med. 1973;79:340–7.
144. Beltran J, Marty-Delfaut E, Bencardino J, et al. Chondrocalcinosis of the hyaline cartilage of the knee: MRI manifestations. Skelet Radiol. 1998;27(7):369–74.
145. Dufauret-Lombard C, Vergne-Salle P, Simon A, Bonnet C, Treves R, Bertin P. Ultrasonography in chondrocalcinosis. Joint Bone Spine. 2010;77(3):218–21.
146. Fodor D, Albu A, Gherman C. Crystal-associated synovitis-ultrasonographic feature, clinical correlation. Orthop Trumatol Rehabil. 2008;10(2):99–110.
147. Filippucci E, Sedie AD, Riente L, et al. Ultrasound imaging for the rheumatologist. XLVII. Ultrasound of the shoulder in patients with gout and calcium pyrophosphate deposition disease. Clin Exp Rheumatol. 2013;31(5):659–64.
148. Frediani B, Filippou G, Falsetti P, et al. Diagnosis of calcium pyrophosphate dihydrate crystal deposition disease: ultrasonographic criteria proposed. Ann Rheum Dis. 2005;64:638–40.
149. Hayes CW, Conway WF. Calcium hydroxyapatite deposition disease. Radiographics. 1990;10:1031–48.
150. Codman EA. The shoulder. Boston: Todd; 1934.
151. Uhthoff HK, Loehr JW. Calcific tendinopathy of the rotator cuff: pathogenesis, diagnosis, and management. J Am Acad Orthop Surg. 1997;5(4):183–91.
152. Gordon B. Observations on periarthritis calcarea. AJR. 1957;77:93–108.
153. Bosworth BM. Calcium deposits in the shoulder and subacromial bursitis: a survey of 12,122 shoulders. JAMA. 1941;116:2477–82.
154. Selby CL. Acute calcific tendinitis of the hand: an infrequently recognized and frequently misdiagnosed form of periarthritis. Arthritis Rheum. 1984;27:337–40.
155. Terkeltaub RA, Ginsberg MH. The inflammatory reaction to crystals. Rheum Dis Clin N Am. 1988;14:353–64.
156. Elferink JGR, Deiekauf M. A biochemical study of hydroxyapatite crystal induced enzyme release from neutrophils. Ann Rheum Dis. 1987;46:590–7.
157. Cho Ns LBG, Rhee YG. Radiologic course of the calcific deposits in calcific tendinitis of the shoulder: does the initial radiologic aspect affect the final results? J Shoulder Elb Surg. 2010;19(2):267–72.
158. Lee SY, Cheng B, Grimmer-Somers K. The midterm effectiveness of extracorporeal shockwave therapy

in the management of chronic calcific shoulder tendinitis. J Shoulder Elb Surg. 2011;20(5):845–54.
159. Mouzopoulos G, Stamatakos M, Mouzopoulos D, et al. Extracorporeal shock wave treatment for shoulder calcific tendonitis: a systematic review. Skelet Radiol. 2007;36(9):803–11.
160. Marder RA, Heiden EA, Kim S. Calcific tendonitis of the shoulder: is subacromial decompression in combination with removal of the calcific deposit beneficial? J Shoulder Elb Surg. 2011;20(6):955–60.
161. Bonavita JA, Dalinka MK, schumacher HR. Hydroxyapatite deposition disease. Radiology. 1980;134:621–5.
162. Bosworth BM. Calcium deposits in the shoulder and subacromial bursitis: a survey of 12,122 cases. J Am Med Assoc. 1941;116:2477–82.
163. Depalma AF, Kruper JS. Long-term study of shoulder joints afflicted with and treated for calcific tendinitis. Clin Orthop. 1961;20:61–72.
164. Mole D, Kempf JF, Gleyze P, Rio B, Bonnomet F, Walch G. Resultat du traitement arthroscopique des tendinopathies non rompues, Il: les calcifications. Rev Chir Orthop. 1993;79:532–41.
165. Faure G, Daculsi G. Calcific tendinitis: a review. Ann Rheum Dis. 1983;42:49–53.
166. Wainner RS, Hasz M. Management of acute calcific tendinitis of the shoulder. J Orthop Sports Phys Ther. 1998;27(3):231–7.
167. Loew M, Sabo D, Wehrle M, et al. Relationship between calcifying tendinitis and subacromial impingement: a prospective radiography and magnetic resonance imaging study. J Shoulder Elb Surg. 1996;5(4):314–9.
168. Hurt G, Baker CL Jr. Calcific tendinitis of the shoulder. Orthop Clin North Am. 2003;34(4):567–75.
169. Cahir J, Saifuddin A. Calcific tendonitis of pectoralis major: CT and MRI findings. Skelet Radiol. 2005;34(4):234–8.
170. Durr HR, Lienemann A, Silbernagl H, et al. Acute calcific tendinitis of the pectoralis major insertion associated with cortical bone erosion. Eur Radiol. 1997;7(8):1215–7.
171. Ikegawa S. Calcific tendinitis of the pectoralis major insertion. A report of two cases. Arch Orthop Trauma Surg. 1996;115(2):118–9.
172. Zubler C, Mengiardi B, Schmid MR, et al. MR arthrography in calcific tendinitis of the shoulder: diagnostic performance and pitfalls. Eur Radiol. 2007;17(6):1603–10.
173. Yang I, Hayes CW, Biermann JS. Calcific tendinitis of the gluteus medius tendon with bone marrow edema mimicking metastatic disease. Skelet Radiol. 2002;31:359–61.
174. Hayes CW, Rosenthal DI, Plata MJ, Hudson TM. Calcific tendinitis in unusual site associated with cortical bone erosion. Am J Roentgenol. 1987;149:967–70.
175. Flemming DJ, Murphey MD, Shekitka KM, Temple HT, Jelinek JJ, Kransdorf MJ. Osseous involvement in calcific tendinitis: a retrospective review of 50 cases. Am J Roentgenol. 2003;181:965–72.
176. Chung CBm Gentili A, Chew FS. Calcific tendinosis and periarthritis: classic magnetic resonance imaging appearance and associated findings. J Comput Assist Tomogr. 2004;28:390–6.
177. Farin PU, Jaroma H. Sonographic findings of rotator cuff calcifications. J Ultrasound Med. 1995;14(1):7–14.
178. Bureau NJ. Calcific tendinopathy of the shoulder. Semin Musculoskelet Radiol. 2013;17(1): 80–4.
179. Le Goff B, Berthelot JM, Guilot P, Glemarec J, Maugars Y. Assessment of calcific tendonitis of rotator cuff by ultrasonography: comparison between symptomatic and asymptomatic shoulders. Joint Bone Spine. 2010;77(3):258–63.
180. McCarty DJ, Halverson PB, Carrera GF, et al. "Milwaukee shoulder": association of microspheroids containing hydroxyapatite crystals, active collagenase, and neutral protease with rotator cuff defects. Arthritis Rheum. 1981;24: 464–73.
181. Halverson PB, McCarty DJ, Cheung HS, et al. Milwaukee shoulder syndrome: eleven additional cases with involvement of the knee in seven (basic calcium phosphate crystal deposition disease). Semin Arthritis Rheum. 1984;14(1):36–44.
182. McCarty DJ. Arthritis associated with crystals containing calcium. Med Clin North Am. 1986;70(2):437–54.
183. McCarty DJ. Milwaukee shoulder syndrome. Trans Am Clin Climatol Assoc. 1991;102:271–83.. (discussion:283-4)
184. Garcia GM, McCord GC, Kumar R. Hydroxyapatite crystal deposition disease. Semin Musculoskelet Radiol. 2003;7(3):187–93.
185. Forster CJ, Oglesby RJ, Szkutnik AJ, Roberts JR. Positive alizarin red clumps in Milwaukee shoulder syndrome. J Rheumatol. 2009;36(12):2853.
186. Epis O, Caporali R, Scire CA, et al. Efficacy of tidal irrigation in Milwaukee shoulder syndrome. J Rheumatol. 2007;34(7):1545–50.

11 Preoperative Planning and Postoperative Imaging of Shoulder Arthroplasty

Jonelle Petscavage-Thomas

11.1 Pertinent Imaging Anatomy

The glenohumeral joint is the articulation between the humeral head and glenoid fossa of the scapula. The humeral head is normally angled 130–140° superomedial to the long axis of the humeral shaft with 30° of retroversion [1]. The lateral protuberance of the humeral head is the greater tuberosity. This is the site of attachment of the supraspinatus, infraspinatus, and teres minor rotator cuff tendons. The greater tuberosity is best seen on externally rotated AP radiographs (Fig. 11.1a) [2]. The lesser tuberosity is a small tubercle anteroinferior to the greater tuberosity and site of the subscapularis tendon attachment. It is best seen on internally rotated radiographs (Fig. 11.1b) [2]. The greater and lesser tuberosities are separated by the bicipital groove. The humeral head is covered by articular cartilage.

The glenoid fossa, or cavity, is a pear-shaped articular surface of the lateral scapula [3] (Fig. 11.1). The fossa accommodates a broad range of motion of the humeral head. The fibrocartilaginous glenoid labrum and synovial-lined joint capsule with glenohumeral ligaments augment and stabilize the osseous glenoid. The myotendinous rotator cuff dynamically stabilizes the glenohumeral joint [3]. The myotendinous rotator cuff occupies the space between the superior humeral head and the undersurface of the acromion. This space is normally greater than 7 mm in diameter [4].

Radiographic evaluation of the glenohumeral joint space and subtle humeral head migration of instability are best seen on the Grashey radiographic view (Fig. 11.1c). The Grashey view is performed with the patient rotated posteriorly 35–45° with the plane of the scapula parallel to the film cassette [5]. The normal glenohumeral joint space is 3–6 mm [6].

11.2 Pathological Conditions

11.2.1 Definition

Approximately two-thirds of shoulder joint replacements are placed for glenohumeral joint osteoarthritis [7]. Osteoarthritis, also known as degenerative arthritis, is a gradual, progressive, and mechanical process of the glenohumeral articular cartilage, bone, and capsule. As the process progresses, there is loss of normal load-bearing surfaces, resulting in pain and disability [8]. Primary osteoarthritis has no specific cause while secondary osteoarthritis may result from shoulder trauma, chronic glenohumeral joint dislocation, and instability, infection, congenital abnormalities, or chronic rotator cuff tears [9]. This last type of secondary osteoarthritis is also termed "cuff-tear arthropathy." The hypothesis is that the rotator cuff tears result in leakage of joint

J. Petscavage-Thomas (✉)
Department of Radiology, Penn State Milton S. Hershey Medical Center, Hershey, PA, USA

J. T. Bencardino (ed.), *The Shoulder*, https://doi.org/10.1007/978-3-030-06240-8_11

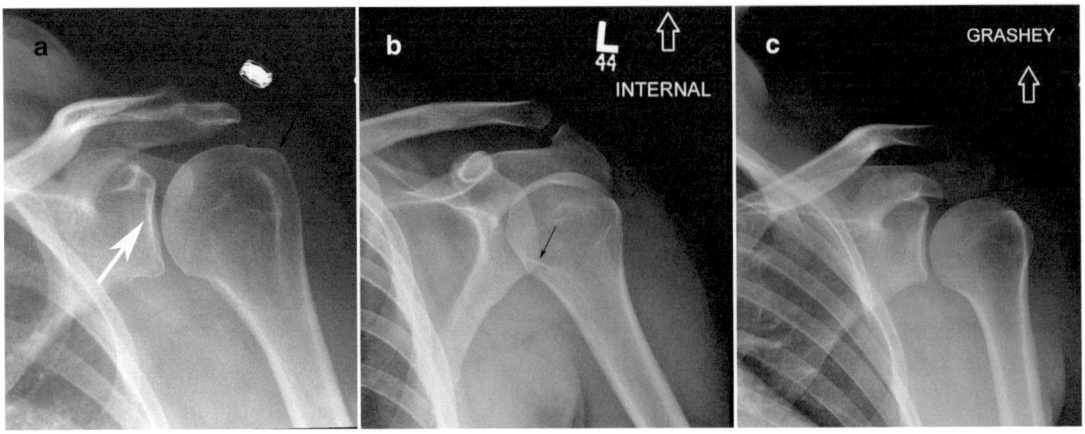

Fig. 11.1 Normal shoulder anatomy. (**a**) AP externally rotated radiograph of the left shoulder shows the greater tuberosity (black arrow) and pear-shaped articular glenoid fossa (white arrow). (**b**) AP internally rotated radiograph of the left shoulder shows the lesser tuberosity (arrow). (**c**) Grashey view of the left shoulder shows normal glenohumeral joint space

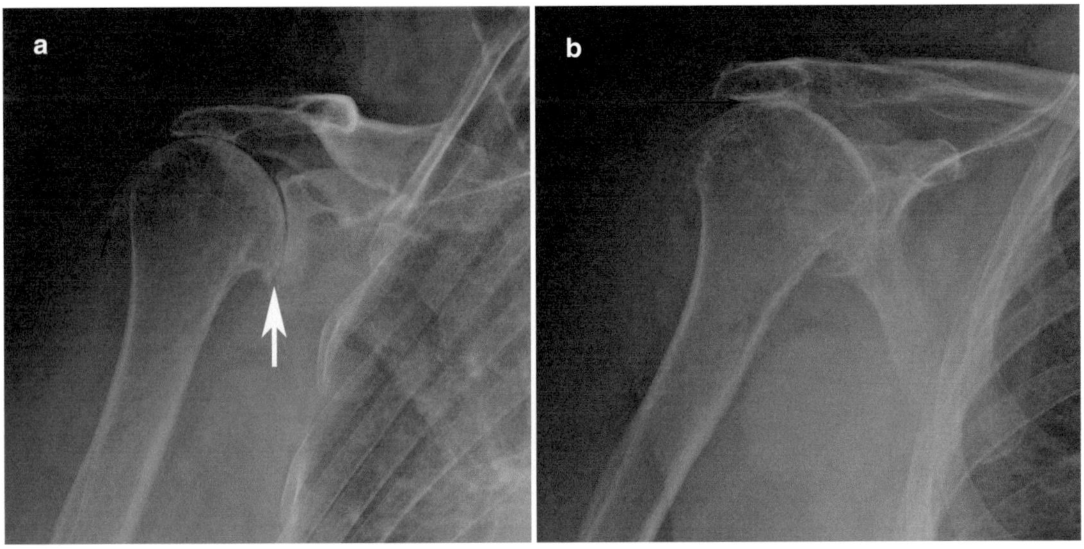

Fig. 11.2 Osteoarthritis. (**a**) Grashey view of the right shoulder shows narrowing of the glenohumeral joint space (white arrow). There is subchondral sclerosis of the articular surfaces with subchondral cysts and osteophytes (black arrow). (**b**) AP view of the right shoulder shows narrowed acromiohumeral distance (black arrow) with superior subluxation of the humeral head

fluid and loss of intra-articular joint pressure. This results in microinstability of the glenohumeral joint and excessive wear and tear on the articular cartilage [10].

Other indications for shoulder arthroplasty are trauma, including proximal humeral fractures and Bankart fractures, rheumatoid arthritis, avascular necrosis, and focal cartilage defects of the humeral head.

11.2.2 Radiographic and CT Findings

Radiographs remain the primary imaging modality for diagnosis and assessment of glenohumeral joint osteoarthritis. Radiographs demonstrate the hallmarks of osteoarthritis, namely osteophyte formation, subchondral sclerosis, subchondral cystic change, and joint-space narrowing (best seen on the Grashey view) (Fig. 11.2a). Massive cuff tear arthropathy is suggested by a narrowed acromiohumeral distance (<7 mm) (Fig. 11.2b) [4] with superior subluxation of the humeral head on AP radiographs. Additional findings include an exaggerated groove between the greater tuberosity and humeral articular surface and remodeling of the undersurface of the acromion. The most specific findings are superior migration of the humeral head with subcortical cystic change of the greater tuberosity [11, 12].

Rheumatoid arthritis, another common indication for shoulder arthroplasty, is seen on radiographs as bilateral symmetric glenohumeral joint-space narrowing. Osseous erosions are most common at the superomedial aspect of the humeral head and acromioclavicular joint. Bones are generally osteoporotic seen [13].

Adequate osseous support for a glenoid component in total shoulder arthroplasty is critical as prior studies have shown that up to 20% of shoulders require grafting due to poor bone stock [14, 15]. Patients with glenohumeral joint osteoarthritis often have a retroverted glenoid due to posterior glenoid rim erosions [16]. Patients with rheumatoid arthritis have also been shown to have a retroverted glenoid [17]. It is imperative for surgeons to correct retroversion to prevent the complications of radiolucency, loosening, humeral head dislocation, and glenoid wear [18–20]. Thus preoperative measurements are useful to determine the amount of anterior reaming or bone grafting needed to correct retroversion.

The glenoid is assessed in several ways. First, axillary radiographs or axial computed tomography (CT) images are used to determine glenoid morphology using the Walch classification (Fig. 11.3) [21]. Type A morphology is a centered humeral head with (A1) minor or (A2) major glenoid erosions. Type B morphology is a posteriorly

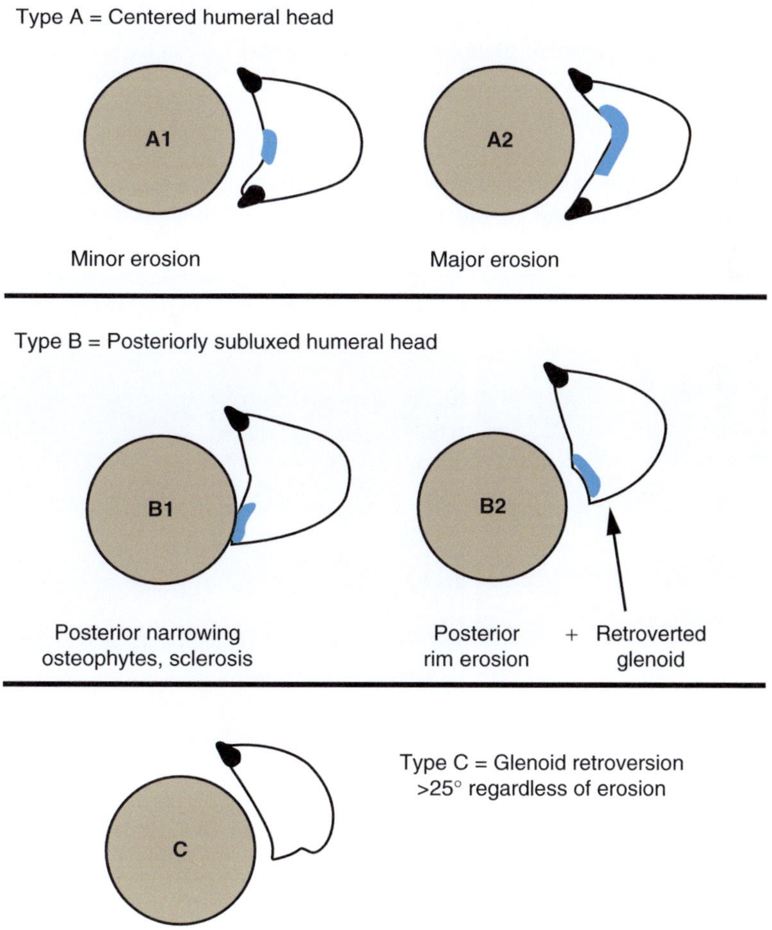

Fig. 11.3 Author's illustration of the Walch classification system of glenoid morphology

subluxed humeral head with (B1) posterior joint-space narrowing and osteophytes or (B2) posterior rim erosions and retroversion. Type C is greater than 25° retroversion. Comparing the two modalities, axillary radiographs have poor inter- and intraobserver reproducibility and have been shown to overestimate the degree of retroversion [22].

Thus, CT is preferred for reproducibility in measurement of glenoid retroversion. On 2-dimensional (2D) CT, version is defined as the angle formed between a line drawn from the medial border of the scapula to the center of the glenoid and the line perpendicular to the face of the glenoid on the axial slice at or just below the tip of the coracoid of the scapula (Fig. 11.4) [23]. Recently, studies have shown 3D CT to be more accurate in detecting posterior glenoid erosion and retroversion [24–26]. To assess retroversion, draw a vertical line on the 3D surface of the glenoid face, centered in the AP direction. A transverse 2D plane is generated perpendicular to the midpoint of the vertical line passing through the scapular axis (center of glenoid and tip of scapular spine) to obtain an image for angle measurement (Fig. 11.5) [11].

Preoperative CT is also used to assess glenoid bone stock. On axial CT images, the glenoid is measured at the level of the upper base of the coracoid, middle, and lower portions [17]. At the upper base, the maximum AP diameter and width of the scapular neck are measured (Fig. 11.6a). The distance between these two is the medial displacement, which reflects the glenoid depth. At the middle and lower glenoid levels, the amounts of supported bone and unsupported anterior and

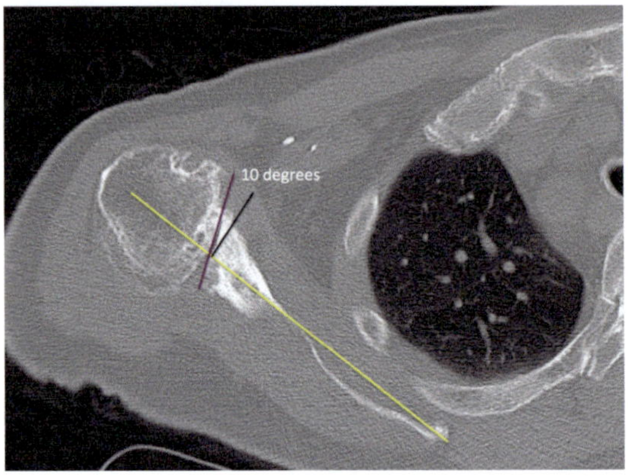

Fig. 11.4 Axial CT in bone windows of the right shoulder shows assessment of glenoid retroversion. The angle is formed between a line perpendicular (black) to a line (yellow) drawn from the medial border of the scapula to the glenoid center and the line (purple) along the glenoid face. In this patient, the glenoid is retroverted by 10°. Also seen is severe narrowing of the glenohumeral joint space with subchondral sclerosis and subchondral cystic change

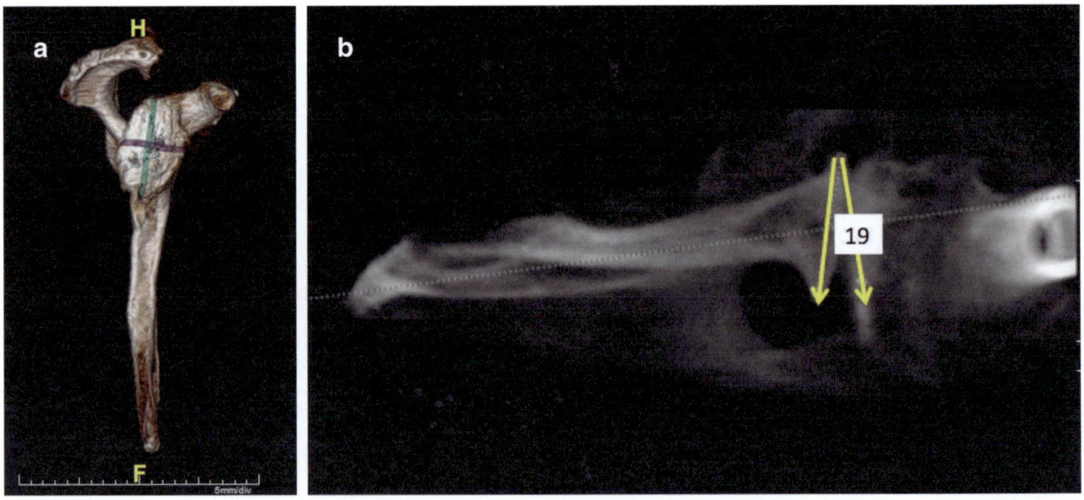

Fig. 11.5 3D CT assessment of glenoid retroversion. (**a**) 3D volume-rendered image of the glenoid face where a vertical line (green) is drawn centered in the anteroposterior direction. A transverse 2D plane is generated perpendicular to the midpoint of the vertical line (purple) to pass through the scapular axis. (**b**) The version angle is then applied at the level of the transverse plane using the Friedman technique for the 2D CT

posterior bone are measured (Fig. 11.6b). Additionally, the medial displacement is measurement at these levels. Both osteoarthritis and rheumatoid shoulders have been shown to have more unsupported bone with greater AP diameters and decreased medial displacement. In rheumatoid arthritis, the significance is that undetected glenoid erosions could lead to medial placement of a glenoid component with inaccurate soft-tissue tension.

A final radiographic or CT preoperative assessment involves lateral humeral offset (LHO). This is the distance between the coracoid base and most lateral part of the greater tuberosity (Fig. 11.7a) [27]. Iannotti showed that LHO correlates with both humeral head size and moment arm [28]. Preoperative LHO should be noted in case it requires surgical correction. Plain films are typically still utilized for LHO assessment but have a projection error of up to 50% [29]. Axial CT has excellent interobserver reliability and intraobserver reproducibility [30]. On CT, LHO is the distance between the medial edge of the base of the coracoid process and the most lateral aspect of the greater tuberosity (Fig. 11.7b).

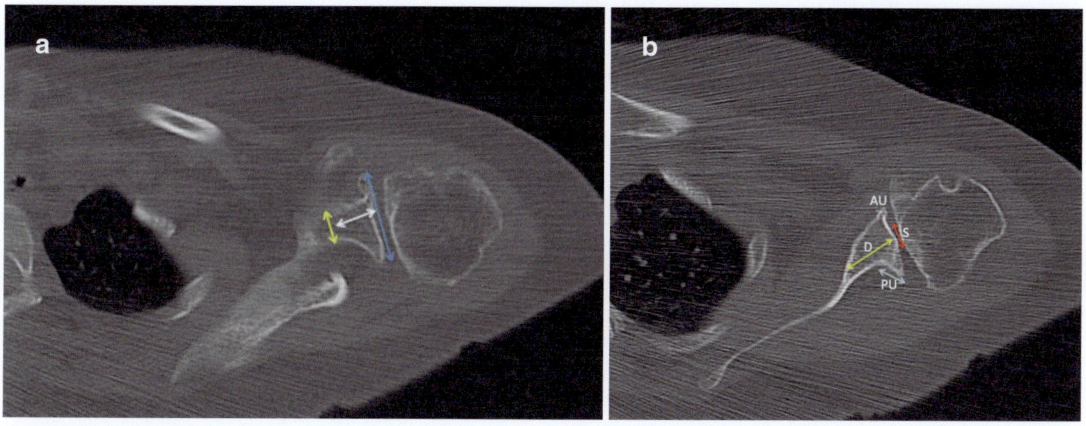

Fig. 11.6 CT assessment of glenoid bone stock. (**a**) Axial image of a left shoulder at the level of the upper glenoid base shows maximum AP diameter (blue line) and width of scapular neck (yellow line). Distance between these (white line) is the glenoid depth. (**b**) Axial image of the middle glenoid shows measurements of unsupported bone anteriorly (AU) and posteriorly (PU) and supported bone (S) as well as glenoid depth (D). Same measurements are performed at the lower glenoid level

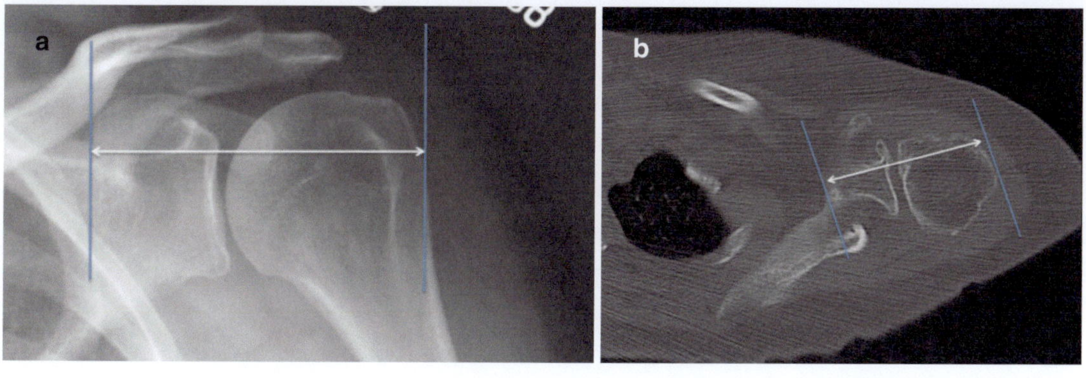

Fig. 11.7 Lateral humeral offset. (**a**) AP radiograph of the left shoulder shows lateral humeral offset as distance (white line) between coracoid base and most lateral part of the greater tuberosity. (**b**) Axial CT image of the same shoulder demonstrates offset as distance between the medial edge of coracoid base and lateral part of greater tuberosity (white line)

11.2.2.1 Ultrasound Findings

Recognition of rotator cuff tears is important in surgical planning. In the absence of tear, the patient may be a candidate for an anatomic total shoulder arthroplasty (ATSA). Irreparable tears or massive tears require a reverse total shoulder arthroplasty (RTSA). Although radiographs can demonstrate findings of massive rotator cuff tear, they do not depict the degree of associated muscle atrophy or retraction and are not as sensitive as other modalities. In equivocal cases, recognition of a rotator cuff tear can be performed with ultrasound. Ultrasound has been shown to have similar accuracy compared to magnetic resonance (MR) imaging for detection of supraspinatus (91.1%), infraspinatus (84.4%), and subscapularis tears (77.8%) [31]. Direct signs of full-thickness tear include non-visualization of the tendon and hypoechoic discontinuity of the tendon. Indirect signs of a full-thickness tear include the double-cortex sign, sagging peribursal fat sign, compressibility, and muscle atrophy [32]. Well-defined hypoechoic or anechoic defects in the tendon involving only the bursal or articular surface indicate a partial-thickness tear. Adjacent cortical pitting and irregularity may be seen in the humeral head. Degree of muscle atrophy should be reported on to provide a full assessment of reparability. Finally, since the deltoid muscle is used as the primary-level arm in RTSA, dehiscence and presence of fatty atrophy should be reported if present.

11.2.2.2 MR Findings

Although the accuracy of ultrasound is comparable to MR, it cannot depict glenohumeral arthrosis and cartilage defects. The bone stock and retroversion with Walch classification of the glenoid can also be performed with MR. Similar to ultrasound, presence of full- versus partial-thickness tears, degree of muscle atrophy as staged by Goutallier, and deltoid muscle status are important findings to report for preoperative assessments.

11.3 Postoperative Imaging

11.3.1 Normal Appearance

11.3.1.1 Anatomic Total Shoulder Arthroplasty

Anatomic total shoulder arthroplasty (ATSA) replaces both glenoid and humeral articular surfaces. The humeral component is a minimally constrained implant with a spherical metal articular surface and a cemented or press-fit metal stem (Fig. 11.8).

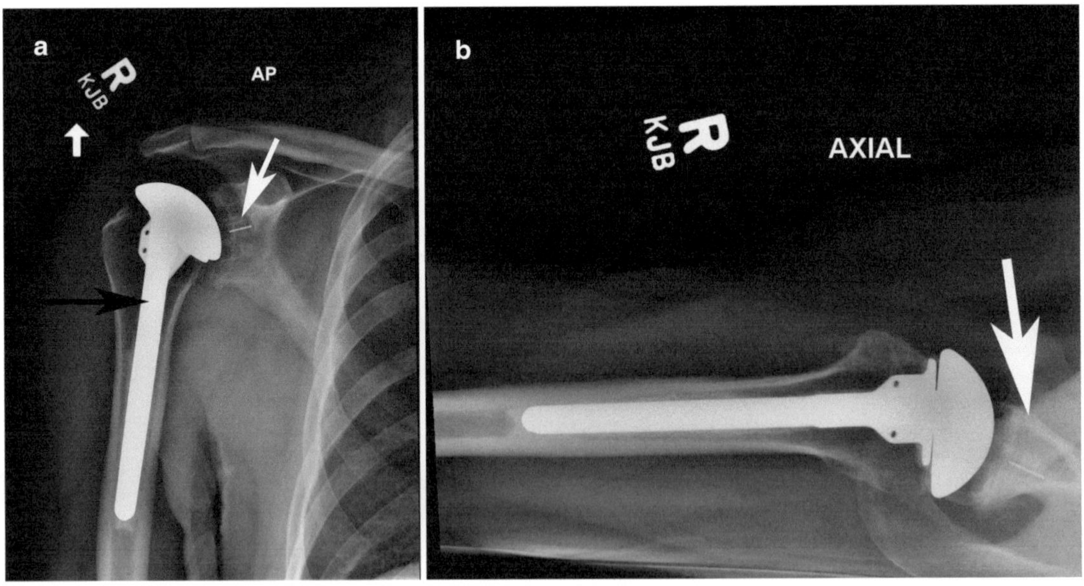

Fig. 11.8 Anatomic total shoulder arthroplasty. (**a**) AP and (**b**) lateral radiographs of the right shoulder show the humeral component of the arthroplasty (black arrow) centered in the humeral shaft. The glenoid component (white arrow) is radiolucent with radiopaque markers for identification

The humeral heads are anatomic or adaptable as they can be adjusted as referenced to the humeral stem in both anteroposterior and mediolateral directions and allow for various degrees of humeral head inclination [33]. Cement is used in patients with poor bone stock, such as rheumatoid arthritis or osteoporosis. An extended-coverage humeral head design (CTA) is an option for patients with rotator cuff tears and narrowed acromial-humeral distance. The head component extends more laterally to cover the greater tuberosity, thereby decreasing impingement [34, 35].

A new trend in ATSA is the use of stemless humeral components (Fig. 11.9). The goal is to preserve humeral bone stock, decrease humeral stem-associated complications, and be less invasive. Preliminary reports show radiographic stability without migration or subsidence at 2- to 3-year minimum follow-up [36].

The glenoid component of ATSA is comprised of radiolucent polyethylene fixed with polymethyl methacrylate. The component is attached to bone by either a central keel or two or more pegs, which have radiopaque markers for identification on radiographs (Fig. 11.8). Lower rates of radiolucency are reported with pegged implants [37]. However, keeled components are required for patients with poor glenoid bone stock [33].

Another trend is ream and run arthroplasty of the glenoid. Here, the glenoid is reamed to have a stabilizing concavity and maximum glenohumeral contact area. It has been shown that the reamed glenoid bone forms new fibrocartilage. This procedure is selected for patients hoping to avoid the risk of glenoid component wear and who are willing to participate in a 2-year daily exercise rehabilitation program [38].

Normal postoperative imaging assessment includes AP internal and external rotation views, Grashey or scapular y views, and axillary views. The humeral stem should be centered in the humeral shaft as more lateral or medial position results in altered stress distribution, cortical bone resorption, and rotator cuff insufficiency [39]. The humeral component height should be between 2 and 5 mm above a line perpendicular to the greater tuberosity (Fig. 11.10). The glenoid component should be centered with the bone with no surrounding radiolucency. Some components

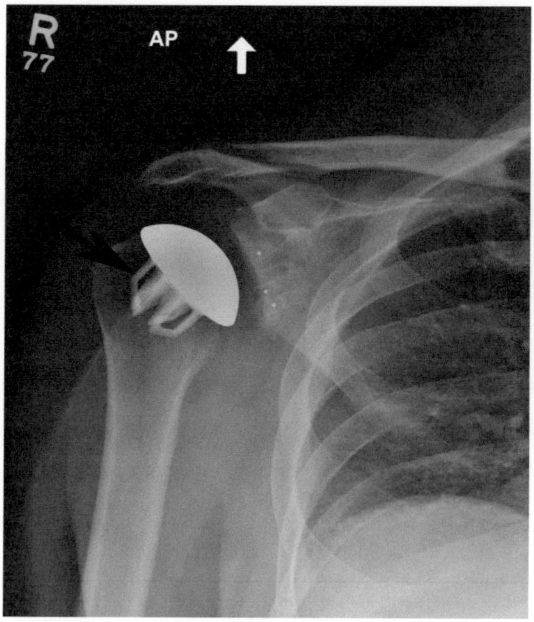

Fig. 11.9 Anatomic total shoulder arthroplasty. AP radiograph of the right shoulder show a stemless humeral component (arrow) and polyethylene glenoid component

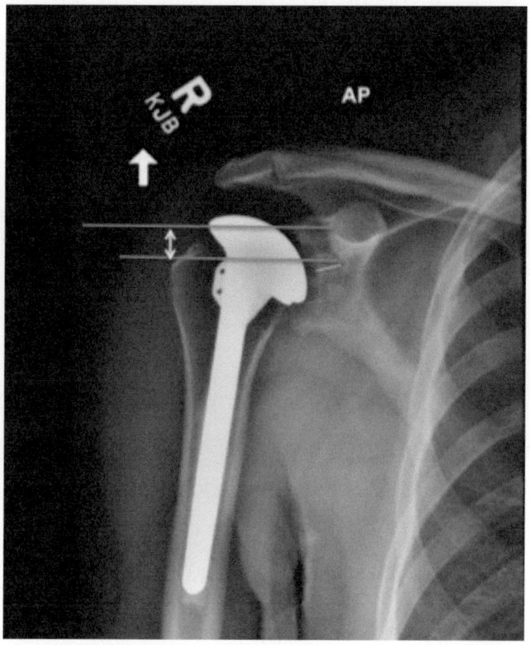

Fig. 11.10 Humeral component height. Distance between the greater tuberosity and humeral head should be 2–5 mm (white line)

have central pegs packed with bone graft for biologic incorporation. Sclerosis around the central peg is a normal finding of graft healing and incorporation.

11.3.1.2 Hemiarthroplasty

Hemiarthroplasty (HA) is replacement of only the humeral articular surface. This usually consists of placement of the stemmed metal humeral component of ATSA (Fig. 11.11a). HA is indicated for severe proximal humerus fractures, arthritis in which glenoid bone stock is inadequate to support a prosthesis, and isolated osteonecrosis or osteoarthritis of the humerus [34, 35].

Two newer hemiarthroplasty options are humeral head resurfacing and partial humeral head resurfacing. Resurfacing was introduced as a cementless, humeral head replacement in young or athletic patients with arthritis, avascular necrosis, instability, or rotator cuff arthropathy [39]. In resurfacing, a humeral osteotomy is not performed and bone stock is preserved for future revisions [40, 41]. The component is a metal-alloy cap with grooved cruciate stem with a hydroxyapatite on growth surface for attaining rotational stability [42]. On radiographs the cap should be flush with the articular surface and humeral head should remain centered on the glenoid (Fig. 11.11b).

Partial humeral head resurfacing is indicated for focal chondral defects as an alterative treatment to autograft or allograft implantation or microfracture. It is also used for patients with focal erosions, such as rheumatoid arthritis [43]. The prosthesis consists of an articular cobalt-chromium alloy surface component with small central peg mated with tapered titanium-alloy-cannulated screw/post. Similar to total humeral head resurfacing, the cap should be flush against bone and centered on the glenoid on the lateral view (Fig. 11.11c).

11.3.1.3 Reverse Total Shoulder Arthroplasty

RTSA is a semiconstrained prosthesis designed to stabilize the glenohumeral center of rotation by moving it more distally and medially, thereby improving length and contraction of the deltoid muscle for motion control over the shoulder [44, 45]. RTSA consists of a metal baseplate, called the metaglene, a glenosphere ball, and a humeral socket (Fig. 11.12) [46]. The metaglene is press-fit with a flat or convex radius of curvature. It is fixed to the glenoid with a central post, keel, or central screw. An additional 1–6 peripheral non-locking or variability angled locking screws are implanted for compressive fixation strength [47]. The glenosphere is a round metal ball attached to the

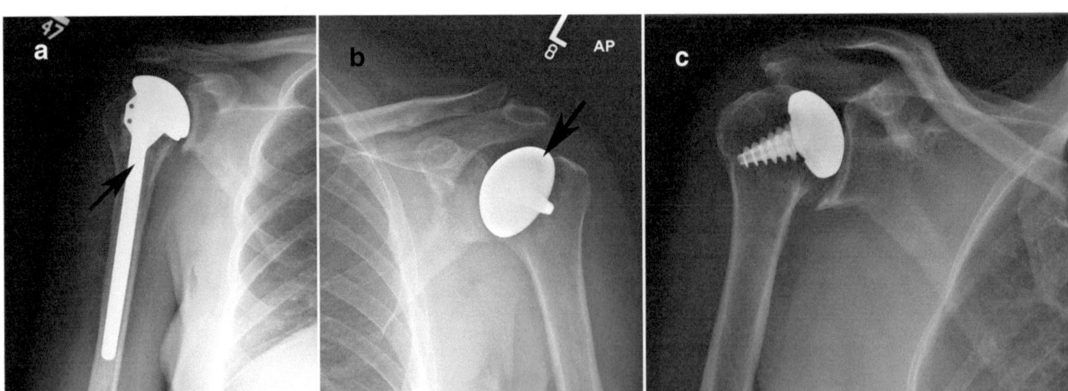

Fig. 11.11 Hemiarthroplasty. (**a**) AP radiograph of the left shoulder shows use of the humeral component of ATSA in hemiarthroplasty. Note no glenoid insert or component. (**b**) AP radiograph of the left shoulder shows the metal cap (black arrow) and stem of a humeral head resurfacing arthroplasty. (**c**) AP radiograph of the right shoulder shows a partial humeral head resurfacing

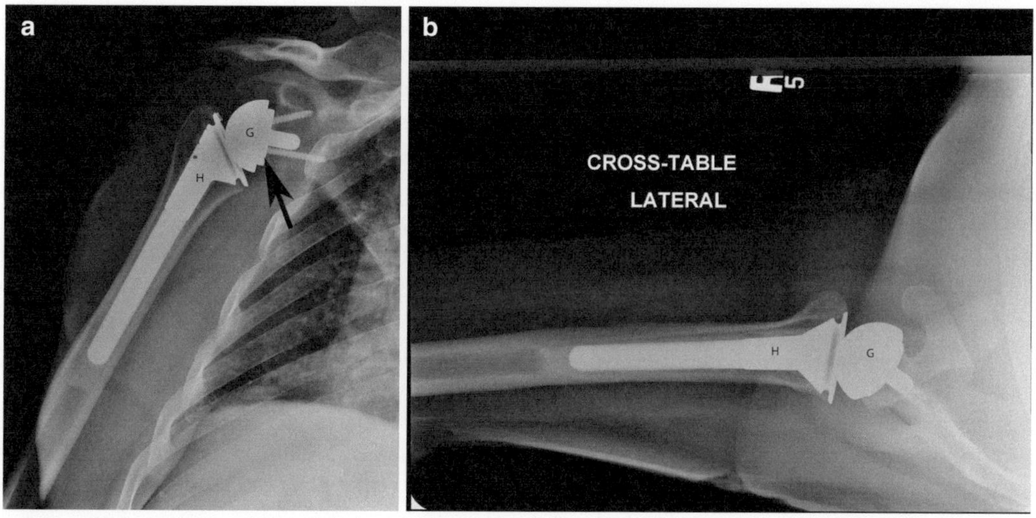

Fig. 11.12 Reverse total shoulder arthroplasty. (**a**) Grashey and (**b**) lateral views of the right shoulder show the metaglene (arrow), glenosphere (G), and humeral stem components (H) of a reverse total shoulder arthroplasty

metaglene. A radiolucent polyethylene insert sits in the humeral component proximal cup-shaped portion as an articulation between the glenosphere and humeral component.

Normal postoperative imaging assessment should be performed with AP, scapular Y, and axillary radiographs. The metaglene should be flush to the glenoid. The glenosphere should be flush to the metaglene. The glenosphere should align with the humeral cup, though thickness can vary depending on polyethylene insert [46]. The humeral socket shaft angle varies between 130 and 150°. However, more varus designs may be used to match native anatomic head neck angle and minimize humeral component notching of the inferior scapula [48].

11.3.1.4 Oncologic Humeral Prostheses

Oncologic humeral components are placed in patients after surgical removal of benign or malignant neoplasms or severe proximal humeral fractures. They may or may not allow for reconstruction of the rotator cuff for additional joint stability. In rotator cuff reconstruction, suture holes are present in the prosthesis for direct attachment or a nylon/Dacron mesh capsuloplasty for indirect attachment [49]. The prostheses consist of an all-metal long-stemmed humeral component (Fig. 11.13).

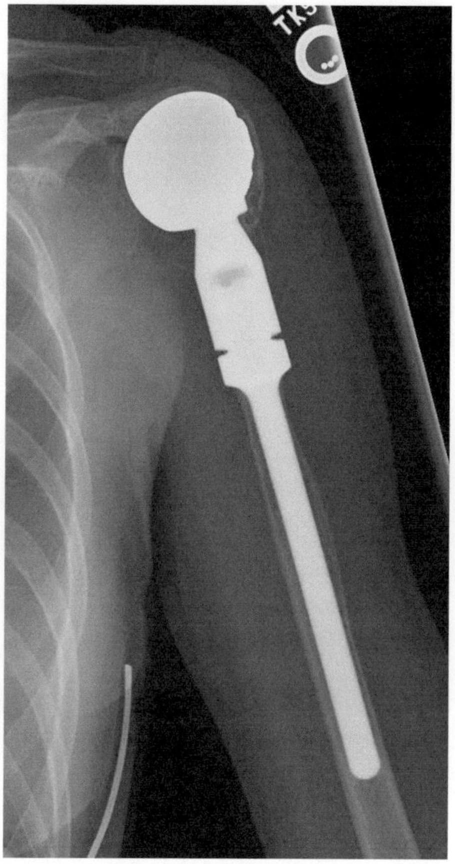

Fig. 11.13 Oncologic shoulder arthroplasty. AP radiograph of the left shoulder shows a long-stemmed humeral component with resection of a large amount of humeral bone stock in a patient with benign bone neoplasm

11.3.2 Complications

11.3.2.1 ATSA

The most common complication of ATSA is glenoid component loosening, occurring in up to one-third of patients [50]. Glenoid component loosening is seen on radiographs as radiolucency at the bone-cement interface (Fig. 11.14a). CT is superior to radiographs for showing osteolysis, showing 19 more lesions than radiographs in a recent study [51]. Thus, CT is recommended when there is suspicion of particle disease (Fig. 11.14b) and radiographs are negative. The Lazarus classification system is used for radiographic and CT description of radiolucency of pegged glenoid components (Fig. 11.14c) [37]. The Franklin classification is used to describe radiolucency surrounding keeled glenoid components (Fig. 11.14d) [52].

Although less commonly a site of loosening, development of progressive radiolucency or radiolucency >2 mm around the humeral component is abnormal (Fig. 11.15a, b). Radiolucency may reflect aseptic loosening, small particle disease, or infection. Radiolucency is reported according to the system of Gruen [53](Fig. 11.15c, d), which divides the humerus into eight regions. Small particle disease occurs when there is wear of the polyethylene components, resulting in a macrophage response with osteolysis.

Presence of the additional findings of periostitis, joint effusion, and soft-tissue swelling suggests that the radiolucency may be due to deep infection (Fig. 11.16a). The incidence of infection is 0–3.9% and most often due to *Staphylococcus aureus* and *Propionibacterium acnes* [54]. Cross-sectional imaging is helpful to further evaluate for joint effusion, soft-tissue collections, bone marrow edema, and periostitis

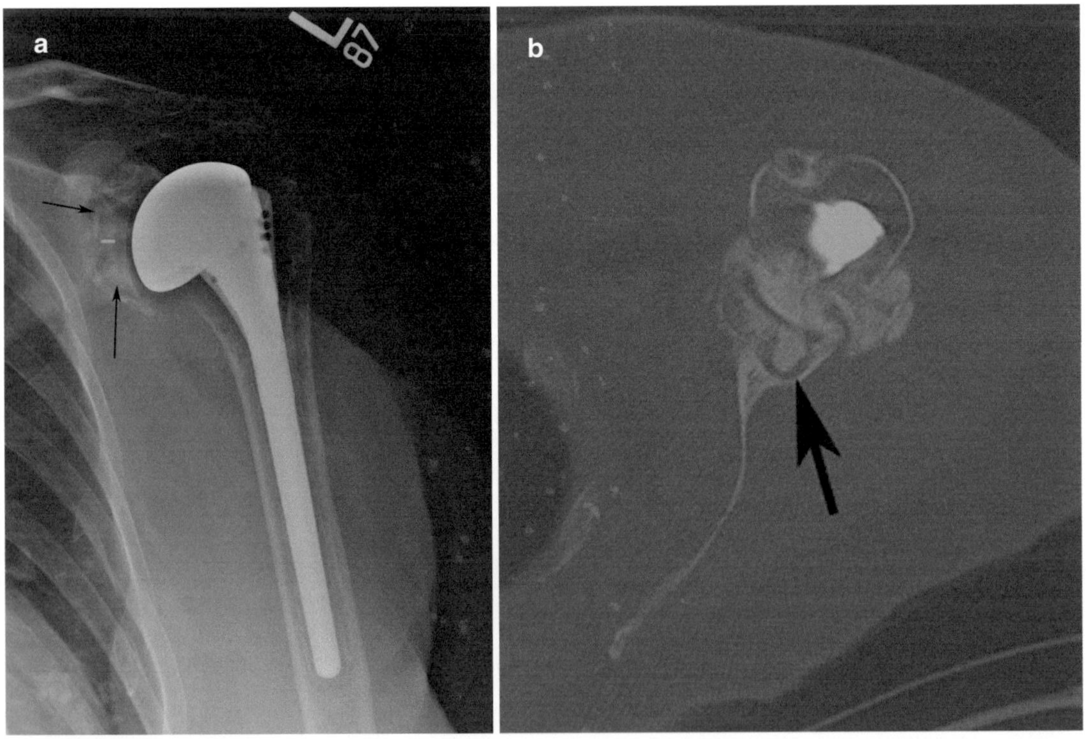

Fig. 11.14 Glenoid component loosening. (**a**) Grashey radiograph of a left shoulder ATSA shows radiolucency surrounding the pegged components (arrows), consistent with polyethylene wear. (**b**) Axial CT image shows radiolucency surrounding the glenoid component and areas of osteolysis (arrow). (**c**) Lazarus classification of pegged glenoid radiolucency. G = glenoid. Yellow indicates radiolucency. (**d**) Franklin classification of keeled glenoid radiolucency. G = glenoid. Yellow indicates radiolucency

Fig. 11.14 (continued)

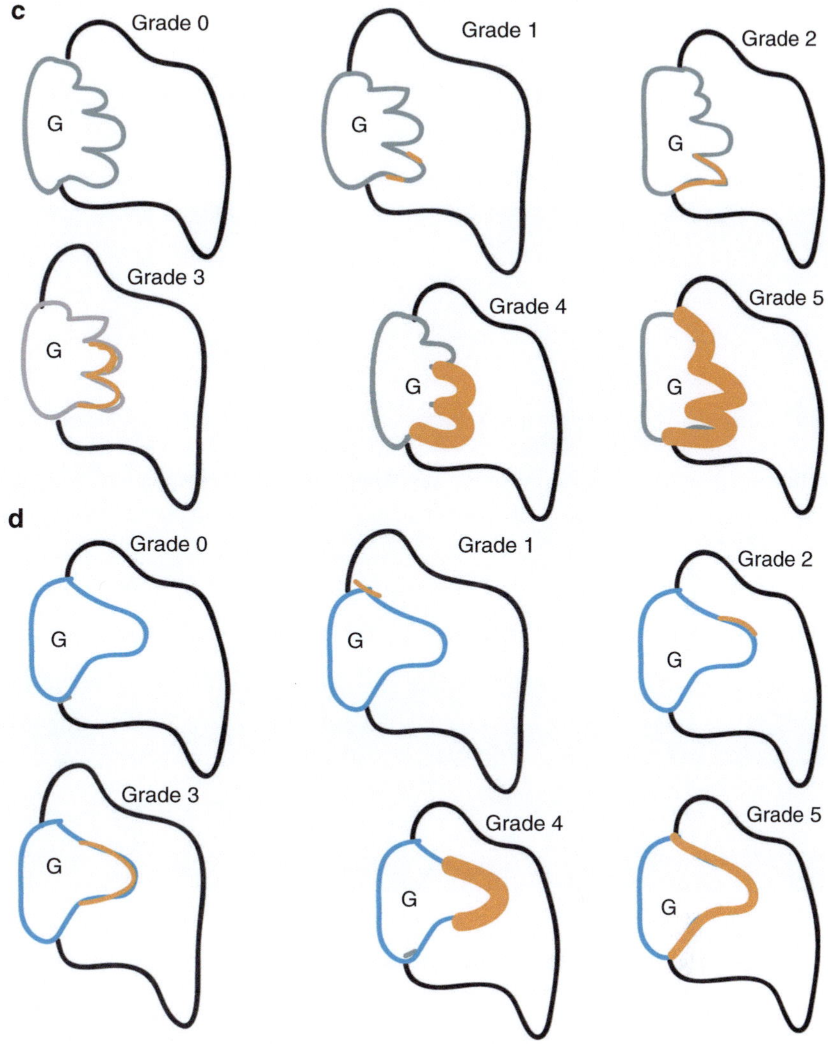

(Fig. 11.16b). Treatment of infected shoulder arthroplasty is explantation of the prosthesis and placement of an antibiotic-impregnated spacer with cement and stabilized by a Steinmann pin (Fig. 11.16c).

A mimic of radiolucency is stress shielding, which occurs in 9% of ATSA and HA. Stress shielding is the long-term adaption of the periprosthetic bone to stresses induced by the humeral component [55]. It is a risk factor for periprosthetic fracture and aseptic loosening. It appears as cortical thinning and increased osteopenia, typically in the region of the greater tuberosity [56] (Fig. 11.17).

Intraoperative periprosthetic fractures occur in 1.2% of primary ATSA [57]. Displaced fractures of the tuberosity (Region 1) are treated with suture fixation of the humeral implant. Region 2 fractures involve the humeral metaphysis, and are treated with cerclage fixation with autologous bone grafting. A longer stemmed humeral component may be placed for fractures of the proximal, mid, or distal humeral diaphysis (Regions 3 and 4). Postoperative fractures (Fig. 11.15a) typically occur due to trauma, at a low rate of 1.6–2.4% [58]. Imaging report should include presence of underlying radiolucency and involvement of the stem.

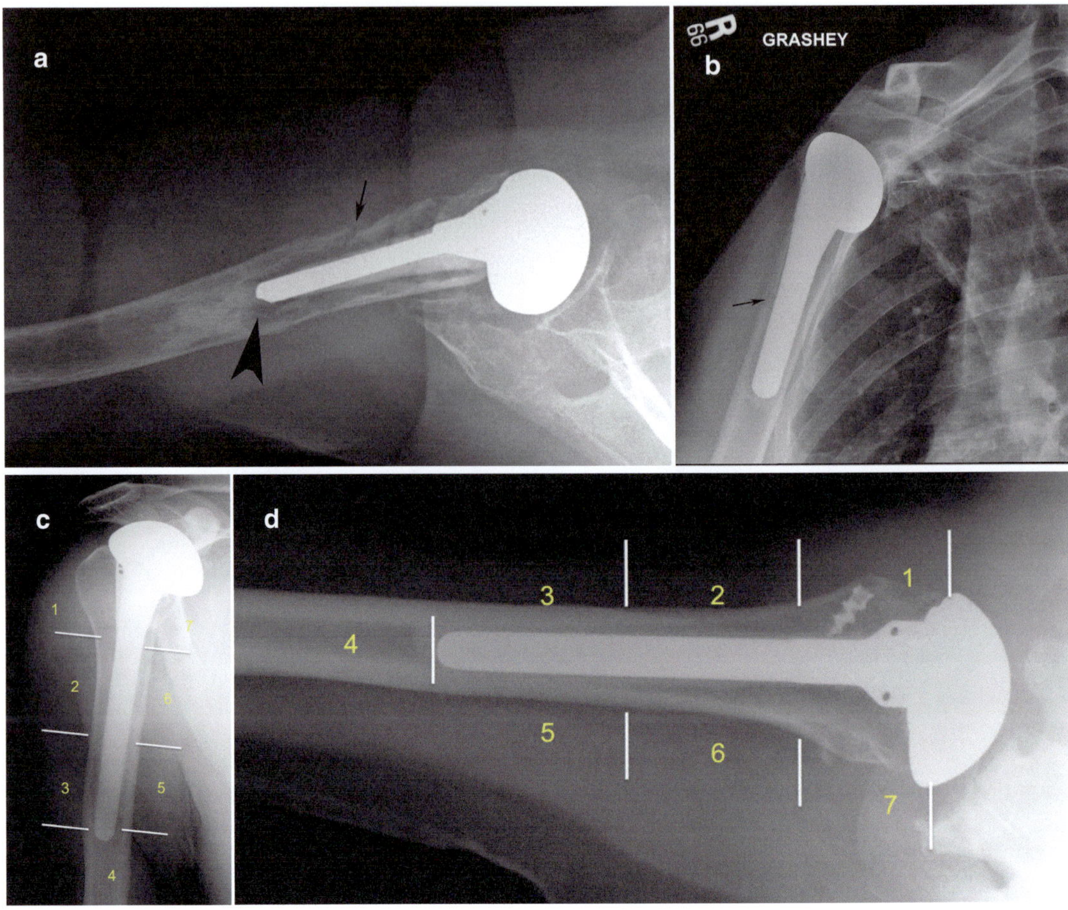

Fig. 11.15 Humeral component radiolucency. (**a**) Lateral radiograph of a right shoulder hemiarthroplasty shows radiolucency greater than 2 mm (arrowhead) around the humeral component and small anterior periprosthetic fracture (arrow) through an area of radiolucency. (**b**) Grashey radiograph of a right ATSA shows focal osteolysis (arrow). (**c**) AP and (**d**) lateral radiographs show eight zones of radiolucency according to Gruen classification

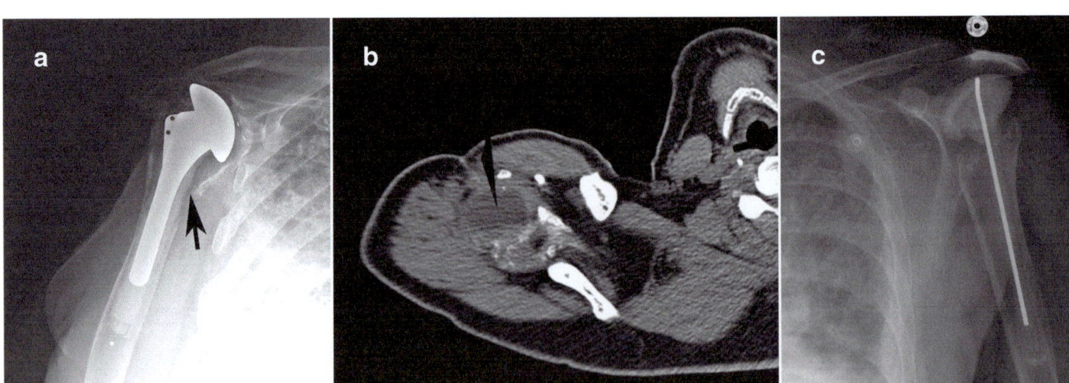

Fig. 11.16 Infection. (**a**) Grashey image of a right total shoulder arthroplasty shows focal erosive change along the proximal humerus (arrow), concerning for infection. (**b**) CT axial image of the right shoulder demonstrates a large glenohumeral joint effusion (arrowhead). This patient's synovial culture showed bacterial infection. (**c**) AP image post-explanation of a left total shoulder arthroplasty shows antibiotic-impregnated cement spacer and pin

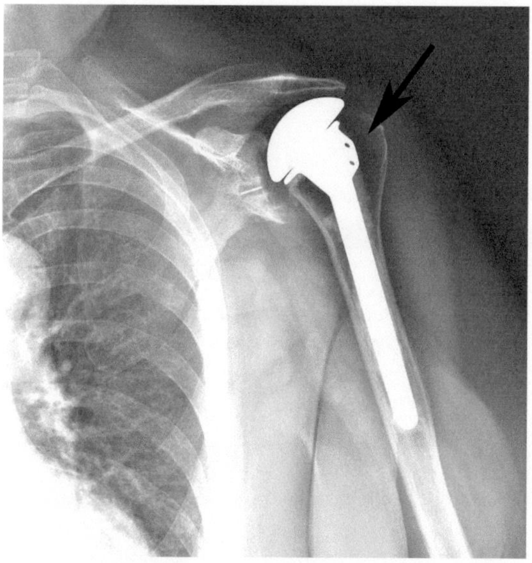

Fig. 11.17 AP radiograph of the left shoulder in a patient with an anatomic total shoulder arthroplasty shows focal osteopenia of stress shielding

Another complication is subsidence, which is axial settling of the humeral component. This is seen on radiographs as a change in vertical distance between the height of the humeral component and the line perpendicular to the greater tuberosity [59](Fig. 11.18a). Abnormal vertical distance may present as narrowing of the acromial humeral distance with superior migration of the humerus (Fig. 11.18b) and suggests new rotator cuff tear, overstuffing from too large of a humeral head component, or subacromial impingement related to acromial spurs [56].

During surgery for shoulder arthroplasty, the subscapularis tendon is divided to allow access to the glenohumeral joint [60]. Postoperative tears can lead to anterior instability, loss of active arm motion, and loosening of the glenoid component [60]. Primary radiographic finding of subscapularis tear is anterior subluxation of the humerus on the

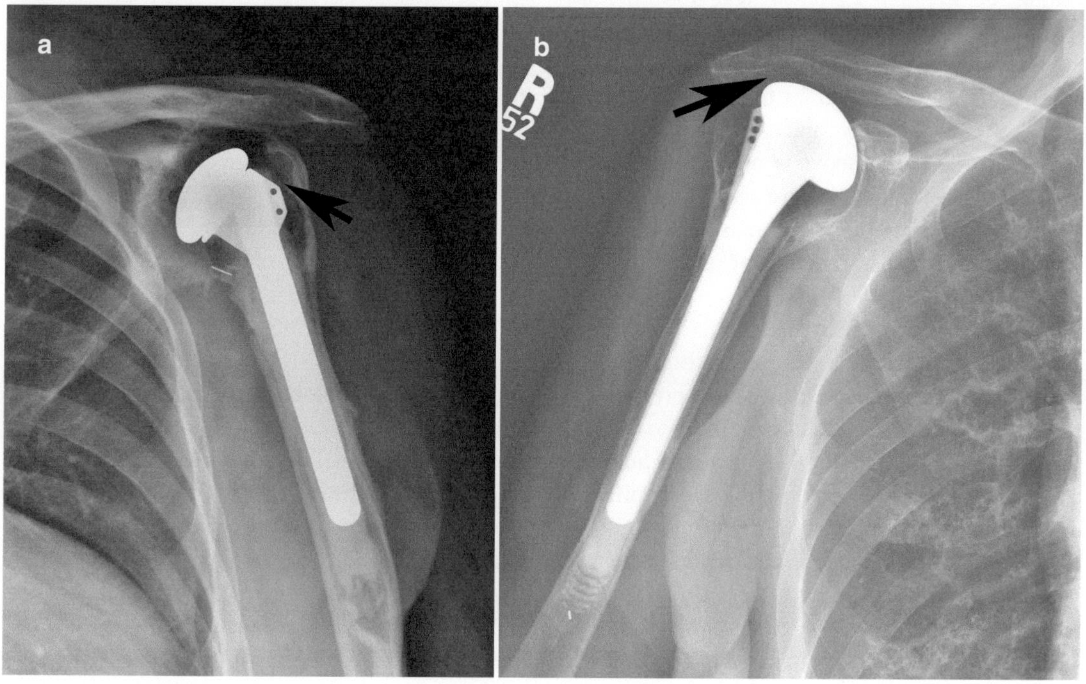

Fig. 11.18 Abnormal vertical distance. (**a**) AP radiograph of a left total shoulder arthroplasty shows abnormal vertical distance with settling of the humeral component (arrow), consistent with subsidence. The radiopaque glenoid marker is also inferiorly dislocated into the glenohumeral joint consistent with glenoid component loosening. (**b**) AP radiograph of a right shoulder hemiarthroplasty shows superior subluxation of the humeral component (arrow) concerning for new rotator cuff tear

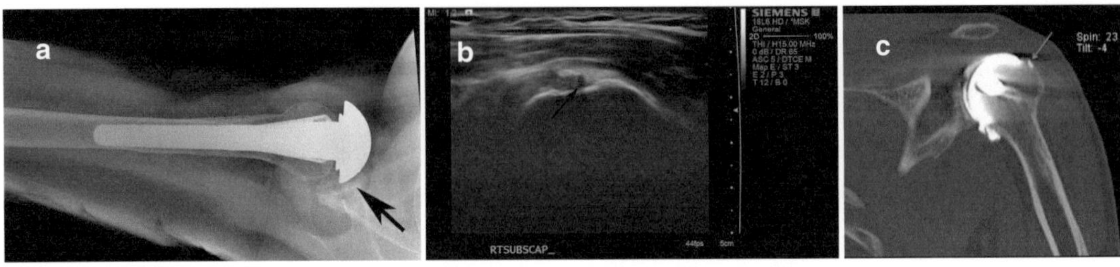

Fig. 11.19 Rotator cuff tear. Lateral radiograph of a patient with a right ATSA shows anterior subluxation of the humeral component in respect to the glenoid. (**b**) Transverse ultrasound image shows hypoechoic defect in the subscapularis tendon (arrow), confirming postoperative tear. (**c**) Coronal CT arthrogram image shows contrast in a defect (arrow) of the infraspinatus tendon

axillary view (Fig. 11.19a). Subluxation of the humeral head is classified as absent, slight (translation <25%), moderate (25–50%), or severe (>50%) [56]. Ultrasound imaging is useful to detect focal hypoechoic defects or full tendon tears (Fig. 11.19b) as it is not limited by metallic susceptibility artifact. CT arthrography can also be used to assess rotator cuff integrity. Although less common, postoperative tearing of the supraspinatus and infraspinatus (Fig. 11.19c) may occur and is seen as narrowing of the acromiohumeral distance. Ultrasound and CT arthrography are preferred for further evaluation of the tear extent, retraction, and associated atrophy.

In addition to the above complications, oncologic humeral components are at risk of failure of allograft incorporation, large areas of heterotopic ossification formation, and tumor recurrence.

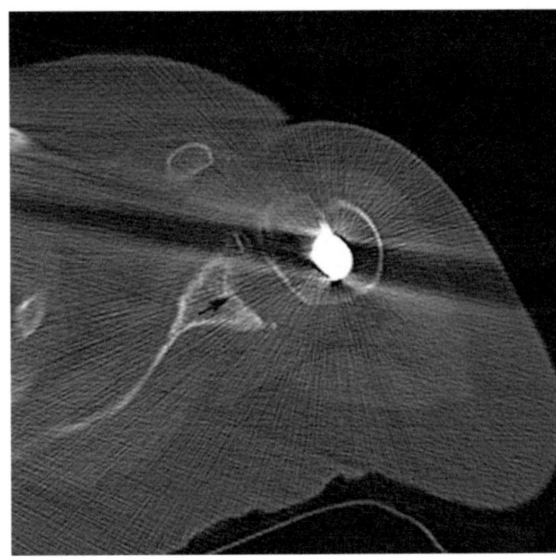

Fig. 11.20 Hemiarthroplasty complication. Axial CT of the left shoulder in a patient with a hemiarthroplasty shows central glenoid erosions and remodeling

11.3.2.2 Hemiarthroplasty

A unique complication to hemiarthroplasty is development of glenoid erosions and progressive glenohumeral arthritis, occurring in up to 64% of patients (Fig. 11.20) [34]. Other humeral component-related complications are similar to those described for ATSA.

The most common reported complication of humeral head resurfacing is superior migration of the humeral head on AP imaging, reported in up to 47% of patients [61]. Other complications include development of glenohumeral arthritis (Fig. 11.21), infection, osteolysis, arthrofibrosis, subscapularis tendon rupture, periprosthetic fracture, instability with subluxation, and loosening [39, 62].

Similar to anatomic hemiarthroplasty and full humeral head resurfacing, the most common complication of partial humeral head resurfacing is progressive glenohumeral arthritis and erosions [62]. A more recent study of 20 shoulders at a mean follow-up of 32.7 months found no radiographics complications [63].

11.3.2.3 RTSA

There are several unique complications to RTSA. Inferior scapular notching (Fig. 11.22) has been reported to occur in 53–67% of cases, although more recent design revisions and varus placement have decreased the incidence [64, 65]. Notching occurs when the humeral socket impinges the inferior scapula as it articulates with the glenosphere [66]. Notching is associated with poorer clinical outcomes and premature baseplate failure [65, 66]. Inferior scapular notching is

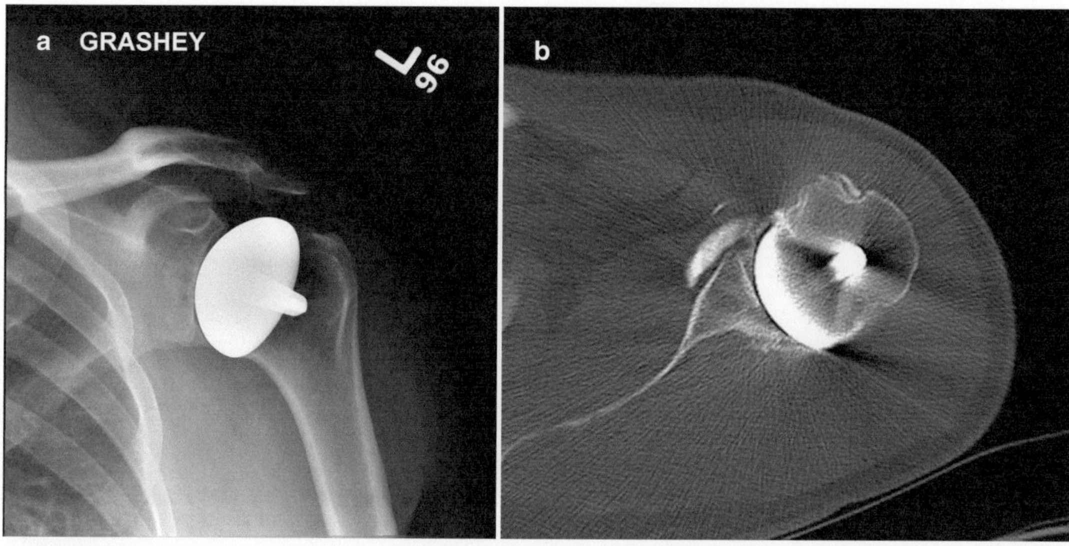

Fig. 11.21 Glenohumeral arthritis post-resurfacing. (**a**) Grashey radiographs and (**b**) axial CT arthrogram images show severe glenohumeral joint-space narrowing, particularly posteriorly, with subchondral sclerosis in a patient with left humeral head resurfacing

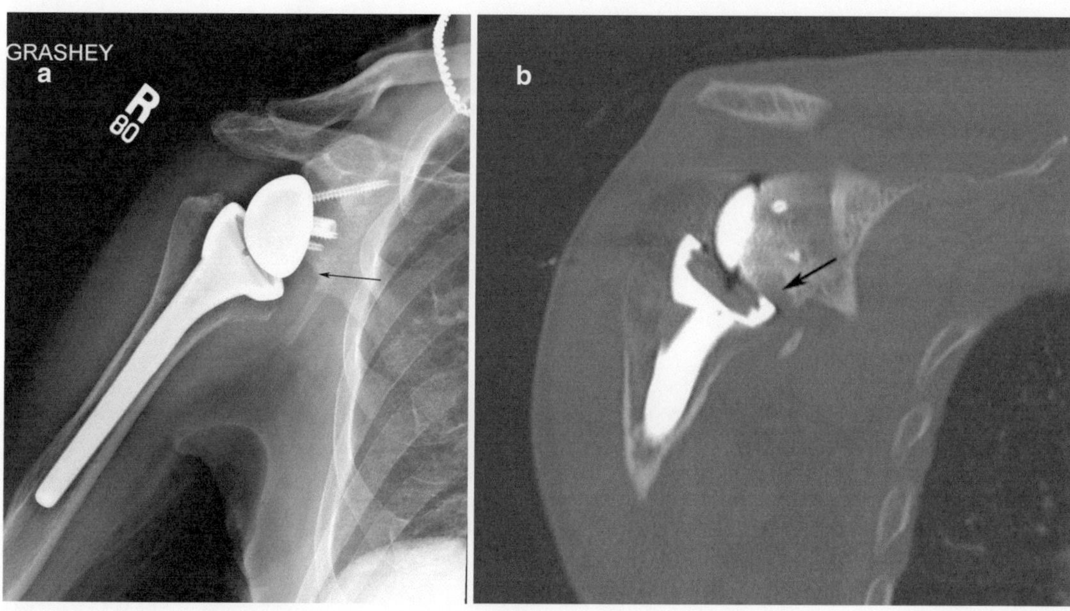

Fig. 11.22 Inferior scapular notching. (**a**) AP radiograph of a right shoulder RTSA shows notching of the inferior scapular (arrow), better seen on (**b**) coronal CT image

graded according to the classification of Sirveaux et al. A defect only involving the pillar is grade 1 severity. Grade 2 severity is present if the defect contacts the inferior baseplate screw, grade 3 if the notch extends over the inferior screw, and grade 4 if the notch extends under the baseplate [67].

Anterior dislocation occurs in up to 20% of cases and is the most common early postoperative complication [46]. Unique to the RTSA, the humeral component dislocates in the anterior-superior direction due to pull of the deltoid muscle (Fig. 11.23) [46].

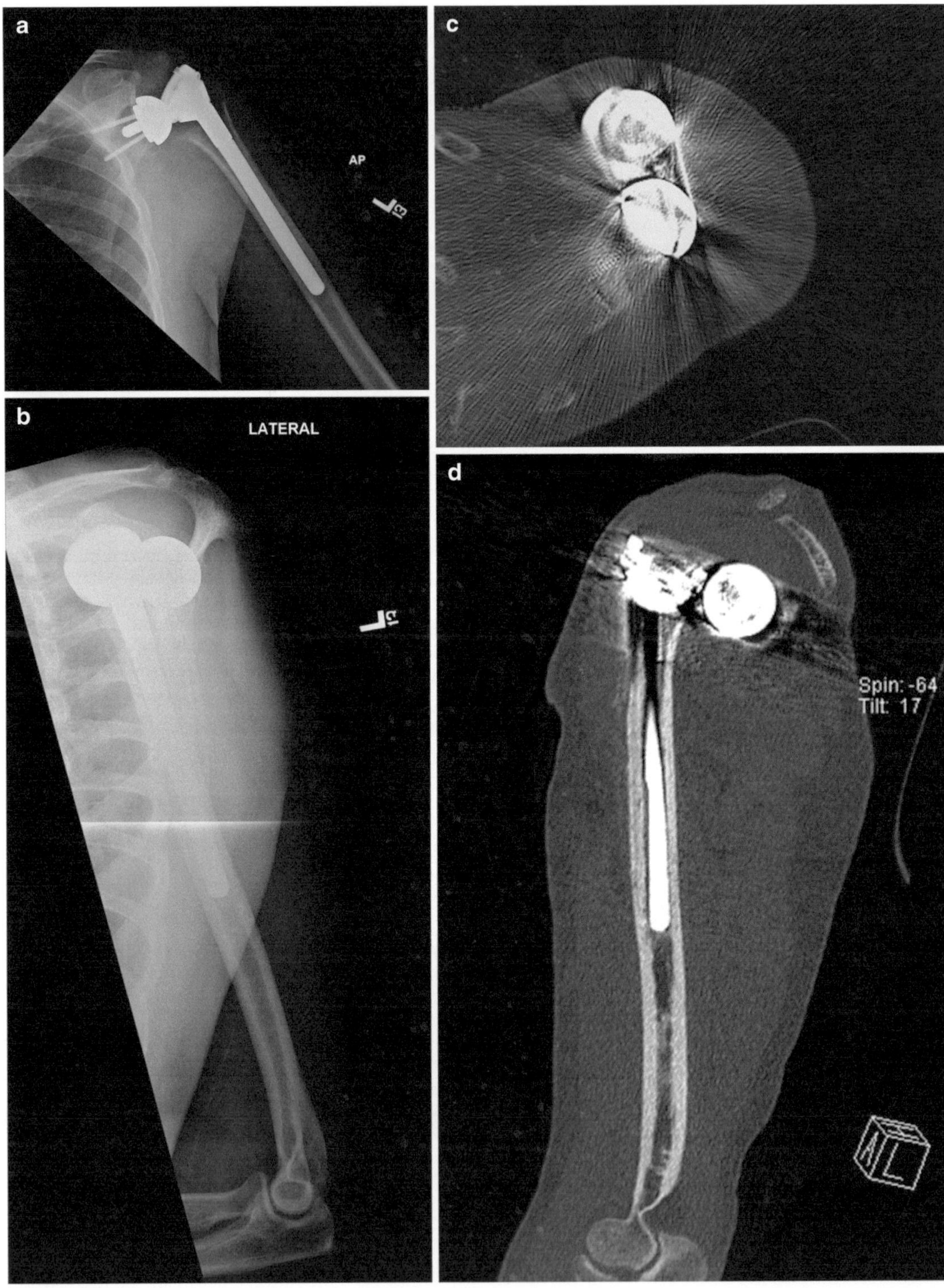

Fig. 11.23 Dislocation. (**a**) AP and (**b**) scapular Y view radiographs of a left shoulder RTSA show anterosuperior displacement of the humeral component of a RTSA. (**c**) Axial and (**d**) sagittal CT images confirm anterosuperior position

Another unique complication of RTSA is acromial fracture (Fig. 11.24), occurring in 5–6.9% of patients [68]. On radiographs, these fractures may appear initially as subtle periosteal reaction and increased sclerosis. These tend to occur in patients with preexisting stiff arthritis with increased stress as glenohumeral motion increases after surgery. For unclear cases, CT can detect subtle fractures and sclerosis related to chronic stress. Scapular fractures occur in three patterns [69]. Type I are small avulsion fractures in the anterior acromion near to or including the footprint of the coracoacromial ligament (2% incidence) [70]. Type II fractures propagate through the anterior acromion just posterior to the AC joint (2.5%). Type III fractures involve the posterior acromion or scapular spine. Acromial insufficiency fracture is another unique complication, possibly resulting from lengthening of the arm and increased tension of the deltoid [71].

Rates of infection for RTSA have recently been shown to be similar to ATSA at 2–3% [72]. Imaging findings of infection are similar to RTSA, including radiolucency, periostitis, and/or joint effusion and soft-tissue swelling.

Other complications of RTSA include mechanical dismantling or fracture of the prosthesis (Fig. 11.25a), glenosphere disengagement

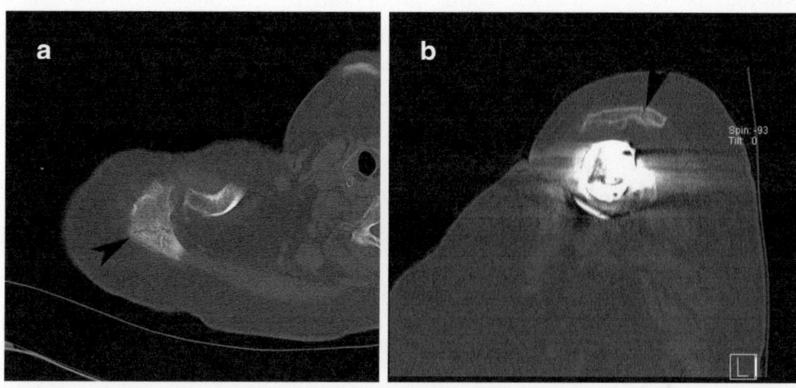

Fig. 11.24 Acromial fracture. (**a**) Axial and (**b**) sagittal CT images of a right shoulder RTSA show fracture line (arrowhead) through the acromion

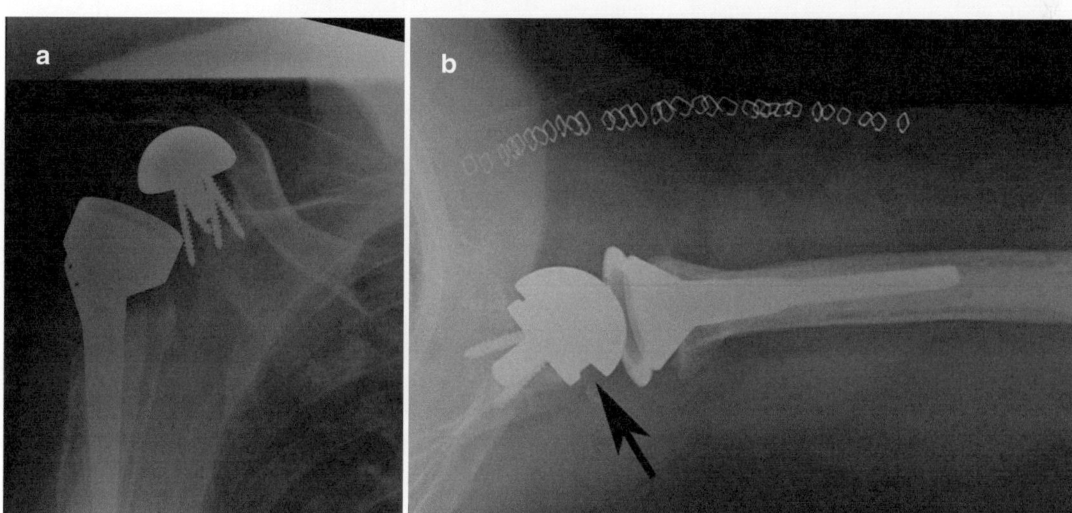

Fig. 11.25 RTSA complications. (**a**) AP radiograph of a right RTSA shows intra-articular metaglene-glenosphere migration. (**b**) Lateral radiograph of a left reverse total shoulder arthroplasty shows asymmetric attachment of the glenosphere to the baseplate (black arrow posteriorly compared to narrower space anteriorly) consistent with glenosphere unseating

(3.2%) (Fig. 11.25b), aseptic loosening with or without intra-articular metaglene migration, and subclinical neuropathy [66]. Subclinical neuropathy occurs more frequently with RTSA due to surgical dissection, exuberant retraction, and/or arm positioning [73]. MR may demonstrate increased signal on fluid-sensitive sequences within the affected portion of the brachial plexus and musculature.

11.4 Conclusion

With the increasing implantation of shoulder prostheses and innovations in hardware design, radiologists will encounter more preoperative and postoperative imaging. Glenoid loosening remains the most common complication of ATSA, while glenoid erosions and progressive glenohumeral osteoarthritis are most commonly seen with HA. Unique complications of RTSA include inferior scapular notching, early dislocation, and scapula fractures.

References

1. Jeong J, Bryan J, Iannotti JP. Effect of a variable prosthetic neck-shaft angle and the surgical technique on replication of normal humeral anatomy. J Bone Joint Surg Am. 2009;91(8):1932–41.
2. Hill HA, Sachs MD. The grooved defect of the humeral head: a frequently unrecognized complication of dislocations of the shoulder joint. Radiology. 1940;35(6):690–700.
3. Sheehan SE, Gaviola G, Gordon R, Sacks A, Shi LL, Smith SE. Traumatic shoulder injuries: a force mechanism analysis–glenohumeral dislocation and instability. AJR Am J Roentgenol. 2013;201(2):378–93.
4. Saupe N, Pfirrmann CWA, Schmid MR, et al. Association between rotator cuff abnormalities and reduced acromiohumeral distance. AJR. 2006;187(2):376–82.
5. Sanders T, Jersey SL. Conventional Radiography of the Shoulder. Semin Roentgenol. 2005;40(3):207–22.. Review
6. Merrill V. Shoulder Girdle. In: Ballinger PW, editor. Merrill's atlas of radiographic positions and radiographic procedures, vol. 1 (ed 6). St. Louis, MO: Mosby; 1986. p. 101–50.
7. Kim SH, Wise BL, Zhang Y, Szabo RM. Increasing incidence of shoulder arthroplasty in the United States. J Bone Joint Surg Am. 2011;93(24):2249–54.
8. Millett PJ, Gobezie R, Boykin R. Shoulder osteoarthritis: diagnosis and management. Am Fam Physician. 2008;78(5):605–11.
9. Kerr R, Resnick D, Pineda C, Haghighi P. Osteoarthritis of the glenohumeral joint: a radiologic-pathologic study. AJR Am J Roentgenol. 1985;144(5):967–72.
10. Neer CS 2nd, Craig EV, Fukuda H. Cuff-tear arthropathy. J Bone Joint Surg Am. 1983;65:1232–44.
11. Kaneko K, Mouy EH, Brunet ME. Massive rotator cuff tears. Screening by routine radiographs. Clin Imaging. 1995;19:8–11.
12. De Smet AA, Ting Y. Diagnosis of rotator cuff tear on routine radiographs. J Can Assoc Radiol. 1977;28:54–7.
13. Resnick D, Niwayama G. Rheumatoid arthritis. In: Resnick D, editor. Diagnosis of bone and joint disorders, vol 2. Philadelphia, PA: Saunders; 1995. p. 866–970.
14. Barrett WP, Franklin JL, Jackins SE, Wyss CR, Matsen FA III. Total shoulder arthroplasty. J Bone Joint Surg Am. 1987;69-A:865–72.
15. McCoy SR, Warren RF, Bade HA, Ranawat CS, Inglis AE. Total shoulder arthroplasty in rheumatoid arthritis. J Arthroplast. 1989;4:105–13.
16. Raymond AC, McCann PA, Sarangi PP. Magnetic resonance scanning vs. axillary radiography in the assessment of glenoid version for osteoarthritis. J Shoulder Elb Surg. 2013;22:1078–83.
17. Mullaji AB, Beddow FH, Lamb GHR. CT measurement of glenoid erosion in arthritis. J Bone Joint Surg (Br). 1994;76-B:384–8.
18. Sabesan V, Callanan M, Ho J, Iannotti JP. Clinical and radiographic outcomes of total shoulder arthroplasty with bone graft for osteoarthritis with severe glenoid bone loss. J Bone Joint Surg Am. 2013;95(14):1290–6.
19. Keller J, Bak S, Bigliani LU, Levine WN. Glenoid replacement in total shoulder arthroplasty. Orthopedics. 2006;29(3):221–6.
20. Neyton L, Walch G. Nov'e-Josserand L, Edwards TB. Glenoid corticocancellous bone grafting after glenoid component removal in the treatment of glenoid loosening. J Shoulder Elb Surg. 2006;15(2):173–9.
21. Walch G, Badet R, Boulahia A, Khoury A. Morphologic study of the glenoid in primary glenohumeral osteoarthritis. J Arthroplast. 1999;14(6):756–60.
22. Nyffeler RW, Jost B, Pfirrmann CW, Gerber C. Measurement of glenoid version: conventional radiographs versus computed tomography scans. J Shoulder Elb Surg. 2003;12(5):493–6.
23. Friedman RJ, Hawthorne KB, Genez BM. The use of computerized tomography in the measurement of glenoid version. J Bone Joint Surg Am. 1992;74(7):1032–7.
24. Hoenecke HR Jr, Hermida JC, Flores-Hernandez C, D'Lima DD. Accuracy of CT-based measurements of glenoid version for total shoulder arthroplasty. J Shoulder Elb Surg. 2010;19(2):166–71.
25. Budge MD, Lewis GS, Schaefer E, Coquia S, Flemming DJ, Armstrong AD. Comparison of standard two-dimensional and three-dimensional cor-

rected glenoid version measurements. J Shoulder Elb Surg. 2011;20(4):577–83.
26. Peyron C, Obert L, Runge M, et al. Evaluation of normal glenoid and humeral landmarks for total glenohumeral arthroplasty. ECR 2013 Scientific Exhibit. C-0471. PDF available at:
27. Takase K, Yamamoto K, Imakiire A, Burkhead WZ Jr. The radiographic study in the relationship of the glenohumeral joint. J Orthop Res. 2004;22(2):298–305.
28. Iannotti JP, Gabriel JP, Schneck SL, Evans BG, Misra S. The normal glenohumeral relationships. An anatomical study of one hundred and forty shoulders. J Bone Joint Surg Am. 1992;74(4):491–500.
29. Rozing PM, Obermann WR. Osteometry of the glenohumeral joint. J Shoulder Elb Surg. 1999;8(5):438–42.
30. Kadum B, Sayed-Noor AS, Perisynakis N, Baea S, Sjoden GO. Radiologic assessment of glenohumeral relationship: reliability and reproducibility of lateral humeral offset. Surg Radiol Anat. 2015;37:363–8.
31. Fischer CA, Weber MA, Neubecker C, et al. Ultrasound vs. MRI in the assessment of rotator cuff structure prior to shoulder arthroplasty. J Orthop. 2015;12(1):23–30.
32. Moosikasuwan JB, Miller TT, Burke BJ. Rotator cuff tears: clinical, radiographic, and Us findings. Radiographs. 2005;25(6):1591–607.
33. Sachez-Sotelo J. Total shoulder arthroplasty. Open Orthop J. 2011;5:106–14.
34. Wiater JM, Fabing MH. Shoulder arthroplasty: prosthetic options and indications. J Am Acad Orthop Surg. 2009;17(7):415–25.
35. Boileau P, Sinnerton RJ, Chuinard C, Walch G. Arthroplasty of the shoulder. J Bone Joint Surg Br. 2006;88(5):562–75.
36. Churchill RS. Stemless shoulder arthroplasty: current status. J Shoulder Elb Surg. 2014;23(9):1409–14.
37. Lazarus MD, Jensen KL, Southworth C, Matsen FA 3rd. The radiographic evaluation of keeled and pegged glenoid component insertion. J Bone Joint Surg Am. 2002;84-A(7):1174–82.
38. Matsen FA III. The ream and run: not for every patients, every surgeon or every problem. Int Orthop. 2015;39:255–61.
39. Copeland SA. Cementless total shoulder replacement. In: Post M, Morrey BF, Hawkins RJ, editors. Surgery of the shoulder. St. Louis: Mosby Year Book; 1990. p. 289–93.
40. Burgess DL, McGrath MS, Bonutti PM, et al. Shoulder resurfacing. J Bone Joint Surg Am. 2009;91(5):1228–38.
41. Widnall JC, Sheerendra SK, MacFarlane RJ, Waseem M. The use of shoulder hemiarthroplasty and humeral head resurfacing: a review of current concepts. Open Orthop J. 2013;7(Suppl 3:M7):334–7.
42. Levy O, Copeland SA. Cementless surface replacement arthroplasty (Copeland CSRA) for osteoarthritis of the shoulder. J Shoulder Elb Surg. 2004;13:266–71.
43. Uribe JW, Botto-van Bemden A. Partial humeral head resurfacing for osteonecrosis. J Shoulder Elb Surg. 2009;18(5):711–6.
44. Jarrett CD, Brown BT, Schmidt CC. Reverse shoulder arthroplasty. Orthop Clin N Am. 2013;44:389–408.
45. Grammont P, Trouilloud P, Laffay JP, Deries X. Concept study and realization of a new total shoulder prosthesis. Rhumatologie. 1987;39:407–18.
46. Roberts CC, Ekelund AL, Renfree KJ, Liu PT, Chew FS. Radiologic assessment of reverse shoulder arthroplasty. Radiographics. 2007;27(1):223–35.
47. Harman M, Frankle M, Vasey M, et al. Initial glenoid component fixation in "reverse" total shoulder arthroplasty: a biomechanical evaluation. J Shoulder Elb Surg. 2005;14:162S–7S.
48. Virani NA, Cabezas A, Gutierrez S, et al. Reverse shoulder arthroplasty components and surgical techniques that restore glenohumeral motion. J Shoulder Elb Surg. 2013;22(2):179–87.
49. Thai DM, Kitagawa Y, Choong PF. Outcome of surgical management of bony metastases to the humerus and shoulder girdle: a retrospective analysis of 93 patients. Int Semin Surg Oncol. 2006;3:5.
50. Bohsali KI, Wirth MA, Rockwood CA Jr. Complications of total shoulder arthroplasty. J Bone Joint Surg Am. 2006;88(10):2279–92.
51. Gregory T, Hansen U, Khanna M, et al. A CT scan protocol for the detection of radiographic loosening of the glenoid component after total shoulder arthroplasty. Acta Orthop. 2014;85(1):91–6.
52. Franklin JL, Barrett WP, Jackins SE, Matsen FA 3rd. Glenoid loosening in total shoulder arthroplasty. Association with rotator cuff deficiency. J Arthroplast. 1988;3(1):39–46.
53. Gruen TA, McNeice GM, Amstutz HC. Modes of failure of cemented stem-type femoral components: a radiographic analysis of loosening. Clin Orthop. 1979;141:17–27.
54. Saltzman MD, Marecek GS, Edwards SL, Kalainov DM. Infection after shoulder surgery. J Am Acad Orthop Surg. 2011;19(4):208–18.
55. Nagels J, Stokdijk M, Rozing PM. Stress shielding and bone resorption in shoulder arthroplasty. J Shoulder Elb Surg. 2003;12(1):35–9.
56. Merolla G, Di Pietto F, Romano S, et al. Radiographic analysis of shoulder anatomical arthroplasty. Eur J Radiol. 2008;68(1):159–69.
57. Athwal GS, Sperling JW, Rispoli DM, Cofield RH. Periprosthetic humeral fractures during shoulder arthroplasty. J Bone Joint Surg Am. 2009;91(3):594–603.
58. Wright TW, Cofield RH. Humeral fractures after shoulder arthroplasty. J Bone Joint Surg Am. 1995;77(9):1340–6.
59. Sanchez-Sotelo J, Wright TW, O'Driscoll SW, Cofield RH, Rowland CM. Radiographic assessment of uncemented humeral components in total shoulder arthroplasty. J Arthroplast. 2001;16(2):180–7.
60. Ives EP, Nazarian LN, Parker L, Garrigues GE, Williams GR. Subscapularis tendon tears: a common sonographic finding in symptomatic postarthroplasty shoulders. J Clin Ultrasound. 2013;41(3): 129–33.

61. Alizadehkhaiyat O, Kyriakos A, Singer MS, Frostick SP. Outcome of Copeland shoulder resurfacing arthroplasty with a 4-year mean follow-up. J Shoulder Elb Surg. 2013;22:1352–8.
62. Delaney RA, Freehill MT, Higgins LD, Warner JJP. Durability of partial humeral head resurfacing. J Shoulder Elb Surg. 2014;23:e14–22.
63. Sweet SJ, Takar T, Ho L, Tibone JE. Primary partial humeral head resurfacing: outcomes with the HemiCAP implant. Am J Sports Med. 2015;43:579.
64. Sirveaux F, Favard L, Oudet D, et al. Grammont inverted total shoulder arthroplasty in the treatment of glenohumeral osteoarthritis with massive rupture of the cuff. Results of a multicenter study of 80 shoulders. J Bone Joint Surg Br. 2004;86(3):388–95.
65. Boileau P, Watkinson D, Hatzidakis AM, et al. The Grammont reverse shoulder prosthesis: results in cuff tear arthritis, fracture sequelae, and revision arthroplasty. J Shoulder Elb Surg. 2006;15(5):527–40.
66. Scarlat MM. Complications with reverse total shoulder arthroplasty and recent evolutions. Int Orthop. 2013;37:843–51.
67. Sirveaux F, Favard L, Oudet D, Huquet D, Walch G, Mole D. Grammont inverted total shoulder arthroplasty in the treatment of glenohumeral osteoarthritis with massive rupture of the cuff: results of a multicentre study of 80 shoulders. J Bone Joint Surg Br. 2004;86(3):388–95.
68. Boileau P, Watkinson DJ, Jatzidakis AM, Balq F. Grammont reverse prosthesis: design, rationale, and biomechanics. J Shoulder Elb Surg. 2005;14(1 suppl S):147S–61.
69. Wahlquist TC, Hunt AF, Braman JP. Acromial base fractures after reverse total shoulder arthroplasty: report of five cases. J Shoulder Elb Surg. 2011;10(7):1178–83.
70. Crosby LA, Hamilton A, Twiss T. Scapula fractures after reverse total shoulder arthroplasty: classification and treatment. Clin Orthop Relat Res. 2011;469(9):2544–9.
71. Walch G, Mottier F, Wall B, et al. Acromial insufficiency in reverse shoulder arthroplasties. J Shoulder Elb Surg. 2009;18(3):495–502.
72. Florschutz AV, Lane PD, Crosby LA. Infection after primary anatomic versus primary reverse total shoulder arthroplasty. J Shoulder Elb Surg. 2015; Epub ahead of print.
73. Ladermann A, Lubbeke A, Melis B, et al. Prevalence of neurologic lesions after total shoulder arthroplasty. J Bone Joint Surg Am. 2011;93:1288–93.
74. Kaback LA, Green A, Blaine TA. Glenohumeral arthritis and total shoulder replacement. Med Health R I. 2012;95(4):120–4.
75. Pritchett JW. Long-term results and patient satisfaction after shoulder resurfacing. J Shoulder Elb Surg. 2011;20(5):771–7.

Part V

Miscellaneous

12 Imaging Diagnosis of Tumors and Tumorlike Conditions of the Shoulder

Eric A. Walker, Matthew J. Minn, and Mark D. Murphey

12.1 Anatomy

Anatomic compartments are defined by natural barriers that also limit the spread of a tumor [1]. Local staging of a malignancy depends on which anatomic compartments are involved and this determination is best accomplished with cross-sectional imaging, preferably magnetic resonance imaging (MRI). Although several staging systems exist, they are all based on the histologic grade of the tumor, the local extent of the lesion, and the presence of metastases. Regarding local extent, lesions confined to one specific compartment are considered intracompartmental. Extracompartmental lesions have spread beyond the compartment of origin [1]. Another consideration requiring knowledge of compartmental anatomy is planning a biopsy path. Resection of the biopsy track is no problem if an amputation is performed but may cause significant difficulties in the case of limb-salvage procedures if inappropriately placed. The radiologist must have a clear understanding of the relevant compartmental anatomy for staging a tumor and avoid unnecessarily contaminating uninvolved anatomic compartments during biopsy. When biopsying a bone or soft-tissue tumor it is advisable to discuss your biopsy approach with the surgeon performing the resection. Failure to do so may result in the biopsy tract within an anatomic region needed for limb-sparing surgery. Different compartments specific to the upper extremity and shoulder include the muscles and fascia covering the dorsal scapula (infraspinatus, teres minor, and rhomboid muscles), the supraspinatus and deltoid compartments, and the anterior and posterior compartments of the upper arm (Fig. 12.1) [1]. The anterior compartment contains the biceps, brachialis, coracobrachialis, and brachioradialis muscles. The posterior compartment is primarily the triceps musculature [2]. More general com-

The authors have nothing to disclose.
The opinions or assertions contained herein are the private views of the authors and are not to be construed as official nor as reflecting the views of the departments of the army, navy, or defense.

E. A. Walker (✉)
Department of Radiology, Milton S. Hershey Medical Center, Hershey, PA, USA

Departments of Radiology and Nuclear Medicine, Uniformed Services University of the Health Sciences, Bethesda, MD, USA
e-mail: ewalker@hmc.psu.edu

M. J. Minn
American Institute for Radiologic Pathology, Silver Spring, MD, USA

M. D. Murphey
American Institute for Radiologic Pathology, Silver Spring, MD, USA

Departments of Radiology and Nuclear Medicine, Uniformed Services University of the Health Sciences, Bethesda, MD, USA

Walter Reed Army Medical Center, Washington, DC, USA
e-mail: mmurphey@acr.org

J. T. Bencardino (ed.), *The Shoulder*, https://doi.org/10.1007/978-3-030-06240-8_12

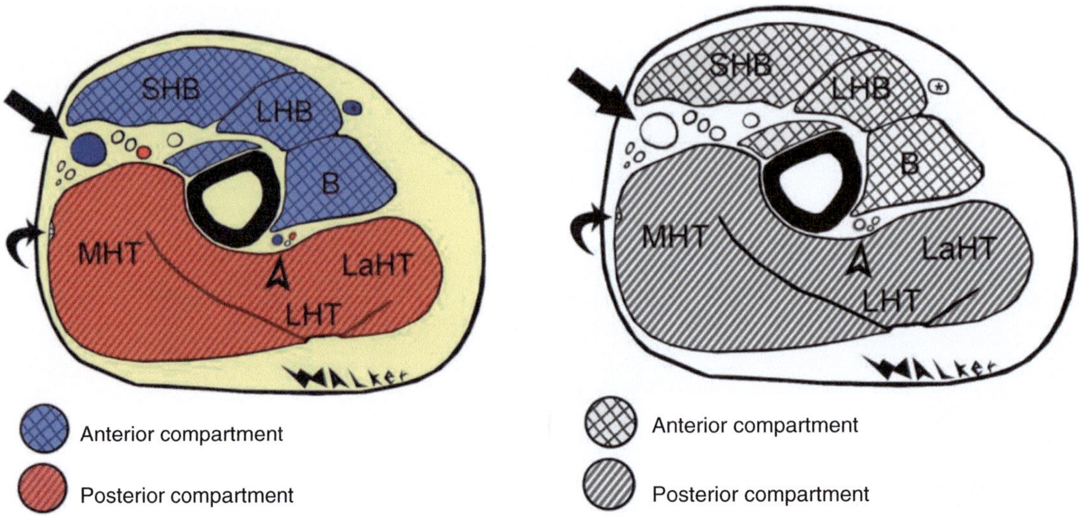

Fig. 12.1 The posterior compartment contains the medial (MHT), lateral (LaHT), and long (LHT) heads of the triceps brachii. The anterior compartment contains the brachialis muscle (B) and long (LHB) and short (SHB) heads of the biceps brachii. Arrow is to the neurovascular bundle containing the median nerve, basilic vein, and brachial artery. Arrowhead is to the neurovascular bundle containing the radial nerve and radial collateral artery and vein. Curved arrow is to the ulnar nerve. Cephalic vein annotated with an asterisk

partments are the skin and subcutaneous fat, the muscle, the nerves and vessels, the parosseous space, the bones, and the joints [2]. When describing a lesion, it is important to note which compartments are involved. When performing a biopsy of the shoulder through the deltoid muscle, the path should be through the anterior deltoid. The axillary nerve innervates the deltoid muscle from posterior to anterior. If a needle track is chosen in the posterior two-thirds of the muscle, the remaining anterior portion of the deltoid may become denervated and functionless after resection of the posterior muscle [2] and may require amputation.

12.2 An Approach to Bone Tumors

The authors value the radiograph as the first and most important diagnostic tool in evaluating a bone tumor and considering a differential diagnosis. Cross-sectional imaging is typically subsequently performed for staging. When considering a lesion and formulating a differential diagnosis, it is important to consider the age and sex of the patient, the lesion location, the lesion margin, the formation of mineralized matrix, and the presence of periosteal reaction (Fig. 12.2a, b). The lesion location includes which bone is involved, the longitudinal location (epiphyseal, metaphyseal, or diaphyseal), and the axial location (central, eccentric, cortical, and juxtacortical/parosteal). Lesions often present within a characteristic location in the skeleton. The lesion margin or zone of transition suggests the aggressiveness or growth rate of the lesion. A geographic 1A lesion is a single well-defined lytic lesion with a sclerotic border and is the least aggressive pattern. The geographic 1B lesion is well defined without a sclerotic border. The growth is likely slow to intermediate. The geographic 1C is an ill-defined single lytic lesion with intermediate growth. Moth-eaten and permeative patterns consist of multiple small lytic foci and suggest a highly aggressive lesion. Mineralized matrix can be characterized as chondroid (ring and arc, honeycomb, or flocculent), osteoid (ivory, solid,

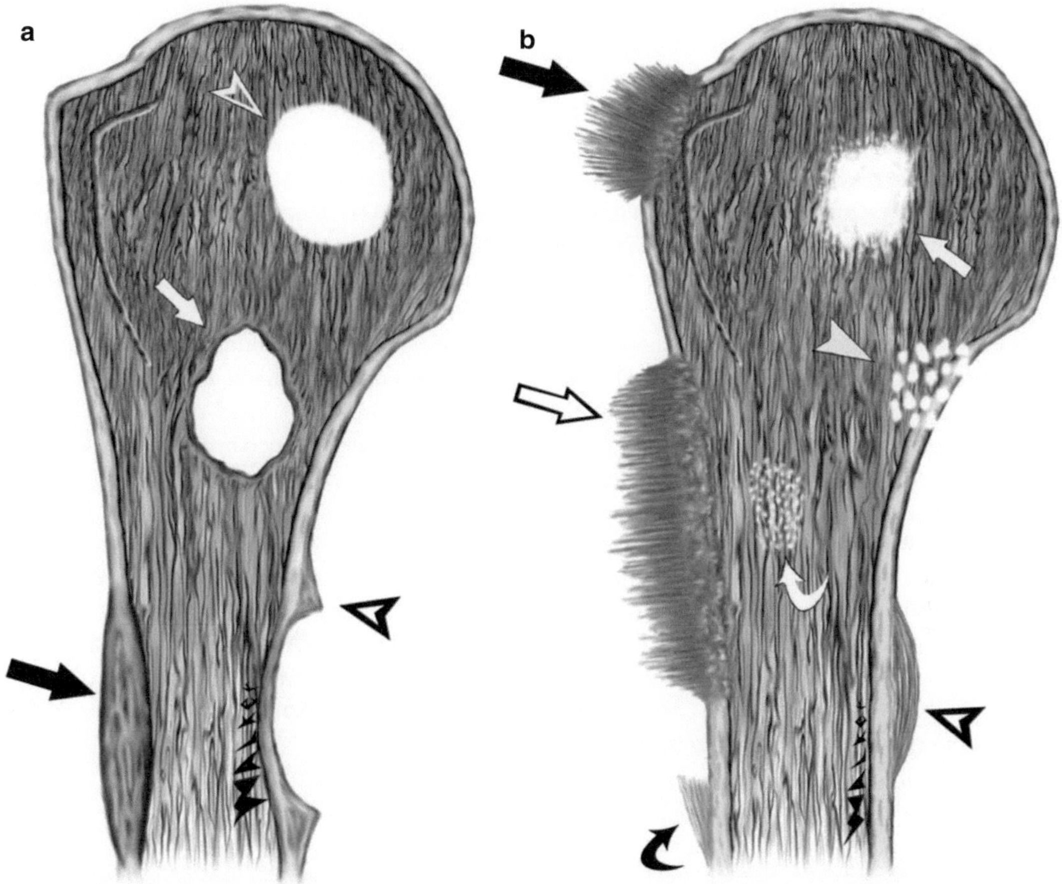

Fig. 12.2 Figure (**a**) represents the margins and periosteal reactions usually associated with nonaggressive lesions. Margins demonstrated are the geographic 1A lesion (white arrow), which is well defined with a sclerotic border and the geographic 1B lesion (white arrowhead) that is well defined without a sclerotic border. The black arrow indicates a solid, slow-growing periosteal reaction and the black arrowhead reveals an area of saucerization with a buttressing periosteal reaction. Figure (**b**) demonstrates the patterns of more aggressive margins and periosteal reactions. A geographic 1C lesion (white arrow) is noted with ill-defined lesion borders. The very aggressive moth-eaten (white arrowhead) and permeative (white curved arrow) patterns are also shown. Aggressive periosteal reactions include the sunburst (black solid arrow), hair-on-end (black hollow arrow), onionskin (black arrowhead), and Codman triangle (black curved arrow)

lumpy, or cloudlike), and ground glass (usually indicating a diagnosis of fibrous dysplasia). Nonaggressive periosteal reactions include solid, buttressing, expansile, and septated. Aggressive periosteal reactions include the Codman triangle, laminated/onion skin, hair on end, and sunburst presentations. Several articles contain a more thorough discussion of bone tumor characteristics [3–7].

12.3 Benign Bone Tumors

12.3.1 Benign Osteoid Lesion: Osteoid Osteoma

Osteoid osteoma is a benign lesion composed of osteoid and woven bone, both of which can be seen as interconnected trabeculae, sheets, or isolated islands with no malignant potential [8]. It is a relatively common skeletal lesion that accounts for nearly 12% of benign skeletal neoplasms [9]. Osteoid osteoma presents in young patients, with approximately 50% presenting between the ages of 10 and 20 years. The lesion is uncommon in patients less than 5 years or greater than 40 years of age. There is a male predilection with a male-to-female ratio of approximately 1.6:1. The presenting symptom is pain, varying in duration from weeks to years. Pain is frequently worse at night, may awaken the patient from sleep, and is often relieved by aspirin or nonsteroidal anti-inflammatory drugs (NSAIDS). Intra-articular lesions often present with nonspecific joint pain. Swelling may be associated with superficial lesions such as those in the fingers and toes [8]. Osteoid osteoma may occur in any bone, but there is a predilection for the lower extremity, with more than 50% occurring in the femur and tibia. The large majority of lesions arise in the cortex of long bones, typically diaphyseal or metadiaphyseal. Only 10–15% of cases of osteoid osteoma occur in the shoulder favoring the proximal end of the humerus or glenoid [10].

On radiograph, the lesion is characterized by a nidus of osteoid tissue less than 1.5–2 cm in diameter surrounded by a larger area of dense fusiform reactive osteosclerosis (solid periosteal reaction). The nidus may be located cortically (70–75%), medullary (25–30%), or subperiosteal and may be radiolucent or contain a variable amount of mineralization [8]. The periosteal reaction may obscure the nidus on plain radiographs. An intra-articular location of the nidus prevents significant periosteal reaction due to differences in the intracapsular periosteum. Computed tomography (CT) is often the best modality to identify the round or oval nidus of decreased attenuation within the surrounding reactive bone. Bone scintigraphy may demonstrate the double-density sign in which there is a small area of focal intense radionuclide activity corresponding to the nidus, superimposed on a second larger area of lesser tracer accumulation related to the surrounding periosteal reaction [8]. The nidus of osteoid osteoma has been described with variable signal characteristics on MRI [11] but most often with low-to-intermediate T1- and high T2-weighted signal. The findings of a round or oval lesion less than 1.5–2 cm in diameter within or adjacent to thickened cortex and marked marrow edema and synovitis of a nearby joint may suggest the diagnosis.

Medical treatment may consist of aspirin or other NSAIDs. Computed tomography (CT)-guided percutaneous radiofrequency ablation is frequently performed at our institutions with an 84–94% cure rate [12].

A reasonable differential diagnosis for an area of mature periosteal thickening includes osteoid osteoma, subacute osteomyelitis (Brodie's abscess), Langerhans cell histiocytosis, and stress fracture.

12.3.2 Benign Chondroid Lesions of Bone (Chondroblastoma, Osteochondroma, Periosteal Chondroma, and Enchondroma)

12.3.2.1 Chondroblastoma

The chondroblastoma (also called Codman tumor) (Fig. 12.3) is a benign, cartilage-producing tumor usually arising in the epiphyses of skeletally immature individuals [13]. The lesion represents approximately 9% of benign bone tumors.

The lesion presents in children and young adults with 90% between age 5 and 25 years. There is a male predilection of 2:1. The clinical presentation of chondroblastoma is typically pain (98%), local tenderness (90%), stiffness (74%), swelling (40%), and joint effusion (4%) [14]. The lesion usually presents in the epiphyses of the long bones, most often the distal femur (20%), proximal humerus (17%), and proximal tibia (17%) [15].

The lesion is often eccentric on radiograph and is usually well defined with a thin sclerotic border (geographic 1A–1B). In 25–50% of lesions, stippled calcifications are present on radiographs [11]. The tumor is classically located adjacent to the growth plate with almost 50% of the cases limited to the epiphysis and many extending for a variable distance into the metaphysis [14].

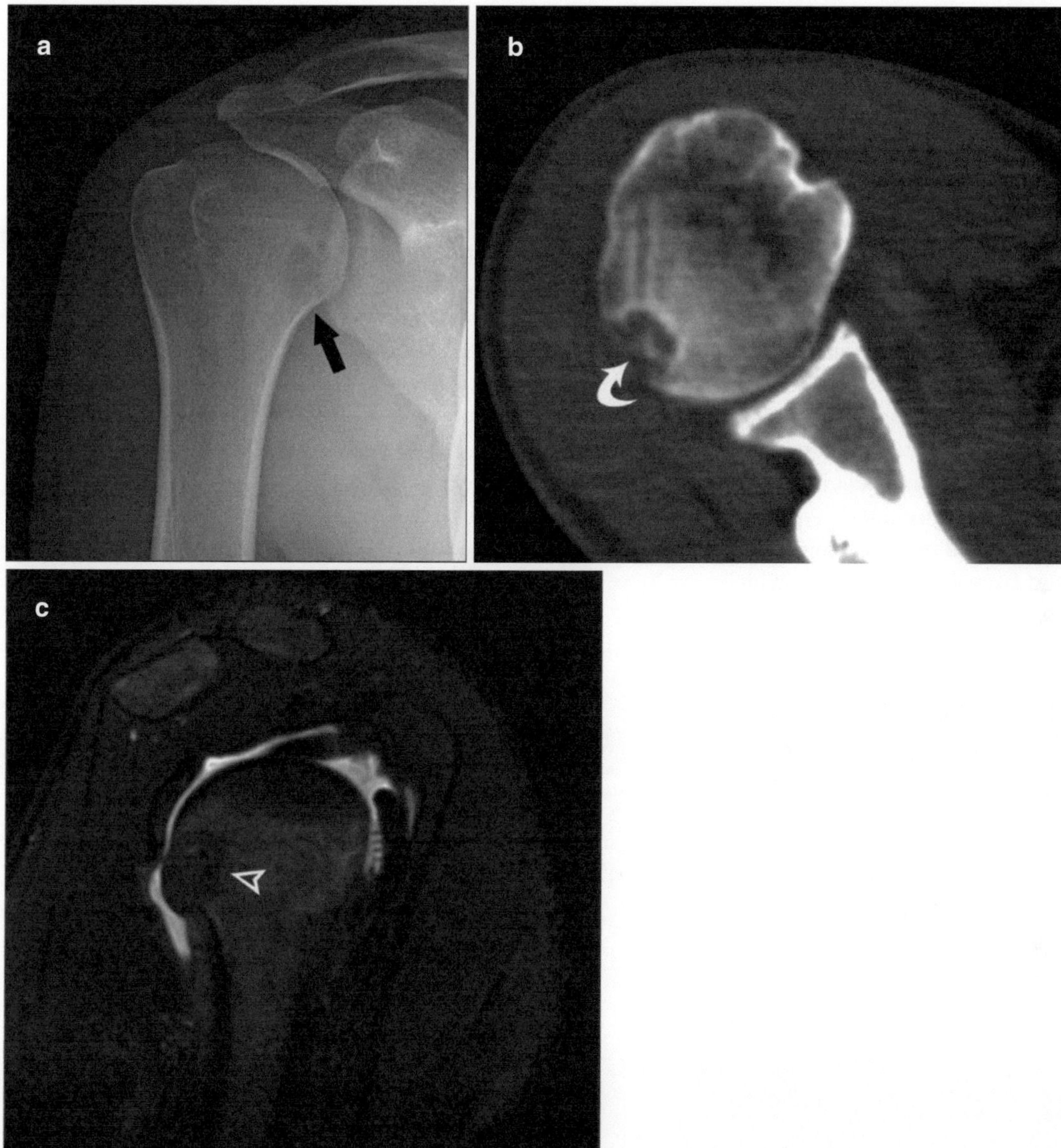

Fig. 12.3 Chondroblastoma: 17-year-old male presents with right-shoulder pain. Radiograph (**a**) demonstrates a geographic 1B lesion (arrow) involving the medial proximal humeral metaphysis adjacent to the physeal scar. Axial CT (**b**) reveals subtle calcifications (curved arrow) within the lesion. T2-weighted (TR4916, TE72) MR (**c**) with fat saturation shows metaphyseal to epiphyseal lesion (arrowhead) extension with low signal and significant surrounding edema. Imaging characteristics favoring the diagnosis of chondroblastoma include epiphyseal extension, lesion mineralization, low T2-weighted signal, and edema surrounding the lesion

Periosteal reaction may be present in 30–62% of cases and is also in the metadiaphysis. CT may be useful for visualizing features such as faint matrix (90–95% with matrix on CT) not seen on radiograph, an extraosseous extension, or a sclerotic margin. A solid or layered periosteal reaction has been described in 50% of cases in one study [16] likely secondary to an inflammatory response. Bone scintigraphy demonstrates uptake on vascular and delayed phases. On MRI, chondroblastoma typically demonstrates intermediate T1-weighted signal intensity and in the majority of cases either complete or partial T2W hypointensity (90–95%), which may be related histologically to abundant immature chondroid matrix, hypercellularity of chondroblasts, calcifications, and hemosiderin deposition [14]. The low lesion signal on fluid-sensitive sequences is a distinguishing feature as it is uncommon in bone tumors. Postcontrast sequences reveal either lobular or peripheral/septal enhancement. The majority of cases (>90%) show marked perilesional bone marrow edema (another distinguishing characteristic). Periostitis, soft-tissue edema, and joint effusion with synovitis are also commonly seen [14]. Fluid levels suggest an aneurysmal bone cyst (ABC) component in 21–77% of lesions.

Chondroblastoma is typically treated with an intralesional curettage and packing of the defect with bone graft or cement, which usually results in an excellent outcome [14]. Radiofrequency ablation has recently been advocated for small lesions.

The benign bone tumors most commonly resulting in bone marrow edema include osteoid osteoma, osteoblastoma, chondroblastoma, and Langerhans cell histiocytosis. Bone metastases and primary malignant bone tumors such as osteosarcoma, Ewing's sarcoma, and chondrosarcoma may also be surrounded by bone marrow edema, particularly if associated with a pathologic fracture [17].

12.3.2.2 Osteochondroma

The osteochondroma (Fig. 12.4) is a benign lesion composed of a cartilage-capped osseous projection on the bone surface. The lesion contains a marrow cavity demonstrating cortical

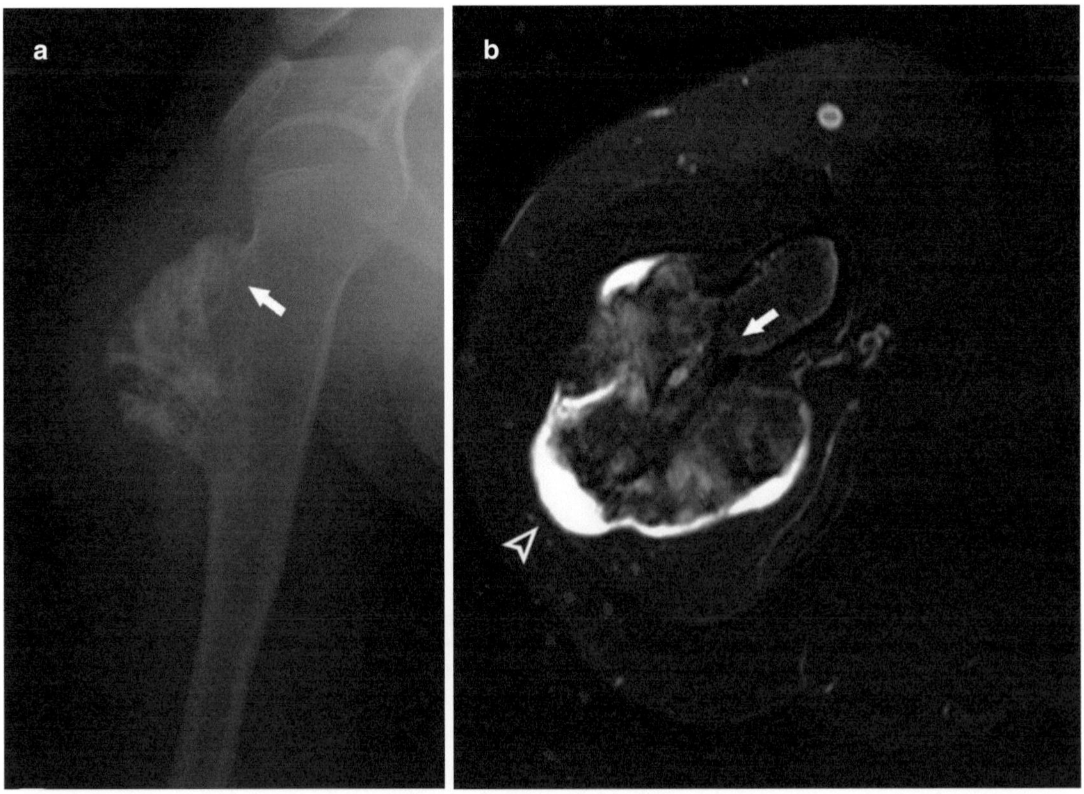

Fig. 12.4 Osteochondroma: 13-year-old male with upper arm pain. Radiograph (**a**) and axial T2-weighted (TR3250, TE70) image (**b**) with fat saturation demonstrate an exophytic mass (sessile osteochondroma) with cortical and medullary continuity (arrows). Typical chondroid matrix is noted in the cartilage cap on the radiograph. The MR best demonstrates the cartilage cap (arrowhead) thickness. This cartilage cap is less than the 2 cm thickness suggestive of malignant transformation

and medullary continuity with the underlying bone. Osteochondroma is the most common bone tumor. It constitutes 20–50% of benign bone tumors and 10–15% of all bone tumors [18]. Osteochondromas may be solitary lesions or multiple, the latter being associated with the autosomal dominant syndrome hereditary multiple exostoses (HME). Osteochondromas are discovered before the age of 20 years in 75–80% of cases. Solitary osteochondroma has a male predilection, from 1.6–3.4 to 1 [18]. The most common symptom related to the osteochondroma is a non-tender, painless deformity related to the slowly enlarging exophytic mass. Additional complications that may cause symptoms include osseous deformity and mechanical impingement, fracture, vascular compromise and pseudoaneurysm, neurologic sequelae, adventitial bursa formation, and malignant transformation. Malignant transformation is observed in approximately 1% of solitary osteochondromas and in 3–5% of patients with HME [18]. The long bones of the lower extremity are most frequently affected (50% of cases), often about the knee (40% of cases). Osteochondromas about the shoulder include humeral involvement (10–20% of cases) and scapula (4% of cases) [18].

The radiographic appearance of solitary osteochondroma is frequently pathognomonic, particularly in long bones. The lesion is composed of cortical and medullary bone arising from and continuous with the underlying bone.

Osteochondromas may be sessile (broad and flat) or pedunculated (narrow with a bulbous tip). Pedunculated lesions usually point away from the nearest joint. Identifying the characteristic cortical and medullary continuity between lesion and parent bone is key for diagnosis. The radiographic appearance of the hyaline cartilage cap is quite variable on radiographs. The chondroid nature of this region is often suggested by the identification of arcs and rings or flocculent calcification. The thickness of the cartilage cap is not well evaluated with radiography unless there is extensive chondroid mineralization. Bone scintigraphy of osteochondroma is variable and is directly correlated with the degree of enchondral bone formation. There is generally more prominent radionuclide uptake in the osteochondromas of younger patients [18]. Cross-sectional imaging may be required to demonstrate cortical and medullary continuity in flat bones or areas of complex anatomy (pelvis, spine, scapula). CT is very useful in depicting the pathognomonic cortical and medullary continuity of the lesion and parent bone. Measurement of hyaline cartilage cap thickness with CT has met with variable success in the literature, and cap mineralization increases the accuracy with CT. The unmineralized cartilage cap is usually lower in attenuation than skeletal muscle, secondary to its high water content [18]. Ultrasound (US) may be more accurate than CT and similar to MR imaging in the evaluation of cartilage cap thickness if the lesion is accessible to US assessment [18]. The cartilage cap on US appears as a hypoechoic layer. Areas of mineralization in the cartilage cap and the underlying osseous component show posterior acoustic shadowing. MR imaging also demonstrates cortical and medullary continuity between the osteochondroma and parent bone. MR imaging (in the authors' opinion) is the best radiologic modality for visualizing the effect of the lesion on surrounding structures and evaluating the hyaline cartilage cap thickness. The cartilage cap demonstrates intermediate to low signal intensity on T1-weighted images and very high signal intensity on T2-weighted or fluid-sensitive sequences [18]. Intravenous administration of gadolinium-based contrast reveals typical chondroid peripheral and septal enhancement (similar to enchondroma or low-grade chondrosarcoma) in the cartilage cap. Cartilage cap thickness of 2 cm or greater in skeletally mature patients is strongly indicative of malignant transformation to secondary chondrosarcoma [19].

The treatment of osteochondroma is follow-ups and only supportive care with small asymptomatic or minimally symptomatic lesions. Larger symptomatic lesions may be surgically resected at their base. Pedunculated lesions are more easily resected. The overall recurrence rate after removal has been estimated at 2%. It is important to entirely resect the overlying perichondrium because inadequate excision of this tissue significantly increases the risk of lesion recurrence [18].

12.3.2.3 Periosteal Chondroma

Periosteal chondroma (Fig. 12.5) is a benign hyaline cartilage neoplasm arising on the surface of a bone beneath the periosteum. Synonyms include juxtacortical chondroma and parosteal chondroma [13]. Histology reveals lobules of immature hyaline cartilage with small chondrocytes interspersed throughout the cartilaginous tissue. Areas of calcification and mucoid degeneration are common [20]. Periosteal chondromas represent less than 2% of bone neoplasms. The lesion is more common in males with a mean age of 27 years at presentation [20]. These lesions have a predilection for the proximal metaphyses or metadiaphyses of the long tubular bones, most com-

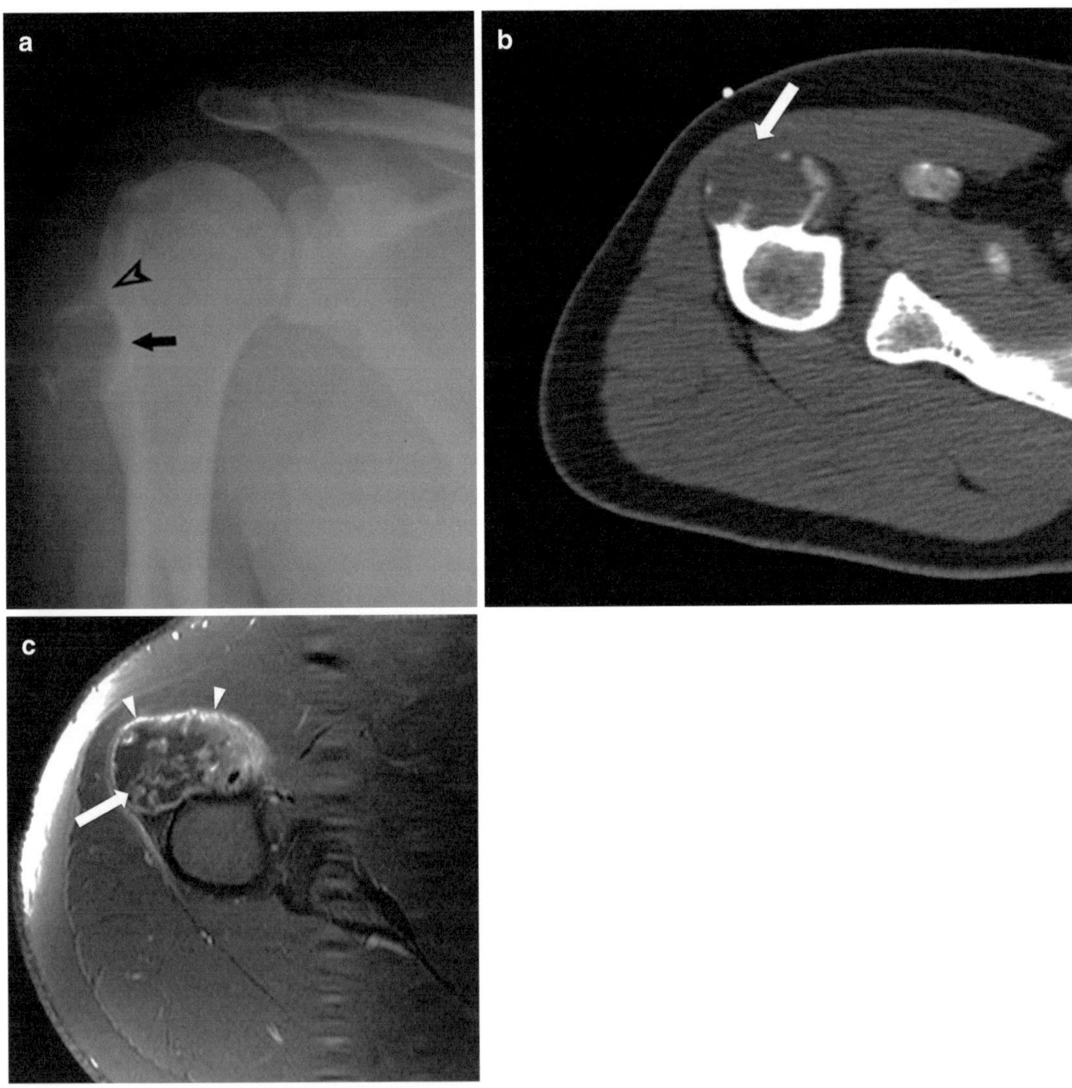

Fig. 12.5 Periosteal chondroma: 19-year-old male with anterior lateral right-shoulder lump for 11 months. Radiograph (**a**) reveals a juxtacortical lesion. There is mild saucerization (arrow) and partial cortical shell. Cortical buttressing is present at the lesion edges (arrowhead). Axial CT (**b**) demonstrates lesion attenuation less than adjacent skeletal muscle (arrow). Axial T1-weighted image (**c**) with fat saturation after gadolinium contrast administration demonstrates the classic peripheral (arrowheads) and septal chondroid enhancement pattern (arrow)

monly the proximal humerus (50%) followed by the femur and tibia. Short tubular bones of the hands and feet are the next most frequent locations [20]. Local swelling, which may be associated with mild pain, is the most common clinical presentation. Lesions are frequently traumatized due to their location on the surface of bone [20].

The classic appearance of periosteal chondroma on radiograph is a small (1–3 cm) area of scalloping (saucerization) of the cortex with adjacent soft-tissue mass. There is usually a well-defined sclerotic margin between the tumor and underlying bone. The outer margin of the lesion may be seen as a thin cortical shell or may be absent on radiographs. Soft-tissue mass with mild-to-moderate amount of cartilaginous mineralized matrix is seen in approximately 50% of cases [20]. Periosteal reaction may present as cortical buttressing at the lesion margins [11]. CT better demonstrates the cortical saucerization and chondroid matrix. The subperiosteal soft-tissue component shows lower attenuation than skeletal muscle. MR imaging demonstrates isointense or low T1 signal and increased T2 signal, with dark foci at areas of mineralized matrix. Postcontrast images reveal peripheral and septal enhancement similar to other chondroid lesions.

Distinguishing between periosteal chondroma and low-grade periosteal chondrosarcoma may be difficult. The best distinguishing characteristic is lesion size. The mean size of a periosteal chondrosarcoma (range 3–14 cm, mean 5.3 cm) is larger than that of periosteal chondroma (range 1–6.5 cm, mean 2.2 cm). Additional imaging findings favoring chondrosarcoma are intramedullary extension, intramedullary edema, soft-tissue edema, and irregular soft-tissue margins on MR imaging [21].

Treatment of these lesions is surgical, with a wide excision performed for periosteal chondrosarcoma and a local excision for periosteal chondroma [21].

12.3.2.4 Enchondroma

Enchondromas (Fig. 12.6) are benign hyaline cartilage neoplasms of medullary bone that are hypocellular and hypovascular with abundant hyaline cartilage matrix [13]. Solitary lesions

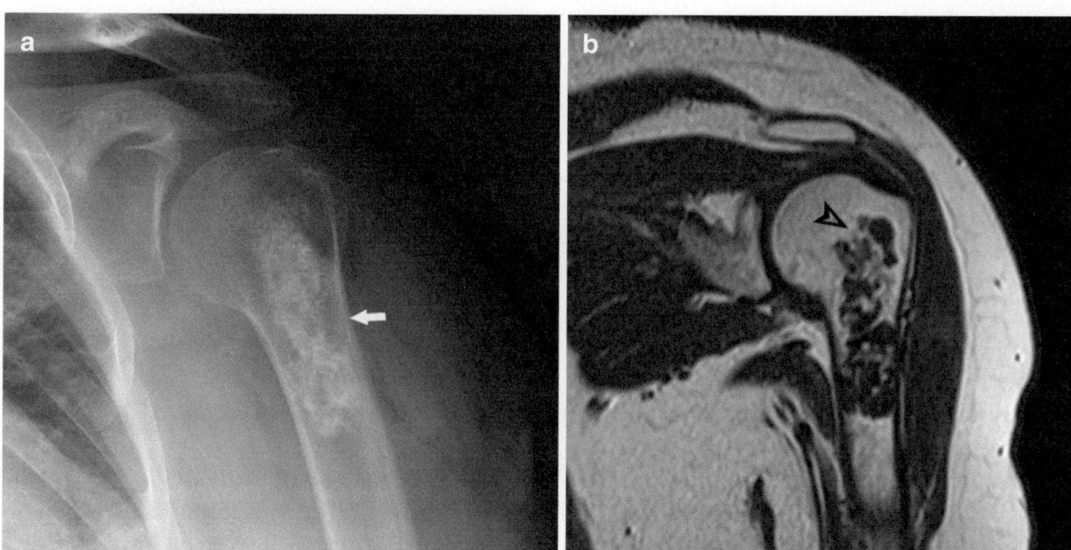

Fig. 12.6 Enchondroma: 58-year-old female with frozen shoulder and failure of 2 months of physical therapy. Grashey view radiograph (**a**) demonstrates ring-and-arc calcifications with central flocculent matrix (arrow). There is no deep endosteal scalloping or cortical remodeling. (**b**) Coronal T1-weighted (TR505, TE16) sequence reveals a central lesion with signal similar to skeletal muscle. The lesion shows lobular growth with fat present between lobules at the proximal margin (arrowhead) "prominent fat trapping"

predominate; however they may be polyostotic. Multiple enchondromas are a feature of Ollier disease and Maffucci syndrome. Enchondromas are quite common and are the second most common benign tumor of bone, representing 10–25% of all benign bone tumors [22]. Because enchondromas usually do not undergo biopsy, the true prevalence is likely underestimated. The lesion may occur at any age but mostly present between the second and fourth decades of life. There is no significant sex predilection. Enchondroma is frequently asymptomatic and is discovered incidentally or after a pathologic fracture through phalangeal lesions. The short tubular bones of the hands and feet (40–65%) are the most common locations followed by the femur, humerus, and tibia [11]. The lesion occurs in the proximal end of the humerus in 10–15% of cases [10].

Radiographs of tubular long bone lesions usually reveal the typical ring and arc chondroid matrix mineralization (95%). Lesions usually present centrally or eccentrically in the metaphysis and diaphysis. Mild (typically much <2/3 of the normal cortical thickness) scalloping of the cortex may be present. The lesion margin is usually well defined to poorly defined (geographic 1B to 1C). Lesion extent may be difficult to characterize accurately on radiographs particularly if mineralization is not prominent. Periosteal reaction, cortical destruction, soft-tissue extension, and extensive cortical remodeling are unexpected findings in long-bone enchondroma [23]. CT is more sensitive in detecting the presence and character of subtle chondroid matrix mineralization and more accurately quantifies the extent of endosteal scalloping than radiography. Enchondromas present as marrow replacement that is low to intermediate in signal on T1-weighted images. Foci of high T1 signal may be noted at the periphery of an enchondroma representing surrounded yellow marrow "trapped fat." The lobular growth of the enchondroma is best revealed on T2-weighted or other fluid-sensitive sequences. The lesion is high (similar to fluid) signal on T2-weighted MR images secondary to the high water content (75–80%) of hyaline cartilage and individual lobules of cartilage may be separated by thin septae that are low in signal. Foci of low signal on T1- and T2-weighted images represent mineralized matrix [23]. MR imaging most reliably determines the absence of a soft-tissue component. Following gadolinium administration, a peripheral and/or septal enhancement pattern is most common. Enchondromas tend to demonstrate homogeneous and mild-to-moderate uptake of radiotracer on whole-body bone scintigraphy in comparison to the anterior iliac spines [23]. Many studies also report positive results regarding the ability of fluorodeoxyglucose-positron-emission tomography (FDG-PET) to differentiate between benign and higher grade malignant cartilaginous lesions [22].

Features that favor the diagnosis of enchondroma over chondrosarcoma include absence of pain, patient age younger than the fourth decade of life, lesion size less than 4 cm, absence of deep endosteal scalloping (typically much <2/3 of the normal cortical thickness), absence of cortical periosteal reaction/thickening/remodeling, absence of soft-tissue extension, a lack of marrow edema surrounding the lesion, prominent fat trapping at the lesion margin on T1 sequences, uptake of radiotracer usually less than the anterior iliac crest on whole-body bone scintigraphy, and lack of hypermetabolic foci on FDG-PET. Involvement of the axial skeleton is very uncommon for a solitary enchondroma [22].

Surgical treatment is frequently unnecessary. Curettage and packing with bone graft material are the typical methods of surgical excision when required. Recurrence is rare.

12.3.3 Non-ossifying Fibroma

Non-ossifying fibroma (NOF) (Fig. 12.7) is a benign fibroblastic proliferative lesion containing osteoclast-type giant cells. The name fibrous cortical defect is used when the lesion is smaller and confined to the bone cortex and the patient is younger. NOF is the term for larger lesions in older patients that extend into the medullary cavity [13]. Some authors prefer the nomenclature

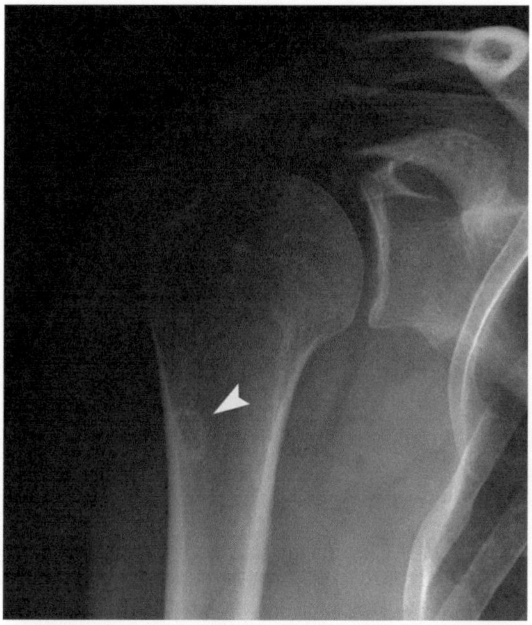

Fig. 12.7 Fibroxanthoma: Lesion incidentally noted in a 40-year-old male with bilateral shoulder pain. Radiograph reveals an eccentric lesion (arrowhead) involving the metaphyseal outer medullary space with a sclerotic (geographic 1A) border. There is no periosteal reaction

fibroxanthoma to refer to both of these lesions. Benign fibrous histiocytoma has the same histologic features but involves the non-metaphyseal region of long bones or the pelvis in older patients [13]. The incidence of NOF is unknown but is stated as the most common fibrous lesion of bone by some authors [11]. It has been estimated that 30–40% of children have one or more occult lesions [13]. There is a 2:1 male predilection and most lesions are identified in the first and second decades of life [11]. Multiple NOF lesions may be present in neurofibromatosis type 1 and Jaffe-Campanacci syndrome. NOF lesions are usually asymptomatic and discovered incidentally unless a pathologic fracture is present. Fibroxanthoma is seen most frequently in the distal femur (38%), proximal tibia, and distal tibia. Less common sites are the humerus (5%) and fibula [11].

Radiographs are often diagnostic. NOF lesions are eccentric elliptical, lucent lesions involving the metaphyseal cortex and much less commonly extending into the medullary space. Lesions are uniloculated or multiloculated (bubbly) and the margin is usually (66%) sclerotic (geographic 1A). During involution they can undergo osteosclerosis [11, 13]. No periosteal reaction is present in the absence of pathologic fracture. CT may better demonstrate cortical thinning and medullary involvement. Hounsfield units within the lesion are higher than normal bone marrow. Scintigraphy reveals minimal to mild increase in radionuclide uptake [11]. With MRI, the lesion shows low signal intensity on T1 compared with that of skeletal muscle. T2-weighted signal is more commonly low, but may be high. T2-weighted signal may decrease as the lesion matures. Enhancement may be diffuse or marginal and septal [24].

Most NOFs heal spontaneously and require no surgical intervention. Treatment is reserved for lesions with atypical radiographs (requiring biopsy) or for symptomatic or larger lesions that require treatment to prevent pathologic fracture [25].

A differential for "bubbly"-appearing lesions of bone includes fibroxanthoma, chondroid lesions, giant-cell tumor, chondromyxoid fibroma, adamantinoma, osteofibrous dysplasia, and desmoplastic fibroma.

12.3.4 Fibrous Dysplasia

Fibrous dysplasia (FD) is a benign, medullary, fibro-osseous lesion, which may involve one bone (monostotic 70–80%) or multiple bones (polyostotic 20–30%). The lesion contains fibrous and osseous tissue present in varying proportions [13]. Syndromes associated with the polyostotic form include McCune-Albright syndrome and Mazabraud syndrome. Fibrous dysplasia most commonly presents in the second and third decades of life. There is an equal distribution between the sexes. The majority of lesions are asymptomatic and incidentally found at radiography. Fibrous dysplasia may present with a pathologic fracture, particularly in the femoral neck [26]. The most common locations affected include the femur (35%), tibia (20%), and ribs (10%). The humerus and skull are also common. A common presentation of fibrous dysplasia is pain related to pathologic fracture. The risk of developing pathologic fracture is accentuated when there is a coexisting aneurysmal bone cyst, further weakening the diseased bone. Malignant degeneration complicates less than 1% of all cases, presenting clinically as pain, rapid growth, and swelling [27].

The radiographic appearance depends on the proportion of osseous to fibrous tissue present. Fibrous dysplasia lesions are intramedullary, expansile, and well defined. Diffuse endosteal scalloping may be present. Lesions show varying degrees of hazy density with a "ground-glass" quality. Occasionally lesions may appear almost completely radiolucent or sclerotic. Greater ossification leads to denser and more sclerotic lesions. Lesions may demonstrate a thick peripheral band of reactive bone or "rind" sign. FD often reveals a nonspecific marked increased uptake of radiotracer on bone scans. Lesion SUV may range from 3 to 19 on FDG-PET. CT and MR cross-sectional imaging are useful for evaluating for soft-tissue components and the extent of a lesion. The MR characteristics are variable, with lesions typically showing intermediate to low signal on T1-weighted images and intermediate to high signal on T2-weighted images. The sclerotic rim (rind sign) presents as a band of low signal on T1- and T2-weighted sequences. Heterogeneous enhancement after the administration of gadolinium is typical [27].

Differential diagnosis for lesions involving multiple bones (polyostotic processes) includes the benign entities of Langerhans cell histiocytosis, enchondromatosis, fibrous dysplasia, hereditary multiple exostoses, osteomyelitis, Paget disease, and angiomatous lesions. Metastases, multiple myeloma, lymphoma, and hemangioendothelioma are polyostotic malignant entities.

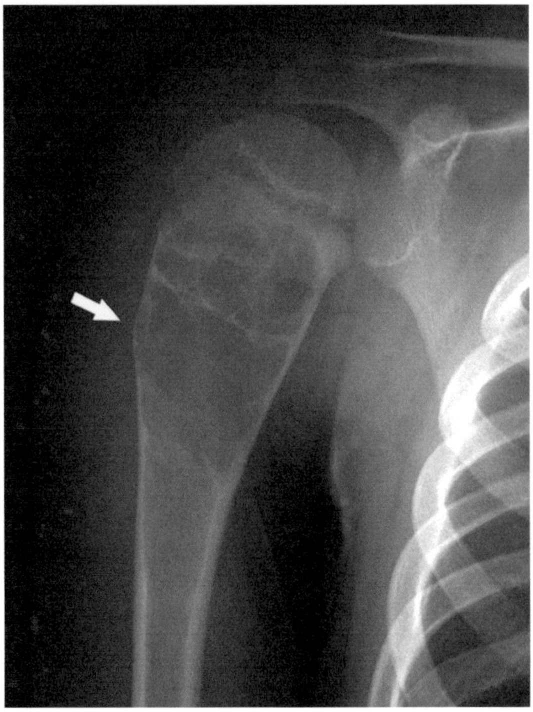

Fig. 12.8 Unicameral bone cyst: 5-year-old male with pathologic fracture and occasional aching pain. Radiograph demonstrates a well-defined, geographic 1A lesion with mild cortical buckling from prior pathologic fracture (arrow). The lesion is located in the central, metaphyseal region of the humerus adjacent to the physis and demonstrates a thin sclerotic rim

12.3.5 Unicameral Bone Cysts

Unicameral bone cysts (UBC) or simple bone cysts (Fig. 12.8) are benign fluid-filled cystic lesions lined by mesothelial cells, which may be unilocular or multilocular with septations [28, 29]. UBCs are thought to be a dysplastic or reactive lesion rather than a true neoplasm. The pathogenesis is believed to be caused by a venous circulation disorder within the cancellous bone, in which a blockage of venous flow leads to increasing pressure and bone resorption [30]. UBC is an uncommon lesion, representing approximately 3% of all primary bone tumors [28, 31]. These lesions typically occur in children and adolescents and traditionally present in the first two decades of life. There is a 2.5:1 male predominance and the lesions are usually solitary without clinical impact [28, 31]. Many lesions are asymptomatic and discovered incidentally when imaging adjacent body parts for various clinical reasons. When symptomatic, a spontaneous fracture of the superior humeral neck and femoral neck is the most common finding. Pathologic fracture occurs in up to 66% of cases [11]. The UBC originates in the metaphyseal region of long bones abutting the epiphyseal plate; however with patient growth it may migrate toward the diaphysis (latent UBC). Based on the distance between the cyst and the growth plate, a UBC is classified as active when the distance is less than 5 mm and latent when greater than 5 mm from the growth plate [32]. These lesions primarily involve the proximal humerus (50–60%), followed by the proximal femur (30%).

On radiographs, UBCs are typically located in the central, metaphyseal region of long bones adjacent to the physis and are well-defined, geographic 1A lesions with a thin sclerotic rim. These may cause mild expansile remodeling of bone with diffuse thinning of the surrounding cortex. The majority of cases demonstrate no periosteal reaction, soft-tissue component, or matrix mineralization [11]. In instances of fracture, an osseous fragment may migrate to the dependent portions of the intracystic fluid. This "fallen fragment sign" is considered pathognomonic for UBC, although it is only seen in about 5% of cases [33]. Bone scintigraphy may be normal or demonstrate increased peripheral uptake with central decreased activity. On FDG-PET imaging the lesions are without hypermetabolic activity [11, 30]. On cross-sectional imaging, UBCs show a thin-walled lesion with the absence of matrix mineralization. CT better characterizes the sclerotic margins and expansile remodeling and may be helpful if the lesion is atypical or located in the pelvis. There may be prominent osseous ridges or trabeculae within the lesion, but most UBCs are made of one contiguous cyst. The attenuation coefficient values (Hounsfield units) can range from 15HU to 20HU within the cysts. MR confirms the cystic components within the lesion with signal characteristics following fluid. An uncomplicated UBC has uniform high signal on T2-weighted sequences and is low to intermediate signal on T1-weighted images. Postcontrast images demonstrate a thin rim of peripheral enhancement without nodular components. Fractured UBCs may contain hemorrhage, fluid levels, and nodular enhancement [30].

UBC is a self-limited benign bone lesion. The purpose of treatment is to prevent pathologic fracture and to manage symptoms, especially pain. Combinations of surgical and nonsurgical techniques ranging among radiological surveillance, intracyst injection (steroids, bone marrow or bone substitutes), cyst wall fenestration with aspiration, intracyst curettage, and internal fixation have been described to treat UBC without a clear treatment consensus. In the setting of fracture, closed treatment (cast or sling immobilization) is the primary treatment, which often is enough to cause resolution and healing of the UBC [34].

12.3.6 Aneurysmal Bone Cyst

Aneurysmal bone cyst (ABC) (Fig. 12.9) is a benign, osteolytic, usually expansile lesion consisting of multiple blood-filled spaces. ABC may arise as a de novo lesion (primary or classical type) or may develop secondarily to a benign bone lesion such as giant-cell tumor (GCT), osteoblastoma, chondroblastoma, chondromyxoid fibroma, FD, or NOF [29]. They may also be secondary to malignant bone lesions (osteosarcoma, fibrosarcoma, chondrosarcoma) as well [11]. ABC is approximately 1% of biopsied primary osseous neoplasms and there may be a slight female predominance. ABC is noted at all ages, but most (75–90% of cases) occur before the age of 20. The most common symptoms of lesions in the long bones are pain and local swelling. Aneurysmal bone cysts can involve any part of the skeleton, but are most common to affect the long bones (67%), spine (15%), and pelvis (9%). The metaphysis is most often involved (80–90%), and the bones most frequently involved are the distal femur, tibia, humerus, and fibula. ABC and UBC affect a similar population and location (proximal humerus, proximal femur) and the aspiration of fluid is nonspecific.

At radiograph, ABC presents as a multicystic, eccentric, osteolytic, expansile, and sometimes trabeculated lesion containing fine-walled cystic cavities. Lesions with marked expansile bone remodeling may have a "blowout" appearance. The lesion has a narrow zone of transition and sometimes a sclerotic margin (geographic

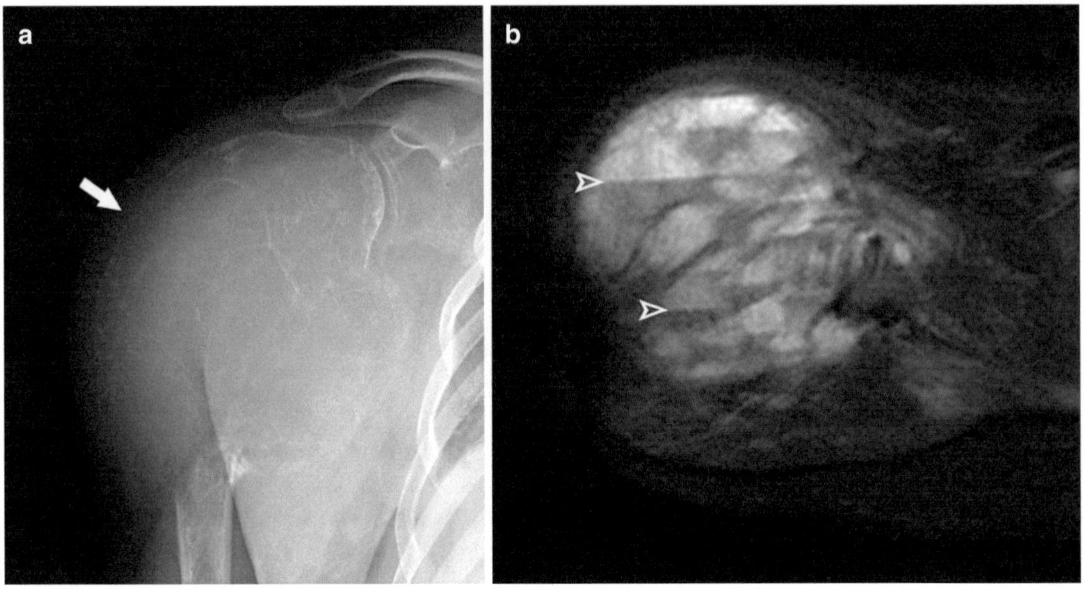

Fig. 12.9 Aneurysmal bone cyst: 22-year-old Latino male with chronic shoulder pain after a fall from horse 6 months prior. Radiograph (**a**) reveals a large multicystic osteolytic lesion (arrow) with a "blownout" appearance. (**b**) Axial STIR sequence (TR5565, TE30) demonstrates multiple cystic spaces with fluid levels (arrowheads)

1A or 1B) at the medullary margin but more aggressive appearance at the cortical margin, which often cannot be seen on radiographs. The cortical or periosteal shell surrounding ABC and lack of soft-tissue extension are better delineated with CT. The attenuation coefficient values (Hounsfield units) can range from 20HU to 75HU [11]. Fluid levels are often appreciated on CT in up to 30% of cases secondary to sedimentation of red blood cells [29]. Bone scintigraphy may show increased radionuclide uptake in a ringlike pattern around the periphery of the lesion (65%). The typical MRI appearance is an expansile lesion either lobular or with septa. Multiple fluid levels present within cystic cavities may be detected on T2-weighted axial sequences. Multiple fluid levels and thin septa without nodularity are highly suggestive of ABC. Postcontrast MR imaging reveals enhancement of the thin and nodular cyst walls and internal septa.

Lesion curettage and filling by graft, cement, or bone substitute may provide good results, but there is a 10–30% risk of local recurrence [29].

12.3.7 Giant-Cell Tumor

Giant-cell tumor (GCT) of bone (Fig. 12.10) is a benign, locally aggressive lesion composed of sheets of neoplastic ovoid mononuclear cells interspersed with uniformly distributed large, osteoclast-like giant cells [13]. These lesions account for approximately 5–10% of primary bone tumors. GCT of bone has the potential for more aggressive behavior "malignant giant-cell tumor" with metastatic pulmonary spread in less than 2% of cases [35, 36]. GCT typically develops in younger adults aged 20–50 years and there is a 2:1 female predominance [11]. Most patients with GCT complain of tenderness or pain at the affected site. The pain can be of months' duration and is sometimes accompanied by warmth, swelling, tenderness, or decreased range of motion [37]. Approximately 50% of all GCTs occur in the knee. In the upper extremity, in decreasing order of frequency, GCT occurs in the radius (distal much more commonly than proximal), humerus (4–8% and proximal much more commonly than distal), phalanges, metacarpals, and ulna (distal much more commonly

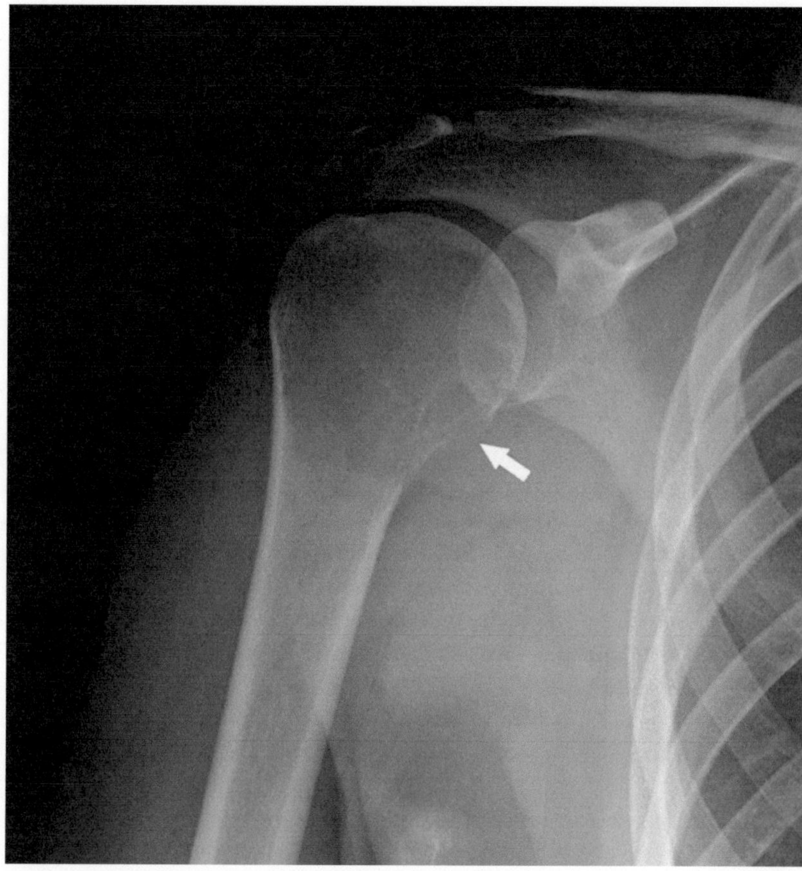

Fig. 12.10 Giant-cell tumor: 28-year-old female with right-shoulder pain for 6 weeks. Radiograph demonstrates a lytic lesion with a geographic 1B margin. Lesion center is near the physeal scar and extends very close to the subchondral bone plate. Probable cortical breakthrough is noted medially (arrow)

than proximal) [37]. Lesions arise in long bones in approximately 60% of cases and almost all extend to the subchondral bone [11].

At radiograph, GCT of bone is most frequently a lytic lesion with a geographic 1B (80–85%) pattern of destruction. Larger lesions may show expansile remodeling of the bone. The lesion arises eccentrically in the metaphysis and expands through the adjacent epiphysis to the subarticular plate [11, 37]. Periosteal reaction is uncommon without pathologic fracture. CT demonstrates similar findings to radiography, but is more sensitive for detecting areas of cortical destruction and soft-tissue extension (33–50%). Bone scintigraphy often demonstrates increased radionuclide activity, which may extend beyond the GCT to involve nearby bones and may be valuable in detecting multicentric GCT. Intense uptake at the periphery and diminished central activity in a pattern resembling a doughnut have been described in approximately 50% of cases [11, 37]. GCT most often reveals a low to intermediate signal on T1- and T2-weighted images (90% of cases). Postcontrast images most often demonstrate heterogeneous enhancement [11].

Intralesional curettage is the mainstay of management for primary GCT of bone. The recurrence rate has declined to approximately 17% with the use of adjuvant treatment such as liquid nitrogen, phenol, hydrogen peroxide, and bone cement [36]. Denosumab is a promising medical treatment to prevent bone destruction and may offer symptom and disease control for patients with limited surgical options [38].

A differential diagnosis for epiphyseal lesions of the proximal humerus includes GCT, chondroblastoma, subchondral cyst, Brodie's abscess, Langerhans cell histiocytosis, and clear-cell chondrosarcoma.

12.4 Malignant Bone Tumors

12.4.1 Multiple Myeloma

Multiple myeloma is a clonal neoplastic proliferation of plasma cells. The process is usually multicentric (polyostotic). A solitary lesion (plasmacytoma) initially lacks systemic manifestations. Synonyms of multiple myeloma include myeloma, plasma cell myeloma, and Kahler disease. Multiple myeloma is the most frequent malignant tumor occurring primarily in bone and accounts for 27% of biopsied bone tumors [13, 26]. Myeloma is rare in patients younger than 40 years and most commonly presents in the sixth and seventh decades of life. Male involvement (68%) is more common than female [26]. Myeloma is often associated with abnormal proteins in the blood and urine and may result in amyloid deposition. Elevated serum calcium levels, anemia, or serum protein electrophoresis may suggest the diagnosis of myeloma before biopsy in a patient with a solitary lesion or unknown diagnosis. The most common presenting symptom is mild and transient pain, worse during the day and increased by weight bearing noted in 75% of patients [39]. Malaise, fatigue, weight loss, fever, bone pain, and pathologic fracture are other commonly encountered symptoms. Myeloma usually arises in bones that contain red marrow. Radiological evidence of skeletal involvement on the skeletal survey is seen in nearly 80% of myeloma patients, most commonly affecting the following sites: vertebrae in 66%, ribs in 45%, skull in 40%, shoulder in 40%, pelvis in 30%, and long bones in 25% [40].

Myeloma may present in a variety of radiographic patterns. Polyostotic well-defined lesions with a geographic 1B margin are the most frequent presentation. A pattern of diffuse osteoporosis particularly in the spine may be present and lead to vertebral compression fracture. Diffuse osteopenia as a result of multiple myeloma cannot be distinguished on radiographs from more common causes of osteopenia, such as senile and postmenopausal osteoporosis (entities noted in a similar age group). The least common pattern is sclerosing myeloma (1%) present in POEMS syndrome (polyneuropathy, organomegaly, endocrinopathy, monoclonal plasmaproliferative disorder, and skin changes) [11, 40]. The sensitivity of radiography versus bone scanning for detecting multiple myeloma has been reported from 75 to 91% for radiography and 46 to 60% for scintigraphy [41, 42]. One of the most significant advantages of FDG-PET/CT imaging is its ability to distinguish between active multiple myeloma (FDG positive) and monoclonal gammopathy of undetermined significance (MGUS) or smoldering disease [40]. Subtle lesions or lesions in areas of complex anatomy such as the spine may require cross-sectional imaging for detection. CT is more sensitive than radiograph for revealing intraosseous extent, cortical disruption, and soft-tissue extension. One negative aspect of CT is that it typically shows persistent bone lesions throughout the course of the disease and, unlike MRI and FDG-PET/CT, it cannot assess continued activity of myeloma in areas of prior bone destruction. MR imaging is more sensitive than CT or radiography in lesion detection. The marrow replacement on MR may be diffuse or focal. T1-weigthed sequences reveal low-signal-intensity lesions. Fluid-sensitive MR sequences demonstrate lesions to be homogeneous and high signal. Lesions generally show enhancement on gadolinium-enhanced images.

The treatment of multiple myeloma may include chemotherapy, bisphosphonates, radiation, biologic therapy, stem cell transplant, and plasmapheresis. Reasons for surgical intervention include an indeterminate lesion, spinal cord compression, and pathologic fracture.

12.4.2 Metastatic Disease

The skeleton is the third most common site of metastases. Metastases are most often located in the red bone marrow. The presentation of a metastatic bone lesion is highly variable and lesions may resemble any malignant or benign primary bone neoplasm, so it is usually prudent to include bone metastases in the differential diagnosis of aggressive or multiple bone lesions in a patient over the age of 40 years. Bone metastases are far more common than primary bone tumors. It is estimated that 2900 new sarcomas of bone are diagnosed in the United States each year. In comparison 169,500 new cases of carcinoma of the lung and 193,700 new cases of breast carcinoma are diagnosed [26]. Malignant bone tumors are metastatic in origin in approximately 70% of cases [11]. Metastatic bone lesions are biopsied at least 35 times more frequently than primary bone tumors. Prostate, breast, kidney, lung, and thyroid (in order of decreasing frequency) make up 80% of all metastatic skeletal lesions. Pain is the most common symptom and present in up to 67% of patients. Pathologic fracture and vertebral compression may occur. Breast carcinoma is most commonly lytic (65%) followed by mixed lytic and blastic on radiography and CT. Prostate carcinoma is the most common cause of bone metastases in men and 75% are osteoblastic on radiography and CT. Lung cancer patients have bone metastases in 15% of cases and the majority (80%) of lesions are lytic on radiography and CT. Renal cell carcinoma and thyroid carcinoma are frequently lytic and highly vascular, with many lesions showing prominent expansile remodeling of bone. Lytic bone metastases may demonstrate geographic (usually 1B or 1C pattern), moth-eaten, or permeative margins. Lesions distal to the knees and elbows (acral metastases) are unusual and likely bronchogenic lung carcinoma (also frequently responsible for "cookie bite" lesions of the cortex). Periosteal reaction is usually absent or limited in response at sites of bone metastases. Prostate carcinoma, gastrointestinal (GI) malignancies, and retinoblastoma are most likely to cause significant periosteal reaction. The radionuclide bone scan is a good screening method for detection of both lytic and sclerotic bone metastases. For evaluating marrow disease, MR is an established technique that is both more sensitive and specific than bone scintigraphy. T1-weighted signal lower than skeletal muscle usually indicates abnormal marrow. FDG-PET is used in the staging of malignancies, for their management, and for monitoring the response to therapy [11, 43–45].

12.4.3 Osteosarcoma (Osteogenic Sarcoma)

Conventional intramedullary osteosarcoma (Fig. 12.11) is a high-grade, malignant neoplasm in which the neoplastic cells produce bone (osteoid). Histologic patterns include osteoblastic (82%), fibroblastic (7%), and chondroblastic (5%). Even if only a minority of the lesion is producing osteoid, it is designated an osteosarcoma. It may be primary or secondary (if the underlying bone is altered by previous radiation, Paget disease, or bone infarct) [13]. Osteosarcoma is the most common primary malignant tumor of bone in children and young adults and second only to multiple myeloma overall. It accounts for approximately 15% of all primary bone tumors. Several subtypes of primary osteosarcoma have been described, including intramedullary lesions (high grade, telangiectatic, low grade, small cell, osteosarcomatosis, and gnathic), surface lesions (intracortical, parosteal, periosteal, and high-grade surface), and extraskeletal osteosarcoma. This chapter focuses on conventional intramedullary osteosarcoma. Patients in the age range of 15–25 years account for 75% of cases of conventional intramedullary osteosarcoma. There is a male-to-female ratio of 1.5–2:1 [46]. Osteosarcoma presents as an enlarging painful mass that may be palpable. The pain is deep-seated and progressive and may be present for several months before diagnosis [35]. High-grade intramedullary osteosarcoma most frequently affects long bones (70–80% of cases), particularly about the knee (50–55%). The humerus is involved in 10–15% of cases [46].

Evaluation of osteosarcoma should begin with the radiograph. A mixed pattern of sclerosis and lytic areas is most frequent. The majority (approximately 90%) of osteosarcomas demonstrate a variable amount of fluffy, cloudlike opacities within the lesion. Identifying osteoid matrix mineralization and other aggressive features is key to diagnosis. The lesion usually violates the cortex without remodeling and demonstrates aggressive periosteal reaction (Codman triangle, laminated, hair-on-end, or sunburst patterns) and soft-tissue masses are present in 80–90% of

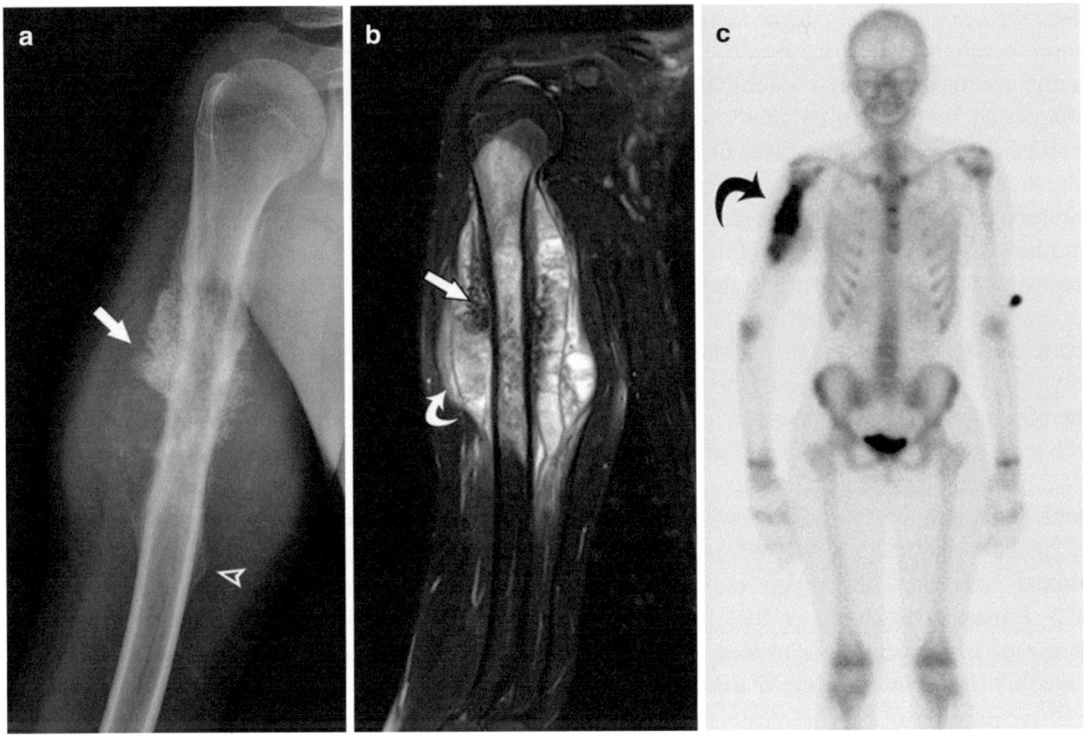

Fig. 12.11 Osteosarcoma: 15-year-old female with right upper extremity mass. Radiograph (**a**) reveals a mixed pattern of sclerosis and lucent areas. Aggressive periosteal reaction is present within the soft-tissue component (arrow). Codman triangles are present distally (arrowhead). (**b**) Coronal T2-weighted (TR2700, TE76) sequence with fat saturation of the entire humerus is performed to look for skip metastases (not present in this case). Note the significant soft-tissue component (curved arrow) and dark areas (arrow) corresponding to osteoid matrix. Whole-body scintigraphy (**c**) is performed to evaluate for distant metastases. The proximal humeral lesion (curved arrow) shows radionuclide uptake greater than the anterior iliac spines. CT of the chest (not shown) should also be performed on the initial workup to evaluate for lung metastases

cases. Lesions are most frequently centered in the metaphysis (90%) of long bones and 75–90% of lesions extend across the epiphyseal plate. Cross-sectional imaging is essential for staging and preoperative planning. CT may help identify mineralized matrix that is not appreciable at radiography and chest CT is utilized to evaluate for lung metastases. At bone scintigraphy, significant uptake of radiotracer is seen on blood flow, blood pool, and delayed images. The major role of scintigraphy is evaluating for distant and skip metastases. Both osseous and extraosseous metastatic diseases may be detected [46]. On MR imaging, tumor is seen primarily as areas of intermediate signal intensity on TI-weighted images and as areas of high signal intensity replacing the normal marrow on T2-weighted images. A large field of view to image the entire bone is essential to identify "skip" metastases. Discontinuous or skip metastases are seen in 1–25% of cases and appear separated from the primary tumor by normal intervening marrow but within the same bone [47]. Areas of low signal intensity on both T1- and T2-weighted MR images are frequent and represent mineralized matrix. Foci of central hemorrhage (high signal intensity with all MR pulse sequences) and areas of necrosis (low signal intensity on T1-weighted images and high signal intensity on T2-weighted MR images) are common in both the intraosseous and soft-tissue tumor components. The lesion margins may be obscured by perilesional edema on MR images obtained with water-sensitive pulse sequences [46]. The use of contrast is valuable in monitoring the response to chemotherapy. In responsive tumors, the intraosseous component may not change in size, but the extraosseous component decreases. Contrast may assist in differentiating viable tissue from nonviable tissue [47].

The chemotherapy regimen may include several or all of the following four drugs: doxorubicin, high-dose methotrexate with leucovorin-rescue, cisplatin, and ifosfamide. Preoperative (neoadjuvant) plus postoperative (adjuvant) polychemotherapy should be used. Surgery should be wide surgical resection and limb salvage or amputation if salvage is not possible [48].

12.4.4 Chondrosarcoma

Chondrosarcoma (Fig. 12.12) is a malignant tumor that produces cartilage matrix. Lesions that arise de novo are called primary chondrosarcoma. A secondary chondrosarcoma may arise in an enchondroma, osteochondroma, Paget focus, radiated bone, or other preexisting lesion. Primary chondrosarcoma is the third most common primary malignant tumor of bone, constituting 20–27% of all primary malignant osseous neoplasms [49]. Numerous types of primary chondrosarcomas have been described, including conventional intramedullary, clear cell, juxtacortical/periosteal, myxoid, mesenchymal, extraskeletal, and dedifferentiated chondrosarcoma. The conventional intramedullary chondrosarcoma is the most frequent type and is discussed in this chapter [49]. Histologic grade is grade 1 (30%), grade II (40%), or grade III (30%). Patients with conventional chondrosarcoma most commonly present in the fourth to fifth decades of life. There is a male predilection of approximately 3:2. Clinical symptoms of chondrosarcoma are nonspecific, with pain being the most frequent, occurring in at least 95% of patients. A palpable soft-tissue mass or fullness may also be a presenting symptom, described in 82% of patients [49]. The most common skeletal location for conventional chondrosarcoma is the long bones (also a common site for solitary enchondroma),

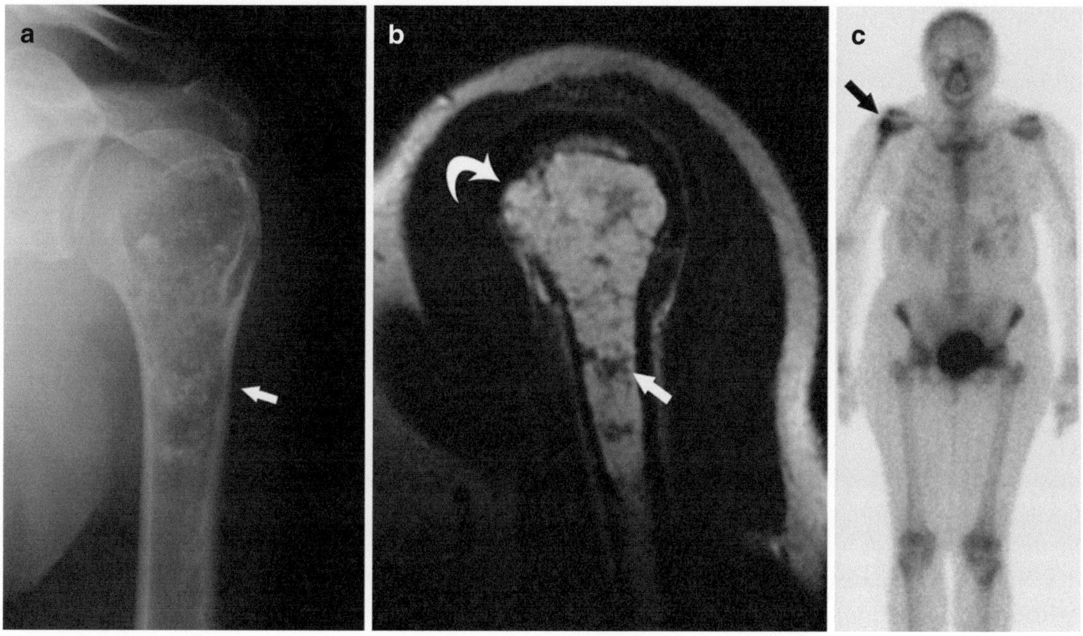

Fig. 12.12 Chondrosarcoma: 38-year-old female with shoulder pain after heavy lifting at work. Radiograph (**a**) demonstrates a proximal humeral lesion with classic chondroid matrix. The lesion shows greater than two-thirds endosteal scalloping (arrow). (**b**) Coronal T2-weighted sequence (TR1800, TE80) demonstrates high signal, similar to water, with lobular growth (curved arrow) and lower signal foci corresponding to mineralized matrix (arrow). Whole-body scintigraphy (**c**) reveals proximal humeral lesion uptake (arrow) of radiotracer greater than the anterior iliac spines

accounting for approximately 45% of cases. The upper extremity is involved in 10–20% of cases, with the proximal humerus being the most frequent location [49].

Radiographs of conventional intramedullary chondrosarcoma typically demonstrate a mixed lytic and sclerotic appearance. The sclerotic foci represent chondroid matrix mineralization and are seen in 60–78% of lesions. The characteristic appearance of chondroid matrix is the "ring-and-arc" pattern of calcification. This mineralized matrix may coalesce to form a more radiopaque flocculent pattern of calcification. Higher grade chondrosarcomas contain relatively less extensive matrix mineralization. The radiolucent component usually reveals geographic (1B or 1C) bone lysis and is multilobulated, directly corresponding to the lobular pattern of growth seen pathologically. More aggressive patterns of bone lysis (moth-eaten and permeative) may be seen with higher grade conventional chondrosarcomas (grade III). Continued lesion growth leads to lobulated endosteal scalloping that eventually produces cortical disruption (57% of long-bone lesions on radiographs) and a soft-tissue component (46% of long-bone lesions on radiographs). In the authors' experience, the depth of endosteal scalloping at its most prominent focus is the best distinguishing feature between long-bone enchondroma and chondrosarcoma. Low-grade chondrosarcoma demonstrates relatively slow growth. The cortex responds to this lobular growth by attempting to maintain the lesion in the medullary canal resulting in cortical expansile remodeling, cortical thickening, and periosteal reaction (usually a less aggressive pattern). The majority (82%) of long-bone chondrosarcomas reveal marked increased radionuclide uptake on bone scintigraphy compared with that in the anterior iliac crest. CT allows optimal detection and characterization of chondroid matrix mineralization, depth of endosteal scalloping, and soft-tissue extension. MR imaging provides the best method for depicting the extent of marrow involvement by conventional intramedullary chondrosarcoma. On T1-weighted MR images, marrow replacement appears as low-to-intermediate signal intensity. Entrapped areas of peripheral yellow marrow may be seen as small speckled punctate regions of high signal intensity (trapped fat) on T1-weighted MR images in long-bone intramedullary chondrosarcomas (35% of lesions) but are much less common than in enchondromas (65%). Fluid-sensitive MR images demonstrate lesion signal similar to fluid (in grade I lesions) and emphasize the lobular growth pattern [49]. Mineralized matrix reveals low signal intensity on all MR pulse sequences. The contrast enhancement pattern of conventional intramedullary chondrosarcoma is typically mild in degree and peripheral and septal in pattern (similar to enchondroma) [49]. In one study, FDG-PET using the combination of SUV and histopathologic tumor grade improved prediction of outcome, allowing identification of patients at high risk for local relapse or metastatic disease [50].

Acceptable oncologic and functional results have been observed in patients with grade I chondrosarcoma treated with curettage and cryosurgery alone, although local recurrence is not unusual if there is inadequate resection [49].

Features that favor the diagnosis of chondrosarcoma as compared to enchondroma in the long bones include the presence of pain, patient age greater than the fourth decade of life, lesion size greater than 4 cm, deeper than 2/3 endosteal scalloping, cortical thickening/remodeling, soft-tissue extension, marrow edema surrounding the lesion on MR fluid-sensitive sequences, uptake of radiotracer usually greater than the anterior iliac crest on whole-body bone scintigraphy, and presence of hypermetabolic foci on FDG-PET [22]. MR imaging findings that support a diagnosis of high-grade chondrosarcoma include intratumoral hemorrhage and soft-tissue mass formation. High-grade and dedifferentiated chondrosarcomas frequently lose the common MR imaging features often seen in low-grade chondrosarcomas of entrapped fat at the tumor margin, internal and outer lobular architecture, characteristic peripheral and septal enhancement pattern after contrast administration, and high signal intensity on water-sensitive sequences [22].

12.4.5 Ewing Sarcoma

The Ewing sarcoma family of tumors includes osseous Ewing sarcoma (Fig. 12.13), extraskeletal Ewing sarcoma, primitive neuroectodermal tumor (PNET), and Askin tumor of the chest wall. Histologically, these lesions demonstrate crowded fields of small round blue cells [51]. Ewing sarcoma accounts for 6–8% of primary malignant bone tumors, and is the second most common bone sarcoma of children and young adults (after osteosarcoma). Ewing sarcoma accounts for approximately 3% of all pediatric malignancies. Ewing sarcoma demonstrates a slight male predominance (1.5:1). Approximately 75% of patients are aged 10–25 years. Common presenting symptoms include pain severe enough to wake the patient (96%), palpable mass (61%), and intermittent fever (21%) [13]. The most common affected bones are the femur (21% of cases), ilium (12–13%), tibia (8–11%), humerus (10%), fibula (7–9%), ribs (8%), and sacrum (6%). While a diaphyseal location of osseous Ewing sarcoma is often stressed, the majority of long-bone lesions are actually metadiaphyseal (44–59%) and pure diaphyseal lesions account for only 33–35% of cases [51].

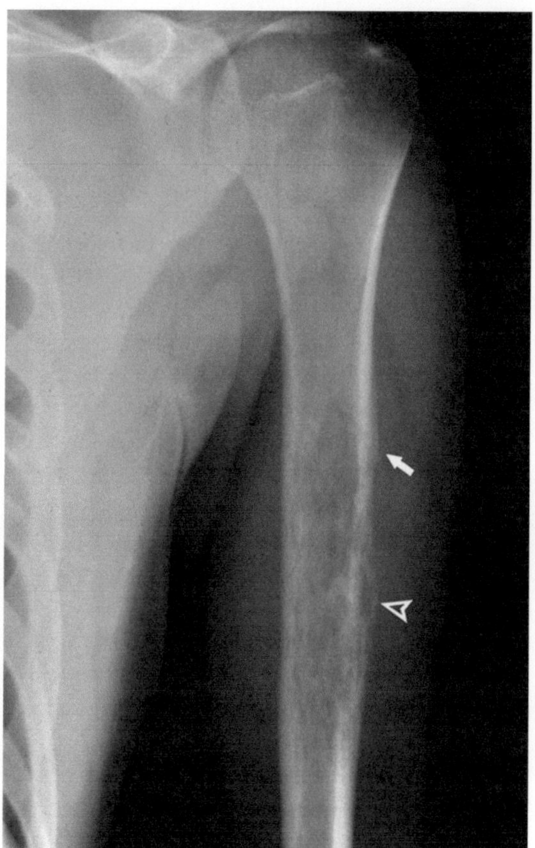

Fig. 12.13 Ewing sarcoma: 20-year-old male with shoulder pain. Radiograph demonstrates a diaphyseal lesion with moth-eaten to permeative (arrowhead) destruction of the cortex and medullary space. There is an aggressive periosteal reaction (arrow)

At radiography, Ewing sarcoma of bone reveals aggressive features, reflecting the high-grade nature of this lesion. Bone destruction with a moth-eaten to permeative pattern is seen in 76–82% of lesions, and a wide zone of transition is identified in 96% of lesions. Cortical destruction (19–42%) with associated soft-tissue extension (56–80%) is also common. Aggressive periosteal reaction is frequent (58–84%) and is usually either lamellated/onionskin (55%) or spiculated (sunburst or hair-on-end pattern) [51]. Nuclear medicine studies show increased radionuclide uptake at both bone scintigraphy and gallium scanning. FDG-PET shows increased metabolic activity in the primary lesion, with a mean maximum standardized uptake value (SUV) ranging from 5.3 (no metastases at presentation) to 11.3 [51]. The appearance of Ewing sarcoma at CT is similar to radiographs, with bone destruction and a large associated soft-tissue mass (96% of cases). The cortical involvement may have a striated appearance within the cortex without focal destruction and continuity between the medullary and soft-tissue component on CT and MR. The soft-tissue component is commonly homogeneous and similar in attenuation to that of skeletal muscle (98% of cases). MR imaging of Ewing sarcoma of bone demonstrates bone marrow replacement (100%) and cortical destruction (92%), with an associated soft-tissue mass in 96% of cases. The signal intensity of Ewing sarcoma is usually homogeneous (73%) and intermediate signal (95%) on T1-weighted images. On T2-weighted images, Ewing sarcoma is typically homogeneous (86%) and low to intermediate in signal intensity (68%). Contrast enhancement is noted in all cases and is usually either diffuse or peripheral nodular in pattern [51].

Therapy primarily involves initial use of neoadjuvant chemotherapy for the purpose of eliminating micrometastases and reducing the size of the primary tumor. Chemotherapy of Ewing sarcoma includes neoadjuvant (before local control) and adjuvant (after local control) therapy over approximately 6 months to 1 year. Chemotherapy agents commonly used in the treatment of Ewing sarcoma include vincristine, doxorubicin, and cyclophosphamide alternated with ifosfamide and etoposide. Surgical treatment of the Ewing sarcoma is often the primary method of local control [51].

The differential diagnosis of a moth-eaten/permeative bone lesion with no matrix mineralization and aggressive periosteal reaction would include Ewing tumor, lymphoma, metastatic lesion, malignant fibrous histiocytoma (MFH)/fibrosarcoma of bone, Langerhans cell histiocytosis, osteomyelitis, and osteosarcoma (10% of osteosarcoma may fail to demonstrate matrix). The presence of a prominent soft-tissue component on cross-sectional imaging would favor Ewing tumor, lymphoma, MFH/fibrosarcoma of bone, and osteosarcoma. Lack of soft-tissue mass and presence of marked edema and fluid collections would favor osteomyelitis.

12.5 Intra-articular Lesions

There is a limited differential diagnosis for intra-articular lesions. The lesions most likely to be encountered in the shoulder include lipoma arborescens, synovial chondromatosis, pigmented villonodular synovitis, and rice bodies secondary to an inflammatory synovial process.

Lipoma arborescens (LA) is thought to be a reactive process and is frequently associated with degenerative joint changes or chronic rheumatoid arthritis. LA is composed of villous lipomatous proliferation of the synovial membrane resulting in prominent fatty fronds. Associated joint effusion is present in all cases and most involved joints (90%) have coexisting degenerative change. The knee is much more commonly involved with rare case reports of lipoma arborescens involving the shoulder. Radiographs often show soft-tissue swelling around the joint that may be radiolucent if the lesion is sufficiently large. CT demonstrates hypertrophied fatty fronds of low attenuation. MR imaging reveals prominent frond-like lipomatous masses within the involved joint. Signal intensity is consistent with fat (high T1, high T2, low T2 fat-suppressed-FS-MR images). Enhancement may be seen in the adjacent inflamed synovium [1].

Pigmented villonodular synovitis (PVNS) (Fig. 12.14a) represents a benign, hypertrophic synovial process characterized by villous, nodular, and villonodular proliferation and pigmentation from hemosiderin [52]. This lesion most often presents in the third and fourth decades. There is an equal sex predilection. Patients most often present with a slowly growing mass. Joint involvement with decreasing frequency includes the knee (75–80% of cases), hip, ankle, shoulder, and elbow [1]. Radiographs may be normal, but erosive bone lesions may develop in tight joints such as the shoulder (75%) and hip (93%). Ultrasound demonstrates a large complex intra-articular mass containing fluid and septations. CT shows an intra-articular soft-tissue mass with increased attenuation (because of the hemosiderin) relative to muscle. Lower attenuation joint effusion may be present [52]. If erosive lesions are present, CT most frequently reveals sharply defined lesions with sclerotic margins. The MR appearance of PVNS is characteristic with a heterogeneous synovial based mass. T1-weighted images show signal intensity similar to or less than skeletal muscle. Low signal intensity predominates on T2-weighted MR images, owing to the preferential shortening of T2 relaxation time caused by hemosiderin, an effect that is accentuated at higher magnet field strength. The characteristic most suggestive of PVNS is enlargement of the low-signal-intensity areas ("blooming") caused by magnetic susceptibility artifact on gradient-echo (GRE) sequences [52]. Intense

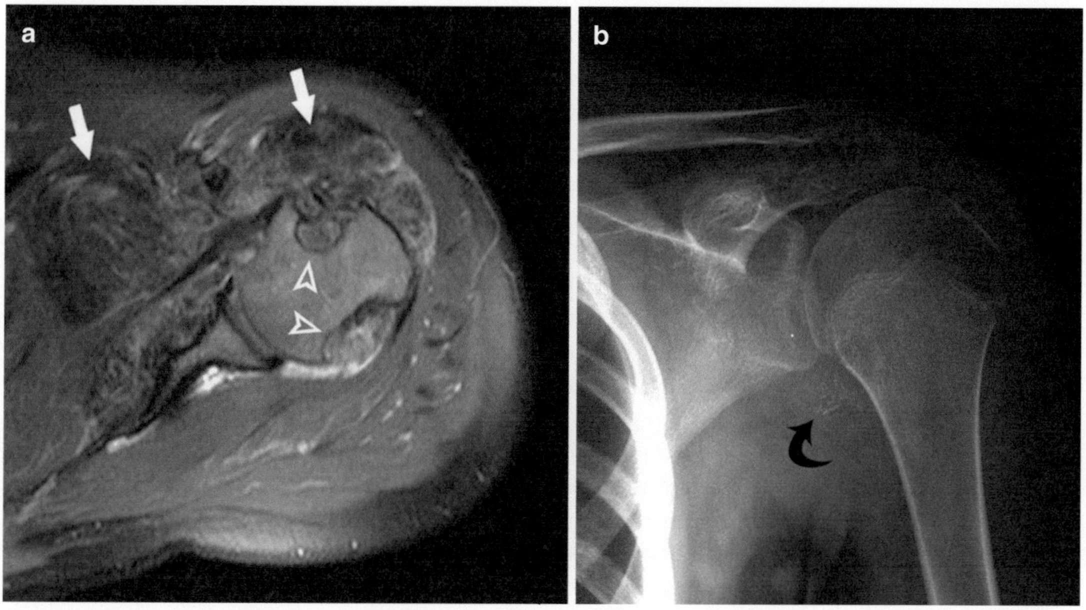

Fig. 12.14 Intra-articular lesions: (**a**) Pigmented villonodular synovitis demonstrated on axial T2-weighted sequence with fat saturation. The mass reveals a predominantly low-signal-intensity lesion (arrows) with preferential shortening of T2 relaxation time caused by hemosiderin. Note the osseous erosions (arrowheads) of the humeral head. (**b**) Synovial chondromatosis on AP radiograph. Note multiple small mineralized nodules of similar size within the axillary recess (curved arrow)

contrast enhancement is typical secondary to significant vascularity. Synovectomy is the treatment of choice [1].

Primary synovial chondromatosis (Fig. 12.14b) is a benign neoplastic process with hyaline cartilage nodules in the subsynovial tissue of a joint, tendon sheath, or bursa. It typically affects patients in the third to fifth decades of life. Men are affected two to four times more frequently than women [53]. Clinical symptoms typically include pain, swelling, and decreased range of motion of the affected joint. The knee is the most frequently affected articulation (50–65% of cases) followed by the hip, elbow, shoulder, and ankle [53]. Radiographs reveal multiple intra-articular calcified bodies in 70–95% of cases, which are typically distributed evenly throughout the joint. The calcified lesions are typically innumerable and very similar in shape. In long-standing disease, individual chondral bodies may coalesce to form a larger, conglomerate, mineralized mass. CT is the optimal imaging modality to both detect and characterize calcification and low-attenuation nonmineralized regions from associated joint fluid [53]. CT is particularly useful for identifying the characteristic ring-and-arc or punctate mineralization and the multiplicity of nodules in cases for which radiographic findings are normal. The most frequent MR appearance is a lobulated intra-articular lesion with homogeneous intermediate signal intensity similar to that of muscle on T1-weighted images, high signal intensity on T2-weighted images, and focal areas of low signal intensity on all pulse sequences representing mineralization. The contrast enhancement pattern of primary synovial chondromatosis is typical of hyaline cartilage lesions, which demonstrate a characteristic peripheral and septal enhancement pattern [53]. The treatment of choice for primary synovial chondromatosis is synovectomy and surgical resection. The recurrence rate for intra-articular disease in larger series appears to range from 3% to 23% [53].

12.6 Benign Soft-Tissue Tumors

12.6.1 Lipoma

The lipoma (Fig. 12.15) is a benign neoplasm composed of mature adipose tissue. It is the most common neoplasm of soft tissue and represents about 50% of all soft-tissue tumors. The incidence of lipoma is approximately 2.1% [54]. Most lipomas are discrete soft-tissue masses categorized by the anatomic location as superficial (subcutaneous) or deep lesions. Deep lesions are much less common and account for approximately 1% of lipomas but are imaged more frequently [54]. Lipomas are rare in the first two decades of life [54]. Superficial lipomas typically present in the fifth to seventh decades, with 80% of lesions in patients aged 27–85 years, and no clear sex predilection [54]. Most lesions are small, with 80% measuring less than 5 cm. Superficial lipomas are most commonly located in the trunk followed by the shoulders, upper arm, and neck. These lesions are unusual in the hands and feet [54]. The superficial lipoma is often difficult to distinguish from surrounding subcutaneous tissue, particularly if the lesion is unencapsulated. For this reason, the authors recommend placing a fiducial marker over superficial lesions, and position the patient so the lesion is not compressed, and comparing the area with the contralateral unaffected side [54]. Deep lipomas include intramuscular and intermuscular lipomatous lesions. These lesions occur most commonly in patients aged 20–60 years. Men are affected more frequently than women. The lesions are located in the shoulder in 12% of cases. The size range of lipoma is large, and lesions can measure up to 20 cm [54]. Both superficial and deep lipomas often present with a painless slow-growing soft-tissue mass. Lipomas may be multiple in 5–15% of patients [54]. In the authors' experience, deep lipomas involving the extremity are most commonly intramuscular lesions [55].

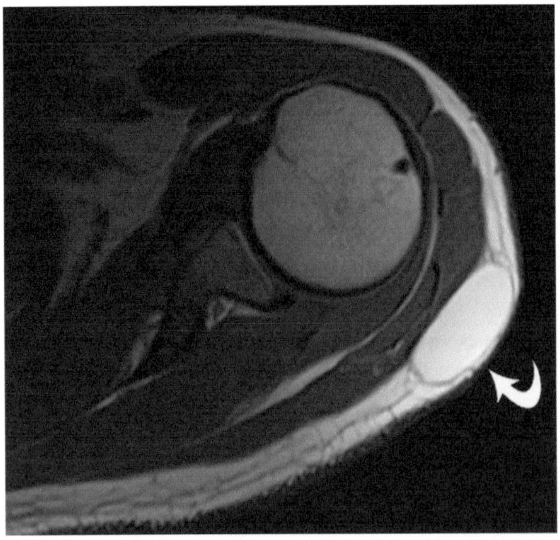

Fig. 12.15 Subcutaneous lipoma: 38-year-old female with shoulder mass. Axial T1-weighted sequence (TR500, TE9.9) reveals an encapsulated subcutaneous lesion of high signal (curved arrow)

Imaging evaluation is diagnostic in up to 71% of cases [55]. Radiographs of superficial lipoma may be unremarkable or demonstrate a mass of fat density. Deep lipoma may reveal a mass with density similar to subcutaneous fat. The sonographic appearance of superficial lipoma is usually an elliptical mass parallel to the skin surface. The lesion is hyperechoic relative to the adjacent skeletal muscle and may contain linear echogenic lines at right angles to the ultrasound beam. They have no increase through transmission and compress with moderate pressure on the transducer [1]. On CT, lipomas appear as a homogeneous mass with attenuation (−65 to −120 Hounsfield units) similar to the subcutaneous fat. The lesion fibrous capsule shows attenuation similar to skeletal muscle when present [51]. Lesions are usually well defined, but lesions may occasionally have infiltrating margins. Lipomas on MR imaging most commonly demonstrate signal isointense to subcutaneous fat on all pulse sequences with high signal on T1-weighted and T2-weighted sequences and thin (<2 mm) septations. However, 28–30% have been reported to have thick septa or nodularity similar to liposarcoma [54]. The authors find it useful to compare the degree of lesion septation to the adjacent normal subcutaneous fat. Lipomas typically reveal septations of no greater thickness or number than this normal tissue. We believe that the use of this comparison can reduce the number of lipomatous lesions that are reported as well-differentiated liposarcoma by imaging. Intramuscular lipomas may have irregular margins, which interdigitate with the adjacent skeletal muscle referred to as infiltrating lipoma. In a 2003 study of 58 lipomatous lesions, lipomas showed no enhancement of septa in 58% of cases and moderate enhancement of the septa in 37% [54]. The fibrous capsule of the lesion often enhances. Calcifications are reported in 11% of benign fatty lesions but are more common in malignant fatty tumors [54].

Treatments described in the literature include steroid injection, liposuction, and surgical excision [56]. The local recurrence rate of these lesions is approximately 4%.

The differential diagnosis for a lipomatous lesion with mild complexity includes lipoma, angiolipoma, myolipoma, chondroid lipoma, lipoblastoma, spindle cell/pleomorphic lipoma, hibernoma, and well-differentiated liposarcoma.

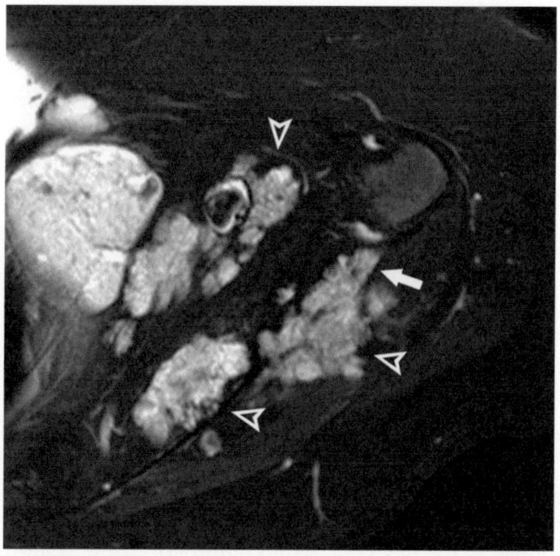

Fig. 12.16 Angiomatosis: 43-year-old female with osseous abnormality of the scapula noted on chest radiograph. T2-weighted image with fat saturation (TR2181, TE60) shows a large lesion with features of serpentine vascular channels (arrowheads) involving multiple compartments and the scapula (arrow)

12.6.2 Hemangioma

The authors prefer to combine hemangiomas and vascular malformations into one category for discussion. Hemangiomas and/or vascular malformations are among the most frequent tumors to involve the soft tissue and comprise 7% of all benign tumors. Hemangioma is the most common tumor in infancy and childhood. It has been estimated that 1–2% of the general population and 10% of Caucasians are affected [57]. Hemangiomas are more common in females with a 3:1 ratio. Lesions may enlarge dramatically during pregnancy. Soft-tissue hemangioma may be superficial or deep, and deep lesions are most frequently intramuscular. Angiomatosis (Fig. 12.16) represents diffuse infiltration by hemangiomas or lymphangiomas with imaging characteristics similar to solitary lesions except for the distribution with involvement of multiple soft-tissue planes (involving several compartments) and prominent longitudinal extension. The clinical presentation is often as a painful lesion that intermittently changes in size. The pain associated with intramuscular hemangiomas is often vague and related to exercise.

Radiographs may be normal or may show a soft-tissue mass and phleboliths. Reactive and pressure changes of bone may occur, particularly when lesions are adjacent to bone, and include a benign periosteal reaction and cortical scalloping (25–30% of cases). The unenhanced CT shows a soft-tissue density mass with or without phleboliths. US reveals a complex mass with acoustic shadowing if phleboliths are present. MR imaging features are often characteristic. The lesion may be well defined or infiltrative. Lesions demonstrate low-to-intermediate signal intensity on T1-weighted images. There may be associated fatty overgrowth due to chronically ischemic muscle in deep-seated lesions, which follows subcutaneous adipose signal. Vascular elements show high signal intensity on T2-weighted images and are typically serpentine in morphology. Enhancement is prominent, and feeding vessels may be evident. In our experience, approximately 90% of deep hemangiomas reveal these pathognomonic features of serpentine vascular channels and fat overgrowth and do not require biopsy for diagnosis.

Management of cavernous hemangioma is dependent on the presence or absence of symptoms. Treatment of these vascular lesions ranges from observation, medical therapy, percutaneous ablation, or surgical excision.

12.6.3 Fibromatosis

The deep fibromatosis that commonly involves the shoulder is extra-abdominal fibromatosis or desmoid-type fibromatosis. These lesions are benign but intermediate in grade with no malignant potential. Fibromatoses are most common in the second and third decades, with a peak incidence in the ages between 25 and 40 years. Lesion incidence is approximately 2–4 people per million with less than 5% seen in the pediatric age group. There is a female predilection in younger patients, which equalizes in older populations [54]. Desmoid-type fibromatosis often presents as a deep, firm, and poorly circumscribed soft-tissue mass, which is slow growing and painless. The most common locations of extra-abdominal fibromatosis are the shoulder/upper arm (28%), chest wall/paraspinal region (17%), thigh (12%), and head and neck (10–23%) [54].

Radiographs are usually normal. On US, lesions are hypoechoic and may be ill defined or well defined. Similar to MR, the fascial tail sign may be noted on US [58]. On CT, the lesion is a nonspecific soft-tissue mass. Unless outlined by fat, the margins of the lesion are poorly defined. The lesion attenuation is variable and may be higher, similar to, or lower than skeletal muscle [58]. MR imaging is the optimal modality for evaluation of deep fibromatosis because of its superior soft-tissue contrast. Lesions are usually centered intermuscular and invasion of the surrounding muscle is frequent. Lesion margins are equally distributed between well-defined or irregular infiltrative. Linear extension along fascial planes (fascial tail sign is seen in up to 80% of cases) is a common manifestation. The signal intensity of desmoid-type fibromatosis is variable, reflecting the relative amounts of collagen and degree of cellularity of the lesion. The most common MR appearance of desmoid-type fibromatosis on MR imaging is intermediate signal intensity on both T1- and T2-weighted images [54]. Immature lesions with marked cellularity reveal higher signal intensity on long TR images. In our experience, these immature lesions are also associated with a higher local recurrence rate after resection. Relatively mature hypocellular areas with abundant collagen reveal lower signal intensity on T1- and T2-weighted sequences often in a band-like morphology (up to 86% of cases) [54].

Primary surgery with negative surgical margins is the most successful primary treatment modality for desmoid tumors. Radiation therapy may be used as a treatment for recurrent disease or as primary therapy to avoid mutilating surgical resection. Pharmacologic therapy with antiestrogens and prostaglandin inhibitors may also be used [59]. A new treatment with sorafenib is also being employed [60].

A reasonable differential diagnosis for soft-tissue lesions with areas of low signal intensity on T1- and T2-weighted sequences includes desmoid-type fibromatosis, densely calcified masses, pigmented villonodular synovitis/giant-cell tumor of tendon sheath (GCTTS), granular cell tumor, and MFH/fibrosarcoma.

12.7 Malignant Soft-Tissue Tumors

Soft-tissue sarcomas occur in the upper extremity in approximately 33% of all cases [61]. The most common soft-tissue sarcoma in adults is undifferentiated pleomorphic sarcoma (UPS, formerly called MFH), which occurs most often in older adults (50–70 years) and 25% occur in the upper extremity. Lesions are typically seen as an intramuscular mass with low-to-intermediate signal intensity on T1-weighted images and intermediate-to-high signal on T2-weighted images. The lesions are heterogeneous on all pulse sequences reflecting variable amounts of collagen, myxoid tissue, necrosis, and hemorrhage [62]. Liposarcoma is the second most common soft-tissue sarcoma [62]. The well-differentiated liposarcoma is the most common subtype of liposarcoma and 14% occur in the upper extremity [62]. The imaging characteristics are very similar to lipoma described earlier. The significant nonadipose components in well-differentiated liposarcoma are seen as prominent thick septa greater than 2 mm and focal nodular regions usually less than 2 cm in size. The septations within a liposarcoma are usually thicker and more numerous than the septa within the normal adjacent subcutaneous tissue. Synovial sarcoma is a soft-tissue malignancy typically occurring in young adults (15 and 35 years). It accounts for approximately 5–10% of soft-tissue sarcomas with an equal male and female predominance. Synovial sarcoma may be associated with faint soft-tissue calcifications, a juxta-articular location, and a high metastatic rate. These lesions may demonstrate the "triple sign" (areas that are hyperintense, isointense, and hypointense on T2-weighted MR) or the "bowl of grapes" (multiloculated with numerous septa) appearance [62]. Fibrosarcoma, leiomyosarcoma, rhabdomyosarcoma, dermatofibrosarcoma protuberans, clear-cell sarcoma, and epithelioid sarcoma (most common sarcoma of the distal upper extremity) are less common soft-tissue malignancies that may be encountered in the shoulder.

Soft-tissue malignancies tend to grow pushing against adjacent structures and form a pseudocapsule as they enlarge, particularly when deep-seated. The pseudocapsule consists of compressed fibrous connective tissue, normal tissue, vascularization, and inflammatory reaction. Malignant lesions tend to respect anatomic compartments and fascial borders until late in their course [57]. Heterogeneous signal may represent mixed tissue types, necrosis, or hemorrhage within the lesion. Only a minority (5%) of benign soft-tissue tumors are greater than 5 cm in diameter and about 1% of benign lesions are deep [57]. Malignant lesions may show increased vascularity at the periphery and high interstitial pressure at their center leading to a high rim-to-center differential enhancement ratio [62]. In general, well-defined, smooth margins, homogenous signal intensity, and small size are seen with benign lesions and heterogeneous signal and large size are indications of malignant lesions. However, unless a specific diagnosis can be determined, a lesion should be considered indeterminate and biopsy should be considered for definitive diagnosis.

12.8 Myxoid Soft-Tissue Lesions

Myxoid soft-tissue lesions are a heterogeneous group of benign and malignant mesenchymal tumors with an abundance of extracellular mucoid material. These lesions may mimic cysts on radiologic evaluation (low attenuation on CT, fluid-like high T2 on MR) because of the high lesion water content. The differential diagnosis of a soft-tissue lesion with signal characteristics and attenuation of fluid include the benign myxoid lesions intramuscular myxoma, synovial cyst, bursa, ganglion, and benign peripheral nerve sheath tumor, including neurofibroma and schwannoma. Malignant myxoid entities include myxofibrosarcoma (formerly myxoid MFH), myxoid liposarcoma, and myxoid chondrosarcoma [63].

12.9 Tumorlike Conditions

12.9.1 Myositis Ossificans

Myositis ossificans (heterotopic ossification within muscle) (Fig. 12.17) is the most common bone-forming lesion of the soft tissues. The anterior musculature of the thigh and arm is most frequently involved. Many patients (approximately 40%) have no history of trauma, and the diagnosis may not be suspected clinically [64].

The initial radiographs may show soft-tissue fullness without calcification. Peripheral calcifications can be recognized on plain radiographs by the third week, although their appearance may vary from 11 days to 6 weeks largely depending on patient age (earlier in younger patients) [64]. Calcification is also present in some soft-tissue sarcomas (soft-tissue osteosarcoma, soft-tissue chondrosarcoma, synovial sarcoma), but is noted diffusely throughout the tumor. In contradistinction, myositis ossificans typically demonstrates a peripheral pattern (zone phenomena) of calcification that becomes more evident as the heterotopic ossification matures. CT is more sensitive than radiography for identifying early mineralization and central low-attenuation zone [64]. MR reveals heterogeneous low signal intensity on T1-weighted images, heterogeneous high signal intensity on T2-weighted images, and enhancement after contrast. The sig-

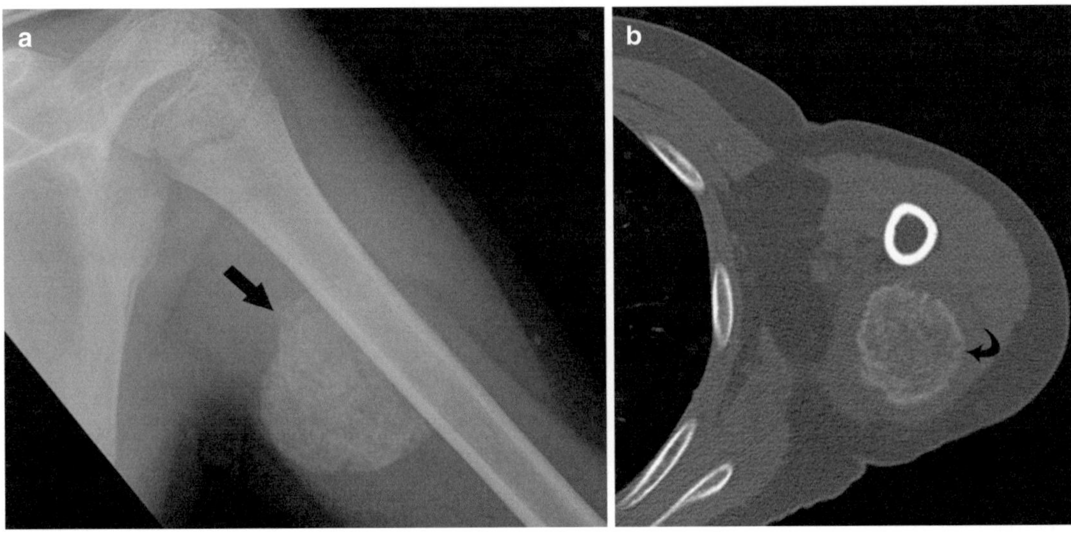

Fig. 12.17 Myositis ossificans: 12-year-old male with left posterior arm mass and 4 months of pain after trauma. Radiograph (**a**) reveals a highly mineralized soft-tissue lesion (arrow). Differential diagnosis would include soft-tissue osteosarcoma, soft-tissue chondrosarcoma, and synovial sarcoma. Myositis ossificans shown on an axial CT (**b**) is distinguished by the typical peripheral pattern (zone phenomena) of calcification (curved arrow) that becomes more evident as the lesion matures

nificant soft-tissue edema surrounding myositis ossificans during the early stages tends to be prominent on CT and MR and is the key to discriminating this lesion from soft-tissue tumors, which usually have little or no surrounding edema [64]. On MR imaging, the calcification is difficult to recognize and the edema may simulate an infiltrative mass.

12.9.2 Paget Disease of Bone

The origin of Paget disease (Fig. 12.18) is unclear, although evidence suggests that an infectious agent (possibly viral) may be the cause. Paget disease is frequently a polyostotic disorder with increased bone turnover. It is most common in people of northwestern European origin and in countries with a large representation by descendants of British emigrants, such as Australia and New Zealand. The prevalence of Paget disease seems to be decreasing in recent decades. It is common in the older population, with an incidence as high as 3–4% in patients older than 50 years [65]. Paget is rarely diagnosed in those younger than 40 years. The most common presentation of Paget disease is of an incidental finding. It may also present with dull pain not related

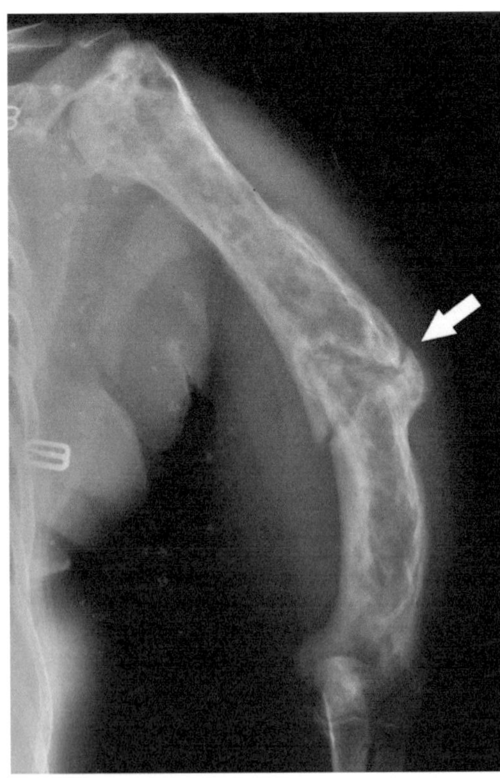

Fig. 12.18 Paget disease: 64-year-old female with pathologic fracture (arrow) through Paget disease. The mixed phase of Paget demonstrates the characteristic radiographic manifestations of osseous expansion and cortical and trabecular thickening

to activity pain, tenderness, and increased warmth (related to lesion hypervascularity). Long-standing disease may be associated with bone deformity (most often the tibia), accelerated osteoarthritis (particularly in the hips), and neurologic symptoms. Pathologic fractures may occur. Secondary sarcoma (usually osteosarcoma) is rare (1% of cases) [65].

Frequent anatomic areas of involvement include the skull (25–65% of cases), the spine (30–75%), the pelvis (30–75%), and the proximal long bones (25–30%).

The early phase of Paget disease is characterized by osteolysis on radiographs. In the long bones, the osteolysis begins as a subchondral area of lucency with an advancing wedge of osteolysis often demonstrating a characteristic sharp radiolucent margin without sclerosis likened to a "blade of grass" or "flame" shape. In the mixed phase of Paget (the majority of cases), the characteristic manifestations seen radiographically are coarsening and thickening of the trabecular pattern and cortex. In the long bones and pelvis, progression to the blastic phase results is areas of bone sclerosis that may be extensive, obscuring areas of previous trabecular thickening. Bone enlargement is prominent in the blastic phase. Bone scintigraphy typically demonstrates marked increased uptake of radionuclide in all phases of Paget disease. CT and MR imaging often show changes similar to those seen radiographically in noncomplicated Paget disease with maintenance of yellow marrow, osseous expansion, and cortical and trabecular thickening.

Medical treatment with bisphosphonates and calcitonin analogues may be useful for metabolically active disease, in preparation for orthopedic surgery, or patients in a state of hypercalcemia or hypercalciuria.

12.10 Summary

It is vital to include compartmental anatomy when describing a bone or soft-tissue tumor to assist in local staging. Before biopsying a bone or soft-tissue tumor, it is advisable to discuss your approach with the surgeon performing the resection. Failure to do so may result in the biopsy tract within an anatomic region needed for limb-sparing surgery. The radiograph is the first and most important diagnostic tool in evaluating a bone tumor and considering a differential diagnosis. Close evaluation of a bone lesion margin and periosteal reaction can reveal if the lesion is slow growing or aggressive. Geographic 1A and 1B margins and solid or buttressing periosteal reaction suggest a less aggressive lesion. It would be very uncommon for a malignant lesion to have a sclerotic margin (geographic 1A) without prior treatment. Geographic 1C, moth-eaten or permeative margins and Codman triangle, onionskin, hair on end, and sunburst periosteal reaction suggest a more aggressive lesion behavior. Identifying the presence of osteoid or chondroid matrix mineralization can help limit and improve your differential diagnosis. Features such as deep endosteal scalloping, cortical thickening/remodeling, and soft-tissue extension favor the diagnosis of chondrosarcoma over enchondroma. The periosteal chondroma is not a common lesion, but 50% present in the shoulder. ABC may develop secondarily to several primary bone lesions. Multiple myeloma is the most frequent malignant tumor occurring primarily in bone and most often has a polyostotic geographic 1B presentation. Myositis ossificans may mimic a mineralized soft-tissue sarcoma such as soft-tissue osteosarcoma, soft-tissue chondrosarcoma, and synovial sarcoma. The key to make this diagnosis is recognizing the peripheral pattern (zone phenomena) of calcification. Lipoma is the most common neoplasm of soft tissue and represents about 50% of all soft-tissue tumors. Subcutaneous lipoma may be difficult to identify on MR without the placement of a fiducial marker over the perceived mass before imaging. Features that favor a malignant rather than benign soft-tissue tumor are lesion size greater than 5 cm, heterogeneous appearance, and a high rim-to-center differential enhancement ratio. Unless a specific diagnosis can be determined, a soft-tissue lesion should be considered indeterminate and biopsy should be considered for definitive diagnosis.

References

1. Kransdorf MJ, Murphey MD. Imaging of soft tissue tumors. 3rd ed. Philadelphia, PA: Wolters Kluwer, Lippincott Williams & Wilkins; 2013.
2. Anderson MW, Temple HT, Dussault RG, et al. Compartmental anatomy: relevance to staging and biopsy of musculoskeletal tumors. AJR Am J Roentgenol. 1999;173(6):1663–71.
3. Madewell JE, Ragsdale BD, Sweet DE. Radiologic and pathologic analysis of solitary bone lesions. Part I: internal margins. Radiol Clin N Am. 1981;19(4):715–48.
4. Miller TT. Bone tumors and tumorlike conditions: analysis with conventional radiography. Radiology. 2008;246(3):662–74.
5. Moser RPJ, Madewell JE. An approach to primary bone tumors. Radiol Clin N Am. 1987;25(6):1049–93.
6. Ragsdale BD, Madewell JE, Sweet DE. Radiologic and pathologic analysis of solitary bone lesions. Part II: periosteal reactions. Radiol Clin N Am. 1981;19(4):749–83.
7. Sweet DE, Madewell JE, Ragsdale BD. Radiologic and pathologic analysis of solitary bone lesions. Part III: matrix patterns. Radiol Clin N Am. 1981;19(4):785–814.
8. Kransdorf MJ, Stull MA, Gilkey FW, et al. Osteoid osteoma. Radiographics. 1991;11(4):671–96.
9. Dahlin DC, Unni KK. Dahlin's bone tumors. 4th ed. Springfield, Ill: Lippincott Williams & Wilkins; 1987.
10. Huvos AG. Bone tumors, diagnosis, treatment, and prognosis. Philadelphia, PA: Saunders; 1979.
11. Greenspan A, Jundt G, Remagen W. Differential diagnosis in orthopaedic oncology. 2nd ed. Philadelphia, PA: Lippincott Williams & Wilkins; 2007.
12. Rosenthal DI, Hornicek FJ, Wolfe MW, et al. Percutaneous radiofrequency coagulation of osteoid osteoma compared with operative treatment. J Bone Joint Surg Am. 1998;80(6):815–21.
13. Fletcher CDM. World Health Organization; International Agency for Research on Cancer. WHO classification of tumours of soft tissue and bone. Lyon: IARC Press; 2013.
14. Qasem SA, DeYoung BR. Cartilage-forming tumors. Semin Diagn Pathol. 2014;31(1):10–20.
15. Dahlin DC, Ivins JC. Benign chondroblastoma. A study of 125 cases. Cancer. 1972;30(2):401–13.
16. Braunstein E, Martel W, Weatherbee L. Periosteal bone apposition in chondroblastoma. Skelet Radiol. 1979;4(1):34–6.
17. James SL, Panicek DM, Davies AM. Bone marrow oedema associated with benign and malignant bone tumours. Eur J Radiol. 2008;67(1):11–21.
18. Murphey MD, Choi JJ, Kransdorf MJ, et al. Imaging of osteochondroma: variants and complications with radiologic-pathologic correlation. Radiographics. 2000;20(5):1407–34.
19. Bernard SA, Murphey MD, Flemming DJ, et al. Improved differentiation of benign osteochondromas from secondary chondrosarcomas with standardized measurement of cartilage cap at CT and MR imaging. Radiology. 2010;255(3):857–65.
20. Robbin MR, Murphey MD. Benign chondroid neoplasms of bone. Semin Musculoskelet Radiol. 2000;4(1):45–58.
21. Robinson P, White LM, Sundaram M, et al. Periosteal chondroid tumors: radiologic evaluation with pathologic correlation. AJR Am J Roentgenol. 2001;177(5):1183–8.
22. Logie CI, Walker EA, Forsberg JA, et al. Chondrosarcoma: a diagnostic imager's guide to decision making and patient management. Semin Musculoskelet Radiol. 2013;17(2):101–15.
23. Flemming DJ, Murphey MD. Enchondroma and chondrosarcoma. Semin Musculoskelet Radiol. 2000;4(1):59–71.
24. Jee WH, Choe BY, Kang HS, et al. Nonossifying fibroma: characteristics at MR imaging with pathologic correlation. Radiology. 1998;209(1):197–202.
25. Arata MA, Peterson HA, Dahlin DC. Pathological fractures through non-ossifying fibromas. Review of the Mayo Clinic experience. J Bone Joint Surg Am. 1981;63(6):980–8.
26. Unni KK. Dahlin's bone tumours. 6th ed. Philadelphia, PA: Lippincott Williams & Wilkins; 2010.
27. Fitzpatrick KA, Taljanovic MS, Speer DP, et al. Imaging findings of fibrous dysplasia with histopathologic and intraoperative correlation. AJR Am J Roentgenol. 2004;182(6):1389–98.
28. Capanna R, Campanacci DA, Manfrini M. Unicameral and aneurysmal bone cysts. Orthop Clin North Am. 1996;27(3):605–14.
29. Mascard E, Gomez-Brouchet A, Lambot K. Bone cysts: unicameral and aneurysmal bone cyst. Orthop Traumatol Surg Res. 2015;101(1 Suppl):S119–27.
30. Cohen J. Simple bone cysts. Studies of cyst fluid in six cases with a theory of pathogenesis. J Bone Joint Surg Am. 1960;42-A:609–16.
31. Dormans JP, Sankar WN, Moroz L, et al. Percutaneous intramedullary decompression, curettage, and grafting with medical-grade calcium sulfate pellets for unicameral bone cysts in children: a new minimally invasive technique. J Pediatr Orthop. 2005;25(6):804–11.
32. Jaffe H, Lichtenstein L. Solitary unicameral bone cyst: with emphasis on the roentgen picture, the pathologic appearance and the pathogenesis. Arch Surg. 1942;44(6):1004–25.
33. Reynolds J. The "fallen fragment sign" in the diagnosis of unicameral bone cysts. Radiology. 1969;92(5):949–53.
34. Kadhim M, Thacker M, Kadhim A, et al. Treatment of unicameral bone cyst: systematic review and meta analysis. J Child Orthop. 2014;8(2):171–91.
35. Fletcher CDM, Unni KK, Mertens F. World Health Organization; International Agency for Research on Cancer. Pathology and genetics of tumours of soft tissue and bone. Lyon: IARC Press; 2002.
36. Raskin KA, Schwab JH, Mankin HJ, et al. Giant cell tumor of bone. J Am Acad Orthop Surg. 2013;21(2):118–26.

37. Moser RPJ, Kransdorf MJ, Gilkey FW, et al. From the archives of the AFIP. Giant cell tumor of the upper extremity. Radiographics. 1990;10(1):83–102.
38. Xu SF, Adams B, Yu XC, et al. Denosumab and giant cell tumour of bone-a review and future management considerations. Curr Oncol. 2013;20(5):e442–7.
39. Dimopoulos MA, Moulopoulos LA, Maniatis A, et al. Solitary plasmacytoma of bone and asymptomatic multiple myeloma. Blood. 2000;96(6):2037–44.
40. Healy CF, Murray JG, Eustace SJ, et al. Multiple myeloma: a review of imaging features and radiological techniques. Bone Marrow Res. 2011; 2011:583439.
41. Ludwig H, Kumpan W, Sinzinger H. Radiography and bone scintigraphy in multiple myeloma: a comparative analysis. Br J Radiol. 1982;55(651): 173–81.
42. Woolfenden JM, Pitt MJ, Durie BG, et al. Comparison of bone scintigraphy and radiography in multiple myeloma. Radiology. 1980;134(3):723–8.
43. Resnick D. Frequency and distribution of skeletal metastasis. Diagnosis of Bone and Joint Disorders. 4th ed. Philadelphia, PA: Saunders; 2002.
44. Rubenstein J. Imaging of skeletal metastases. Tech Orthop. 2004;19(1):2–8.
45. Söderlund V. Radiological diagnosis of skeletal metastases. Eur Radiol. 1996;6(5):587–95.
46. Murphey MD, Robbin MR, McRae GA, et al. The many faces of osteosarcoma. Radiographics. 1997;17(5):1205–31.
47. Jaffe N, Bruland OS, Bielack S. Pediatric and adolescent osteosarcoma. Boston, MA: Springer; 2010.
48. Ritter J, Bielack SS. Osteosarcoma. Ann Oncol. 2010;21(Suppl 7):vii320–5.
49. Murphey MD, Walker EA, Wilson AJ, et al. From the archives of the AFIP: imaging of primary chondrosarcoma: radiologic-pathologic correlation. Radiographics. 2003;23(5):1245–78.
50. Brenner W, Conrad EU, Eary JF. FDG PET imaging for grading and prediction of outcome in chondrosarcoma patients. Eur J Nucl Med Mol Imaging. 2004;31(2):189–95.
51. Murphey MD, Senchak LT, Mambalam PK, et al. From the radiologic pathology archives: Ewing sarcoma family of tumors: radiologic-pathologic correlation. Radiographics. 2013;33(3):803–31.
52. Murphey MD, Rhee JH, Lewis RB, et al. Pigmented villonodular synovitis: radiologic-pathologic correlation. Radiographics. 2008;28(5):1493–518.
53. Murphey MD, Vidal JA, Fanburg-Smith JC, et al. Imaging of synovial chondromatosis with radiologic-pathologic correlation. Radiographics. 2007;27(5):1465–88.
54. Walker EA, Fenton ME, Salesky JS, et al. Magnetic resonance imaging of benign soft tissue neoplasms in adults. Radiol Clin N Am. 2011;49(6):1197–217.
55. Murphey MD, Carroll JF, Flemming DJ, et al. From the archives of the AFIP: benign musculoskeletal lipomatous lesions. Radiographics. 2004;24(5):1433–66.
56. Salam GA. Lipoma excision. Am Fam Physician. 2002;65(5):901–4.
57. Walker EA, Song AJ, Murphey MD. Magnetic resonance imaging of soft-tissue masses. Semin Roentgenol. 2010;45(4):277–97.
58. Walker EA, Petscavage JM, Brian PL, et al. Imaging features of superficial and deep fibromatoses in the adult population. Sarcoma. 2012;2012:215810.
59. El-Haddad M, El-Sebaie M, Ahmad R, et al. Treatment of aggressive fibromatosis: the experience of a single institution. Clin Oncol (R Coll Radiol). 2009;21(10):775–80.
60. Gounder MM, Lefkowitz RA, Keohan ML, et al. Activity of Sorafenib against desmoid tumor/deep fibromatosis. Clin Cancer Res. 2011;17(12):4082–90.
61. Rockwood CAJ, Matsen FA III, Wirth MA, et al. Tumors and related conditions. The shoulder. 4th ed. Philadelphia, PA: Elsevier; 2009.
62. Walker EA, Salesky JS, Fenton ME, et al. Magnetic resonance imaging of malignant soft tissue neoplasms in the adult. Radiol Clin N Am. 2011;49(6):1219–34.
63. Petscavage-Thomas JM, Walker EA, Logie CI, et al. Soft-tissue myxomatous lesions: review of salient imaging features with pathologic comparison. Radiographics. 2014;34(4):964–80.
64. Walker E, Brian P, Longo V, et al. Dilemmas in distinguishing between tumor and the posttraumatic lesion with surgical or pathologic correlation. Clin Sports Med. 2013;32(3):559–76.
65. Smith SE, Murphey MD, Motamedi K, et al. From the archives of the AFIP. Radiologic spectrum of Paget disease of bone and its complications with pathologic correlation. Radiographics. 2002;22(5):1191–216.

13 Imaging of Pediatric Disorders of the Shoulder

Jorge Delgado and Diego Jaramillo

13.1 Introduction

The skeletal development of the shoulder influences the imaging appearance of congenital, infectious, and inflammatory diseases in children. Additionally, as competitive sports are being practiced at an earlier age and at a higher level, the number of pediatric patients requiring shoulder imaging is continuously increasing. Understanding the normal development of the shoulder is essential to appropriately interpret imaging findings.

13.2 Development of the Normal Pediatric Shoulder

At birth, the diaphysis of the clavicle, the body and spine of the scapula, and the proximal humeral diaphysis are ossified, whereas the proximal humeral epiphysis, the glenoid, the coracoid process, the acromion, the vertebral border and the inferior angle of the scapula, and the lateral epiphysis of the clavicle are composed of hyaline cartilage [1]. The medial clavicular physis, which closes at 22–25 years of age, is responsible for most of the longitudinal growth of this bone [1], and the lateral clavicular physis, which is not always present, can often be confused with a fracture [2].

Throughout osseous maturation, multiple secondary ossification centers arise from the cartilaginous epiphyses and apophyses of the shoulder. Bone growth from secondary ossification centers occur by endochondral ossification [3]. The appearance and growth of each secondary ossification center occur at a different age, which modifies the appearance of the shoulder at different stages of development (Table 13.1).

13.2.1 Anatomy

13.2.1.1 Proximal Humerus

The proximal humeral epiphysis has three ossification centers: the head of the humerus, the greater tuberosity, and the lesser tuberosity. At the moment, there is debate about the lesser tuberosity secondary ossification center being an independent entity or being part of the humeral head ossification center [4]. Before the appearance of the ossification centers in the proximal humerus, a progression of changes that begins with chondrocyte hypertrophy and is followed by central vascularization leads to the formation of ill-defined, small, low-to-intermediate T1, high T2 signal intensity (SI) foci called preossification centers, which should not be mistaken for intraepiphyseal abnormalities. After the formation of early osteoid

J. Delgado (✉)
Department of Radiology, Harvard Medical School, Massachusetts General Hospital, Boston, MA, USA

D. Jaramillo
Department of Radiology, Columbia University Medical Center, New York, NY, USA

J. T. Bencardino (ed.), *The Shoulder*, https://doi.org/10.1007/978-3-030-06240-8_13

Table 13.1 Approximate age of appearance and fusion of the multiple ossification centers of the shoulder [1, 2, 6, 9]

Bone structure	Ossification center	Age of appearance	Age of fusion
Proximal humerus	Head of the humerus	1–6 months	3–5 years
	Greater tuberosity	9–12 months	
	Lesser tuberosity	12–16 months	
Scapula: glenoid	Subcoracoid	8–10 years	14–17 years
	Centers in the inferior two-thirds of the glenoid	14–15 years	17–18 years
Scapula: coracoid process	Center of the coracoid process	3 months	15–17 years
	Base of the coracoid process	8–10 years	
Scapula: acromion	Acromial secondary ossification centers	14–16 years	18–25 years
Scapula	Vertebral border	14–20 years	22 years
	Inferior angle		

matrix within the preossification centers, this foci become of intermediate SI in both T1- and T2-weighted images (WI) consistent with the normal appearance of hematopoietic bone marrow [4]. These areas rapidly become fatty bone marrow [3]. The ossification center at the head of the humerus is the first to appear approximately at 1–6 months of age, followed by the greater tuberosity ossification center and the lesser tuberosity ossification center at 9–12 and 12–16 months of age, respectively. The presence of an ossification center in the head of the humerus can be expected in up to 20% of full-term newborns. Eventually, all ossification centers within the humeral head fuse together at 3–5 years of age, creating a single epiphyseal ossification center [5]. After fusion, the osseous margins of the proximal humeral epiphysis may be irregular, with a fragmented appearance on coronal images and a posterior notch on axial images [1]. As growth continues, the surface of the structure becomes smoother, abutting the proximal humeral physis [1].

During the first 3 months of life, the proximal humeral physis is smooth and has a flat or slightly arched shape. After this period it becomes progressively angulated, with a tented contour that can be seen in the lateral aspect of the proximal humerus (Fig. 13.1). The physeal closure begins in its central portion at approximately 14 and 15 years of age, and ends with the fusion of its posterolateral aspect at approximately 16 and 17 years of age for boys and girls, respectively. Asymmetric widening of the physis and irregularity of the metaphyseal border suggest proximal humeral fracture or proximal humeral epiphysiolysis ("little league shoulder") [6].

13.2.1.2 Coracoid

The coracoid process usually has two ossification centers. These centers appear in the middle point in the first year, and at the base of the coracoid process at 10 years of age. A third ossification center located in the tip of the coracoid process is an uncommon anatomical variant that may mimic a fracture [2].

13.2.1.3 Acromion

At birth, the acromion is a cartilaginous replica of the ossified adult acromion. With growth, ossification occurs from the primary ossification center, located posteriorly, toward the anterolateral border of the bone, and multiple distal secondary ossification centers ossifying the most anterolateral segment of the cartilaginous acromion [6]. The age range for the appearance and fusion of these ossification centers is quite broad, with these processes expected to occur between 14–16 and 18–25 years of age, respectively. Failure of fusion of the distal acromial ossification centers may be mistaken for an avulsion fracture [6]. The failure of fusion between any of the different ossification centers of the acromion has been described as the cause of os acromiale [7]. The most common form of os acromiale consists of a large triangular meso-acromion that is separated from the rest of the acromion by an irregular cartilaginous layer with bone marrow edema visualized along the bone-to-bone interphase. Recently,

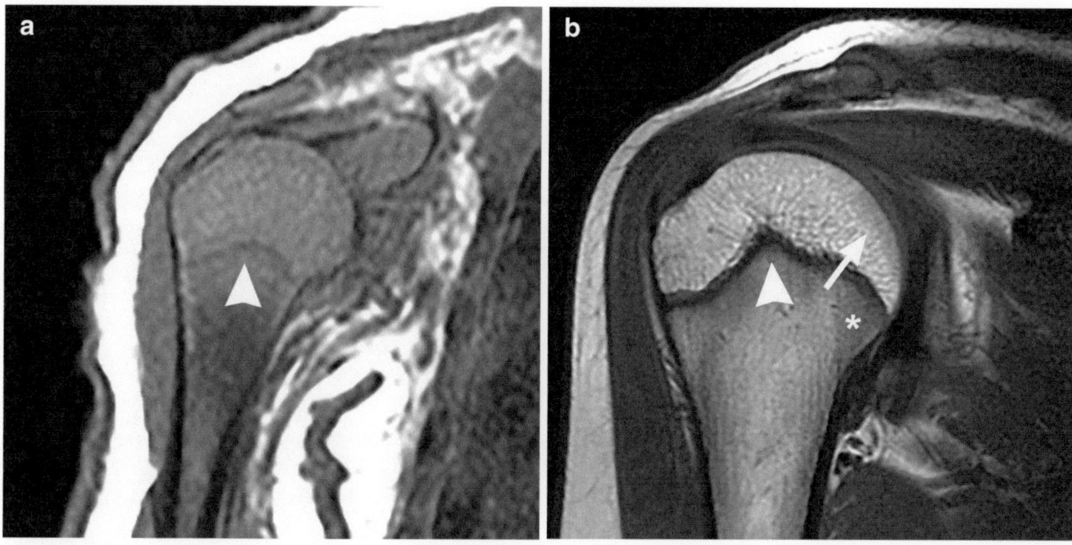

Fig. 13.1 Normal change in the angulation of the proximal humeral physis. (**a**) Coronal T1-WI in a newborn boy with a history of distal humeral fracture. The proximal humeral physis has a smooth and slightly arched shape (arrowhead), which is normal for this age group. No ossification center in the proximal humeral epiphysis is visualized. (**b**) Coronal T1-WI in a 12-year-old girl with a history of shoulder injury. The proximal humeral physis has a tented contour (arrowhead) with the most superior angle located in the midsection of the physis. Additionally, residual hematopoietic bone marrow is seen as a rim of low SI in the medial border of the epiphysis (arrow) and as low SI vertical stripes (asterisk) in the proximal humeral metaphysis

os acromiale has been described as a sequela of acromial apophysiolysis [8]. Os acromiale is usually asymptomatic, but may be related to impingement, instability, and pain that may require surgical treatment [6, 8].

13.2.1.4 Glenoid Fossa

At birth, the subchondral bone of the glenoid has a convex appearance on plain radiographs; nonetheless, MR images show that newborns have a cartilaginous glenoid fossa with a similar contour to the concave adult glenoid [1]. As growth occurs, the subchondral bone of the glenoid becomes flattened. At this stage, the osseous surface can have multiple undulations that may mimic osteochondral injuries [1, 6]. The concave osseous glenoid fossa develops in its superior third from the subcoracoid (or infracoracoid) ossification center, whereas the inferior two-thirds develop from multiple ossification centers around the glenoid rim that coalesce to form a horseshoe-like ossification center. The subcoracoid ossification center is the first to appear at approximately 8–10 years of age, fusing with the scapula at 14–17 years of age. A zone of cartilage located between the primary coracoid center and the primary scapular center acts as a bipolar physis with growth toward the body of the scapula (posterolateral) and the distal end of the coracoid (anteromedial). There is normally a tongue of ossification within the cartilage. In the absence of bone marrow edema, this normal ossification pattern should not be confused with a superior glenoid avulsion fracture [9] (Fig. 13.2). The multiple ossification centers located in the inferior two-thirds of the glenoid begin to form at 14–15 years of age and fuse by 17–18 years of age [9]. It is important not to mistake the inferior glenoid ossification centers with traumatic lesions [9]. Another common finding in the glenoid articular surface consists of a well-circumscribed small focus of T2 hyperintensity at its center called "bare spot of the glenoid" [9, 10]. This is most likely an acquired finding that may be related to shoulder instability and should not be interpreted as osteochondritis dissecans (ODC) or glenolabral articular cartilage disruption (GLAD) (Fig. 13.3) [9–11].

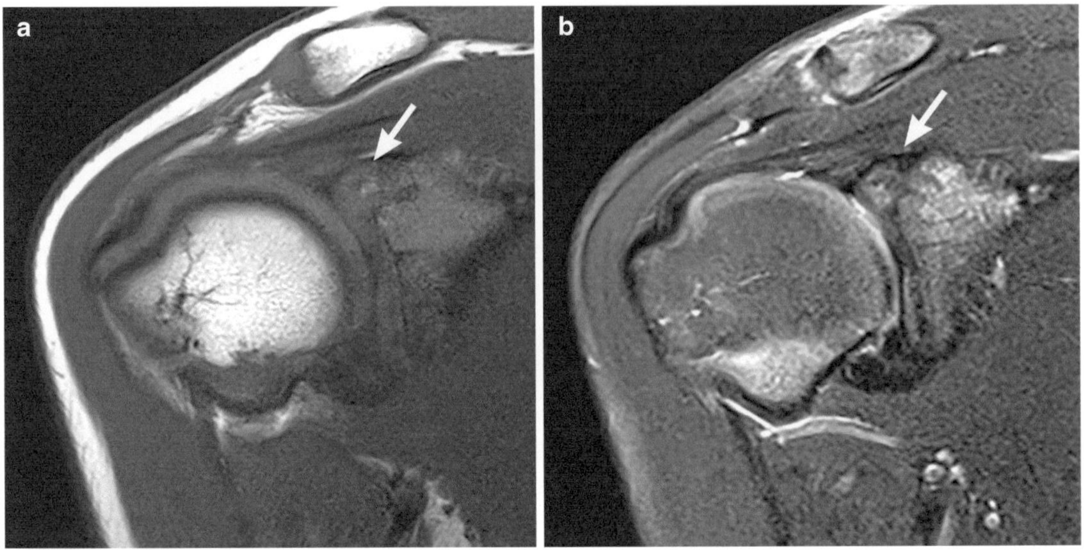

Fig. 13.2 Subcoracoid ossification center in a 10-year-old boy with a history of shoulder trauma. (**a**) Coronal T1-WI and (**b**) coronal T2-WI of the right shoulder showing a small tongue of ossification located in the anterior-superior aspect of the glenoid (arrows). In the absence of edema, this finding should not be confused with a superior glenoid avulsion fracture

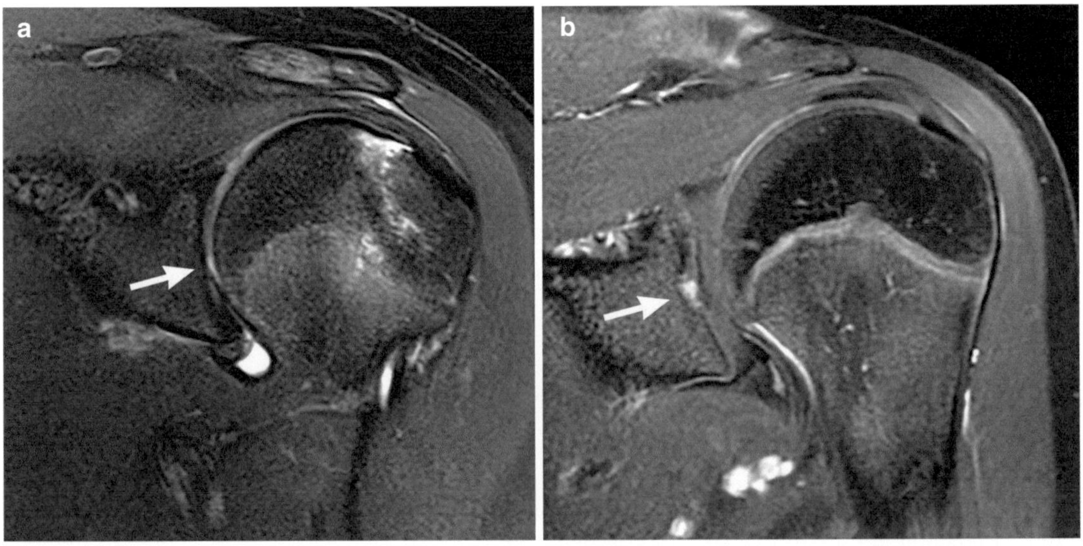

Fig. 13.3 Differences in the appearance of a bare spot of the glenoid (**a**) and an OCD of the glenoid (**b**). (**a**) Coronal T2-WI of the shoulder in a 13-year-old girl with a history of shoulder dislocation. A regular, well-defined, bare spot located in close proximity to the isocenter of the glenoid without adjacent bone marrow edema is seen (arrow). (**b**) Coronal gadolinium-enhanced fat-suppressed T1-WI of the shoulder in an 11-year-old girl during workout for a focal bony lesion previously seen on plain films. Intense enhancement of an irregular lesion located in the central sublabral region of the glenoid consistent with the appearance of an OCD of the glenoid is seen (arrow)

13.2.1.5 Vertebral Border and Inferior Angle of the Scapula

Two ossification centers are apparent in the vertebral border and the inferior angle of the scapula. Both appear at puberty and fuse with the scapula approximately at 22 years of age [2].

13.2.1.6 Bone Marrow Transformation

Transformation from hematopoietic bone marrow (red marrow) to fatty bone marrow (yellow marrow) occurs in a predictable and organized fashion [3]. At birth, the bone marrow throughout the body is hematopoietic and, accordingly, has a low SI on T1-WI and a high SI of fat-suppressed fluid-sensitive sequences. In the upper extremities, bone marrow transformation begins distally and continues proximally (from the fingers to the shoulder) [3]. In the humerus, marrow conversion occurs first in the epiphyses, followed by central diaphysis, and then continues proximally and distally until complete conversion of the metaphyseal marrow results (Fig. 13.4). Residual hematopoietic bone marrow can be found in the proximal humeral metaphysis as vertically oriented stripes with well-delimited margins, in the humeral head as a halo of low T1, high T2 SI in the medial border of the epiphysis, and in the distal clavicle and distal acromion until late adolescence and early adulthood [1, 6, 12] (Fig. 13.2).

13.2.1.7 Metaphyseal Stripes

The most inner layer of the periosteum called the cambium of the periosteum or metaphyseal stripe is a highly vascularized tissue that is responsible for the appositional growth of long bones. It is seen on MR imaging as a 1–2 mm symmetric rim of intermediate SI on T1-WI and high SI of fluid-sensitive sequences that surrounds the low-SI bone cortex and is in direct contact with the low-SI periosteum (Fig. 13.5). This layer is seen in the proximal humeral metaphysis, and less commonly in the distal clavicular metaphysis and acromion in patients aged 5 months to 14 years. After this age, it slowly disappears, being almost always imperceptible by the age of physeal closure [4, 6, 13]. This normal finding on MR

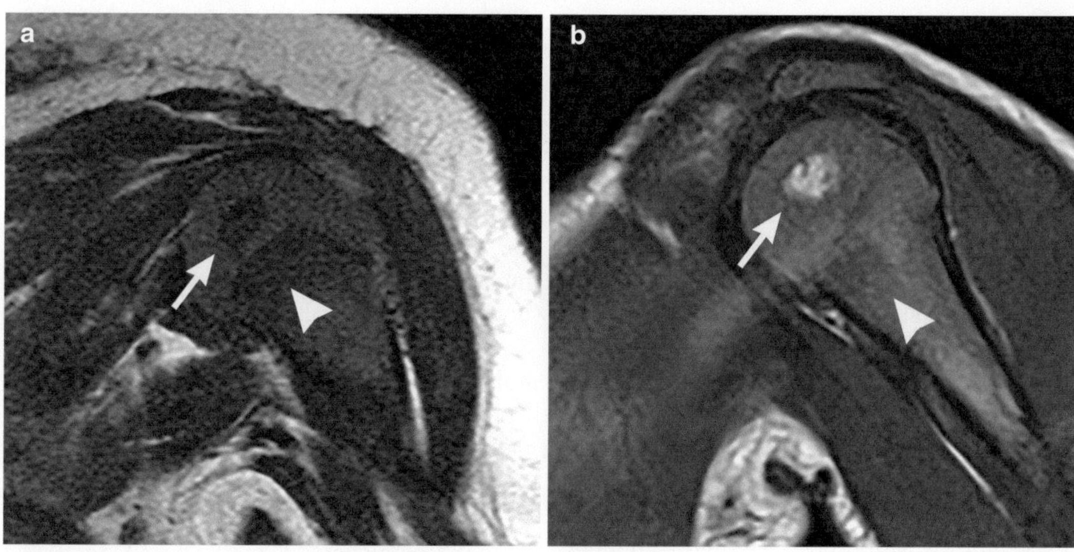

Fig. 13.4 Bone marrow transformation. Sagittal T1-WI of the shoulder in (**a**) a 4-month-old girl, and (**b**) a 15-month-old girl. (**a**) The humeral head ossification center (arrow) and the proximal humeral metaphysis (arrowhead) at 4 months of age have a low SI on T1-WI consistent with the normal appearance of hematopoietic bone marrow. (**b**) At 15 months of age the humeral head ossification center (arrow) and the humeral mid-diaphysis have high SI on T1-WI consistent with the normal appearance of fatty bone marrow. The proximal humeral metaphysis (arrowhead) still has SI characteristics of hematopoietic bone marrow. The imaging findings seen correspond to the predictable and organized transformation of bone marrow during the childhood

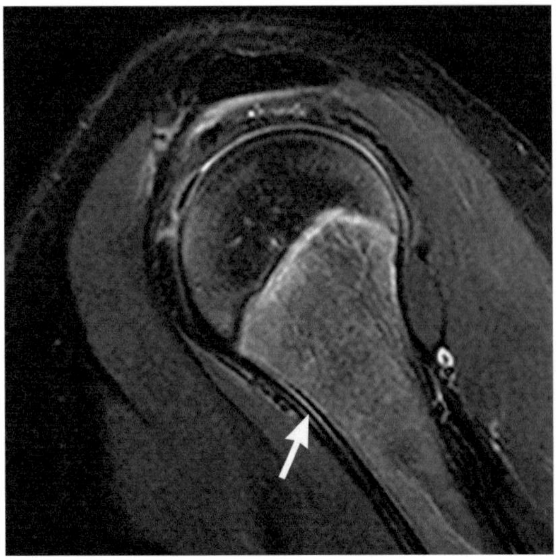

Fig. 13.5 Sagittal T2-WI of the right shoulder in a 10-year-old girl with concern for internal derangement following trauma. A high-SI line in between the low SI bone cortex and the low-SI periosteum consistent with a metaphyseal stripe (arrow) is visualized

imaging should not be confused with periosteal reaction seen in pathologic processes such as osteomyelitis, fracture, or tumors [4].

13.3 Diseases

13.3.1 Congenital Diseases

13.3.1.1 Brachial Plexus Palsy

Neonatal brachial plexus palsy results from the traction of the brachial plexus during birth, when the neonate shoulder becomes locked by the pubic symphysis of the mother and opposite traction is performed by the labor attendant [14, 15]. The prevalence of this complication has been reported as 1–3 cases per 1000 live births [15, 16]. Risk factors include shoulder dystocia, exceptionally large baby (>4.5 Kg), and forceps or vacuum extraction [15]. The most common pattern of injury, seen in 80% of the cases, involves injury of the vertebral roots at levels C5 and C6 [14]. These cases have a good prognosis with spontaneous recovery in approximately 90% of patients. When injury of the nerve roots C5, C6, and C7 occurs, the rate of spontaneous recovery is about 65%. Rarely, injury of the nerve roots C5, C6, C7, C8, and T1 occurs. With this pattern of injury spontaneous recovery occurs in approximately 50% of cases if the Horner triad is not seen, whereas it almost never occurs when the Horner triad is present [17, 18].

Although surgical exploration is recognized as the reference standard for determination of nerve injuries, studies have shown the feasibility of demonstrating intraductal nerve root injures with CT myelography [19] and, more recently, with high-resolution MR imaging, by obtaining heavily T2-WI using steady-state free precession sequences [14].

Up to one-third of affected children will have some residual dysfunction, most commonly weakness in the shoulder external rotators (teres minor and infraspinatus), shoulder abductors, and shoulder forward elevators. As a result, there is a contracture of the subscapularis and pectoralis major muscles, and capsuloligamentous contracture of the shoulder may lead to cartilaginous and bone deformities. The formation of a hypoplastic humeral head and posterior humeral head displacement ultimately leads to subluxation, dislocation, or a fixed articular deformity [20].

Plain radiographs are inadequate to evaluate the extent of bone deformity, as ossification of the humeral head is delayed until puberty [1]. In children younger than 1 year of age, ultrasonography has demonstrated to be a useful modality for the detection of posterior subluxation of the humeral head. A posterior approach, obtaining images in the axial plane from the posterior aspect of the shoulder to demonstrate the humeral head ossification centers and the posterior aspect of the scapula, results in more reproducible and interpretable images in comparison to images obtained in the axial plane from the lateral aspect of the shoulder. Additionally, the posterior approach is less affected by the ossification of the humeral head. With the posterior approach, shoulder posterior subluxation or dislocation is seen as a posteriorly located center of the humeral head ossification center in relation to the posterior scapular line, whereas in the normal shoulder the center of the humeral head

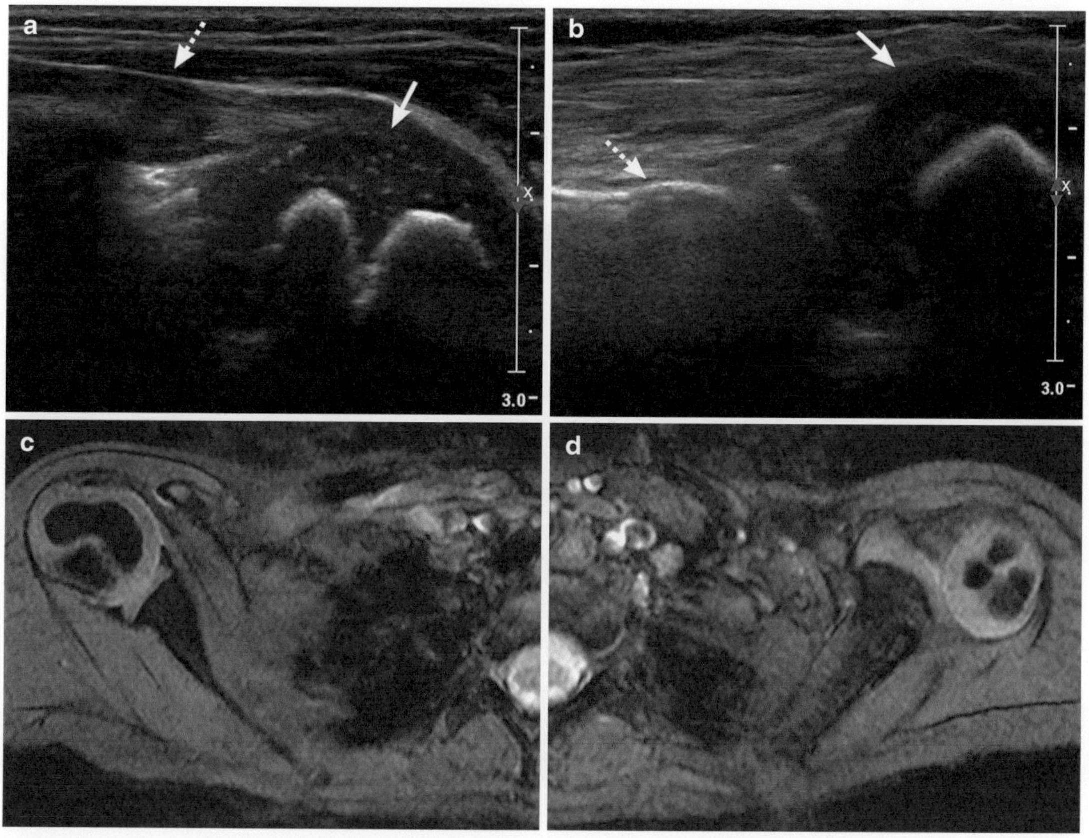

Fig. 13.6 Comparison of the right (**a** and **c**) and left (**b** and **d**) shoulders in a girl with brachial plexus palsy of the left shoulder. At 10 months of age US imaging of the right shoulder shows (**a**) the humeral head ossification center (arrow) in normal relation to the posterior scapular line (dashed arrow). (**b**) Note the posterior location of the humeral head ossification center (arrow) in relation to the posterior scapular line (dashed arrow) consistent with posterior subluxation of the left shoulder. At 2 years of age, GRE MR imaging shows a (**d**) dysplastic left humeral head with posterior sloping, posterior subluxation, and a poorly defined acetabular labrum in comparison to a (**c**) normal right humeral head and labrum

ossification is located anterior with respect to the same line [21] (Fig. 13.6).

In children from 1 to 5 years of age, MR imaging of the affected shoulder with comparative imaging of the contralateral shoulder is the best imaging approach. The protocol should include bilateral shoulder imaging using high-resolution, 3 mm thick, axial and oblique coronal GRE sequences to evaluate the glenoid version angle, the shape of the humeral head, the degree of glenoid hypoplasia, and the incongruity of the glenohumeral joint [22]. In children younger than 5 years, high SI on GRE imaging in the physis and the cartilaginous glenoid and low SI in the labrum are seen [1]. The glenoscapular angle, described as the angle obtained between a line located from the anterior and posterior margins of the cartilaginous glenoid fossa and a second line from the central point of the glenoid fossa to the medial tip of the scapula, can be measured to determine the degree of glenoid version [23]. Retroversion of the humeral head leads to thinning of the posterior aspect of the glenoid, and in more severe cases thinning of the superior aspect of the glenoid cartilage, posterior displacement of the posterior labrum and humeral head, and subsequent subluxation or dislocation. Muscle atrophy and intramuscular fatty replacement may be evident in the subscapularis muscle and to a lesser extent in the infraspinatus and supraspinatus muscles. Changes observed in the subscapularis muscle are of paramount importance as they have been related to a greater degree of glenoscapular deformity [23, 24].

In all patients with brachial plexus palsy, rehabilitation therapy should be the center of intervention with the aim of avoiding contracture formation, improving muscle strength, and preventing compensatory movement patterns [17]. In older children, surgery is restricted to capsular release, extra-articular tendon transfers and glenoid osteotomy to restore external rotation, or salvage procedures such as humeral external derotational osteotomy for the correction of advanced glenohumeral deformity [25].

13.3.2 Trauma and Sport-Related Injuries

Most pediatric osseous injuries occur at the chondro-osseous junctions of the physes and apophyses, especially during the growth spurt in adolescence, due to physeal thickening and abrupt increase in muscle strength. More than half of all high school students participate in competitive sports in the United States, and there has been a significant increase in the number and severity of shoulder injuries among this age group [26]. The risk of an acute shoulder injury while participating in sports is estimated to be 2 per 10,000 athlete exposures, being substantially higher in boys, during competition in comparison to practice, and in contact sports including football and wrestling [26]. Chronic sport-related shoulder injuries are more commonly seen in baseball and tennis [1]. In contrast to adults, in whom full-thickness rotator cuff tears, biceps pathology, and osteoarthritis account for most disease, in children and adolescents, labral disease involving primarily the anterior labrum and the superior labrum (superior labrum anterior posterior lesions (SLAP)) are responsible for about four of every five injuries seen by shoulder arthroscopy. In adolescents, partial supraspinatus tendon avulsions located in the insertional zone are more common than full-thickness supraspinatus tears located in the critical zone [27].

13.3.2.1 Fractures

The most common fracture of the shoulder involves the clavicle, usually in the midshaft, caused by direct trauma or fall with an extended upper extremity [25]. A thick periosteal layer acts as a barrier for the displacement of the fractured bone segments, especially in children younger than 10 years of age. Although most cases can be treated conservatively, there is increasing controversy in the indications for operative management [28]. Almost all cases of clavicular fractures can be evaluated using conventional radiographs and additional imaging is almost never required.

Less commonly, fractures of the proximal humerus and scapula can be observed. In children under 10 years of age, with extensive remodeling capabilities, nonoperative treatment is usually the recommended option. Beyond 13 years of age, remodeling capabilities are similar to the adult, and more aggressive surgical treatment is recommended. Patients between 10 and 13 years should be evaluated in a case-by-case basis. In neonates and infants, complete separation of the proximal humeral epiphysis following obstetric, accidental, or non-accidental trauma can be seen. Due to the absence of ossification centers in the proximal humeral epiphysis up to 6 months following birth, sonography of the shoulder is the best diagnostic modality. It can be performed on the patient bedside without the need of sedation, and images are usually superior to MR imaging (Fig. 13.7) [29].

Physeal fractures of the shoulder are uncommon, comprising about 3% of all physeal fractures. Due to the transformation of the proximal humeral physis from a flat structure in infants to a tented contour in adolescents, Salter-Harris Type I fractures are more common in younger children, whereas Salter-Harris Type II fractures occur more frequent in older children and adolescents. The prognosis of physeal fractures in this location is excellent and surgical treatment is almost never required [30].

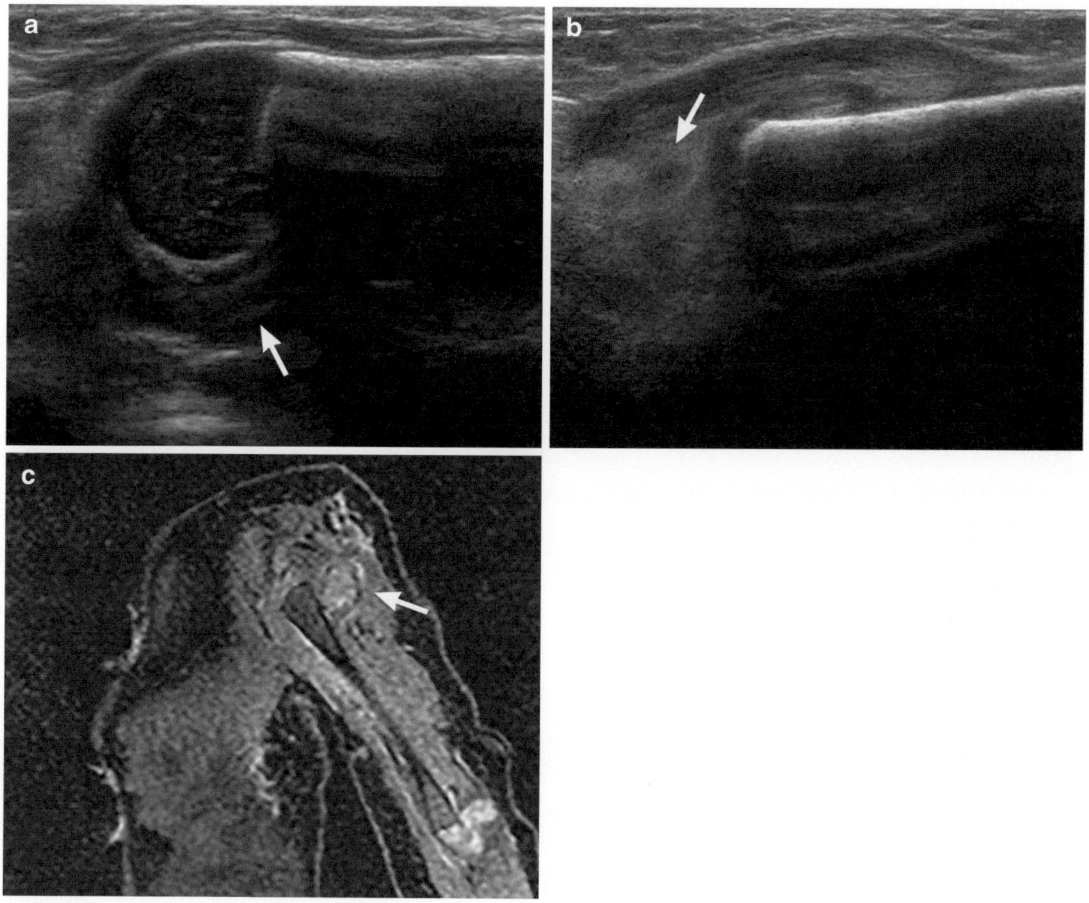

Fig. 13.7 Anterior US imaging of the (**a**) right and (**b**) left proximal humeri in a 3-day-old girl with a history of left-shoulder dislocation following shoulder dystocia. (**a**) The right proximal non-ossified humeral head (arrow) is well positioned following the contour of the ossified humeral diaphysis. (**b**) Absence of the left proximal humeral head (arrow) on top of a well-demarcated left humeral diaphysis. This finding is similar to a scoop of ice cream slipping off the top of a cone. (**c**) MR imaging of the same patient performed 1 day after the US images showing a posterolateral subluxation of the humeral head (arrow)

13.3.2.2 Dislocations

Children with anterior shoulder dislocation following low-energy trauma have a much lower incidence of proximal humeral fractures in comparison to adults, and thus do not require prereduction radiographs [31]. Postreduction radiographs are still recommended.

The pathophysiology and imaging findings of anterior dislocations of the shoulder are the same for older children than for adults and thus will not be discussed.

13.3.2.3 Little Leaguer's Shoulder

Repetitive microtrauma sustained by adolescent athletes involved in repetitive overhead throwing may result in disruption of endochondral ossification and an increase in the number of chondrocytes remaining in the metaphysis seen as physeal thickening and irregularity [32]. The clinical presentation is characterized by chronic pain in the lateral aspect of the shoulder and tenderness to palpation. Radiographs and MR imaging are characteristic for physeal widening and irregularity.

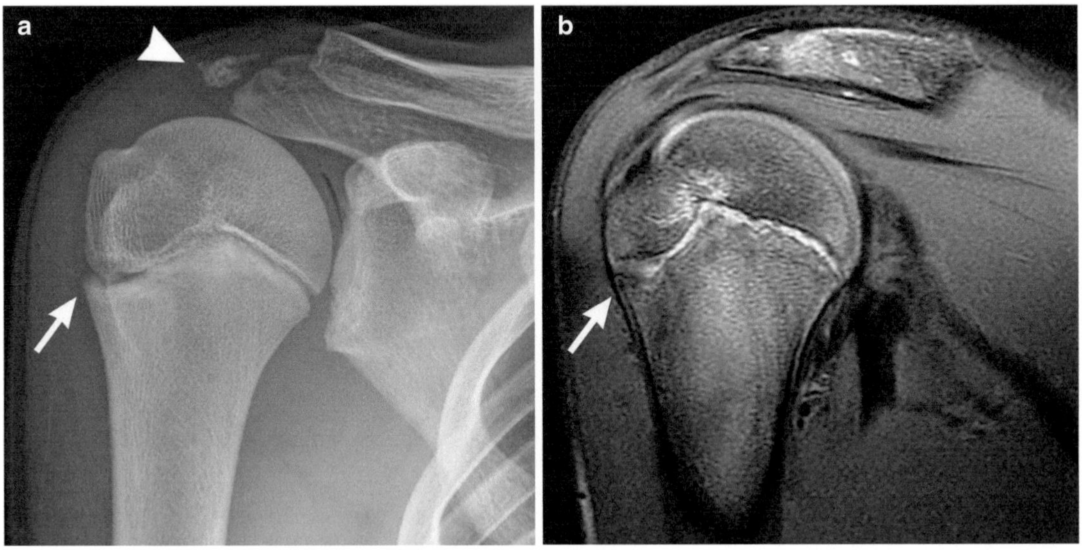

Fig. 13.8 (**a**) AP radiograph and (**b**) coronal PD image of the right shoulder in a 13-year-old boy who is a baseball pitcher. (**a**) Physeal widening and irregularity in the lateral proximal humeral physis are visualized (arrow). Note the well-corticated acromial ossification center (arrowhead), which should not be confused with an avulsion fracture. (**b**) On MR images, physeal widening and irregularity are also seen; additionally, bone marrow edema and effacement of the zone of provisional calcification are visualized (arrow). Findings are consistent with a little leaguer's shoulder

On MR imaging increased metaphyseal SI on water-sensitive sequences and effacement of the zone of provisional calcification in all sequences is also visualized (Fig. 13.8). The treatment of this disease consists of cessation of sport activities to avoid the formation of bony bridges [33].

13.3.2.4 Acromial Apophysiolysis

Acromial apophysiolysis is a disease that can occasionally be seen on baseball or softball pitchers in their late adolescence, especially males who have a pitch count higher than 100 pitches per week. On MR images, it is characterized by incomplete fusion and bone marrow edema on the meta-acromial and meso-acromial ossification centers (Fig. 13.9). It presents clinically as pain and tenderness to palpation at the superior shoulder. Patients who present at some point of their lives with acromial apophysiolysis are at increased risk of having full-thickness rotator cuff tears and meta-acromion-meso-acromion-type os acromiale. The association between this type of stress injury and the presence of os acromiale suggest that the latter may not be an anatomical variant, but a sequela of repetitive apophyseal injury [8].

13.3.3 Infectious Diseases

13.3.3.1 Acute Osteomyelitis

The humerus is the site of involvement in 13% of pediatric hematogenous osteomyelitis cases. It may be seen rarely (<1% of total cases), in the clavicle or the scapula [34]. The metaphyses of long bones are more vascularized in the pediatric population in comparison to adults, making them more susceptible to infection by hematogenous spreading, usually following subclinical bacteremia. Microtrauma or emboli may occlude these slow-flowing vessels creating a nidus for infection.

Just like in other bones of the growing skeleton, infections are more commonly due to *Staphylococcus aureus*, *Streptococcus pyogenes*, and *Streptococcus pneumoniae*. Due to the improvement in culture techniques, *Kingella kingae,* a gram-negative organism, is now recognized as a significant causative agent of osteomyelitis in children younger than 4 years of age. Although less commonly, fungi and parasites can also be the causative organisms for osteomyelitis in children [35].

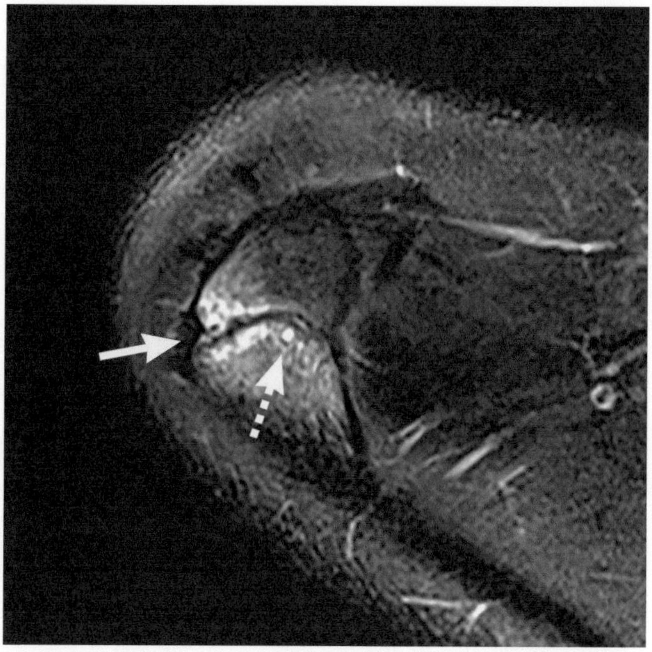

Fig. 13.9 Acromial apophysiolysis. Axial PD MR image of the right shoulder in a 15-year-old girl who is a softball pitcher. Incomplete fusion of the meso-acromion and meta-acromion, bone marrow edema (arrow), and cystic changes (dashed arrow) are visualized

The clinical presentation consists of fever, pseudoparalysis of the arm, and pain with passive motion. Imaging should focus on detecting the presence of infection, excluding additional foci of osteomyelitis, and detecting drainable collections. Radiographs should be the first step in the workout for osteomyelitis. Nevertheless, findings suggestive of osseous infection will be seen in less than 20% of patients; thus, its use must be focused on excluding differential diagnoses such as trauma or tumors [34]. MR imaging is the best modality to depict acute osteomyelitis. The protocol should include T1-weighted sequences, fat-suppressed water-sensitive sequences, and gadolinium-enhanced sequences. The infected area appears as having a low SI on T1-WI, a high SI on water-sensitive sequences, and an increased heterogeneous bone marrow enhancement on postcontrast imaging. Postcontrast imaging is of special value in the evaluation of suspected osteomyelitis in the non-ossified epiphyseal cartilage (Fig. 13.10). It is important to differentiate the normal appearance of hematopoietic bone marrow in the growing skeleton from the findings seen on osteomyelitis. The SI of normal hematopoietic marrow on T1-WI is never lower than the SI of the adjacent musculature [3]. In children, it is common to see subperiosteal collections elevating the periosteum and stopping at the perichondrial junction (Fig. 13.11). MR imaging is also valuable to detect complications of osteomyelitis such as chronic osteomyelitis and bony bridging across the physis [1].

13.3.3.2 Septic Arthritis

The shoulder accounts for 5% of all septic arthritis in children [36]. Most cases occur in boys under the age of 2 years, particularly in neonates in the intensive care unit [37]. Similarly to osteomyelitis, most cases in the pediatric population are caused by hematogenous spreading or by direct extension into the joint space from infections located in the soft tissues or adjacent metaphyses. The latter is a specific phenomenon seen more commonly in children under the age of 18 months [38].

The most common causative organisms of septic arthritis are the same as for osteomyelitis. *Neisseria gonorrhoeae* can be found in neonates and sexually active adolescents, and *type B Haemophilus influenzae* may be occasionally cultivated in unvaccinated children.

In 85% of cases, the symptoms are monoarticular and the presence of multiple joint involvement

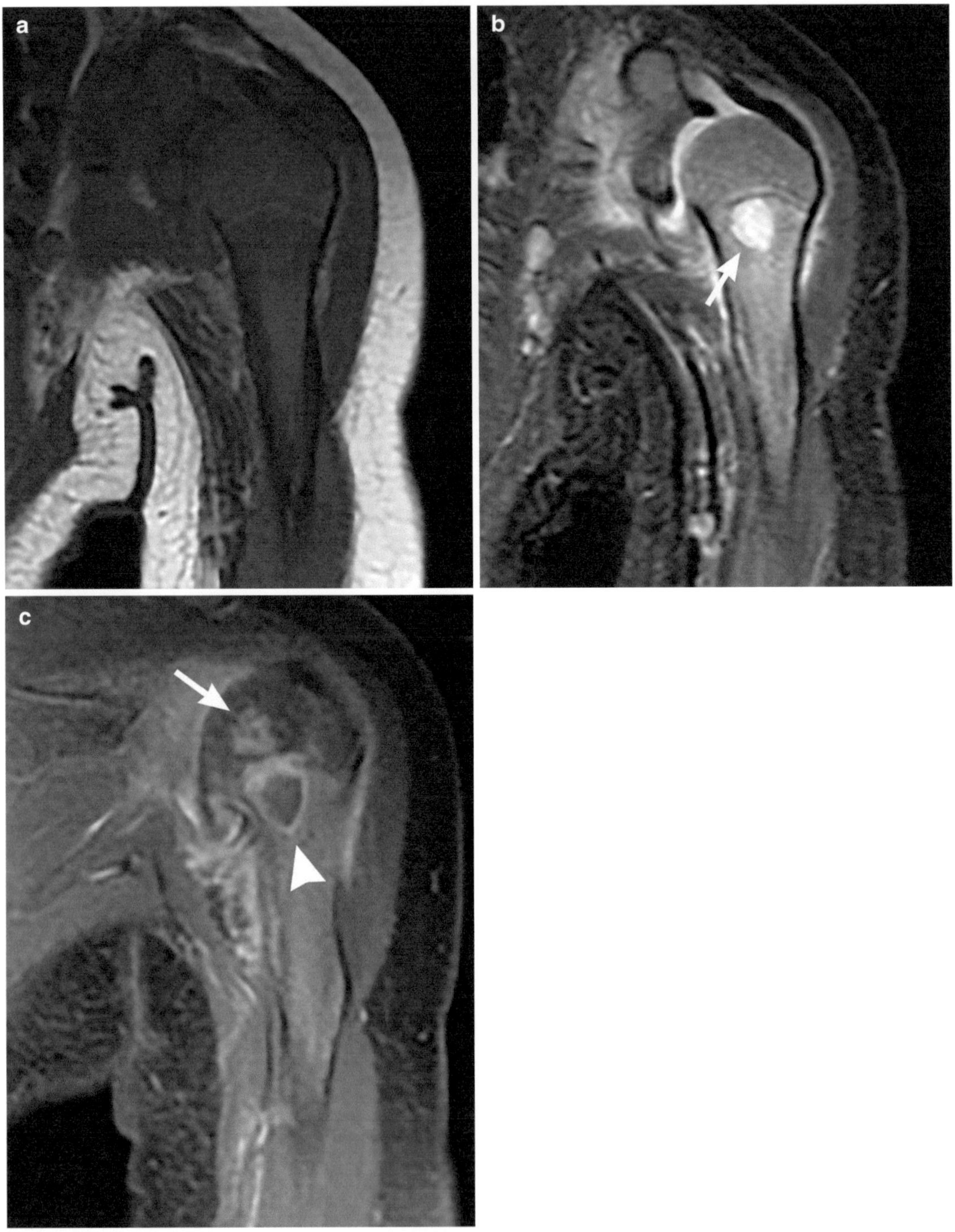

Fig. 13.10 Coronal MR imaging of the left shoulder in a 2-month-old boy with osteomyelitis. (**a**) T1-WI shows homogeneous low SI in the proximal humeral epiphysis and metaphysis. The high content of hematopoietic bone marrow in young infants makes the diagnosis of osteomyelitis especially difficult. (**b**) T2-WI showing a fluid collection in the proximal metaphysis (arrow). No apparent extension into the epiphysis is visualized. (**c**) Gadolinium-enhanced fat-suppressed T1-WI showing rim enhancement of the fluid collection located in the proximal metaphysis (arrowhead) and a focus of enhancement in the non-ossified proximal humeral epiphysis (arrow). These findings are consistent with osteomyelitis extension from the metaphysis into the proximal epiphysis thru the nutrient metaphyseal capillaries

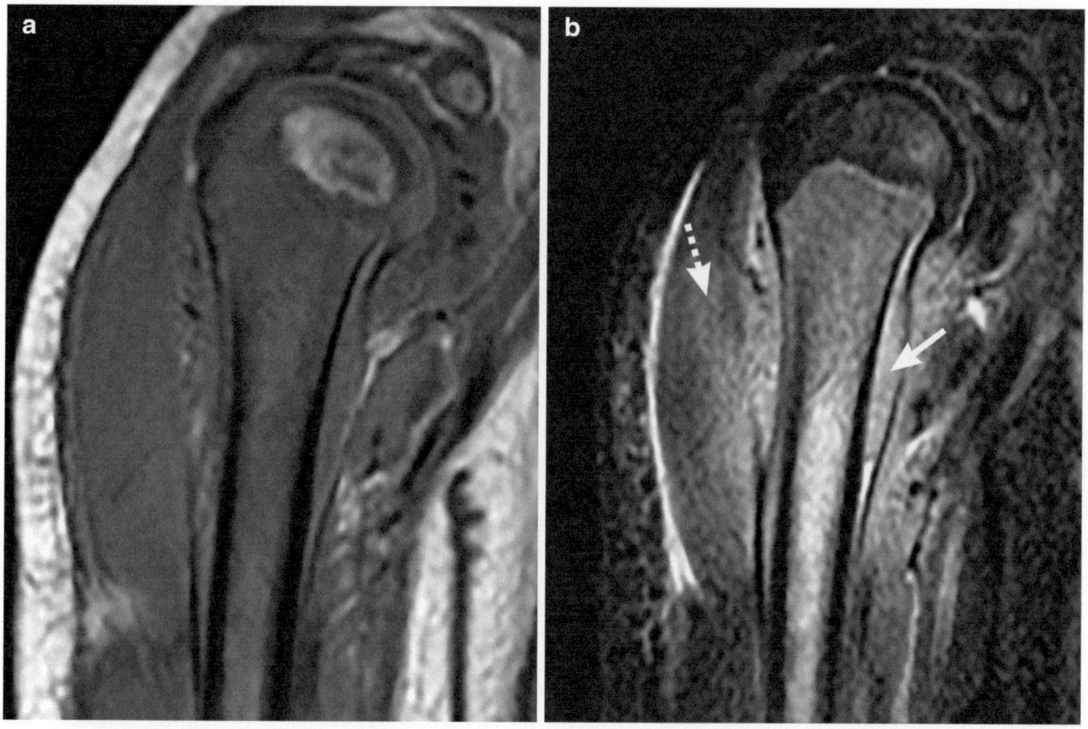

Fig. 13.11 Coronal MR imaging of the right humerus in a 3-year-old boy with a history of 8 days of fever and 1 day of pain and pseudoparalysis of the right arm. (**a**) T1-WI shows decreased bone marrow SI which corresponds to the area of bone marrow edema seen on the (**b**) T2-WI; additionally, a large subperiosteal collection (arrow) and extensive myositis (dashed arrow) involving the deltoid muscle are visualized

must raise doubts on the infectious etiology of the case [39]. Radiographs add little to the diagnosis but should be ordered to exclude trauma as the cause for the patient's symptoms. US is useful to detect joint fluid and to guide joint aspiration, but does not help to differentiate infected from noninfected fluid [40]. MRI is the imaging method of choice for this disease. Findings include effusion, reactive edema within the adjacent bone, and synovial enhancement of gadolinium-enhanced images. The use of postcontrast subtraction imaging may be of great use to depict subtle changes in the blood flow of the epiphyses and synovium [1]. In any case of suspected septic arthritis, joint aspiration with cytology and microbiology is the cornerstone of diagnosis [40].

The sequelae depend on the age of presentation, virulence of the infecting pathogen, and appropriate treatment onset. In children under 12 months of age, in whom secondary ossification centers of the proximal humeral epiphysis have not developed, septic arthritis results in a delayed appearance of small and irregular secondary ossification centers with final deformity of the humeral head. In cases in which delayed or inappropriate treatment is performed, proximal humeral physis involvement may occur. As 80% of the humeral length depends on the proximal physis, this may cause significant shortening of the extremity [41].

13.3.4 Inflammatory Diseases

13.3.4.1 Juvenile Idiopathic Arthritis

The shoulder is affected late in the course of the disease, and involvement occurs more often in subjects with polyarticular disease or enthesitis-related arthritis (positive HLA-B27) [42, 43]. At the onset, about 5% of patients present with shoulder involvement, whereas after 5 years of having JIA approximately 21% of subjects will have shoulder involvement [42].

US and MRI are superior to clinical examination in the detection of joint inflammation and should be considered in the diagnosis and follow-up of JIA. Both techniques are also superior to radiographs for the evaluation of structural abnormalities such as erosions, joint-space narrowing, and deformity [44]. US is also helpful to detect enthesitis-related arthritis, especially at the insertions of the quadriceps, the common extensor, and the Achilles tendon [45]. MRI is the best imaging modality to evaluate JIA. It detects disease extent and progression and evaluates response to treatment. Fat-suppressed PD and gradient-echo sequences can best evaluate glenohumeral cartilage abnormalities. Hypertrophic synovium may appear as a thickened and irregular structure with low SI on T1-WI and high SI on fat-suppressed T2-WI. Other important imaging findings include erosions and deep cartilage loss extending into the subchondral bone that may cause internal joint derangement and rice bodies which are small aggregates of mononuclear cells and fibrin seen in the synovial fluid or bursae suggestive of severe synovial inflammation (Fig. 13.12) [46]. In some cases it is impossible to differentiate a fibrotic synovium from a highly vascularized inflammatory hypertrophic synovium, or from a joint effusion, and thus contrast-enhanced imaging is recommended. Postcontrast imaging should be performed within 5 min after the administration of gadolinium to avoid the diffusion of contrast media from the synovium into the joint space, creating the illusion of a thickened synovium and gradual enhancement of the joint fluid [1, 43, 47].

13.3.4.2 Chronic Recurrent Multifocal Osteomyelitis

Chronic recurrent multifocal osteomyelitis (CRMO) is an idiopathic inflammatory noninfectious disease affecting multiple bones of the skeleton, showing acute, subacute, and chronic patterns of inflammation in the affected areas. It occurs mostly in the late childhood and early adolescence with an incidence peak between 7 and 12 years of age. Girls are affected twice more often than boys [48, 49]. For staging, whole-body MR imaging is replacing scintigraphy as the method of choice to depict clinically occult sites of disease. Whole-body MR imaging is done by using STIR sequences that may show evidence of

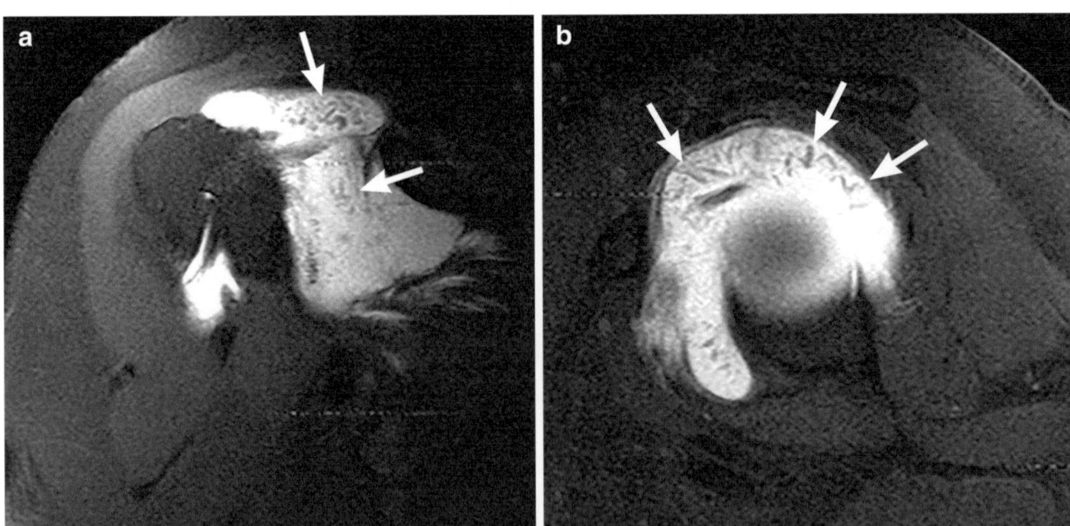

Fig. 13.12 MR arthrogram of the right shoulder in a 17-year-old girl with a history of persistent shoulder pain. (**a**, **b**) A significant number or low-T1-SI bodies within the distended articular space following intra-articular injection of gadolinium are seen (arrows). These bodies are aggregates of mononuclear cells and fibrin secondary to severe synovial inflammation usually seen in JIA

foci of high SI, which must be confirmed by seeing low SI in these same areas on T1-WI. Although most of the literature describes lesions seen in CRMO as symmetric, there is usually lack of temporal symmetry, making lesions to appear at different stages and being even inexistent on imaging. During the active phase diffuse inflammation, small joint effusions, and periosteal inflammation may be seen; nevertheless, the presence of large fluid collections, sequestrum, or a sinus tract makes the diagnosis of CRMO less likely, favoring a bacterial etiology [1]. Later in the course of the disease, radiographs may reveal osteolytic lesions with a sclerotic border [50]. Usually the metaphyses and metaphyseal equivalents are the most common locations, but involvement of the clavicle is fairly common accounting for up to 30% of CRMO lesions (Fig. 13.13) [51]. Lesions in the clavicle usually manifest with local pain and swelling located in the medial third of the bone. Additionally, lytic lesions and onionskin-like periosteal reaction, which can be better evaluated on CT imaging, are apparent. The cycle of healing-relapse leads to progressive hyperostosis and sclerosis of the medial aspect of the clavicle without involvement of the sternoclavicular joint. Rarely the scapula may be affected [52]. In the humerus, patients are at greatest risk for the formation of bony-bridging leading to growth disturbance [53].

13.3.5 Benign Tumors

13.3.5.1 Simple Bone Cysts

Simple bone cysts, also known as unicameral bone cysts or solitary bone cysts, are uncommon lesions that represent 3% of all primary bone tumors. The peak of incidence occurs between 9 and 15 years of age [54]. About 50% of these lesions occur in the proximal humeral metaphysis. On radiographs, these tumors are characterized as cystic lesions in the central area of the metaphysis without periosteal reaction [55]. A fallen fragment may be seen following pathologic fractures [56]. These tumors are usually described as being painless; however, they are commonly associated with pathologic fractures. On MR imaging its SI is described as intermediate on T1-WI and high on T2-WI. Noncomplicated fluid-filled cysts are often visualized; however, following pathologic fractures, fluid-fluid levels may appear. On gadolinium-enhanced imaging, nodular and thick perilesional enhancement is usually visualized.

13.3.5.2 Chondroblastoma

Chondroblastomas are uncommon cartilaginous benign tumors that account for about 2% of all primary bone tumors, but about 20% of them occur in the proximal humerus [57]. They present twice more commonly in boys compared to girls

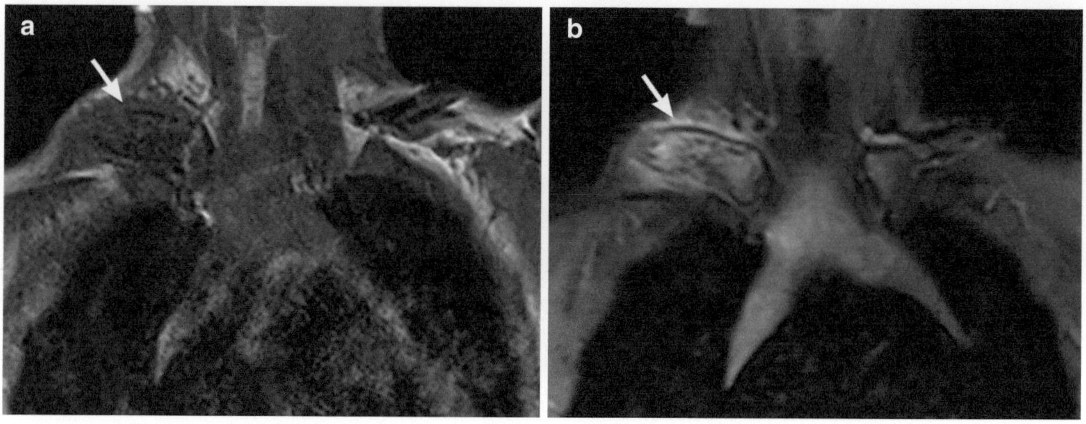

Fig. 13.13 Clavicular CRMO in a 9-year-old female. Coronal T1-WI (**a**) of the chest showing low-SI bone marrow in the right clavicle (arrow) which corresponds to an area of high SI within the bone marrow on T2-WI (**b**) (arrow). There is adjacent soft-tissue edema, but large fluid collections, sequestrum, and sinus tracts are absent

with a peak incidence in the adolescence and early adulthood [32, 58]. Chondroblastomas originate from the secondary ossification centers of the epiphyses and apophyses, with the most common affected bones being the proximal tibial epiphysis and the proximal humeral epiphysis. The clinical presentation includes severe pain, limitation in the range of motion of the adjacent joint, local tenderness, and swelling. On plain radiographs, these lesions have a lytic appearance with well-defined sclerotic margins. Calcification may be seen in up to 60% of cases [55]. On MR imaging these tumors are seen as an intraosseous lobulated mass with low-to-intermediate SI on T1-WI and intermediate-to-high SI on water-sensitive sequences surrounded by a halo of bone marrow edema. A thin low T1, low T2 SI rim that corresponds to the sclerotic border, is seen in almost all lesions. Fluid-fluid levels may be seen in 20–30% of patients [32] (Fig. 13.14).

13.3.6 Malignant Tumors

Osteosarcoma and Ewing sarcoma are the most common bone malignancies in the childhood, accounting for 6% of all malignancies in this age group [56]. The proximal humeral metaphysis is the third most common location for osteosarcoma, which occurs twice more commonly in boys compared to girls. Ewing sarcoma usually occurs in the pelvis followed by the metaphyses of the femur, tibia, and humerus in respective order, and boys are equally affected as girls [56, 59]. Children with either tumor can have deep

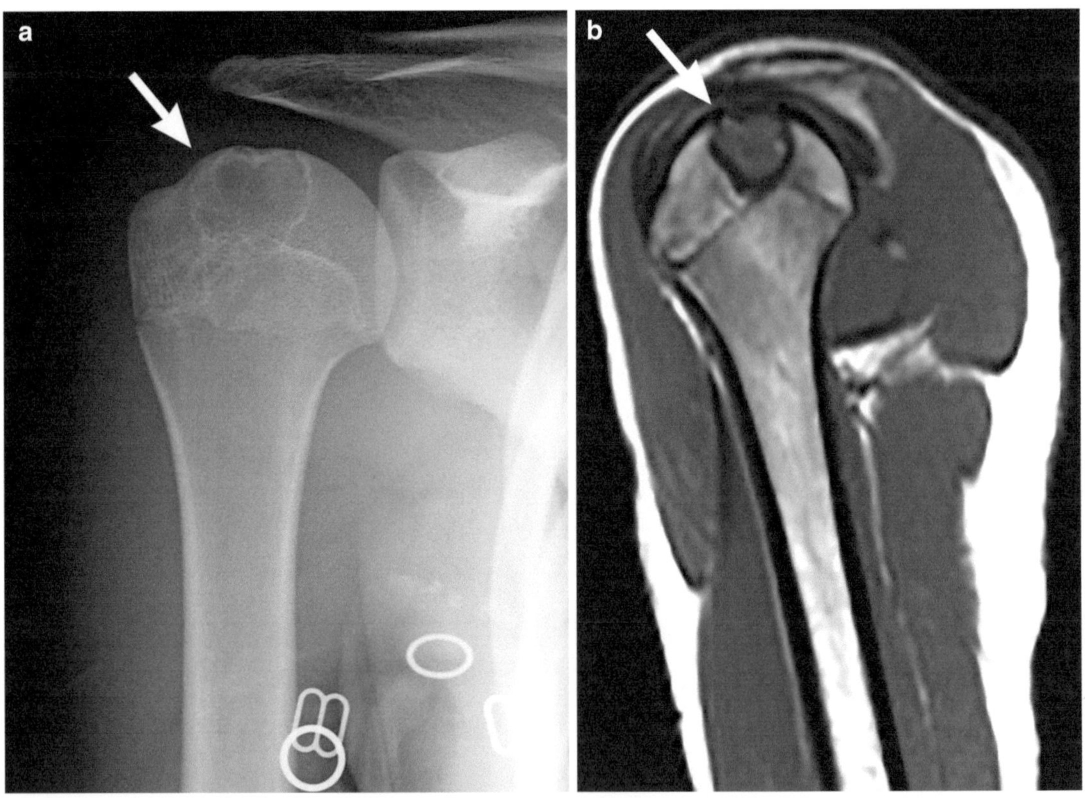

Fig. 13.14 Chondroblastoma in a 15-year-old girl with a history of crepitus and pain in the right shoulder. (**a**) AP radiographs show a well-demarcated lytic lesion with sclerotic borders in the proximal humeral metaphysis (arrow). No periosteal reaction is seen. (**b**) Sagittal T1-WI shows low-to-intermediate-SI mass surrounded by a low-SI rim of sclerosis (arrow). (**c**) Coronal STIR image shows a high-SI lesion surrounded by a low-SI rim and diffuse bone marrow edema (arrow)

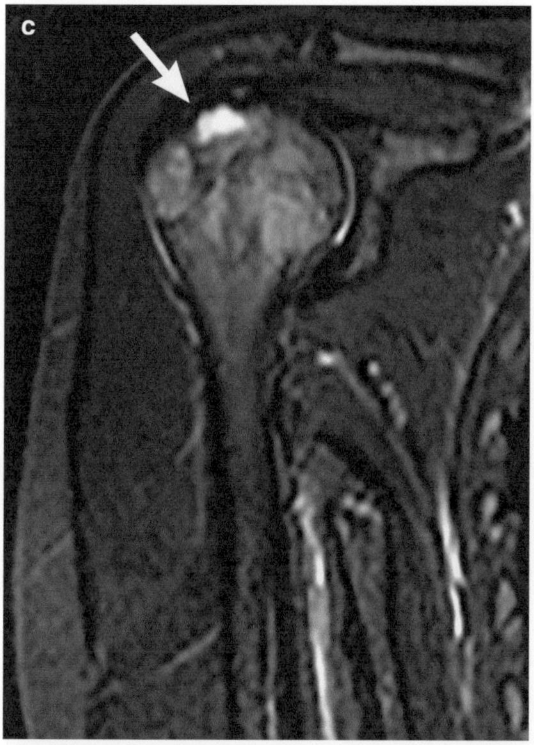

Fig. 13.14 (continued)

pain lasting for several months, which is increased with activity or motion of the adjacent joint [59]. Additionally, for Ewing sarcoma systemic symptoms can include fever, anemia, leukocytosis, and elevated erythrocyte sedimentation rate. The goal of imaging is to define the extent of the primary lesion in relation to adjacent joints, bones, blood vessels, and nerves, and the presence of metastases. Initial imaging usually consists of conventional radiographs, which are used to determine the aggressiveness of the tumor and suggest malignancy. It is useful to perform longitudinal imaging primarily on the sagittal plane in order to avoid phase-encoding artifacts from the thoracic structures. On MR imaging, osteosarcomas and Ewing sarcoma are seen as having low SI on T1-WI and high SI on water-sensitive sequences. The infiltrated bone has low SI in all sequences and in T1-WI the SI is lower than the one of the surrounding muscles (Fig. 13.15). In both tumors, extensive bone marrow edema and soft-tissue edema are seen [56]. Following gadolinium injection, avid heterogeneous enhancement is present for both tumors [56].

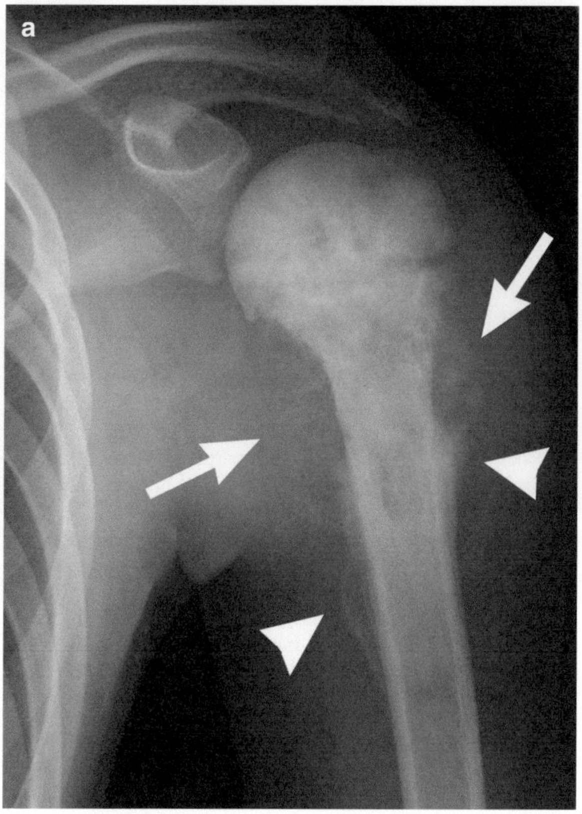

Fig. 13.15 Osteosarcoma in a 13-year-old boy. (**a**) AP radiographs of the left shoulder show poor defined borders of the lesion and aggressive speculated periosteal reaction (arrows) with the presence of Codman triangles (arrowheads). (**b**) Sagittal T1-WI shows infiltrated, low-SI bone marrow in the proximal humeral metaphysis (asterisk). Note that the SI of the bone marrow is lower than the one seen on the adjacent muscles; additionally, a significant soft-tissue component with disruption of the normal anatomy and diffuse disruption of the bone cortex is visualized (arrow). (**c**) Sagittal gadolinium-enhanced fat-suppressed T1-WI shows intense heterogeneous enhancement of the soft-tissue component (arrow)

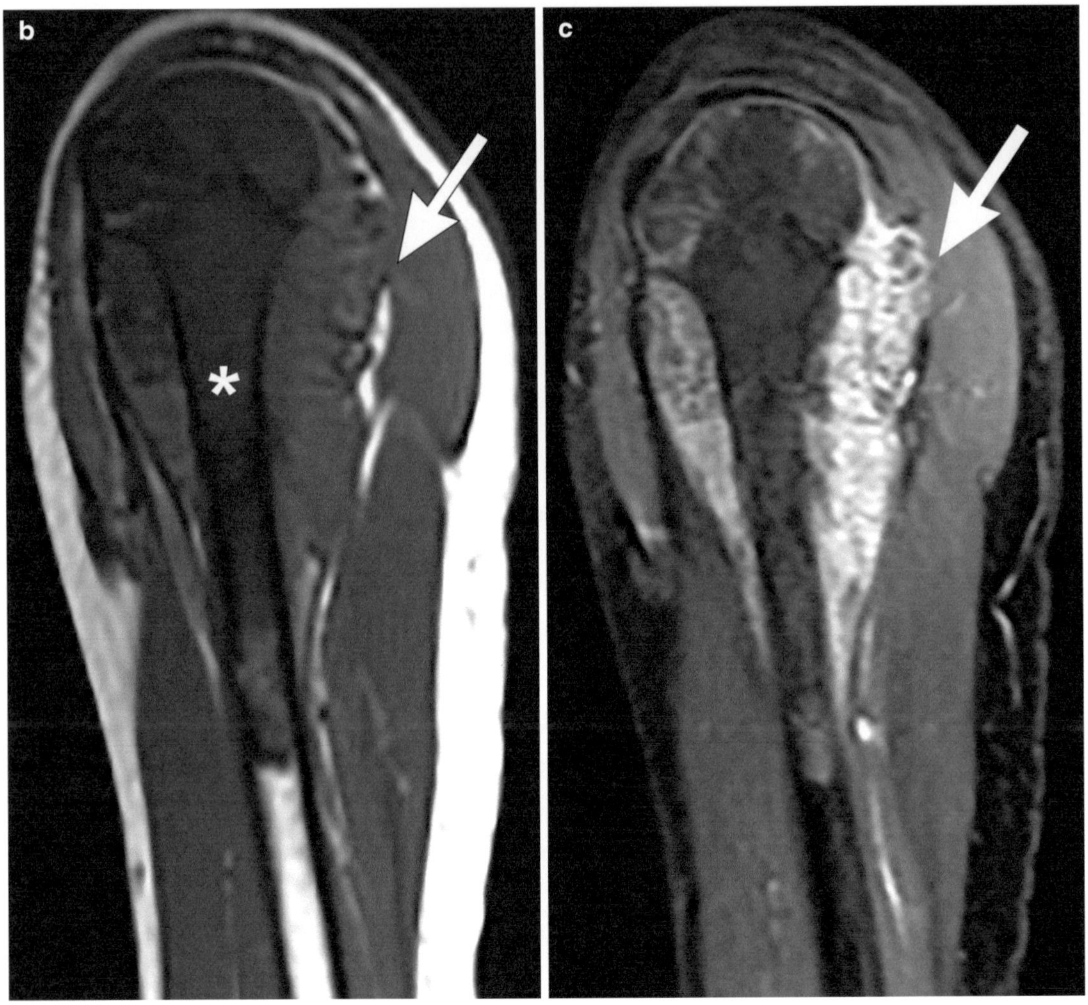

Fig. 13.15 (continued)

References

1. Chauvin NA, Jaimes C, Laor T, Jaramillo D. Magnetic resonance imaging of the pediatric shoulder. Magn Reson Imaging Clin N Am. 2012;20(2):327–47.. xi
2. Rockwood CA. The shoulder. Philadelphia, PA: Saunders/Elsevier; 2009.. http://hdl.library.upenn.edu/1017.12/1337257 Connect to full text
3. Laor T, Jaramillo D. MR imaging insights into skeletal maturation: what is normal? Radiology. 2009;250(1):28–38.
4. Kwong S, Kothary S, Poncinelli LL. Skeletal development of the proximal humerus in the pediatric population: MRI features. AJR Am J Roentgenol. 2014;202(2):418–25.
5. Clarke SE, Chafetz RS, Kozin SH. Ossification of the proximal humerus in children with residual brachial plexus birth palsy: a magnetic resonance imaging study. J Pediatr Orthop. 2010;30(1):60–6.
6. Zember JS, Rosenberg ZS, Kwong S, Kothary SP, Bedoya MA. Normal skeletal maturation and imaging pitfalls in the pediatric shoulder. Radiographics. 2015;35(4):1108–22.
7. Johnston PS, Paxton ES, Gordon V, Kraeutler MJ, Abboud JA, Williams GR. Os acromiale: a review and an introduction of a new surgical technique for management. Orthop Clin North Am. 2013;44(4):635–44.
8. Roedl JB, Morrison WB, Ciccotti MG, Zoga AC. Acromial apophysiolysis: superior shoulder pain and acromial nonfusion in the young throwing athlete. Radiology. 2015;274(1):201–9.
9. Kothary S, Rosenberg ZS, Poncinelli LL, Kwong S. Skeletal development of the glenoid and glenoid-coracoid interface in the pediatric population: MRI features. Skelet Radiol. 2014;43(9):1281–8.

10. Kim HK, Emery KH, Salisbury SR. Bare spot of the glenoid fossa in children: incidence and MRI features. Pediatr Radiol. 2010;40(7):1190–6.
11. Ly JQ, Bui-Mansfield LT, Kline MJ, DeBerardino TM, Taylor DC. Bare area of the glenoid: magnetic resonance appearance with arthroscopic correlation. J Comput Assist Tomogr. 2004;28(2):229–32.
12. Zawin JK, Jaramillo D. Conversion of bone marrow in the humerus, sternum, and clavicle: changes with age on MR images. Radiology. 1993;188(1):159–64.
13. Bedoya MA, Jaimes C, Khrichenko D, Delgado J, Dardzinski BJ, Jaramillo D. Dynamic gadolinium-enhanced MRI of the proximal femur: preliminary experience in healthy children. AJR Am J Roentgenol. 2014;203(4):W440–6.
14. Somashekar D, Yang LJ, Ibrahim M, Parmar HA. High-resolution MRI evaluation of neonatal brachial plexus palsy: a promising alternative to traditional CT myelography. AJNR Am J Neuroradiol. 2014;35(6):1209–13.
15. Foad SL, Mehlman CT, Ying J. The epidemiology of neonatal brachial plexus palsy in the United States. J Bone Joint Surg Am. 2008;90(6):1258–64.
16. Pondaag W, Malessy MJ, van Dijk JG, Thomeer RT. Natural history of obstetric brachial plexus palsy: a systematic review. Dev Med Child Neurol. 2004;46(2):138–44.
17. Yang LJ. Neonatal brachial plexus palsy--management and prognostic factors. Semin Perinatol. 2014;38(4):222–34.
18. Narakas AO. Injures to the brachial plexus. In: Bora FWJ, editor. The pediatric upper extremity. Philadelphia: W.B. Saunders Co; 1986. p. 247–58.
19. Steens SC, Pondaag W, Malessy MJ, Verbist BM. Obstetric brachial plexus lesions: CT myelography. Radiology. 2011;259(2):508–15.
20. Hogendoorn S, van Overvest KL, Watt I, Duijsens AH, Nelissen RG. Structural changes in muscle and glenohumeral joint deformity in neonatal brachial plexus palsy. J Bone Joint Surg Am. 2010;92(4):935–42.
21. Moukoko D, Ezaki M, Wilkes D, Carter P. Posterior shoulder dislocation in infants with neonatal brachial plexus palsy. J Bone Joint Surg Am. 2004;86-A(4):787–93.
22. Waters PM, Smith GR, Jaramillo D. Glenohumeral deformity secondary to brachial plexus birth palsy. J Bone Joint Surg Am. 1998;80(5):668–77.
23. Poyhia TH, Nietosvaara YA, Remes VM, Kirjavainen MO, Peltonen JI, Lamminen AE. MRI of rotator cuff muscle atrophy in relation to glenohumeral joint incongruence in brachial plexus birth injury. Pediatr Radiol. 2005;35(4):402–9.
24. Kozin SH. Correlation between external rotation of the glenohumeral joint and deformity after brachial plexus birth palsy. J Pediatr Orthop. 2004;24(2):189–93.
25. Emery KH. MR imaging in congenital and acquired disorders of the pediatric upper extremity. Magn Reson Imaging Clin N Am. 2009;17(3):549–70.. vii
26. Robinson TW, Corlette J, Collins CL, Comstock RD. Shoulder injuries among US high school athletes, 2005/2006-2011/2012. Pediatrics. 2014;133(2):272–9.
27. Zbojniewicz AM, Maeder ME, Emery KH, Salisbury SR. Rotator cuff tears in children and adolescents: experience at a large pediatric hospital. Pediatr Radiol. 2014;44(6):729–37.
28. Caird MS. Clavicle shaft fractures: are children little adults? J Pediatr Orthop. 2012;32(Suppl 1): S1–4.
29. Goldfisher R, Amodio J. Separation of the proximal humeral epiphysis in the newborn: rapid diagnosis with ultrasonography. Case Rep Pediatr. 2015;2015:825413.
30. Pahlavan S, Baldwin KD, Pandya NK, Namdari S, Hosalkar H. Proximal humerus fractures in the pediatric population: a systematic review. J Child Orthop. 2011;5(3):187–94.
31. Reid S, Liu M, Ortega H. Anterior shoulder dislocations in pediatric patients: are routine prereduction radiographs necessary? Pediatr Emerg Care. 2013;29(1):39–42.
32. Jaimes C, Chauvin NA, Delgado J, Jaramillo D. MR imaging of normal epiphyseal development and common epiphyseal disorders. Radiographics. 2014;34(2):449–71.
33. Obembe OO, Gaskin CM, Taffoni MJ, Anderson MW. Little Leaguer's shoulder (proximal humeral epiphysiolysis): MRI findings in four boys. Pediatr Radiol. 2007;37(9):885–9.
34. Krogstad P. Osteomyelitis. In: Feigin RD, Cherry JD, Demmler-Harrison GJ, Kaplan SL, editors. Textbook of pediatric infectious diseases. 7th ed. Philadelphia: Saunders; 2014. p. 711–27.
35. Peltola H, Paakkonen M. Acute osteomyelitis in children. N Engl J Med. 2014;370(4):352–60.
36. Krogstad P. Septic arthritis. In: Feigin RD, Cherry JD, Demmler-Harrison GJ, Kaplan SL, editors. Textbook of pediatric infectious diseases. 7th ed. Philadelphia: Saunders; 2014. p. 711–27.
37. Blickman JG, van Die CE, de Rooy JW. Current imaging concepts in pediatric osteomyelitis. Eur Radiol. 2004;14(Suppl 4):L55–64.
38. Ogden JA. Pediatric osteomyelitis and septic arthritis: the pathology of neonatal disease. Yale J Biol Med. 1979;52(5):423–48.
39. Caksen H, Ozturk MK, Uzum K, Yuksel S, Ustunbas HB, Per H. Septic arthritis in childhood. Pediatr Int. 2000;42(5):534–40.
40. Devauchelle-Pensec V, Thepaut M, Pecquery R, Houx L. Managing monoarthritis in children. Joint Bone Spine. 2015;83:25.
41. Lejman T, Strong M, Michno P, Hayman M. Septic arthritis of the shoulder during the first 18 months of life. J Pediatr Orthop. 1995;15(2):172–5.
42. Hemke R, Nusman CM, van der Heijde DM, Doria AS, Kuijpers TW, Maas M, et al. Frequency of joint involvement in juvenile idiopathic arthritis during a 5-year follow-up of newly diagnosed patients: implications for MR imaging as outcome measure. Rheumatol Int. 2015;35(2):351–7.

43. Johnson K, Gardner-Medwin J. Childhood arthritis: classification and radiology. Clin Radiol. 2002;57(1):47–58.
44. Colebatch-Bourn AN, Edwards CJ, Collado P, D'Agostino MA, Hemke R, Jousse-Joulin S, et al. EULAR-PReS points to consider for the use of imaging in the diagnosis and management of juvenile idiopathic arthritis in clinical practice. Ann Rheum Dis. 2015;74(11):1946–57.
45. Weiss PF, Chauvin NA, Klink AJ, Localio R, Feudtner C, Jaramillo D, et al. Detection of enthesitis in children with enthesitis-related arthritis: dolorimetry compared to ultrasonography. Arthritis Rheumatol. 2014;66(1):218–27.
46. Martini G, Tregnaghi A, Bordin T, Visentin MT, Zulian F. Rice bodies imaging in juvenile idiopathic arthritis. J Rheumatol. 2003;30(12):2720–1.
47. Harty MP, Mahboubi S, Meyer JS, Hubbard AM. MRI of the pediatric shoulder: nontraumatic lesions. Eur Radiol. 1997;7(3):352–60.
48. Ferguson P, Laxer RM. Autoinflammatory bone disorders. In: Cassidy and Petty's textbook of pediatric rheumatology [Internet]. 7th ed. Philadelphia: Elsevier; 2015. p. 627–41.
49. Walsh P, Manners PJ, Vercoe J, Burgner D, Murray KJ. Chronic recurrent multifocal osteomyelitis in children: nine years' experience at a statewide tertiary paediatric rheumatology referral centre. Rheumatology (Oxford). 2015;54(9):1688–91.
50. Ferguson PJ, Sandu M. Current understanding of the pathogenesis and management of chronic recurrent multifocal osteomyelitis. Curr Rheumatol Rep. 2012;14(2):130–41.
51. Beretta-Piccoli BC, Sauvain MJ, Gal I, Schibler A, Saurenmann T, Kressebuch H, et al. Synovitis, acne, pustulosis, hyperostosis, osteitis (SAPHO) syndrome in childhood: a report of ten cases and review of the literature. Eur J Pediatr. 2000;159(8):594–601.
52. Khanna G, Sato TS, Ferguson P. Imaging of chronic recurrent multifocal osteomyelitis. Radiographics. 2009;29(4):1159–77.
53. Manson D, Wilmot DM, King S, Laxer RM. Physeal involvement in chronic recurrent multifocal osteomyelitis. Pediatr Radiol. 1989;20(1–2):76–9.
54. O'Brien SJ, Neves MC, Arnoczky SP, Rozbruck SR, Dicarlo EF, Warren RF, et al. The anatomy and histology of the inferior glenohumeral ligament complex of the shoulder. Am J Sports Med. 1990;18(5):449–56.
55. Helms CA. Benign lytic lesions. In: Fundamentals of skeletal radiology [Internet]. 4th ed. Philadelphia: Saunders; 2014. p. 7–31.
56. Wootton-Gorges SL. MR imaging of primary bone tumors and tumor-like conditions in children. Magn Reson Imaging Clin N Am. 2009;17(3):469–87, vi
57. Schuppers HA, van der Eijken JW. Chondroblastoma during the growing age. J Pediatr Orthop B. 1998;7(4):293–7.
58. Jee WH, Park YK, McCauley TR, Choi KH, Ryu KN, Suh JS, et al. Chondroblastoma: MR characteristics with pathologic correlation. J Comput Assist Tomogr. 1999;23(5):721–6.
59. Yaw KM. Pediatric bone tumors. Semin Surg Oncol. 1999;16(2):173–83.

Imaging Diagnosis of Nerve Entrapments in the Shoulder

14

Alireza Eajazi, Miriam A. Bredella, and Martin Torriani

14.1 Introduction

Nerve injuries are an unusual source of shoulder pain. They can result from several causes including trauma, neoplasia, infection, neuropathy, autoimmune disease, and iatrogenic conditions [1]. Neuropathies of the shoulder are frequently considered entrapment syndromes and account for about 2% of cases of shoulder pain [2]. However, this frequency is likely to be underestimated because these conditions have been overlooked in the past [3]. As a result of increased familiarity regarding these conditions, they are diagnosed with growing frequency in patients with symptoms suggestive of nerve pathology.

The most commonly affected nerves in the shoulder region are the suprascapular nerve, axillary nerve, long thoracic nerve, cervical accessory nerve, and dorsal scapular nerve. These nerves may be involved in patients engaging in vigorous overhead activity, with massive rotator cuff tears, tears accompanied by fatty infiltration and/or atrophy of muscle, labral tear and paralabral cyst formation, and space-occupying lesions [3]. Muscle weakness with or without associated sensory deficit, sharp burning pain, and paresthesias over a localized skin area are a few signs and symptoms of entrapment neuropathies. Most of these cases are related to physical circumstances leading to a nerve being stretched or compressed into a fibrous or osteofibrous space. Particularly in neuropathy of the suprascapular nerve, the clinical diagnosis is often delayed because of nonspecific symptoms [4–6].

In this chapter, we review anatomic structures and landmarks of the most important nerves around the shoulder. We also discuss the pathologic conditions causing entrapment neuropathies such as compression, stretching, or iatrogenic lesions and outline different diagnostic imaging modalities. Finally, we review specific shoulder neuropathies and explain their MRI characteristics.

14.2 Pertinent Anatomy

14.2.1 Suprascapular Nerve

The suprascapular nerve originates from the upper trunk of the brachial plexus, with contributions from C5, C6, and sporadically C4 nerve root (Fig. 14.1). It is responsible for motor innervation of two rotator cuff muscles: the supraspinatus and infraspinatus. The nerve travels posterior to the clavicle and obliquely traverses towards the superior border of the scapula

A. Eajazi · M. A. Bredella · M. Torriani (✉)
Division of Musculoskeletal Imaging and Intervention, Department of Radiology, Massachusetts General Hospital and Harvard Medical School, Boston, MA, USA
e-mail: mbredella@mgh.harvard.edu; mtorriani@mgh.harvard.edu

J. T. Bencardino (ed.), *The Shoulder*, https://doi.org/10.1007/978-3-030-06240-8_14

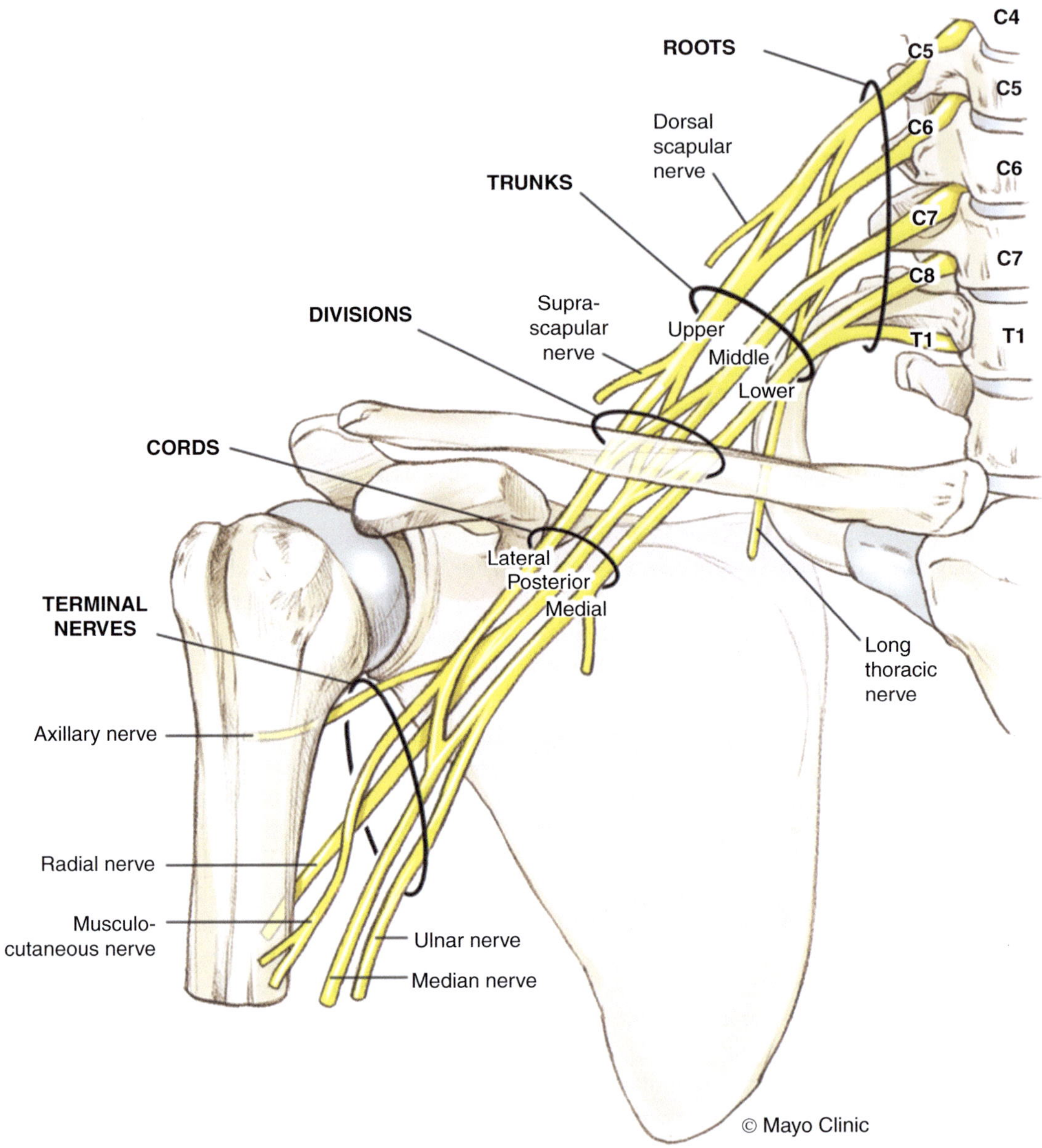

Fig. 14.1 Schematic representation of the anatomy of brachial plexus and its branches. Used with permission of Mayo Foundation for Medical Education and Research. All rights reserved

(Fig. 14.2). The nerve then passes through the suprascapular notch in an anterior-to-posterior direction. Generally, the nerve travels beneath the transverse scapular ligament in the suprascapular notch, while its associated artery passes over the ligament. Branches to the supraspinatus muscle emanate posterior to the suprascapular notch. The nerve continues towards the spinoglenoid notch of the scapula, where it travels beneath the spinoglenoid ligament (inferior transverse ligament) to provide branches to the infraspinatus muscle.

The presence of these two anatomical notches and the awareness of local muscle innervation patterns can assist the physician in diagnosing specific conditions. The role of these notches in entrapment neuropathies was first suggested by Aiello et al. [7] who discriminated between

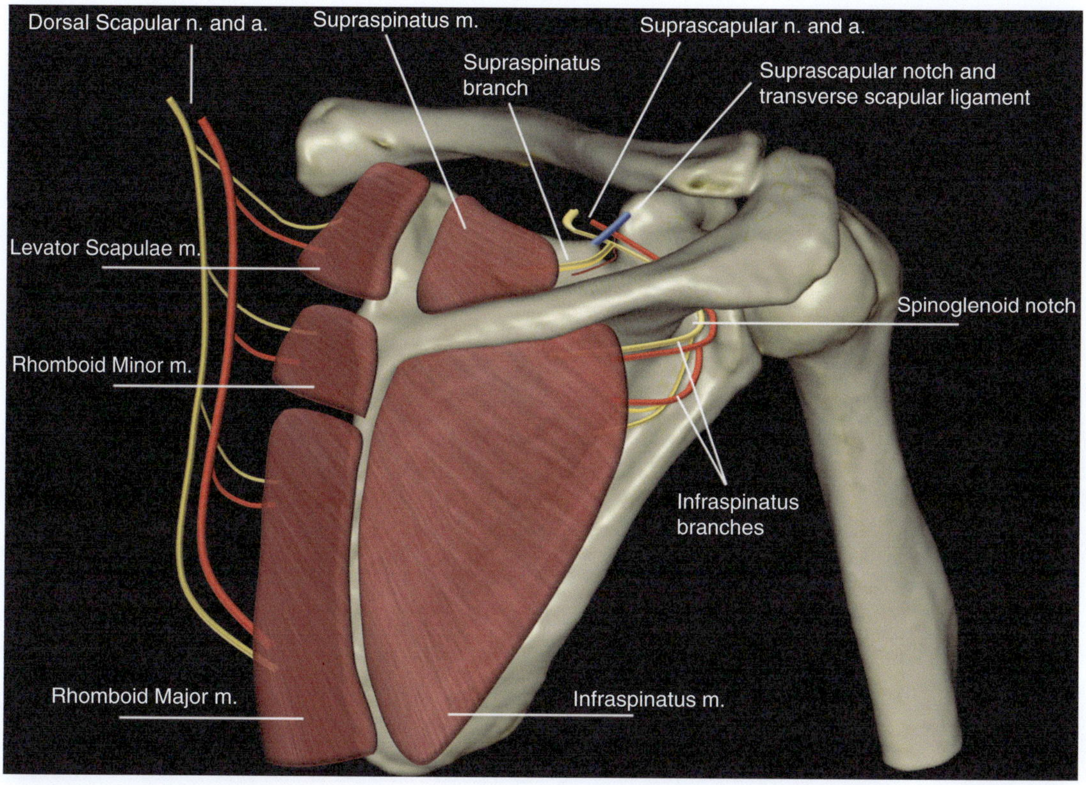

Fig. 14.2 Schematic representation of shoulder nerves and branches. Note the relationship between the suprascapular nerve with the suprascapular and spinoglenoid notches

entrapment of the nerve at the suprascapular notch and entrapment at the spinoglenoid notch. Although the suprascapular nerve has been considered a pure motor nerve, cadaveric studies have indicated sensory branches to the glenohumeral joint, acromioclavicular joint, coracoacromial ligament, and skin [8, 9]. Improved anatomic recognition of the sensory contributions of the suprascapular nerve helped to clarify the associated pain resulting from injury or traction of this nerve. Up to 70% of the sensation of the shoulder may be provided by the suprascapular nerve [10], and studies have shown improved postoperative pain after suprascapular nerve block in patients who had shoulder surgery [11, 12].

The suprascapular nerve and its concomitant vessels, well delineated by fat, are originally best identified on oblique coronal T1-weighted MRI showing the suprascapular notch, at the junction of the glenoid with the scapular neck, just medial to the superior glenoid rim. As the suprascapular neurovascular bundle arrives in the spinoglenoid notch, it can be seen on axial MRI images. A noticeable suprascapular vein, which occasionally is responsible for compressive neuropathy, is in some instances noted in the proximity of the nerve.

14.2.2 Axillary Nerve

The axillary nerve is a final branch of the posterior cord of the brachial plexus and originates from the ventral rami of C5 and C6 (Fig. 14.1). The first portion of the axillary nerve is located lateral to the radial nerve, posterior to the axillary artery, and anterior to the subscapularis muscle. It continues in an oblique direction across the inferolateral border of the subscapularis. It then travels through the quadrilateral space associated with the posterior humeral circumflex artery (Fig. 14.3). The quadri-

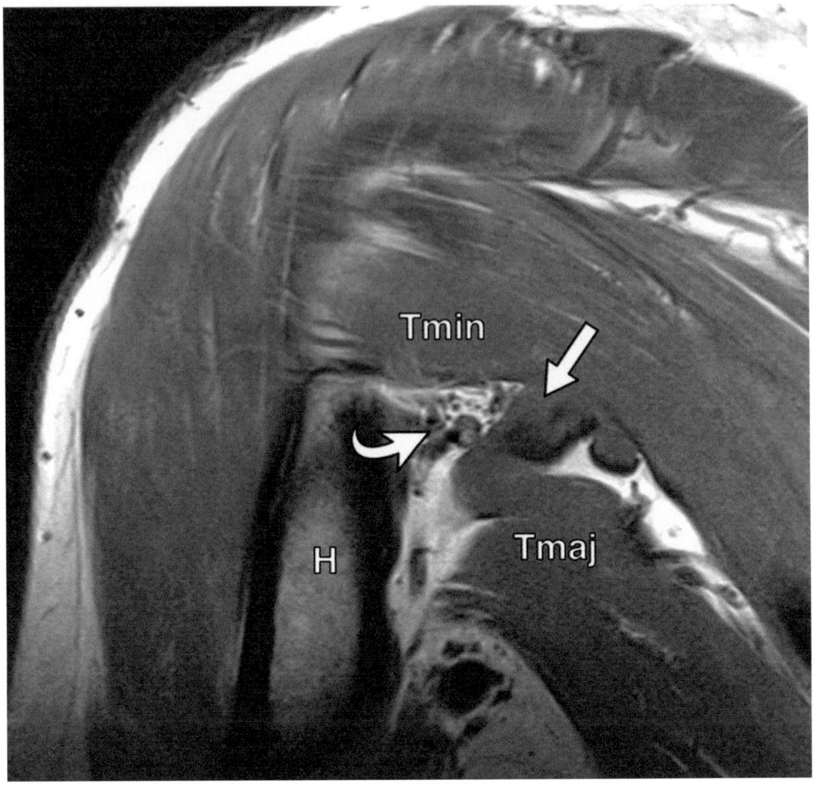

Fig. 14.3 Coronal oblique T1-weighted image of the right shoulder showing the teres major (Tmaj), teres minor (Tmin), triceps (arrow), and humerus (H) delimiting the quadrilateral space (curved arrow), where the posterior circumflex vessels and axillary nerve are identified

lateral space is a rectangular cuboid, located inferoposterior to the glenohumeral joint, with mean dimensions of about 2.5 × 1.5 cm [13, 14]. It is bordered superiorly by the teres minor muscle, inferiorly by the teres major muscle, medially by the long head of the triceps, and laterally by the surgical neck of the humerus [15]. The axillary nerve is the most superior structure in this space [13], where the nerve divides into its anterior (superior) and posterior (inferior) branches [14]. The anterior branch takes a circuitous route around the surgical neck of the humerus and provides branches for the anterior and middle parts of the deltoid muscle. The posterior branch supplies the subscapular muscle, the teres minor muscle, and often the posterior portion of the deltoid, as well as sensory innervation of the posterolateral shoulder.

The axillary neurovascular bundle is best identified on oblique sagittal T1-weighted MRI of the shoulder. It is well highlighted by surrounding fat and is seen below the inferior glenoid rim passing through the space between the teres minor and the teres major muscles. The quadrilateral space is best depicted next to the medial humeral cortex and lateral to the long head of the triceps muscle on oblique coronal images oriented along the humeral shaft.

14.2.3 Long Thoracic Nerve

The long thoracic nerve is a pure motor nerve particularly responsible for innervation of the serratus anterior muscle. Anatomically, it originates from C5 to C7 and occasionally C8 (8%) (Fig. 14.1) [16]. After advancing anteriorly to the posterior scalene muscle, it travels distally and laterally to pass below the clavicle and under the first and the second ribs. Distally, the nerve descends along the chest wall in the midaxillary line to the outer border of the serratus anterior, sending branches to each of the digitations of this muscle (Fig. 14.4) [16]. The serratus anterior muscle originates from the costomedial border of the scapula and inserts on the first through ninth ribs, forming the medial wall of the axilla and functioning as a scapular protractor.

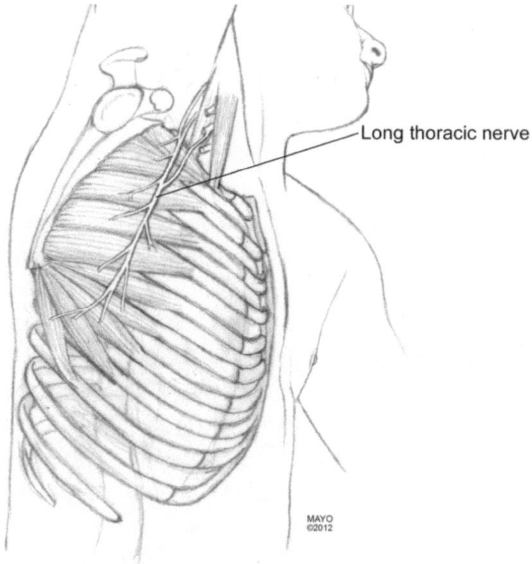

Fig. 14.4 Topographical anatomy of the long thoracic nerve, overlying the serratus anterior muscle. Used with permission of Mayo Foundation for Medical Education and Research. All rights reserved

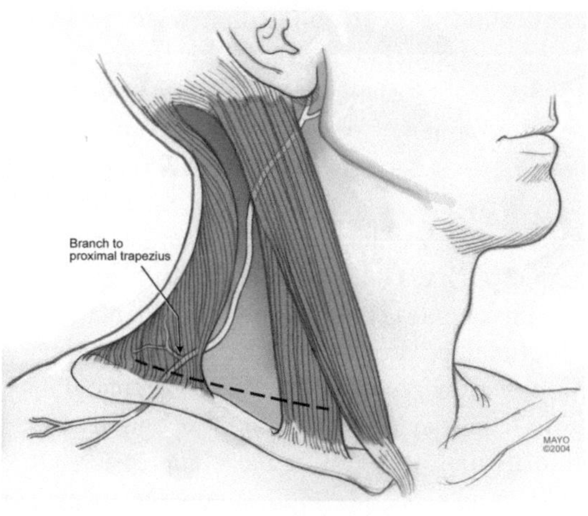

Fig. 14.5 Topographical anatomy of the accessory nerve as it travels along the posterolateral neck. Used with permission of Mayo Foundation for Medical Education and Research. All rights reserved

14.2.4 Spinal Accessory Nerve

The spinal accessory nerve is a cranial nerve (CN XI) originating from the upper segments of the spinal cord, ultimately supplying motor fibers to the sternocleidomastoid (SCM) and trapezius muscles (Fig. 14.5), being included in the gamut of shoulder nerves [17]. It is a pure motor nerve originating from C1 to C4 cervical segments and ascends through the foramen magnum, and returns through the jugular foramen. After providing motor innervation to SCM muscle, it enters the posterior triangle of the neck and eventually innervates the trapezius muscle. Additionally, the nerve proceeds caudally and dorsally in the subcutaneous tissue along the posterior triangle of the neck.

14.2.5 Dorsal Scapular Nerve

The dorsal scapular nerve is a motor nerve that arises from the C5 nerve root, with usual contribution from C6 (Fig. 14.1). After its origin, it runs in close proximity of the upper trunk of the brachial plexus, then traversing the middle scalene muscle and traveling posteriorly to innervate the levator scapula muscle. The nerve also reaches the deep surfaces of rhomboid major and minor, supplying both muscles that have a role in moving the scapula medially (Fig. 14.2) [13].

14.3 Pathologic Conditions

14.3.1 Definition

The term entrapment neuropathy refers to an isolated peripheral nerve injury at a specific location where a mechanical constriction occurs, most commonly from a fibrous or fibro-osseous tunnel, or by a fibrous band. However, there are cases in which the nerve is injured by chronic direct compression by space-occupying lesions (such as a cyst), or by chronic deformation, angulation, or stretching forces causing mechanical damage. Finally, iatrogenic causes can result in the nerve injury, including direct nerve injury or by means of deformation induced by postsurgical scarring.

14.3.1.1 Nerve Compression

Entrapment neuropathies of the shoulder secondary to nerve compression by mechanical or dynamic forces could be a cause of upper extremity weakness and pain in the athlete. Structurally narrow tunnels make individual nerves susceptible to entrapment neuropathies. Dynamic changes within these narrow passages during repetitive athletic activity can create further compression of a nerve with only minimal anatomic variation [18]. Nerve compression may also be produced by space-occupying lesions such as cysts, tumors, and inflammatory processes or by posttraumatic conditions such as hematoma, myositis ossificans, and scar formation. Direct compression occurs mainly because a space-occupying lesion evolves in the proximity of the nerve, which can also develop if local anatomy has been altered by a fracture. Other causes for nerve compression are associated with hormonal alterations and systemic diseases, such as pregnancy, oral contraceptive ingestion, diabetes mellitus, and hypothyroidism.

14.3.1.2 Nerve Stretching

Along the trajectory of nerves, there are fixed points limiting its mobility potentially predisposing to focal deformation that exceeds its mechanical properties. Specific repetitive movements can create excess nerve traction, causing strain injuries at these fixed points, evolving with inflammation that impairs normal nerve conduction. Additional factors, such as fibrous bands or small arterial branches crossing a nerve, can create additional fixed points and also be the basis for entrapments.

14.3.1.3 Iatrogenic Lesions

Iatrogenic lesions from surgery can also be a source for shoulder neuropathies. For example, the spinal accessory nerve may be injured after biopsies of a cervical lymph node. Neurologic symptoms are present after approximately 0.2–3% of shoulder arthroscopic procedures, 4% of arthroplasties, and 8% of open surgeries for the treatment of instability [19–21]. The majority of these injuries are minor cutaneous nerve lesions and transient neurapraxias [22–25]. Permanent sequelae and injuries that require secondary surgical intervention are rare, and the long-term outcomes of patients with nerve injury from shoulder surgery have been rarely reported. These situations are less diagnostically challenging.

14.3.2 Radiographs and Computed Tomography

The decision on the timing and modality of shoulder imaging is based on multiple factors, including the acuity of the injury, the suspected tissue and nerve involved, the age of the patient, and demands that the patient applies on the shoulder. In general, acute traumatic injuries are imaged with plain films to exclude fracture or dislocation. For several bone and joint problems, radiographs are often the only required imaging study, being noninvasive and rather inexpensive compared to other imaging studies. They should be obtained to rule out likely osseous causes of nerve entrapment and to evaluate concomitant shoulder conditions, such as glenohumeral subluxation or osteoarthritis. Several views of the shoulder are necessary for comprehensive visualization of the osseous and articular anatomy. A Stryker notch view allows evaluation of the suprascapular notch and may display complete ossification or near obliteration of its foramen. A suprascapular notch view (X-ray beam directed 15–30° cephalad) allows visualization of osseous notch variants. Anteroposterior radiographs directly show superior migration of humeral head suggestive of chronic rotator cuff disease. Appropriate evaluation of conventional radiographs often encourages selection of higher level imaging studies. In situations in which osseous abnormalities are speculated to be the primary purpose of nerve injury, a computed tomography (CT) scan may be beneficial in recognizing specific regions of likely nerve compression [26]. Radiographs are not well suited for suspected nerve injuries of insidious onset given their preferential involvement of soft tissues.

CT scans allows for excellent detail regarding osseous pathology in addition to reliable identification of muscular fatty degeneration and atrophy. Although CT has limitations in directly assessing shoulder nerves, this method provides excellent visualization of suprascapular and spinoglenoid notches. In addition, CT arthrography can help diagnose paralabral cysts, in particular those communicating with the glenohumeral joint, as well as identify rotator cuff tears as a potential source of shoulder pain. A low-dose CT scan can concurrently analyze the position of the scapula and the attached muscles and look for signs of denervation (fatty degeneration, etc.) and dynamic 3-dimensional (4D) reconstructions obtained with a large detector CT scanner can demonstrate scapular kinematics in suspected scapular winging [2, 27].

14.3.3 Ultrasound

Ultrasound is an excellent imaging modality to assess muscle, ligament, and tendon anatomy, with the unique advantage of allowing for dynamic imaging studies. In the shoulder, ultrasound has consistently demonstrated high levels of accuracy to detect rotator cuff pathology. However, this modality still has a limited role in comprehensively assessing the shoulder for entrapment neuropathies, given the difficulty in reliably demonstrating variable levels of muscle edema and directly showing the challenging anatomy of shoulder nerves throughout their entire course. Nevertheless, shoulder ultrasound can be used as a first intention modality for shoulder pain to rule out confounding symptoms. Although the initially suspected diagnosis is often a rotator cuff tendon tear, the radiologist must not ignore differential diagnoses that could relate to a neuropathy, particularly when no cuff tendon abnormality has been identified. For this reason, beyond the standard assessment for rotator cuff and biceps tendons, it is suggested to systematically include the following items in a shoulder ultrasound examination [28]:

A- *Suprascapular and spinoglenoid notches to assess for a space-occupying lesion.* A paralabral cyst can be readily differentiated from dilated suprascapular veins by combining color Doppler and compression of the structure; veins are filled with colored Doppler flow signal and collapse under pressure, whereas cysts do not.

B- *Supraspinatus and infraspinatus muscles compared to contralateral side.* Muscle atrophy can be readily determined with asymmetry of muscle volume, along with fatty degeneration that causes increased echogenicity. This can be done rapidly at the end of ultrasound examination while evaluating the posterior aspect of the glenohumeral joint.

Although this methodology only relates to suprascapular neuropathy, it can be valuable since this nerve can account for up to 97% of shoulder entrapment neuropathies. A direct search for specific nerves can be performed as needed but access can be limited by the complex nerve trajectory, depth, and overlapping osseous anatomy [29].

14.3.4 Magnetic Resonance Imaging

Besides providing direct visualization of a nerve and surrounding tissues, MRI is able to illustrate intrinsic signal abnormalities within the nerve and is considered superior in defining the associated indirect signs from muscle denervation [30, 31]. The signal intensity of a normal nerve on MRI is intermediate to low on T1-weighted sequences being slightly higher on T2-weighted and other fluid-sensitive sequences [31, 32]. Enlargement with obvious increase in T2 signal is regarded as an abnormal MRI appearance [32]. Additionally, a hyperintense signal of the denervated muscle is commonly seen when entrapment is acute, and fatty infiltration and muscle atrophy are signs of long-standing neuropathy in chronic cases [30–32]. Recognizing muscular denervation (muscular edema, atrophy, and fatty degeneration) in a neural distribution pattern is essential to the diagnosis of entrapment neuropathies. MRI is the only imaging modality that can reliably detect muscular edema, which is the earliest abnormality to appear in entrapment neuropathies. MRI also allows an assessment of the severity of the disease and the search for its etiology, being valuable in excluding differential diagnoses. The

MRI protocol should be adjusted to each situation: in case of suspected suprascapular or axillary neuropathy, the field of view (FOV) has to be centered on the glenohumeral joint, while in case of scapular winging the FOV needs to be enlarged to cover both scapulae and their attaching posterior and medial muscles.

14.3.4.1 Building an MRI Protocol

The most important pulse sequence is fast spin-echo T2-weighted imaging with fat suppression, carried out in the axial plane. This imaging allows the recognition of muscular edema, using echo times ≥45 ms for sufficient T2 weighting [2]. T1-weighted sequences without fat suppression are also important for the diagnosis of muscle fatty degeneration. Acquisition in the sagittal plane may be supplementary to grant better comparisons between the different muscles, particularly if the signal abnormalities are slight. It is reasonable to increase the gap between the slices to cover the total volume of the muscles, given that shoulder muscle may be partially involved with edema or chronic atrophy, depending on the site of entrapment. Typically, intravenous injection of gadolinium injection is not required for the assessment of shoulder neuropathies. However, denervated muscles frequently show contrast enhancement, making such images comparable to those obtained with T2-weighted fat-suppressed pulse sequences [1, 27].

The edema observed in entrapment neuropathies has many specific features [2]: it involves only the denervated muscles, being homogeneous in intensity and affecting the muscle diffusely. Muscle edema from neuropathies is an early phenomenon. Clinical studies report it to be detectable in the second week after trauma or at the onset of electromyography (EMG) abnormalities, but in experimental studies it manifests earlier, up to a few days after trauma [33]. Neuropathic muscle edema is also isolated because of the lack of other intramuscular abnormalities. The intensity of edema relies upon the severity and duration of the primary lesion. Experimental studies show that muscle edema peaks 2–4 weeks after the primary trauma but its intensity increases with the severity of lesions [33]. In sports-related shoulder neuropathy, this anomaly can be seen beyond 6 months [5].

Denervated muscle atrophy typically progresses slower than edema. Atrophy is best shown on sagittal T1-weighted images due to the optimal contrast between muscle and surrounding fat. The sagittal plane grants a comparison among scapular muscles, which are visualized along their short axes, allowing for an estimation of their bulk. The degree of atrophy can be assessed by examining the muscle surfaces, which are normally convex but turn flat and ultimately concave in the later stages [5]. Atrophic pseudohypertrophy has been described in which the afflicted muscle paradoxically enlarges in response to denervation; however it is diffusely infiltrated by adipose tissue [1]. However, unlike true muscle hypertrophy in which the signal is normal on all MRI sequences, the pseudohypertrophied muscle loses its normal signal intensity because of edema and fatty replacement. Fatty degeneration initiates during the subacute phase and is a hallmark of chronic muscle denervation [30]. Rotator cuff muscle fatty degeneration can be measured on sagittal T1-weighted images using the Bernageau and Goutallier classification method [34].

14.3.5 Specific Shoulder Neuropathies and Related MRI Features

14.3.5.1 Suprascapular Nerve Neuropathies

Suprascapular Nerve Syndrome

The suprascapular nerve can be injured by several mechanisms. These include repetitive overhead sports or activities and associated nerve traction [35–38], compression from a space-occupying lesion such as a cyst [39–41], trauma

[42–45], and rotator cuff tears [46]. Athletes who perform repetitive overhead activities such as tennis and volleyball have been described to experience neuropathy secondary to traction and microtrauma [35, 47, 48]. The mechanism is increased pressure on the nerve by the spinoglenoid ligament when the shoulder is in a position of overhead throwing [49]. Traction injury can also happen in the presence of a retracted superior or posterior rotator cuff tear. The secondary traction of the nerve is created at the suprascapular notch or around the base of the scapular spine. Repetitive adduction and internal rotation of the shoulder can stretch the nerve below the spinoglenoid ligament [50]. Ossification of the transverse scapular ligament or spinoglenoid ligament at the suprascapular or spinoglenoid notch, respectively, may increase the risk of suprascapular neuropathy [36, 51–54]. This may create stretching and compression of the suprascapular nerve and its branches below the suprascapular ligament. Nerve compression may also happen at either the suprascapular or the spinoglenoid notch by soft-tissue or bone tumor, or a cyst secondary to a labral or capsular injury [39–41].

The association between labral tears and paralabral cysts causing suprascapular neuropathy is well determined in both radiographic and clinical investigations [55–59].

Paralabral cysts are usually associated with tears of the superior and posterior glenoid labrum (from 8- to 11-o'clock positions), related to the passage of joint fluid into the cyst through a thin pedicle [60, 61]. During their growth, paralabral cysts may spread into the spinoglenoid notch, the suprascapular notch, or both, possibly causing nerve entrapment and muscle denervation. Ultrasound and MRI can identify the cyst and recognize secondary changes of nerve damage, including loss in bulk and echotextural or signal intensity changes in the innervated muscles due to edema and fatty replacement [62]. A direct correlation has been found between the size of paralabral cysts and the onset of denervation symptoms [60]. Due to their deep location, depiction of paralabral cysts requires a careful scanning technique with ultrasound [63]. Varicose veins in the spinoglenoid notch are the main differential diagnosis. Although enlarged spinoglenoid notch veins look like a cyst because they appear as fluid-filled images, they change their shape, collapsing in internal rotation of the arm and dilating maximally in external rotation [64].

Historically, suprascapular neuropathy was speculated as a diagnosis of exclusion; however several studies have shown multifactorial causes of suprascapular neuropathy. Other sources of suprascapular neuropathy include intimal damage to the suprascapular artery resulting in microemboli in the vasa nervorum [37], glenohumeral dislocation [43–45], fractures around the shoulder girdle [42, 65, 66], and penetrating injury to the shoulder or surgical procedures using a posterior approach to the scapula [67]. The clinical and imaging characteristics of entrapment neuropathies of the suprascapular nerve and its branches differ, depending on the location of compression, traction, or injuries. Entrapment of the suprascapular nerve at the scapular notch leads to supraspinatus and infraspinatus muscle denervation, while distal entrapment at the spinoglenoid notch typically causes isolated involvement of the infraspinatus muscle [68].

MRI is a valuable diagnostic modality in patients who have suprascapular nerve entrapment. The MRI characteristics of compressive neuropathy consist of direct signs involving the nerve and indirect signs pertaining to muscle denervation. Abnormalities in the signal intensity, size, and position of the affected nerve are direct signs of peripheral nerve entrapment [6]. The structural causes may be displayed including space-occupying lesions, such as ganglia and tumors, or osseous abnormalities, such as bony spurs, fracture fragments, and callus. Ganglia are isointense or hypointense in comparison with muscle on T1-weighted images, are homogeneously hyperintense on T2-weighted sequences, and show thin peripheral enhancement with

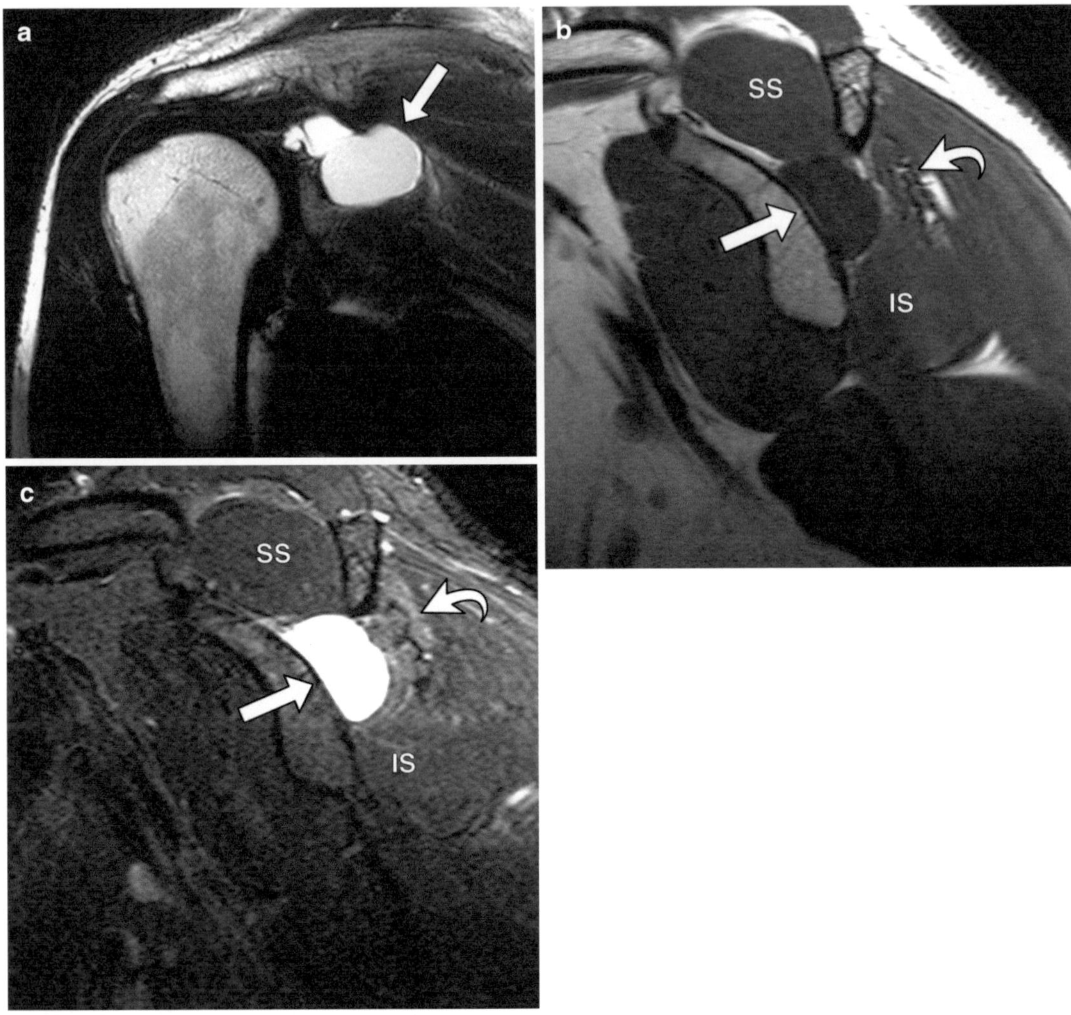

Fig. 14.6 30-Year-old male: (**a**) Coronal oblique T2 fast spin echo showing a hyperintense large cyst occupying the spinoglenoid notch (arrow). (**b**) T1-weighted sagittal oblique image shows the cyst as a low/isointense mass (arrow) and mild atrophy of the upper infraspinatus muscle. The supraspinatus muscle (SS) appears normal suggesting involvement of the infraspinatus branch of the suprascapular nerve. (**c**) STIR sagittal oblique image shows the cyst (arrow) in spinoglenoid notch with secondary edema of the upper portion of infraspinatus muscle (IS, curved arrow)

gadolinium (Figs. 14.6 and 14.7). The pattern of muscle denervation provides information about the duration of entrapment and can identify the location of neurologic compromise. Acute denervation is demonstrated as hyperintensity of the supraspinatus and infraspinatus or infraspinatus muscle alone on fluid-sensitive sequences. Chronic compression is displayed as a reduction in muscle bulk and fatty infiltration of the involved muscles. Involvement of both the supra- and infraspinatus muscles indicates compression at the suprascapular notch, while isolated involvement of infraspinatus reflects compression at the spinoglenoid notch [6].

14.3.5.2 Axillary Nerve Neuropathies

Axillary neuropathy can be secondary to stretching injures or extrinsic compression in the quadrilateral space induced by humeral fractures, improper use of crutches, casts, fibrous bands, space-occupying lesions, and inferior paraglenoid cysts [16, 69]. Iatrogenic nerve injury during

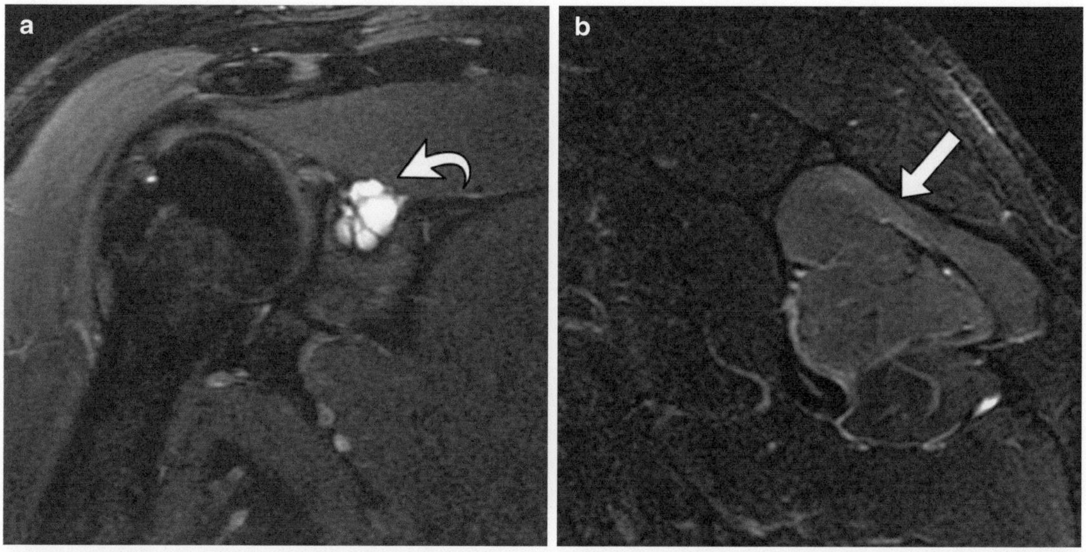

Fig. 14.7 39-Year-old male showing (**a**) coronal oblique T2-weighted FSE fat-suppressed image in which a multiloculated cyst (curved arrow) involves the suprascapular notch. (**b**) Sagittal oblique STIR image shows diffuse neurogenic edema involving the infraspinatus muscle (arrow)

arthroscopic procedures around the coracoid or by posterior surgical arthroscopic portals has also been described [16]. When entrapment of the axillary nerve happens in the quadrilateral space, there is isolated denervation of the teres minor muscle because the anterior branch of the nerve (supplying the deltoid) is spared (Fig. 14.8). Axillary neuropathy may be identified incidentally during routine MRI of the shoulder, since clinically this may not be apparent because the action of teres minor cannot be definitely separated from the contribution of infraspinatus. When symptomatic, axillary neuropathy appears with ambiguous, often nonspecific posterior shoulder pain, sensory disturbances over the external aspect of the shoulder, and weakness aggravated by overhead activity and heavy lifting. Even without any noticeable soft-tissue abnormality along the nerve course, the imaging diagnosis of axillary neuropathy is based on the signs of volume loss and signal alteration of the affected muscles in the absence of a tendon tear [6].

Quadrilateral Space Syndrome

Quadrilateral space syndrome is a rare condition referring to an isolated compressive neuropathy of the axillary nerve. The syndrome was first explained by Cahill and Palmer [70] in 1983 in which the neurovascular bundle, containing the axillary nerve and posterior humeral circumflex artery, is compressed by fibrous bands as it travels through the quadrilateral space. It commonly occurs in young athletes between the ages of 25 and 35 years without a history of serious trauma. The syndrome is determined clinically by poorly localized anterolateral shoulder pain and is aggravated by forward flexion, abduction, and external rotation of the humerus. This pain is typically associated with point tenderness over the posterior shoulder, near the teres minor insertion site. Skin paraesthesia in the sensory distribution of the axillary nerve (overlying the deltoid muscle) and atrophy or weakness of the teres minor and deltoid may occur as well [71]. The development of fibrous bands in the quadrilateral space sounds to be related to microtrauma due to repeated overhead activity such as throwing [72, 73]. Although extrinsic compression by fibrous bands is the most common cause of the syndrome, various other causes have now been discussed in the literature. Robinson et al. [74] were the first to report a case of quadrilateral space syndrome caused by a paralabral cyst.

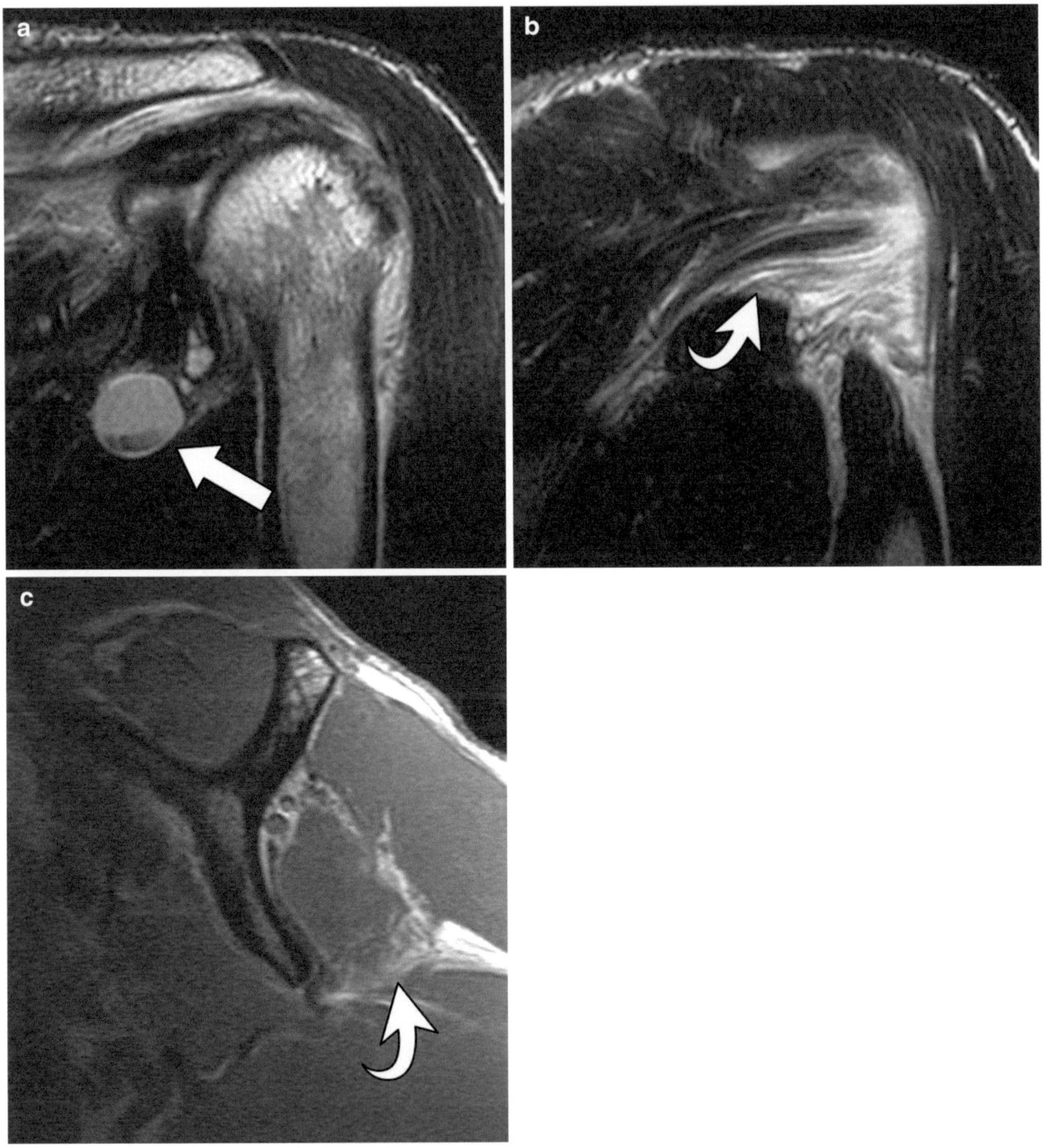

Fig. 14.8 43-Year-old male showing (**a**) coronal oblique T2-weighted FSE images with multiloculated cyst that dissected towards the quadrilateral space (arrow) and secondary edema of the teres minor muscle (**b**) (curved arrow). (**c**) Sagittal T1-weighted image shows loss of bulk of the teres minor muscle with fatty infiltration (curved arrow)

Juxta-articular cysts are a typical entity occurring next to large joints and are a well-established reason of compressive suprascapular neuropathy in the shoulder. Glenòid labral cysts are thought to arise from extrusion of joint fluid via labrocapsular tears. They develop most commonly in the superior and posterior aspects and are infrequent in the inferior region of the joint [75]. When large, inferior labral cysts can create mass effect on the neurovascular bundle in the tightly constrained quadrilateral space. Quadrilateral space masses such as soft-tissue tumors and hematomas have also been described to result in this syndrome. Other reported cases of axillary nerve injury include trauma (humeral neck or scapular fractures), acute translational incidents such as glenohumeral subluxation or anterior dislocation, and surgical or arthroscopic intervention [76–78]. The relatively fixed position of the quadrilateral space makes it particularly susceptible, and such injuries usually affect both the teres minor and deltoid muscles due to the level at which the axillary nerve injury happens [79, 80].

The diagnosis of quadrilateral space syndrome may be difficult on the basis of clinical examinations alone and is typically one of exclusion. Generally poorly localized shoulder pain may be confused with a rotator cuff injury or impingement. When a clear structural lesion such as fibrous bands or a mass is discovered on imaging, diagnosis can be relatively easy. MRI is superior to ultrasound to display any space-occupying lesion in the quadrilateral space, such as paralabral cysts extending off the inferior aspect of the glenoid in association with a tear of the inferior labrum [63, 76, 81]. However, MRI generally shows no structural abnormality within the quadrilateral space but may display secondary features of denervation myopathy. These characteristics include atrophy of the teres minor and, less frequently, of the deltoid, which is seen as a reduction in muscle volume and fatty degeneration with chronic compression [71]. Fatty degeneration is best observed on T1-weighted sequences but can also be viewed as abnormal signal intensity within the muscle belly on T2-weighted images (Fig. 14.8). Quadrilateral space syndrome is a potentially reversible cause of shoulder pain. It should be considered when selective atrophy or a signal change of teres minor with or without involvement of the deltoid is observed in the appropriate clinical setting. Other diagnoses producing muscle atrophy or neurogenic edema in the absence of a clear cause, such as traumatic injury to the axillary nerve, brachial plexus, or nerve roots, must also be considered [81].

Posttraumatic Axillary Nerve Injury

Up to 45% of shoulder dislocation cases may have associated nerve injury [44]. The axillary nerve is most commonly involved, because it has a relatively tethered course within the quadrilateral space. The risk for axillary nerve and brachial plexus injury is higher if the shoulder is not reduced within 12 h. In spite of the high prevalence of axillary nerve injury following shoulder dislocation, only a few reports in the radiological literature address the association of teres minor atrophy with prior dislocation [76, 82]. Traction and compression of the axillary nerve and subscapularis muscle can be induced by the dislocated humeral head or during manipulative reduction in which traction with rotation or abduction is concurrently performed. Posttraumatic injury to the axillary nerve can also be secondary to proximal humeral fracture [66], and seldom due to a direct blow to the deltoid muscle. The clinical diagnosis of axillary nerve injury may be difficult because the signs and symptoms are often ambiguous. Because branches to the lateral cutaneous innervation and to teres minor muscle are closest to the glenoid rim, they are most vulnerable to posttraumatic injuries [83]. Injury to the infraspinatus muscle, however, may be clinically overlooked.

MRI may illustrate signs suggestive of teres minor denervation injury with increased signal on water-sensitive images or atrophy of the muscle. Unlike EMG studies, which can directly assess the function of nerves, MRI provides indirect indicators of nerve injury by finding changes in fat and water composition of muscle. Effects to T1 and T2 prolongation can be recognized within 15 days post-injury [69, 84]. Most typically, isolated fatty atrophy of the teres minor muscle is incidentally identified (Fig. 14.9). The diagnosis of teres minor atrophy in the absence of quadrilateral space lesions should prompt accurate assessment for signs suggestive of posttraumatic glenohumeral instability and prior dislocation [76, 82, 85].

14.3.5.3 Scapular Winging

Entrapments of the long thoracic, accessory, or dorsal scapular nerves directly prevent scapular movements due to the muscles involved. These entrapments account for the static or dynamic scapular prominence recognized as scapular winging. This clinical condition is distinct from suprascapular and axillary nerve entrapment

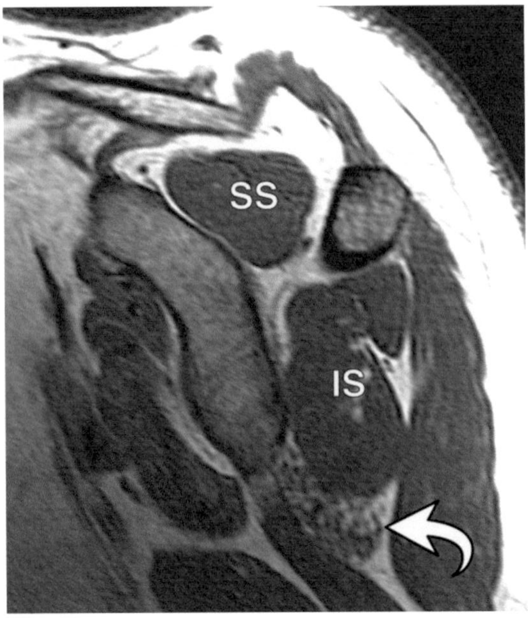

Fig. 14.9 36-Year-old male T1-weighted sagittal oblique image showing isolated atrophy of the teres minor muscle (curved arrow). SS, supraspinatus muscle, IS infraspinatus muscle

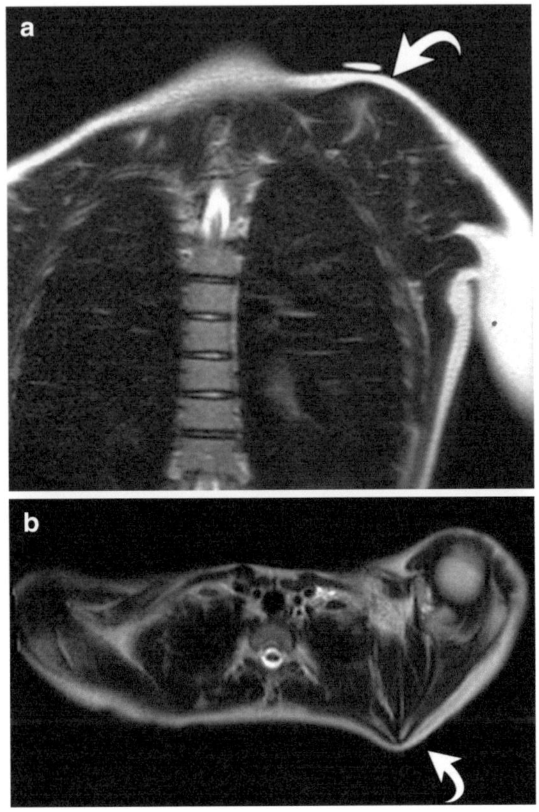

Fig. 14.10 13-Year-old female with clinical evidence of left scapular winging after a fall. Coronal (**a**) and axial (**b**) T2-weighted images show left scapular winging (curved arrow) characterized by deformity and scapular malalignment without muscle edema

Table 14.1 Classification of scapular winging [2, 96]

Primary scapular winging	
Neurologic origin	Spinal accessory nerve (trapezius palsy)
	Long thoracic nerve (serratus anterior palsy)
	Dorsal scapular nerve (rhomboids palsy)
Osseous origin	Osteochondromas
	Fracture, malunions
Soft-tissue origin	Contractural winging
	Muscle avulsion or agenesis
	Scapulothoracic bursitis
Secondary scapula winging	Accompanies glenohumeral disorders and should resolve once that disorder has been addressed
Voluntary scapula winging	

because there is a clinical abnormality suggestive of it, which can be identified on physical examination (Fig. 14.10). The patient is likely to be referred for the exploration of this abnormality [27] (Table 14.1).

The MRI protocol should be adjusted in case of scapular winging. In this case the FOV has to be expanded to include both scapulae, covering the posterior and medial muscles attaching to them. The serratus anterior, the rhomboid muscles, and the trapezius should be inspected (Fig. 14.11). Because this coverage is beyond the reach of a dedicated shoulder coil, a multichannel phased array body coil should be used and the whole width of the scapular girdle must be viewed. Craniocaudally, the investigation must range from the upper edge of the shoulder to the tip of the scapula. This allows a comparison between both sides, which can be helpful when dealing with subtle abnormalities. T2-weighted images with fat suppression and T1-weighted images are performed in the axial and sagittal planes.

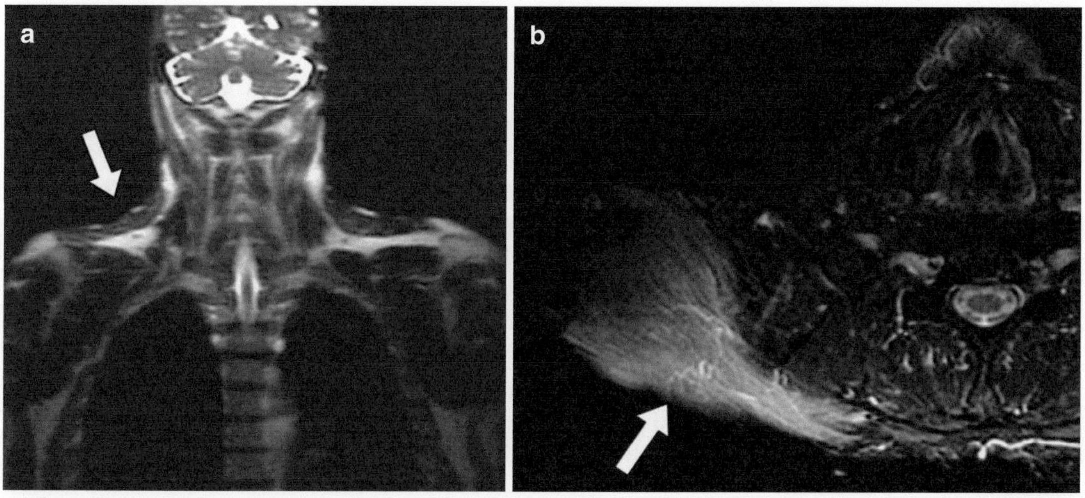

Fig. 14.11 45-Year-old male with right-shoulder pain and weakness with scapular winging for a month. (**a**) Axial STIR and (**b**) coronal T1-weighted MRI show diffuse neurogenic edema involving right trapezius muscle (arrow)

Long Thoracic Nerve Neuropathy

Long thoracic neuropathy most often results from repeated microtrauma due to stretching injury. This usually occurs in athletes (e.g., throwing sports such as javelin, baseball, or when serving or spiking a tennis or volleyball ball) when the head is tilted and rotated laterally away from the affected extremity and the arm is elevated overhead [16]. Direct trauma over the upper anterior chest and whiplash injury may also cause nerve compression [86]. Nontraumatic causes consist of compression by enlarged bursae, such as the subcoracoid bursa or the subscapularis recess. Irrespective of mechanism, it is still unknown where the injury occurs along the course of the nerve. Injury to the long thoracic nerve paralyzes the anterior serratus muscle, which causes medial winging of the scapula and a deficit in active forward flexion, which is more common than lateral winging. The scapular asymmetry (diagnosed by comparing the distance between the spinal processes and the medial edge of the scapula on both sides) may be clinically evident on physical examination. It can be aggravated more on forward flexion of both arms or by the wall push-up test. In the most severe cases, thorough elevation of the arm may be impossible [87]. Physical examination shows an obvious clinical picture with scapular winging, especially when the patient extends his or her arms and pushes against a wall [88]. Direct assessment of the long thoracic nerve is possible only in part and for limited segments with ultrasound. The diagnosis basically will be confirmed by EMG or MRI, which demonstrates signs of denervation (edema, atrophy) of the serratus anterior muscle. The serratus anterior muscle is sometimes outside the usual scope of exploration of the shoulder and standard joint examination may miss the anomaly. A shoulder coil with a large field is sufficient in thin patients. A spine coil and a multielement body coil will give satisfactory results in larger subjects. MRI also allows for elimination of alternative causes of scapular winging.

Accessory Nerve Neuropathy

Spinal accessory nerve neuropathy most frequently follows a stretch injury associated with lifting, heavy load bearing on the shoulders, whiplash, or trauma [89]. It has also been referred to skull deformities, infiltrative lesions, and radiation fibrosis [90]. Moreover, it may follow operations involving the head and neck in which the dissection of a lymph node occurs. Patients present with mild shoulder droop, weakness of shoulder elevation, and scapular winging during shoulder abduction. Atrophy of the trapezius muscle causes scapular instability and painful shoulder abduction [17]. Lateral scapular winging is always present [91]; however only more severe types like the "droopy shoulder" may be observed, associated with trapezius atrophy, shoulder drop, and lateral winging. Abduction and external rotation against resistance aggravate the scapular displacement, while forward flexion reduces the deformation because of serratus anterior contraction [29]. MRI is indicated in difficult cases to confirm the diagnosis. Focused on the trapezius and anterior serratus muscles, it shows classic signs of denervation affecting the trapezius and allows for exclusion of long thoracic neuropathy.

Dorsal Scapular Nerve Neuropathy

The dorsal scapular nerve supplies the rhomboids and is rarely injured in isolation, being generally involved with a C5 radiculopathy. Reports have been made of injury of the dorsal scapular nerve due to muscle hypertrophy in bodybuilders [92]. Neuropathies of the dorsal scapular nerve are uncommon but their frequency is perhaps underestimated because their impact is generally minor [93]. They result in denervation of the rhomboids, which clinically leads to discomfort or pain in these muscles, minimal scapular winging, and difficulty on arm elevation. The location of nerve compression is unclear, but could be a specific form of thoracic outlet syndrome in the scalene space [94]. One article reports diagnostic confirmation of damage to this nerve by MRI [95], the positive finding being thinner rhomboid muscles on MRI of the thorax. In addition, T2-weighted images may show an increase of pathologic signals suggestive of muscular denervation [95].

14.3.5.4 Polyneuropathies (Parsonage-Turner Syndrome)

Parsonage-Turner syndrome is an uncommon, self-limiting disorder characterized by immediate onset of nontraumatic shoulder pain accompanied with progressive weakness of the shoulder girdle musculature. It was first recognized in 48 patients by Spillane in 1943 [97] and then by Parsonage and Turner [98] in 1948 who described the condition in 136 servicemen, which they called "neuralgic amyotrophy" or "shoulder-girdle syndrome." Afterwards, the pathology has commonly been referred to as Parsonage-Turner syndrome or acute brachial neuritis, although the terms "brachial plexus neuropathy" [99], "acute brachial radiculitis" [100, 101], and "paralytic brachial neuritis" [102, 103] have all been used to describe the entity. Clinical diagnosis may be difficult because symptoms can simulate those of more common disorders such as cervical spondylosis, rotator cuff tears, impingement syndrome, adhesive capsulitis, and calcific tendinitis [97–99, 104]. The exact cause of Parsonage-Turner syndrome is unclear, although viral neuritis [99, 105], immunization [102], autoimmune mechanisms [106], trauma, strenuous exercise, and surgery [107] have all been noted. Prior infection has been reported in up to 25% of cases [99]. The overall incidence has been estimated at 1.64 per 100,000 individuals in one population [108]. The age range of affected patients is very wide, with most patients presenting in the third to seventh decades of life [104, 109]. Males are mostly affected; bilateral involvement is observed in up to one-third of patients [99, 108]. Originally the long thoracic nerve was thought to be the most commonly involved in Parsonage-Turner syndrome [98]. However, future studies showed that the most frequently involved muscles are those innervated by the suprascapular nerve (supraspinatus and infraspinatus) [109], although the entire brachial plexus can be affected. In a study of 27 patients with Parsonage-Turner syndrome, Gaskin and Helms [110] found that the suprascapular nerve was involved in 97% of the subjects and the axillary nerve in 50% [80].

Imaging Findings

There is no specific test for the diagnosis of Parsonage-Turner syndrome. EMG, nerve conduction studies, and MRI must be interpreted in light of the patient's clinical history. MRI is the modality of choice in patients with shoulder pain and weakness, being sensitive for changes indicating denervation injury. The studies by Gaskin and Helms [110] and Scalf et al. [104] are the

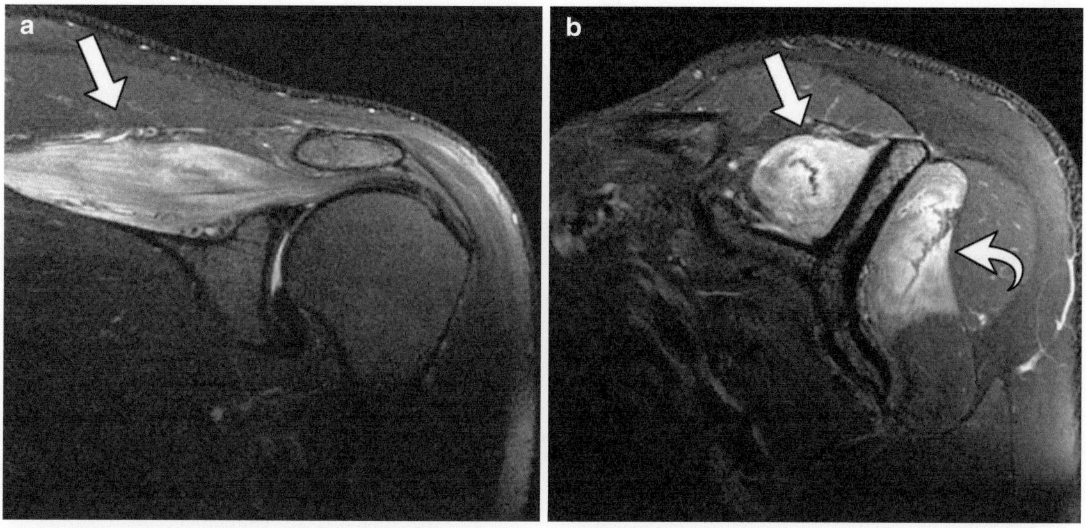

Fig. 14.12 37-Year old male sagittal T2-weighted fat-suppressed coronal (**a**) and sagittal (**b**) oblique showing diffuse neurogenic edema of supraspinatus (arrow) and infraspinatus (curved arrow) muscles. The patient had no history of trauma or other pathology and no evidence of compressive lesions in the suprascapular notch or rotator cuff tear (not shown)

largest reported series describing the MRI features of Parsonage-Turner syndrome to date. The diagnosis is proposed when there is an abnormality of muscles innervated by the brachial plexus in the absence of history of excessive overhead activity, trauma, or morphologic cause at MRI. The earliest recognizable change in denervated muscles is diffusely high signal on fluid-sensitive sequences such as STIR or T2-weighted images (because of increase in extracellular water content) and normal signal on T1-weighted sequences [1]. After a few weeks in the subacute to chronic phase, the denervated muscle may decrease in volume with increased T1 signal because of fatty infiltration (Fig. 14.12) [104]. Intramuscular signal may return to normal several months after the chronic phase; however, in complete muscle denervation (>1 year after injury), changes are irreversible [111].

MRI is also helpful in excluding intrinsic shoulder abnormalities that can create symptoms equivalent to Parsonage-Turner syndrome such as rotator cuff tears, impingement syndrome, and labral tears. MRI can display structural lesions that may produce similar denervation changes in the rotator cuff musculature such as cuff tears or masses compressing the brachial plexus or peripheral nerves and other causes of intramuscular high signal including myositis, rhabdomyolysis, inflammatory myopathies, compartment syndrome, and tumor involvement of muscle [112, 113].

References

1. Kamath S, Venkatanarasimha N, Walsh M, Hughes P. MRI appearance of muscle denervation. Skelet Radiol. 2008;37:397–404.
2. Blum A, Lecocq S, Louis M, Wassel J, Moisei A, Teixeira P. The nerves around the shoulder. Eur J Radiol. 2013;82:2–16.
3. Boykin RE, Friedman DJ, Higgins LD, Warner JJ. Suprascapular neuropathy. J Am Acad Orthop Surg. 2010;92:2348–64.
4. Lorei MP, Hershman EB. Peripheral nerve injuries in athletes. Sports Med. 1993;16:130–47.
5. Ludig T, Walter F, Chapuis D, Molé D, Roland J, Blum A. MR imaging evaluation of suprascapular nerve entrapment. Eur Radiol. 2001;11:2161–9.
6. Bencardino JT, Rosenberg ZS. Entrapment neuropathies of the shoulder and elbow in the athlete. Clin Sports Med. 2006;25:465–87.
7. Aiello I, Serra G, Traina G, Tugnoli V. Entrapment of the suprascapular nerve at the spinoglenoid notch. Ann Neurol. 1982;12:314–6.
8. Bigliani LU, Dalsey RM, McCann PD, April EW. An anatomical study of the suprascapular nerve. Arthroscopy. 1990;6:301–5.

9. Warner J, Krushell R, Masquelet A, Gerber C. Anatomy and relationships of the suprascapular nerve. J Bone Joint Surg Am. 1992;74:36–45.
10. Brown D, James D, Roy S. Pain relief by suprascapular nerve block in gleno-humeral arthritis. Scand J Rheumatol. 1988;17:411–5.
11. Matsumoto D, Suenaga N, Oizumi N, Hisada Y, Minami A. A new nerve block procedure for the suprascapular nerve based on a cadaveric study. J Shoulder Elb Surg. 2009;18:607–11.
12. Ritchie ED, Tong D, Chung F, Norris AM, Miniaci A, Vairavanathan SD. Suprascapular nerve block for postoperative pain relief in arthroscopic shoulder surgery: a new modality? Anesth Analg. 1997;84:1306–12.
13. Tubbs RS, Tyler-Kabara EC, Aikens AC, et al. Surgical anatomy of the axillary nerve within the quadrangular space. J Neurosurg. 2005;102:912–4.
14. Apaydin N, Tubbs RS, Loukas M, Duparc F. Review of the surgical anatomy of the axillary nerve and the anatomic basis of its iatrogenic and traumatic injury. Surg Radiol Anat. 2010;32:193–201.
15. McClelland D, Paxinos A. The anatomy of the quadrilateral space with reference to quadrilateral space syndrome. J Shoulder Elb Surg. 2008;17:162–4.
16. Safran MR. Nerve injury about the shoulder in athletes, part 2: long thoracic nerve, spinal accessory nerve, burners/stingers, thoracic outlet syndrome. Am J Sports Med. 2004;32:1063–76.
17. Wiater JM, Bigliani LU. Spinal accessory nerve injury. Clin Orthop. 1999;368:5–16.
18. Pecina M, Krmpotic-Nemanic J, Markiewitz A. Tunnel syndromes in the upper extremities; 1991. p. 11–84.
19. Ho E, Cofield RH, Balm MR, Hattrup SJ, Rowland CM. Neurologic complications of surgery for anterior shoulder instability. J Shoulder Elb Surg. 1999;8:266–70.
20. Lynch NM, Cofield RH, Silbert PL, Hermann RC. Neurologic complications after total shoulder arthroplasty. J Shoulder Elb Surg. 1996;5:53–61.
21. Small NC. Complications in arthroscopic surgery performed by experienced arthroscopists. Arthroscopy. 1988;4:215–21.
22. Rodeo SA, Forster RA, Weiland AJ. Neurological complications due to arthroscopy. J Bone Joint Surg Am. 1993;75:917–26.
23. Segmüller HE, Alfred SP, Zilio G, Saies AD, Hayes MG. Cutaneous nerve lesions of the shoulder and arm after arthroscopic shoulder surgery. J Shoulder Elb Surg. 1995;4:254–8.
24. Boardman ND, Cofield RH. Neurologic complications of shoulder surgery. Clin Orthop. 1999;368:44–53.
25. Marecek GS, Saltzman MD. Complications in shoulder arthroscopy. Orthopedics. 2010;33:492.
26. Piasecki DP, Romeo AA, Bach BR Jr, Nicholson GP. Suprascapular neuropathy. J Am Acad Orthop Surg. 2009;17:665–76.
27. Budzik J, Wavreille G, Pansini V, Moraux A, Demondion X, Cotten A. Entrapment neuropathies of the shoulder. Magn Reson Imaging Clin N Am. 2012;20:373–91.
28. Bianchi S, Martinoli C. Shoulder. In: Anonymous ultrasound of the musculoskeletal system. Berlin: Springer; 2007. p. 189–331.
29. Canella C, Demondion X, Abreu E, Marchiori E, Cotten H, Cotten A. Anatomical study of spinal accessory nerve using ultrasonography. Eur J Radiol. 2013;82:56–61.
30. Kim S, Hong SH, Jun WS, et al. MR imaging mapping of skeletal muscle denervation in entrapment and compressive neuropathies. Radiographics. 2011;31:319–32.
31. Beltran J, Rosenberg ZS. Diagnosis of compressive and entrapment neuropathies of the upper extremity: value of MR imaging. AJR Am J Roentgenol. 1994;163:525–31.
32. Petchprapa CN, Rosenberg ZS, Sconfienza LM, Cavalcanti CFA, La Rocca Vieira R, Zember JS. MR imaging of entrapment neuropathies of the lower extremity: part 1. The pelvis and hip 1. Radiographics. 2010;30:983–1000.
33. Yamabe E, Nakamura T, Oshio K, Kikuchi Y, Ikegami H, Toyama Y. Peripheral nerve injury: diagnosis with MR imaging of denervated skeletal muscle—experimental study in rats 1. Radiology. 2008;247:409–17.
34. Goutallier D, Postel JM, Bernageau J, Lavau L, Voisin MC. Fatty infiltration of disrupted rotator cuff muscles. Rev Rhum Engl Ed. 1995;62:415–22.
35. Ferretti A, Cerullo G, RUsso G. Suprascapular neuropathy in volleyball players. J Bone Joint Surg Am. 1987;69:260–3.
36. Holzgraefe M, Kukowski B, Eggert S. Prevalence of latent and manifest suprascapular neuropathy in high-performance volleyball players. Br J Sports Med. 1994;28:177–9.
37. Ringel SP, Treihaft M, Carry M, Fisher R, Jacobs P. Suprascapular neuropathy in pitchers. Am J Sports Med. 1990;18:80–6.
38. Witvrouw E, Cools A, Lysens R, et al. Suprascapular neuropathy in volleyball players. Br J Sports Med. 2000;34:174–80.
39. Lee BC, Yegappan M, Thiagarajan P. Suprascapular nerve neuropathy secondary to spinoglenoid notch ganglion cyst: case reports and review of literature. Ann Acad Med Singap. 2007;36:1032.
40. Semmler A, von Falkenhausen M, Schroder R. Suprascapular nerve entrapment by a spinoglenoid cyst. Neurology. 2008;70:890.
41. Yi JW, Cho NS, Rhee YG. Intraosseous ganglion of the glenoid causing suprascapular nerve entrapment syndrome: a case report. J Shoulder Elb Surg. 2009;18:e25–7.
42. Solheim LF, Roaas A. Compression of the suprascapular nerve after fracture of the scapular notch. Acta Orthop Scand. 1978;49:338–40.
43. Travlos J, Goldberg I, Boome RS. Brachial plexus lesions associated with dislocated shoulders. J Bone Joint Surg Br. 1990;72:68–71.

44. Visser C, Coene L, Brand R, Tavy D. The incidence of nerve injury in anterior dislocation of the shoulder and its influence on functional recovery a prospective clinical and EMG study. J Bone Joint Surg Br. 1999;81:679–85.
45. Yoon TN, Grabois M, Guillen M. Suprascapular nerve injury following trauma to the shoulder. J Trauma. 1981;21:652–5.
46. Mallon WJ, Wilson RJ, Basamania CJ. The association of suprascapular neuropathy with massive rotator cuff tears: a preliminary report. J Shoulder Elb Surg. 2006;15:395–8.
47. Lajtai G, Pfirrmann CW, Aitzetmuller G, Pirkl C, Gerber C, Jost B. The shoulders of professional beach volleyball players: high prevalence of infraspinatus muscle atrophy. Am J Sports Med. 2009;37:1375–83.
48. Cummins CA, Anderson K, Bowen M, Nuber G, Roth SI. Anatomy and histological characteristics of the spinoglenoid ligament. J Bone Joint Surg Am. 1998;80:1622–5.
49. Plancher KD, Luke TA, Peterson RK, Yacoubian SV. Posterior shoulder pain: a dynamic study of the spinoglenoid ligament and treatment with arthroscopic release of the scapular tunnel. Arthroscopy. 2007;23:991–8.
50. Demirhan M, Imhoff AB, Debski RE, Patel PR, Fu FH, Woo SL. The spinoglenoid ligament and its relationship to the suprascapular nerve. J Shoulder Elb Surg. 1998;7:238–43.
51. Bayramoğlu A, Demiryürek D, Tüccar E, et al. Variations in anatomy at the suprascapular notch possibly causing suprascapular nerve entrapment: an anatomical study. Knee Surg Sports Traumatol Arthrosc. 2003;11:393–8.
52. Cummins CA, Messer TM, Nuber GW. Current concepts review-suprascapular nerve entrapment*. J Bone Joint Surg. 2000;82:415–24.
53. Rengachary SS, Neff JP, Singer PA, Brackett CE. Suprascapular entrapment neuropathy: a clinical, anatomical, and comparative study: part 1: clinical study. Neurosurgery. 1979;5:441–6.
54. Ticker JB, Djurasovic M, Strauch RJ, et al. The incidence of ganglion cysts and other variations in anatomy along the course of the suprascapular nerve. J Shoulder Elb Surg. 1998;7:472–8.
55. Abboud JA, Silverberg D, Glaser DL, Ramsey ML, Williams GR. Arthroscopy effectively treats ganglion cysts of the shoulder. Clin Orthop. 2006;444:129–33.
56. Fehrman DA, Orwin JF, Jennings RM. Suprascapular nerve entrapment by ganglion cysts: a report of six cases with arthroscopic findings and review of the literature. Arthroscopy. 1995;11:727–34.
57. Moore TP, Fritts HM, Quick DC, Buss DD. Suprascapular nerve entrapment caused by supraglenoid cyst compression. J Shoulder Elb Surg. 1997;6:455–62.
58. Tirman PF, Feller JF, Janzen DL, Peterfy CG, Bergman AG. Association of glenoid labral cysts with labral tears and glenohumeral instability: radiologic findings and clinical significance. Radiology. 1994;190:653–8.
59. Westerheide KJ, Dopirak RM, Karzel RP, Snyder SJ. Suprascapular nerve palsy secondary to spinoglenoid cysts: results of arthroscopic treatment. Arthroscopy. 2006;22:721–7.
60. Tung GA, Entzian D, Stern JB, Green A. MR imaging and MR arthrography of paraglenoid labral cysts. Am J Roentgenol. 2000;174:1707–15.
61. O'Connor EE, Dixon LB, Peabody T, Stacy GS. MRI of cystic and soft-tissue masses of the shoulder joint. Am J Roentgenol. 2004;183:39–47.
62. Van Es H. MRI of the brachial plexus. Eur Radiol. 2001;11:325–36.
63. Martinoli C, Bianchi S, Pugliese F, et al. Sonography of entrapment neuropathies in the upper limb (wrist excluded). J Clin Ultrasound. 2004;32:438–50.
64. Martinoli C, Gandolfo N, Perez MM, et al. Brachial plexus and nerves about the shoulder. Semin Musculoskelet Radiol. 2010;14:523.
65. Huang K, Tu Y, Huang T, Hsu RW. Suprascapular neuropathy complicating a Neer type I distal clavicular fracture: a case report. J Orthop Trauma. 2005;19:343–5.
66. Visser CP, Coene L, Brand R, Tavy DL. Nerve lesions in proximal humeral fractures. J Shoulder Elb Surg. 2001;10:421–7.
67. Wijdicks CA, Armitage BM, Anavian J, Schroder LK, Cole PA. Vulnerable neurovasculature with a posterior approach to the scapula. Clin Orthop Relat Res. 2009;467:2011–7.
68. Fritz RC, Helms CA, Steinbach LS, Genant HK. Suprascapular nerve entrapment: evaluation with MR imaging. Radiology. 1992;182:437–44.
69. Bredella M, Tirman P, Fritz R, Wischer T, Stork A, Genant H. Denervation syndromes of the shoulder girdle: MR imaging with electrophysiologic correlation. Skelet Radiol. 1999;28:567–72.
70. Cahill BR, Palmer RE. Quadrilateral space syndrome. J Hand Surg. 1983;8:65–9.
71. Sanders TG, Tirman PF. Paralabral cyst: an unusual cause of quadrilateral space syndrome. Arthroscopy. 1999;15:632–7.
72. Redler MR, Ruland LJ 3rd, FC MC 3rd. Quadrilateral space syndrome in a throwing athlete. Am J Sports Med. 1986;14:511–3.
73. Schulte KR, Warner JJ. Uncommon causes of shoulder pain in the athlete. Orthop Clin North Am. 1995;26:505–28.
74. Robinson P, White L, Lax M, Salonen D, Bell R. Quadrilateral space syndrome caused by glenoid labral cyst. Am J Roentgenol. 2000;175:1103–5.
75. Tirman PF, Bost FW, Steinbach LS, et al. MR arthrographic depiction of tears of the rotator cuff: benefit of abduction and external rotation of the arm. Radiology. 1994;192:851–6.
76. Sofka CM, Lin J, Feinberg J, Potter HG. Teres minor denervation on routine magnetic resonance imaging of the shoulder. Skelet Radiol. 2004;33:514–8.
77. Perlmutter GS. Axillary nerve injury. Clin Orthop. 1999;368:28–36.

78. Bryan WJ, Schauder K, Tullos HS. The axillary nerve and its relationship to common sports medicine shoulder procedures. Am J Sports Med. 1986;14:113–6.
79. Wilson L, Sundaram M, Piraino DW, Ilaslan H, Recht MP. Isolated teres minor atrophy: manifestation of quadrilateral space syndrome or traction injury to the axillary nerve? Orthopedics. 2006;29: 447–50.
80. Yanny S, Toms AP. MR patterns of denervation around the shoulder. Am J Roentgenol. 2010;195:W157–63.
81. Cothran RL Jr, Helms C. Quadrilateral space syndrome: incidence of imaging findings in a population referred for MRI of the shoulder. Am J Roentgenol. 2005;184:989–92.
82. Tuckman GA, Devlin TC. Axillary nerve injury after anterior glenohumeral dislocation: MR findings in three patients. AJR Am J Roentgenol. 1996;167:695–7.
83. Price MR, Tillett ED, Acland RD, Nettleton GS. Determining the relationship of the axillary nerve to the shoulder joint capsule from an arthroscopic perspective. J Bone Joint Surg Am. 2004;86:2135–42.
84. Fleckenstein JL, Watumull D, Conner KE, et al. Denervated human skeletal muscle: MR imaging evaluation. Radiology. 1993;187:213–8.
85. Bencardino J, Petchprapa C, Rybak L, Hassankhani A, Palmer W. Teres minor atrophy: a sign of axillary denervation injury following shoulder trauma. Radiology. 2002;225:371.
86. Omar N, Alvi F, Srinivasan M. An unusual presentation of whiplash injury: long thoracic and spinal accessory nerve injury. Eur Spine J. 2007;16: 275–7.
87. McFarland EG, Garzon-Muvdi J, Jia X, Desai P, Petersen SA. Clinical and diagnostic tests for shoulder disorders: a critical review. Br J Sports Med. 2010;44:328–32.
88. Wiater JM, Flatow EL. Long thoracic nerve injury. Clin Orthop. 1999;368:17–27.
89. Sahin F, Yilmaz F, Esit N, Aysal F, Kuran B. Compressive neuropathy of long thoracic nerve and accessory nerve secondary to heavy load bearing. Eura Medicophys. 2007;47:71–4.
90. O'Dell M, Stubblefield M, O'Dell M, Stubblefield M. Cancer rehabilitation: principles and practice. New York: Demos Medical Publishing; 2009.
91. Martin RM, Fish DE. Scapular winging: anatomical review, diagnosis, and treatments. Curr Rev Musculoskelet Med. 2008;1:1–11.
92. Toth C, McNeil S, Feasby T. Peripheral nervous system injuries in sport and recreation. Sports Med. 2005;35:717–38.
93. Tubbs RS, Tyler-Kabara EC, Aikens AC, et al. Surgical anatomy of the dorsal scapular nerve. J Neurosurg. 2005;102:910–1.
94. Chen D, Gu Y, Lao J, Chen L. Dorsal scapular nerve compression. Atypical thoracic outlet syndrome. Chin Med J. 1995;108:582–5.
95. Akgun K, Aktas I, Terzi Y. Winged scapula caused by a dorsal scapular nerve lesion: a case report. Arch Phys Med Rehabil. 2008;89:2017–20.
96. Kuhn JE, Plancher KD, Hawkins RJ. Scapular Winging. J Am Acad Orthop Surg. 1995;3:319–25.
97. Spillane J. Localised neuritis of the shoulder girdle: a report of 46 cases in the MEF. Lancet. 1943;242:532–5.
98. Parsonage M, Aldren Turner J. Neuralgic amyotrophy the shoulder-girdle syndrome. Lancet. 1948;251:973–8.
99. Tsairis P, Dyck PJ, Mulder DW. Natural history of brachial plexus neuropathy: report on 99 patients. Arch Neurol. 1972;27:109–17.
100. Turner JA. Acute brachial radiculitis. Br Med J. 1944;2:592–4.
101. Dixon GJ, Dick T. Acute brachial radiculitis course and prognosis. Lancet. 1945;246:707–8.
102. Magee KR, DeJong RN. Paralytic brachial neuritis: discussion of clinical features with review of 23 cases. JAMA. 1960;174:1258–62.
103. Weikers NJ, Mattson RH. Acute paralytic brachial neuritis. A clinical and electrodiagnostic study. Neurology. 1969;19:1153–8.
104. Scalf RE, Wenger DE, Frick MA, Mandrekar JN, Adkins MC. MRI findings of 26 patients with Parsonage-Turner syndrome. Am J Roentgenol. 2007;189:W39–44.
105. Pellas F, Olivares J, Zandotti C, Delarque A. Neuralgic amyotrophy after parvovirus B19 infection. Lancet. 1993;342:503–4.
106. Suarez GA, Giannini C, Bosch EP, et al. Immune brachial plexus neuropathy: suggestive evidence for an inflammatory-immune pathogenesis. Neurology. 1996;46:559–61.
107. Ryan M, Twair A, Nelson E, Brennan D, Eustace S. Whole body magnetic resonance imaging in the diagnosis of Parsonage Turner syndrome. Acta Radiol. 2004;45:534–9.
108. Beghi E, Kurland LT, Mulder DW, Nicolosi A. Brachial plexus neuropathy in the population of Rochester, Minnesota, 1970–1981. Ann Neurol. 1985;18:320–3.
109. Helms CA, Martinez S, Speer KP. Acute brachial neuritis (Parsonage-Turner syndrome): MR imaging appearance--report of three cases. Radiology. 1998;207:255–9.
110. Gaskin CM, Helms CA. Parsonage-Turner Syndrome: MR Imaging Findings and Clinical Information of 27 Patients 1. Radiology. 2006;240:501–7.
111. Sallomi D, Janzen DL, Munk PL, Connell DG, Tirman PF. Muscle denervation patterns in upper limb nerve injuries: MR imaging findings and anatomic basis. AJR Am J Roentgenol. 1998;171:779–84.
112. Uetani M, Hayashi K, Matsunaga N, Imamura K, Ito N. Denervated skeletal muscle: MR imaging. Work in progress. Radiology. 1993;189:511–5.
113. May DA, Disler DG, Jones EA, Balkissoon AA, Manaster B. Abnormal signal intensity in skeletal muscle at MR imaging: patterns, pearls, and pitfalls 1. Radiographics. 2000;20:S295–315.

MIX
Papier aus verantwortungsvollen Quellen
Paper from responsible sources
FSC® C105338

If you have any concerns about our products,
you can contact us on
ProductSafety@springernature.com

In case Publisher is established outside the EU,
the EU authorized representative is:
Springer Nature Customer Service Center GmbH
Europaplatz 3, 69115 Heidelberg, Germany

Printed by Libri Plureos GmbH
in Hamburg, Germany